*Generalist Medicine and the U.S. Health System*

# Generalist Medicine and the U.S. Health System

Stephen L. Isaacs, James R. Knickman, Editors

Foreword by Risa Lavizzo-Mourey

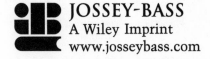

JOSSEY-BASS
A Wiley Imprint
www.josseybass.com

Published by Jossey-Bass
A Wiley Imprint
989 Market Street, San Francisco, CA 94103-1741   www.josseybass.com

Jossey-Bass books and products are available through most bookstores.
To contact Jossey-Bass directly call our Customer Care Department within the
U.S. at (800) 956-7739, outside the U.S. at (317) 572-3986 or fax (317) 572-4002.
Jossey-Bass also publishes its books in a variety of electronic formats. Some
content that appears in print may not be available in electronic books.

Credit lines for Abstracts from the Literature start on page 672.

**Library of Congress Cataloging-in-Publication Data**

Generalist medicine and the U.S. health care system/
Stephen L. Isaacs, James R. Knickman, editors.—1st ed.
p.; cm.
Includes bibliographical references and index.
ISBN 0-7879-7245-2 (alk. paper)
1. Medical care—United States. 2. Family medicine—United States.
3. Physicians (General practice)—United States.
[DNLM: 1. Delivery of Health Care—United States. 2. Family Practice—
United States. 3. Physicians, Family—United States. W 84 AA1 G326 2004]
I. Isaacs, Stephen L. II. Knickman, James.
III. Robert Wood Johnson Foundation.
RA395.A3G44 2004
362.1'0973—dc22
                                    2004001317

Printed in the United States of America
FIRST EDITION

*PB Printing*    10 9 8 7 6 5 4 3 2 1

# CONTENTS

## SECTION FIVE: QUALITY AND COST

# SOURCES

Chapter Three: White KL, Williams TF, Greenberg BG. The ecology of medical care. *N Engl J Med.* 1961;265:885–893.

Chapter Four: Engel GL. The need for a new medical model: a challenge for biomedicine. *Science.* 1977;196(4286):129–136.

Chapter Five: Ad Hoc Committee on Education for Family Practice of the Council on Medical Education. *Meeting the Challenge of Family Practice.* Chicago: American Medical Association; September 1966:2–13, 57.

Chapter Six: Pellegrino ED. The generalist function in medicine. *JAMA.* 1966;198(5):127–131.

Chapter Seven: Larson EB. General internal medicine at the crossroads of prosperity and despair: caring for patients with chronic diseases in an aging society. *Ann Intern Med.* 2001;134:997–1000.

Chapter Eight: Geyman JP, Bliss E. What does family practice need to do next? A cross-generational view. *Fam Med.* 2001;33:259–267.

Chapter Nine: Perkoff GT. Should there be a merger into a single primary care specialty for the 21st century? An affirmative view. *J Fam Pract.* 1989;29(2): 185–190.

Chapter Ten: Rosenblatt RA, Hart LG, Baldwin LM, Chan L, Schneeweiss R. The generalist role of specialty physicians: is there a hidden system of primary care? *JAMA*. 1998;279:1364–1370.

Chapter Eleven: Starfield B. Primary care and health: a cross-national comparison. *JAMA*. 1991;266(16):2268–2271.

Chapter Twleve: Sandy LG, Schroeder SA. Primary care in a new era: disillusion and dissolution? *Ann Intern Med*. 2003;138:262–267.

Chapter Thirteen: Isaacs SL, Sandy LG, Schroeder SA. Improving the health care workforce: perspectives from twenty-four years' experience. *To Improve Health and Health Care 1997: The Robert Wood Johnson Foundation Anthology* (Chap. 2). San Francisco: Jossey-Bass, 1997.

Chapter Fourteen: Council on Graduate Medical Education. *Third Report: Improving Access to Health Care Through Physician Workforce Reform: Directions for the 21st Century*. Rockville, Md: U.S. Department of Health and Human Services; 1992.

Chapter Fifteen: Institute of Medicine. *A Manpower Policy for Primary Health Care* (Chap. 1, pp 1–14). Washington, DC: National Academy Press; 1978.

Chapter Sixteen: Kindig DA, Cultice JM, Mullan F. The elusive generalist physician: can we reach a 50% goal? *JAMA*. 1993;270:1069–1073.

Chapter Seventeen: Cooper RA, Getzen TE, McKee HJ, Laud P. Economic and demographic trends signal an impending physician shortage. *Health Aff*. 2002;21(1):140–154.

Chapter Eighteen: Grumbach K. The ramifications of specialty-dominated medicine. *Health Aff*. 2002;21:155–157.

Chapter Nineteen: Rosenthal MP, Diamond JJ, Rabinowitz HK, et al. Influence of income, hours worked, and loan repayment on medical students' decision to pursue a primary care career. *JAMA*. 1994;271(12):914–917.

Chapter Twenty: Rosenblatt RA, Hart LG. Physicians and rural America. *West J Med*. 2000;173:348–351.

Chapter Twenty-One: Wielawski, IM. Practice sights: state primary care development strategies. *To Improve Health and Health Care, Vol. VI: The Robert Wood Johnson Foundation Anthology* (Chap. 3), San Francisco: Jossey-Bass, 2002.

Chapter Twenty-Two: Citizens' Commission on Graduate Medical Education. *The Graduate Education of Physicians*. Chicago: American Medical Association; 1966:33–56.

Chapter Twenty-Three: Alpert JJ, Charney E. *The Education of Physicians for Primary Care*. Washington, DC: U.S. Department of Health, Education and Welfare; 1973:5–9, 49–63. HRA 74–3113.

Chapter Twenty-Four: Schroeder SA, Showstack JA, Gerbert B. Residency training in internal medicine: time for a change? *Ann Intern Med.* 1986;104(4):554–561.

Chapter Twenty-Five: Charney E. The education of pediatricians for primary care: the score after two score years. *Pediatrics.* 1995;95:270–272.

Chapter Twenty-Six: Inui TS, Williams WT Jr, Goode L, et al. Sustaining the development of primary care in academic medicine. *Acad Med.* 1998;73:245–257.

Chapter Twenty-Seven: Sandy LG, Reynolds R. Influencing academic health centers: The Robert Wood Johnson Foundation experience. *To Improve Health and Health Care, 1998–1999* (Chap. 5), San Francisco: Jossey-Bass, 1999.

Chapter Twenty-Eight: Donohoe MT. Comparing generalist and specialty care: discrepancies, deficiencies, and excesses. *Arch Intern Med.* 1998;158:1596–1608.

Chapter Twenty-Nine: Sox HC Jr. Quality of patient care by nurse practitioners and physician's assistants: a ten-year perspective. *Ann Intern Med,* 1979;91:459–468.

Chapter Thirty: Mundinger MO, Kane RL, Lenz ER, et al. Primary care outcomes in patients treated by nurse practitioners or physicians: a randomized trial. *JAMA.* 2000;283:59–68.

Chapter Thirty-One: Keenan T. Support of nurse practitioners and physician assistants. *To Improve Health and Health Care, 1998–1999: The Robert Wood Johnson Foundation Anthology* (Chap. 11). San Francisco: Jossey-Bass, 1999.

# THE AUTHORS

Joel J. Alpert, M.D., professor of pediatrics and public health (law) at Boston University School of Medicine and former chair of the Department of Pediatrics at Boston University and Boston Medical Center (1972–1993).

Thomas Bodenheimer, M.D., M.P.H., adjunct professor of family and community medicine, University of California, San Francisco.

Evan Charney, M.D., professor and chair emeritus (retired), Department of Pediatrics, University of Massachusetts Medical Center, Worcester, Massachusetts.

Jack M. Colwill, M.D., professor emeritus, Department of Family and Community Medicine, School of Medicine, University of Missouri, Columbia, Missouri.

Richard A. Cooper, M.D., director of the Health Policy Institute, Medical College of Wisconsin, Milwaukee.

Martin T. Donohoe, M.D., FACP, medical director, Old Town Clinic, and adjunct lecturer, Department of Community Health, Portland State University, Lake Oswego, Oregon.

George L. Engel, M.D., former professor emeritus, University of Rochester School of Medicine and Dentistry, Rochester, New York (*deceased*).

John P. Geyman, M.D., professor emeritus, University of Washington School of Medicine, Seattle.

Kevin Grumbach, M.D., professor and chair, Department of Family and Community Medicine, University of California, San Francisco, and chief, Family and Community Medicine, San Francisco General Hospital, San Francisco.

Thomas S. Inui, Sc.M., M.D., president and CEO, Regenstrief Institute, Sam Regenstrief Professor of Health Services Research, associate dean for Health Care Research, and professor of medicine, Indiana University School of Medicine, Indianapolis.

Terrance Keenan, senior program consultant to The Robert Wood Johnson Foundation. He originally joined the Foundation as vice president in 1972.

David A. Kindig, M.D., Ph.D., professor emeritus, emeritus vice chancellor, Department of Population Health Sciences, Madison, Wisconsin.

Eric B. Larson, M.D., M.P.H., director, Group Health Cooperative, Center for Health Studies, professor of internal medicine, and adjunct professor of health services, University of Washington Medical Center, Seattle.

Risa Lavizzo-Mourey, M.D., M.B.A., is The Robert Wood Johnson Foundation's current president and chief executive officer.

Mary O. Mundinger, Dr.PH., dean, School of Nursing, Columbia University, New York.

Edmund D. Pellegrino, M.D., professor emeritus of medicine and medical ethics, senior research scholar of the Kennedy Institute of Ethics, and adjunct professor of philosophy at Georgetown University, Washington, D.C.

Gerald T. Perkoff, M.D., curators professor emeritus, Department of Family and Community Medicine, University of Missouri School of Medicine, Columbia, Missouri.

Roger A. Rosenblatt, M.D., M.P.H., professor and vice chair, Department of Family Medicine, RUOP faculty director, University of Washington, Seattle.

Michael P. Rosenthal, M.D., clinical professor and vice chair, Academic Programs, Department of Family Medicine, Jefferson Medical College, Thomas Jefferson University, Philadelphia.

Lewis G. Sandy, M.D., M.B.A., vice president and executive vice president of The Robert Wood Johnson Foundation 1991–2003; currently executive vice president, Clinical Strategies and Policy, United Healthcare Group, Minnetonka, Minnesota.

Steven A. Schroeder, M.D., president and CEO of The Robert Wood Johnson Foundation 1990–2002; currently distinguished professor of health and health care, Department of Medicine, University of California, San Francisco.

Harold C. Sox Jr., M.D., MACP, editor, *Annals of Internal Medicine,* American College of Physicians, Philadelphia.

Barbara Starfield, M.D., Ph.D., University Distinguished Professor, The Johns Hopkins University Medical Institutions, Baltimore, Maryland.

Kerr L. White, M.D., former professor of health care organization, The Johns Hopkins University, and retired deputy director of health sciences, The Rockefeller Foundation.

Irene M. Wielawski, evaluator of The Robert Wood Johnson Foundation's Reach Out Program and freelance journalist specializing in health care.

# THE EDITORS

**Stephen L. Isaacs, J.D.**, is the president of Health Policy Associates and a principal in the consulting firm of Isaacs/Jellinek, both of which are located in San Francisco. A former professor of public health at Columbia University and founding director of its Development Law and Policy Program, he has written extensively for professional and popular audiences. He is co-editor of the *To Improve Health and Health Care: The Robert Wood Johnson Foundation Anthology* series. His book *The Consumer's Legal Guide to Today's Health Care* was reviewed as "the single best guide to the health care system in print today." His articles have been widely syndicated and have appeared in law reviews and health policy journals. He also provides technical assistance internationally on health law, civil society, and social policy. A graduate of Brown University and Columbia Law School, Isaacs served as vice president of International Planned Parenthood's Western Hemisphere Region, practiced health law, and spent four years in Thailand as a program officer for the U.S. Agency for International Development.

**James R. Knickman, Ph.D.**, is vice president for research and evaluation at The Robert Wood Johnson Foundation. He oversees a range of grants and national programs supporting research and policy analysis to better understand forces that can improve health status and delivery of health care. In addition, he is in charge of developing formal evaluations of national programs supported by the Foundation. He also has played a leadership role in developing grant-making strategies in the area of chronic illness during his tenure at the Foundation. During the 1999–2000 academic year, he held a Regents' Lectureship at the University of California, Berkeley. Previously, Knickman was on the faculty of the Robert Wagner Graduate School of Public Service at New York University. At NYU, he was the founding director of a university-wide research center focused on urban health care. His publications include research on a range of health care topics, with particular emphasis on issues related to financing and delivering long-term care. He is co-editor of the *To Improve Health and Health Care: The Robert Wood Johnson Foundation Anthology* series. He has served on numerous health-related advisory committees at the state and local levels and spent a year working at New York City's Office of Management and Budget. Currently, he chairs the board of trustees of Robert Wood Johnson University Hospital. He completed his undergraduate work at Fordham University and received his doctorate in public policy analysis from the University of Pennsylvania.

# FOREWORD

As president and chief executive officer of the nation's fifth-largest foundation, I believe we have an obligation to share with the field, and the public at large, information about the programs we fund and what we have learned from them. We try to meet this obligation by publishing an annual report and a newsletter, *Advances;* by maintaining a Web site; by producing grant results reports for the Web site; and by editing the book series, *To Improve Health and Health Care: The Robert Wood Johnson Foundation Anthology,* published annually by Jossey-Bass.

As excellent as these communications vehicles may be, we can always do better. About two years ago, an informal working group consisting of Frank Karel, then the Foundation's vice president for communications, and Stephen Isaacs and Jim Knickman, editors of *The Robert Wood Johnson Foundation Anthology,* began discussing with staff members other ways in which the Foundation could get the word out about what it does and what it has learned.

The staff members consulted—which included the Foundation's senior management—observed that the publications and Web site tend to focus inward on the Foundation and its grantees. Although this was deemed appropriate, they felt that there was a need for a new communications vehicle that would (1) look beyond the Foundation by offering an in-depth exploration of the fields in which the Foundation had made substantial investments over many years and (2) highlight, without being self-aggrandizing, the Foundation's work in those fields.

This turned out to be quite a challenge, and this new book series, The Robert Wood Johnson Foundation Series on Health Policy, represents our attempt to meet it. Each volume of the series will attempt to provide—through one or two original review articles by leading experts, reprints of key articles, and abstracts from the literature—a comprehensive examination of the field. At the same time, it will highlight—through reprints of relevant chapters from The Robert Wood Johnson Foundation's *Anthology* and grant results reports—the Foundation's contribution to the field. *Generalist Medicine and the U.S. Health System* is the first book of the series.

Although one never knows in advance how a book will be received or used, it is our hope that *Generalist Medicine and the U.S. Health System* will make a contribution in a number of ways: as a text that will be used in medical schools, schools of public health, and other schools offering courses in primary health care or generalist practice; as a tool that will give individuals working in government the knowledge on which to base policies and programs; as a manual for health professionals working in or entering the field; as an aid to researchers and scholars; and as a guide for foundation officials striving to bring about social change.

This book series represents something of an experiment for the Foundation. Our plan is do three volumes; the following two will explore school-based health care and tobacco policy research. If the reaction to the first three volumes is positive and The Robert Wood Johnson Foundation Series on Health Policy does meet a need, the series will become an additional way for the Foundation to share information with the public and better carry out is mission of improving the health and health care of all Americans.

*Princeton, New Jersey*
*January 2004*

Risa Lavizzo-Mourey
*President and CEO*
*The Robert Wood Johnson Foundation*

# EDITORS' INTRODUCTION

s Risa Lavizzo-Mourey noted in the Foreword, The Robert Wood Johnson
Foundation Series on Health Policy is an attempt to offer a comprehensive
examination of fields in which The Robert Wood Johnson Foundation has
made significant investments over many years and to signal the work of the
Foundation in them. The first book in the series, *Generalist Medicine and the
U.S. Health System*, examines a topic that has been a priority of The Robert
Wood Johnson Foundation since its establishment as a national philanthropy in
1972. Indeed, in the Foundation's very first annual report, president David
Rogers wrote, "The uneven availability of continuing medical care of acceptable
quality is one of the most serious problems we face today. . . . We need to better provide health services of the right kind, at the right time, to those who need
it. Therefore, in its initial years, the Foundation will try to identify and encourage efforts to expand and improve the delivery of primary, frontline care."
Although the Foundation's efforts focused largely on physicians, it was also a
leader in the effort to develop nurse-practitioners and physician's assistants as
providers of primary care.

We have chosen to present the material in a unique way. To enable readers
to grasp the field as a whole, we commissioned two comprehensive review articles by preeminent experts in generalist medicine and have followed them by
reprints of important and influential articles and by abstracts of nearly three
hundred journal articles and reports. To provide an understanding of The Robert
Wood Johnson Foundation's role, we have reprinted relevant chapters from *The*

*Robert Wood Johnson Foundation Anthology* and reports prepared by the Foundation's grant-reporting unit. By including original articles and an extensive annotated bibliography, in addition to reprints, we have gone beyond the bounds of a normal "reader."

The book is organized into five sections. Section One contains original contributions by three preeminent authorities. The first, by Jack Colwill, provides a chronological history of the growth of generalist medicine since the 1950s, intertwined with the author's own journey from medical student to generalist medicine leader. The second, by Kevin Grumbach and Thomas Bodenheimer, examines the challenges facing primary care and generalist medicine in the twenty-first century. Taken together, these chapters offer a comprehensive overview of the philosophy behind and practice of generalist medicine and the challenges it faces.

Section Two looks at the need for and role of generalist physicians. It explores the models of care on which generalist medicine is based, the growth of three disciplines that claim to provide primary care to patients (general internists, family physicians, and pediatricians), the role of specialists in providing primary care, and important issues in the provision of generalist medicine.

Section Three addresses the supply and distribution of generalist physicians. It examines whether there are too few generalist physicians and too many specialists and how to achieve a proper balance (if one is desirable)—issues that have been the subject of considerable controversy since the 1960s. The chapters in this section examine as well the question of how to induce physicians to practice in underserved areas, particularly in rural locations.

Section Four focuses on the education and training of generalist physicians. Most of the chapters in this section discuss the inappropriateness of medical school education (particularly residencies) and suggest how academic medicine could be changed to prepare physicians more effectively for the practice of primary care.

Section Five examines one of the most heated issues in the field: who provides higher-quality and less expensive health care—generalist physicians, physicians in specialty practices, or nurse practitioners? The chapters in this section compare, first, the cost and the quality of the care provided by generalist physicians with that provided by specialists. Second, they compare the quality of care offered by generalist physicians with that provided by nurse practitioners. With health care costs again rising and concern about quality of care, these issues have taken on increasing importance.

Each section, other than the first (which contains the two original articles) is structured in an identical manner.

*Reprints of key articles and reports.* We have selected articles and reports widely recognized to be especially important or influential, or ones that offer an outstanding examination of a critical issue. To give as comprehensive view as possible, we have reprinted trailblazing articles and reports from years past—going back to the 1960s and 1970s in some cases. Beyond reprinting materials that provide a historical context, we have chosen to reprint more recent articles that illuminate the present and the future. These reprints give readers the opportunity to consider the original words of many of the field's leading thinkers.

Opinions differ about which articles and reports are the most important or influential. In making our selections, we have received the guidance of experts in the field: Thomas Bodenheimer, Jack Colwill, Kevin Grumbach, Richard Reynolds, Lewis Sandy, Jonathan Showstack, and Steven Schroeder. Space considerations limited the number of articles and reports that could be reprinted, and we were ultimately forced to choose among many worthy pieces. Despite what will almost certainly be differences of opinion about which articles and reports should have been included or omitted, we believe that the ones we have chosen to reprint do include many of the finest that have been written.

*Abstracts from the Literature.* All told, we have abstracted nearly three hundred articles, reports, and books. The bibliography does not annotate every piece that has ever been written on generalist medicine and the U.S. health system, but it does annotate a great many of those written from the 1960s to the present.

The reprints of key reports and articles (many of which emerged from grants funded by The Robert Wood Johnson Foundation) and the annotated bibliography attempt to capture primary care and the education of generalist physicians as a whole. They are followed by materials that focus specifically on The Robert Wood Johnson Foundation's role in developing the field of generalist medicine—one that has been, as noted earlier, a priority for the Foundation since the 1970s. These materials include the following:

> Reprints of relevant chapters from *To Improve Health and Health Care: The Robert Wood Johnson Foundation Anthology* series. This book, published annually by Jossey-Bass, examines the investments made by The Robert Wood Johnson Foundation and lets readers know what the Foundation did, why it did it, and what it learned.

> Summaries of reports examining the results of grants made by The Robert Wood Johnson Foundation. The complete reports, which are produced by the Foundation's Grant Results Reporting Unit, can be found on the Foundation's Web site, http://www.rwjf.org.

We share Dr. Lavizzo-Mourey's hopes that this book will make a contribution to a number of different audiences. Certainly, it should provide interested readers with a comprehensive view of a field that The Robert Wood Johnson

Foundation has invested heavily in over the years and that has the potential to be the backbone of a rational system of care.

*San Francisco*                                Stephen L. Isaacs
*Princeton, New Jersey*                         James R. Knickman
*January 2004*                                 Editors

# ACKNOWLEDGMENTS

This book would not have been possible without the dedication and hard work of a great many people. We would like to acknowledge their contributions.

Susan Godstone, a writer, researcher, and editor, did a breathtaking amount of work tracking down books and articles and then capturing their main points in clear and understandable abstracts. Her contribution has been enormous.

David Morse served as our partner throughout the process of putting this book together. His comments were always thoughtful, and his suggestions improved the book immeasurably.

Frank Karel, David Morse's predecessor as vice president for communications of The Robert Wood Johnson Foundation, was an original proponent of the idea of a reader series. He guided us through the beginning and middle stages of this book until his retirement in December 2001.

Jack Colwill has been a source of wisdom. His knowledge of the field is unsurpassed. In addition to writing a splendid chapter, he has been extremely generous in sharing his knowledge with us.

Jonathan Showstack, too, has been a wise counselor on primary care. The conference he organized on the future of primary care, held in Glen Cove, New York, in 2001, provided us with one of the articles we have chosen to reprint, as well as many ideas on the future of primary care.

Kevin Grumbach and Thomas Bodenheimer not only wrote a thoughtful chapter but also offered us a great deal of helpful advice on the practice of primary care.

Steven Schroeder, Lewis Sandy, and, Richard Reynolds—all experts in primary care and the education of generalist physicians—guided us in the structure of the book and took the time to review at various times our choices of articles to be reprinted and abstracted.

C. Pat Crow did an outstanding job of editing both the editors' introductions and the two original contributions that make up Section One.

Paul Moran and Deborah Malloy provided important administrative support at The Robert Wood Johnson Foundation, and Jim Ingram guided us through contractual issues. Also at The Robert Wood Johnson Foundation, Molly McKaughan and Marion Bass helped with structural issues and provided relevant grant results reports.

Elizabeth Dawson and Greta McKinney at Health Policy Associates deserve our thanks for their help in handling administrative and financial aspects.

At Jossey-Bass, Andy Pasternack was, once again, very professional and a pleasure to work with.

S.L.I.
J.R.K.

SECTION ONE

# PRIMARY CARE AND THE EDUCATION OF GENERALIST PHYSICIANS

*Past, Present, and Future*

# Editors' Introduction to Section One

In this section, three of the field's leading thinkers and practitioners provide an overview of primary care and the education of generalist physicians.

Chapter One is written by Jack M. Colwill. Colwill began his medical education in the 1950s and participated in the development of the generalist movement in medicine for half a century. His professional career has been spent in academic medicine, first as an internist and then as a family physician. He chaired the Department of Family and Community Medicine at the University of Missouri-Columbia (where he is now professor emeritus) and served as director of The Robert Wood Johnson Foundation–funded Generalist Physician Initiative during the 1990s. In these capacities, he could follow the growth of generalism in internal medicine and pediatrics as well.

In his chapter, "Primary Care Medicine and the Training of Generalist Physicians," Colwill provides a memoir that weaves his personal experience as a family practitioner and the evolution of primary care in the United States generally and medical education specifically. He offers a sweeping chronological overview of the field. Colwill's emphasis is on family medicine, but readers will see that the functions, goals, and aspirations of all three generalist disciplines—family medicine, general internal medicine, and general pediatrics—have much in common, even though they come from different traditions.

Chapter Two, "Reconstructing Primary Care for the Twenty-First Century," written by Kevin Grumbach and Thomas Bodenheimer, examines five critical issues that will determine whether or not primary care "can emerge as a reju-venated and energized sector of American health care." Grumbach is professor of family and community medicine and health policy at the University of California, San Francisco, and is chief of family and community medicine at San Francisco General Hospital/Community Health Network. He is one of the nation's leading researchers and analysts on the physician workforce, primary care, and health policy, was named a Robert Wood Johnson Foundation Generalist Physician Faculty Scholar, and, in 1997, was elected a member of the Institute of Medicine of the National Academy of Sciences. Bodenheimer, who has been in the private practice of internal medicine for more than two decades, is clinical professor of family and community medicine at the University of California, San Francisco. Bodenheimer and Grumbach are coauthors of a textbook, *Understanding Health Policy*.

The two chapters are complementary. Colwill intertwines his personal odyssey with the development of generalist medicine in the second half of the twentieth century; Grumbach and Bodenheimer target issues that will affect the future of primary care in the twenty-first century. Together, the two chapters provide a comprehensive look at the past, present, and future of primary care and the education of generalist physicians in the United States.

# CHAPTER ONE

# Primary Care Medicine and the Education of Generalist Physicians

## *A Personal Perspective*

Jack M. Colwill, M.D.
2003

In this chapter, I intertwine my personal experience in internal and family medicine with the development of the generalist movement over the past half a century.

## THE 1950s AND 1960s

I entered medical school at the University of Rochester in 1953. Although A. E. Hertzler's *Horse and Buggy Doctor* helped cement my decision to enter medicine,[1] I don't recall having any particular personal sense of mission. What I did have was a vague sense that I wanted to take care of people. Having been healthy all my life and blessed with a healthy family, I knew little of medical practice and had no role models. But I did understand that the foundation of American medicine had been the general practitioner and that specialization signaled his demise. Indeed, the concept of the general practitioner as a caring physician who was committed to the needs of his patient and was willing to make house calls any time of the day or night seemed not to exist in the medical schools, where he had come to be seen as the person who had the least amount of training but did the most to people—not a positive view.

The only comprehensive physicians I had contact with as a medical student were practicing general internists and pediatricians who provided continuing care for patients in both the office and the hospital. They were superb clinicians who volunteered part of their time as teaching attending physicians. The relatively small full-time internal medicine faculty was made up of specialists who devoted their lives to teaching, research, and a modest clinical practice. They worked in small subspecialty divisions, which were expanding rapidly as funding increased, mainly from the nascent but growing National Institutes of Health, the NIH. At that time, approximately 40 percent of the nation's physicians were general practitioners, but I completed four years of medical school and a residency in internal medicine without ever meeting a general practitioner.

I did not then grasp the effect that specialization in medical schools would have on the delivery of health care. Medical schools were considered to be at the cutting edge of medicine and had already created a culture that led medical students and residents to specialize. These graduates went on to establish specialized practices in their communities. Faculty members also helped further specialization through their leadership of specialty organizations, accreditation bodies, and specialty boards. In many ways, the medical schools defined the composition of the medical workforce; the market seems to have had little to do with it.

As a medical student at Rochester, I did not yet realize that the trend toward medical specialization was already more than half a century old. In 1900, the physician-to-population ratio was approximately 173 physicians per 100,000 people, and about 90 percent of those doctors were general practitioners.[2] Physicians had already begun limiting their practices to a single area of interest, and some people even expressed concern about the dangers of specialization.[3]

In 1900, the quality of medical education was poor.[4] Most medical schools had not followed the Johns Hopkins model—one that was soon to change the face of medical education—but instead were proprietary mills with few faculty members and little in the way of resources. Medical education was didactic, and students received little or no experience in caring for patients; there were no internships or residencies to speak of. Public outcry led to the closing or merger of ninety-two medical schools between 1904 and 1915, and the number of graduates declined by more than half. (The demand for reform was given significant support in 1910 with the publication of Abraham Flexner's report on medical education.[5]) All but a few remaining schools joined universities, required a college education for admission, and adopted a four-year curriculum. Laboratory-based education in the first two years was followed by two years of clerkships at the bedside and in the clinic. Most faculty members became full-time salaried professors. By 1920, American medical education had been transformed into the best in the world. Medical faculty members were scholars committing themselves to the development of laboratory-based science, which became the underpinning of medical education and practice and would be a driving force in the move toward clinical specialization.

By this time, more and more general practitioners were limiting their practices to areas of specialization, and specialty organizations began to form, among them the American College of Surgeons and the American College of Physicians. Ophthalmologists initiated the first specialty board in 1917, and subsequently many other specialties established certifying boards in the mid-1930s. By 1940, some 38 percent of the nation's practicing physicians described themselves as specialists.[6] The number of general practitioners had fallen to 83 per 100,000 population. Internists and pediatricians were beginning to serve as primary care physicians in urban areas, but their numbers were small—only 4 internists and 2 pediatricians per 100,000.[6]

Before World War II, most medical school graduates entered general practice after a one-year rotating internship, but after the war virtually all medical school graduates entered a medical specialty.[7] Two-year general practice residencies were developed in the 1950s and 1960s in an effort to keep the GP from becoming a dying breed, but there were few applicants, and this effort failed to stem the decline.

By 1960, the number of general practitioners had declined to about 30 per 100,000 and has remained at that level almost to the present, even after the development of family practice residencies. Thus over the past century, the ratio of general practitioners to population has fallen by more than 80 percent. This decline had an enormous impact, especially on rural health care. In cities, internists and pediatricians provided care formerly given by general practitioners, but few internists and few pediatricians settled in rural areas. The shortage of rural physicians became a national issue in the 1940s and has remained a problem to this day.

When I began studying medicine, a small number of faculty members in many medical schools were worried about a curriculum that focused on the underlying mechanisms of disease but had little or no focus on the whole patient in the context of his or her social, psychological, and economic environment. As a result, many medical schools developed educational programs to help their students better understand human behavior. These programs were usually led by departments of psychiatry and frequently had a psychoanalytical orientation. For my class, George Engel, an internist with psychoanalytic training, taught a course in which he provided extraordinary insights into the behavioral aspects of patients and their illnesses.[8] Through weekly interviews with patients using one-way mirrors, he highlighted the behavioral components of each individual's illness and thereby helped medical students develop a behavioral approach to patient care. Engel's teachings became the basis for his biopsychosocial model, which has provided a conceptual basis for understanding patients' illnesses in each of the primary care disciplines.[9] Other institutions appointed sociologists and anthropologists to their faculties to help their students understand patients' illnesses and illness behavior.[10]

I well remember my own dilemma in selecting a specialty. George Engel had been a mentor and had strengthened my interest in understanding people. Leonard Fenninger, an associate dean and internist who was intellectually committed to comprehensive care, also influenced me greatly, pushing me toward internal medicine. I did consider general practice, but the specialty-oriented culture of the medical school led me away from that choice. In 1957, I began an internship in internal medicine at Washington University's Barnes Hospital, followed by three years of residency—including the chief residency—at the University of Washington in Seattle. The learning environment was intellectually and physically demanding. With the vast majority of our work on hospital wards, we learned through hands-on experience and untold hours of reading. We were expected to provide intense patient care while we developed a scholarly understanding of the mechanisms and therapeutic approaches to disease. During our internship and part of our residency, we were on duty every other night. As interns, we hardly sat down when we were on call, and when we were off call, we collapsed into bed. I remember feeling an intense jealousy toward the senior residents who went off to read about our patients after morning rounds, leaving me with the "scut" work. We seldom saw patients after they were discharged. My teachers were all subspecialists in internal medicine. Although they were compassionate physicians, they had limited their own care of patients to those with problems in the organ system of their subspecialty and frequently expressed discomfort in dealing with clinical problems outside their specialty.

One day when I was chief resident at the University of Washington, I had a discussion with my chief, Robert Williams, who was the founding chairman of the Department of Medicine and a leading scholar in diabetes. He asked what I wanted to do after my residency, and I replied that I wanted to enter academic medicine. He then asked what subspecialty I planned to enter. When I answered, "None," he responded, "What would you do?" I had thought a great deal about this question and told him that I would be happy to serve as a permanent ward-attending physician in a job that subspecialty faculty members no longer seemed to enjoy doing. Williams saw a real possibility in the proposal and asked me to present it at a departmental meeting. A lot of discussion ensued, but the idea proved to be highly threatening to those faculty members who thought of themselves first as general internists and second as subspecialists. Thirty years later, a doctor filling the position that I had proposed would be called a "hospitalist."

In the spring of 1961, Larry Young, the chairman of the Department of Medicine at Rochester, called me with a job offer. A hematologist himself, he recognized that programs in internal medicine were preparing residents to enter subspecialties, rather than preparing them to be comprehensive general internists.[11] He feared that the comprehensive internist diagnostician would gradually disappear from the medical landscape and asked me to return to Rochester to head the medical outpatient department and to help carry out his vision of restructuring the Rochester residency to educate comprehensively trained internists who could provide high-quality general care for adults. He obviously also wanted Rochester to continue emphasizing the subspecialties as the focus of its academic future.

When I returned to Rochester, I found that the school had initiated a Combined Clinic to teach medical students comprehensive patient care. Each student attended this clinic for half a day each week in his senior year and, supervised by a faculty member, cared for a small number of patients over time. Similar programs evolved in other medical schools.[12] The Combined Clinic was developed with admirable purpose, but it had fatal flaws. The patients seen by the students were usually indigent and had enormous social and economic problems in addition to their medical problems. A typical patient was alcoholic, had resultant hepatic cirrhosis, and had no source of income and no family. Such patients were daunting for even the most skilled clinician. Any gratification that students might have received from caring for them was either delayed or nonexistent. The medical student and the faculty both felt torn between their responsibilities in other areas and their responsibilities in the Combined Clinic. The effort was noble, but this program and others like it faltered and eventually died.

My new role at Rochester proved to be exciting and productive. My responsibility was to supervise residents in the clinic, to direct the clinic, and to practice medicine. I could double my $11,000 salary through my own practice—an experience that proved to be particularly illuminating. Patients complained of low back pain, menstrual disorders, middle-ear infection, fatigue, depression, chronic hypertension, shoulder pain, and many other things that I had not encountered in my hospital-based residency. In contrast to the residency, my practice was 90 percent ambulatory and only 50 percent internal medicine. I was seeing adult patients for all problems, a high proportion of which I had not been trained to treat. Clearly, my education had not reflected the content of my current practice. At that time, Kerr White and colleagues had just published their classic article on the "ecology" of medical care.[13] Using population data, they estimated that in any one month, 750 of 1,000 people would report one or more illnesses, 250 would see a doctor, 9 would be hospitalized, and only 1 would be referred to a university medical center. Obviously, my education had been based on that 1-in-1,000 patient, not on the common illnesses for which most patients sought care.

I came to appreciate the degree to which social, psychological, and economic factors influenced the symptoms and the disease. Many times people were "ill," but I could not identify a disease. In the hospital, I had dealt with the certainty of disease. In the ambulatory setting, I faced the ambiguity of illness. I found myself repeatedly evaluating patients for adrenal insufficiency or collagen vascular disease until I came to realize that common diseases occur commonly and rare diseases occur rarely. I began to learn the diagnostic and therapeutic value of tincture of time. Patients with chronic illnesses were a particular problem for me. They kept returning with the same symptoms. Gradually, I learned the concept of limited goals, and my frustrations frequently became gratifications.

We set out to transform the residency in internal medicine to better prepare general internists. My responsibilities lay in the medical outpatient department. The clinic, a hated place, was referred to as "the pit." Residents saw patients at random, without continuity, and with minimal or no faculty supervision. The residents found their patients' problems overwhelming and their own efforts hopeless. Because there was no continuity, there was no opportunity to know and understand the human being and no way to understand the institutional and community resources necessary to assist in the patient's care.

To change this situation, we started a weekly continuity clinic for the residents where they took ongoing care of their own patients throughout the three years of residency. To emphasize the behavioral aspects of illness, each resident completed a two-month rotation in psychiatry. A liaison group led by George Engel held behavioral medicine rounds weekly on each inpatient service. Finally, to gain broader experience, each intern in the emergency room saw patients without regard to age or the clinical problem under supervision by residents in other specialties. Elective rotations were also developed in ENT (ear, nose, and throat) and gynecology.

As a very junior assistant professor, I knew little of what was happening at other medical schools, but one memory does stand out. In 1964, I met a young faculty member at Case Western Reserve University who was serving on the staff of a new committee funded by the Carnegie Foundation and sponsored by the American Medical Association. It was called the Citizens' Commission for Graduate Medical Education, and its chairman was John Millis, the president of Case Western Reserve University. He told me that this committee was concerned about the shortage of physicians who could take care of patients over time. I was fascinated that such a group existed and looked forward to its report.

In 1964, Robert Haggarty, who was already viewed as the father of primary care pediatrics and community pediatrics, became the chairman of the Department of Pediatrics at Rochester and enticed Evan Charney, a young general pediatrician and subsequent national leader in general pediatrics, to join him.[14,15] The Department of Pediatrics already had strong links to practicing pediatricians doing practice-based research, and under their guidance, it became a leader in general and community pediatrics. They created a continuity clinic for residents and a larger community-based research program and played a key role in initiating a neighborhood health center. Their program became a national model.

In the mid-1960s, Rochester also recruited Gene Farley from practice to establish a new type of residency called family practice. His program, one of the early leaders in family practice, pioneered a community-oriented approach to family practice training.

Such was the commitment of one medical school in the 1960s to giving general internists, pediatricians, and family physicians an education that would more closely mirror their practice. At Rochester, I learned a great deal about patient care and had an incredibly gratifying educational experience.

In 1964, I moved to the University of Missouri at Columbia as assistant dean for admissions and student affairs with academic appointments in the Department of Community Health and Medical Practice and in the Department of Internal Medicine. The mission of the medical school was to serve rural Missouri, and my new mentor, Dean Vernon Wilson, was committed to the new specialty of family practice. He told me that some family practice residencies already existed and that Lynn Carmichael, a former fellow of Bob Haggarty's, had started the first one at the University of Miami. I discovered that Vernon Wilson was a member of The Willard Committee, an American Medical Association committee that was soon to recommend establishing family practice as a new specialty. I was skeptical. My background as an internist had led me to believe that internal medicine was the solution to the need for general practitioners. At the time, I antagonized at least one colleague by making the offhand comment that "internists are the 'Brahmins' of medicine."

Missouri had a single full-time general practitioner on the faculty: A. Sherwood Baker. Vernon Wilson had recruited him from practice in 1962 to start a general practice residency based in the Department of Community Health and Medical Practice. Several of its graduates went on to become leaders in medicine in Missouri, but the number of positions and of applicants was small, as was true across the country. In no way could this one department be expected to meet the state's need for rural doctors.

The Academy of General Practice, the practice organization for general practitioners, had long been concerned about the declining numbers of general practitioners. In the 1950s, some leaders in general practice were advocating the development of family practice as a new specialty. Others within the academy were concerned with maintaining the surgical aspects of general practice. The proposal to develop a new specialty failed several times in the academy's Congress of Delegates but did ultimately pass in 1965.[16]

The timing of the academy's decision was propitious. In the mid-1960s, there was great public concern that the nation needed a new type of comprehensive physician. In 1966, the reports of three commissions were published. The report of the Citizens' Commission headed by John Millis described the increasing specialization and fragmentation of an individual's health care when a number of specialists were involved.[17] The report said the nation needed physicians trained in comprehensive continuing care to accept long-term responsibility for patients. These doctors would be called primary physicians and would need new educational programs.

The Willard Committee Report, sponsored by the Council on Medical Education of the AMA and titled *Meeting the Challenge for Family Practice,* called for a "new kind of specialist in family medicine educated to provide comprehensive personal healthcare, because of the complexity of modern medicine and the healthcare system."[18] The Report of the National Commission on Community Health Services, *Health Is a Community Affair,* called for the education of a "personal physician who is the central point for integration and continuity of all medical and medically related services to the patient."[19]

These three reports, crystallizing national concern, catalyzed the development of primary care education in the nation's medical schools. Forty new medical schools were opened during the 1960s and 1970s, and the majority of these announced that their mission was to produce primary care physicians. In 1969, the American Board of Family Practice (ABFP) was established under the charismatic leadership of Nicholas Pisacano.[16] A residency review committee was formed, and sixteen already established family practice residencies received approval. At this time, there was also ferment within internal medicine and pediatrics, and a number of institutions initiated primary care tracks within their internal medicine and pediatrics residencies. In addition, the American Board of Internal Medicine and the American Board of Pediatrics supported the development of combined residencies in internal medicine and pediatrics, requiring two years of formal training in each specialty.

# THE 1970s

Largely as a result of vigorous crusades by the American Academy of Family Physicians, legislature after legislature passed laws funding family practice residencies. Many legislatures also mandated the establishment of departments of family medicine in their state-supported medical schools. Stimulated by these mandates, most medical schools and virtually all state-supported schools initiated departments of family medicine.

The federal government also committed itself to financial support. In the early 1970s, the Bureau of Physician Manpower began providing a limited number of contracts to support the development of family practice residencies and primary care tracks in internal medicine and pediatrics residencies. In 1976, Congress markedly expanded this activity through passage of Title VII of the Public Health Service Act (the Health Professions Educational Assistance Act), authorizing support for residency training, undergraduate education, departmental development and faculty development in family practice, and primary care residency tracks in internal medicine and pediatrics.

The number of residency programs in family practice grew from 21 in 1969 to 382 by 1980, and the number of physicians completing family practice residencies rose to 2,500 a year in the early 1980s. Medical student interest increased throughout the 1970s. When young faculty members commented to laypeople that they were faculty members in family practice residencies, the typical response was one of admiration and appreciation for their efforts to correct the nation's shortage of primary care physicians.

In the medical schools, the reception was less enthusiastic. Many people in the schools were frankly hostile. Their culture was specialty and consultative medicine, and even though the nation clearly needed primary care physicians, negative images of the general practitioner made the development of family practice anathema for the members of most medical school faculties. They resented legislative mandates requiring the development of departments of family medicine in medical schools. Such activity was seen as a direct threat to their autonomy. For the first time, educational programs were being imposed on academic medicine rather than initiated by it.

Family practice led the movement to educate primary care physicians; it was but one part of a national movement in the 1970s. Change was occurring in internal medicine and pediatrics as well, frequently as an alternative to the family practice movement. John Stoeckle, a Harvard internist, developed a primary care residency in internal medicine at the Massachusetts General Hospital, which made a heavy commitment to a continuity practice and provided about half of the residency experience in the ambulatory setting.[20] Joel Alpert, chair of pediatrics at Boston University, developed a community-oriented primary care pediatrics residency track and demonstrated that the graduates of this program were more likely to become primary care pediatricians than traditional-track residents.[21] Larry Young, following his retirement as chairman at Rochester, developed a community-based residency at Genesee and Rochester general hospitals to educate practicing general internists.[22] I first thought it would be a mistake to move to a community hospital. This was in essence putting the residency out to pasture. I came to realize, however, that the program's success resulted from its being outside Strong Memorial Hospital, Rochester's tertiary care–oriented teaching hospital. The Robert Wood Johnson Foundation helped fund Young's program and sponsored other primary care residency tracks in internal medicine and pediatrics at other medical schools.

Because of a more welcoming environment, most residency programs in family practice were established in community hospitals rather than within the university. Even so, most of these programs were university-affiliated, with the degree of affiliation varying widely. Most faculty members were drawn from the practice community, but many of the new family medicine departments in medical schools also drew sympathetic internists and pediatricians to their faculties. One, the Medical University of South Carolina, appointed a neurologist, Hiram Curry, as chairman of what became a leading department of family practice.

The new family practice residency programs had as their core a model clinic in which each resident provided longitudinal and comprehensive care for a group of patients over three years of residency. The residency requirements emphasized the need for doctors to be educated in the behavioral aspects of patient care and mandated experience in several specialty areas to provide experience in the breadth of common problems typically handled by a family physician. More than half of the residency was typically in ambulatory settings.

At Missouri, Sherwood Baker changed the general practice residency to a family practice residency in 1970, but the medical school faculty was still not fully committed to family practice. In 1971, a committee was established to speed the development of family practice; this committee recommended that the program be institutionwide and that it be run by an associate dean, assisted by an advisory committee made up of members from each of the clinical disciplines. When the committee's preferred candidate for the associate dean's position turned us down, the role fell to me.

Beginning with three family physicians, we succeeded in attracting Paul Young, who had started the first family practice residency in Missouri. He subsequently became chairman of family medicine at the University of Nebraska and then at the University of Texas Medical Branch at Galveston before becoming executive director of the American Board of Family Practice. Our goal for the residency program was to prepare physicians for rural health care and for academic medicine—the areas of greatest need. Ingeborg Mauksch, a well-known nursing academician and nurse practitioner, also joined us. We all believed that family physicians and nurse practitioners in collaborative practice might truly relieve the shortage of physicians in rural areas.

Even though the medical school faculty members realized that family physicians were needed, the bias against the family practitioner remained strong. Initially, the chairman of internal medicine even insisted on personally interviewing all applicants for the family practice residency, to be sure they were qualified to rotate on his medical wards. He abandoned this idea after we met jointly with the dean.

Following the requirements of the residency review committee, we developed a model family practice center, in which both faculty members and residents under faculty supervision practiced. Partnerships of two residents and a collaborating nurse practitioner provided continuing care for patients. Residents spent two, three, and then four half-days weekly in their continuity practice during each of the three years. They were also responsible for keeping track of their patients on the family practice inpatient service. The remainder of each resident's time was spent on rotations in other specialties. In aggregate, less than half of the residents' time was spent with hospitalized patients.

Our faculty members and residents were excited by the pioneering effort. We wrestled with how to reduce the inevitable conflicts that residents faced with joint responsibilities for patients both on hospital rotations in other specialties and in their continuity practices in family medicine. Ultimately, we developed a partnership of two residents modeled after Gene Farley's at Rochester, in which two residents shared responsibility for patients in their continuity practice as well as for patient care on inpatient services. Though other departments were initially skeptical that the partnership would work, it has become a central part of our residency over the years, and our residents value it highly.

In those early days of conflict, hospital privileges were a problem for us as well as for many other programs across the country. Even today, some academic departments of medicine, pediatrics, and obstetrics strongly oppose inpatient privileges for family physicians at the tertiary care centers. The expressed concern has always been quality, but the underlying issues are territorial. In our relatively amenable university environment, we created a hospital department of family practice and provided inpatient credentialing. Level 1 obstetrical privileges initially required the approval by the Department of Obstetrics, but they later became the responsibility of our department.

We knew that an educational program based entirely within an academic health center was unlikely to encourage graduates to seek rural practice. Consequently, in 1975, we started a continuity practice for our residents in Fulton, Missouri, a small college town twenty-five miles east of Columbia. Then, in 1980, we established a second rural practice in Fayette, twenty-five miles west of Columbia. Full-time faculty members moved to these communities to supervise residents both in the office and in the local hospital. Residents in these rural settings, practicing at a distance from consulting specialists, learned the importance of knowing when to consult and when to make a referral. Along with the residency program, we initiated a certificate-level family nurse practitioner program in 1976, directed by Ingeborg Mauksch, with the assistance of a grant from the Kellogg Foundation. Our goal was to prepare nurse practitioners for practice in collaboration with physicians in rural Missouri. The program was quite successful but was initially opposed by the School of Nursing—a development similar to the medical schools' resistance to the growth of family practice. Many of our nurse practitioner graduates are still serving rural populations. The certificate program closed in 1982 as Kellogg support ended and a master's level program in nursing was created.

Over time, in each of the three primary care disciplines, the need for an academically prepared faculty became paramount. The Robert Wood Johnson Foundation's Clinical Scholars Program started out to prepare academic internists and was broadened to include young physicians in other specialties, but the number from other specialties remained small. In the late 1970s, the Foundation also started programs to train academic faculty members in general pediatrics and family medicine. At Missouri, with the help of Robin Blake, a graduate of North Carolina's Clinical Scholars Program, we successfully competed for one of ten Robert Wood Johnson Foundation family practice fellowship programs, which provided support through much of the 1980s. Serendipitously, Jerry Perkoff, a professor of internal medicine at Washington University and a nationally known biomedical and health services researcher, came as a visiting professor. As a cofounder of the Medical Care Group, a prepaid group practice in Saint Louis, he was committed to furthering the development of primary care and confided in me that he was considering academic chairmanships in family practice. Our visions for the future turned out to be identical, and Perkoff ultimately agreed to join our department as curators' professor, associate chairman, and head of the Robert Wood Johnson fellowship program. His intellectual leadership was central to our academic development in the 1980s.

For me, the 1970s constituted an incredibly exhilarating and challenging decade. The switch from internal medicine to family practice was eye-opening. As an internist heading a family practice residency program, I bore the brunt of a lot of humorous banter. I had last seen a baby delivered when I was a medical student. I became a family practitioner but was never comfortable with the care of sick children and vowed never to enter the delivery room. In the ambulatory setting, I found that while I was quite competent in the classical areas of internal medicine, I could not hold a candle to my colleagues in the areas of musculoskeletal medicine, ENT medicine, women's diseases, and sick children. Indeed, I found myself seeking the advice of my colleagues two to three times as often as they sought mine. In our practice, we shared common values and a common vision of the primary physician, but I often wished that I had had a residency that more closely paralleled my responsibilities as a family physician.

As a medical student, I had avoided general practice because I had been led to believe that no individual could embrace the entire scope of medicine. As a clinician, I learned that we develop competence in the areas where we have the most experience. A key component of competence for both the generalist and the specialist is to recognize when a problem is beyond the scope of one's own expertise and then to seek consultation. Perhaps the most difficult but most important aspect of deciding when to obtain consultative assistance is recognizing when one doesn't know what one doesn't know.

I came to realize that the most fundamental difference between a generalist and a specialist lies not so much in the scope of clinical knowledge as in the responsibility assumed. A good friend who is the head of a section of general internal medicine commented that the generalist is inclusive, whereas the specialist is exclusive. That is, specialists handle problems within their disciplinary area, while generalists assume responsibility for all the problems patients bring to them, handling those problems that they can and seeking help when the problems are outside the scope of their own expertise.[10]

Most movements have their philosophers. During the 1960s and 1970s, no one better articulated for me the responsibilities of the primary care physician and the consulting specialist than Ed Pellegrino, at that time the founding chairman of internal medicine at the University of Kentucky.[23] Others saw issues of power and control, while Pellegrino talked of moral responsibility, service to the patient, and the ways in which primary care physicians and consultants could best work together. Richard Magraw, a psychiatrist and subsequently the founding dean at Eastern Virginia Medical School, published *Ferment in Medicine* in 1966.[24,25] This book, which had an enormous readership nationally, described issues in the doctor-patient relationship, a rapidly evolving specialty-oriented workforce, and the need to educate generalist practitioners to coordinate patient care. Within family medicine, the writings of Gayle Stephens, the founder of one of the earliest family practice residencies at Wichita, and Ian McWhinney, head of the Department of Family Practice at Western Ontario, stood out.[26,27] Gayle Stephens's writing on the "intellectual basis of family practice" was especially helpful.[28] Family practice had been questioned as a discipline on the basis that it did not have a unique body of knowledge. As Stephens eloquently put it, no clinical discipline has a body of knowledge that is not shared at least to a degree. The uniqueness of family medicine lies in its function rather than its content. Finally, Joel Alpert and Evan Charney, pediatricians at Boston University and at Rochester, respectively, jointly published a monograph titled *The Education of Physicians for Primary Care* that gave a history of primary care and suggested directions for education in this field.[10] They attempted to reduce the ambiguity in defining primary care, social medicine, comprehensive medicine, and community medicine. They noted that the anchoring points of primary care were first contact care, longitudinal responsibility for the patient, and coordination of care. The efforts of these individuals and others did much to help the education of physicians for primary care evolve in the 1970s.

# THE 1980s

The 1980s were years of consolidating gains and enhancing the quality of developing programs. At the medical schools, the three primary care disciplines sought to strengthen educational programs and to develop the research and intellectual basis of their disciplines. It was not an easy period. The excitement of the national movement toward primary care of the 1970s dimmed somewhat during the 1980s. The nation became more conservative and elected a Republican president, Ronald Reagan. The public focus seemed to shift from primary care to concern about health care costs, which were increasing at double the rate of inflation.

Physicians in each of the primary care disciplines still had a great sense of mission. Most medical schools now had a department of family practice, and virtually all departments of medicine and pediatrics had developed divisions of general internal medicine and general pediatrics. But the generalist disciplines were still small. Faculty in internal medicine and pediatrics frequently felt dominated by their subspecialty faculty. And while the three disciplines shared common goals and aspirations, each had strong ties to its parent discipline, and each lived administratively in a separate organizational silo. Unfortunately, in many schools, competitiveness between the disciplines limited cooperation.

The foremost responsibility of the generalist faculty was the education of medical students and residents. Those in internal medicine and pediatrics usually maintained a practice and supervised residents in the general clinics. They valued their time as inpatient attending physicians on the general medical and pediatric hospital services. Faculty members in family medicine practiced and supervised residents in their ambulatory clinics, which were usually at community hospitals. Required clerkships in family medicine were developing in medical schools across the nation, frequently with the support of federal training grants. These clerkships, usually based in the office of community physicians, had defined objectives in the curriculum, thus taking the rotation beyond a preceptoral experience. In many schools, third-year clerkships in internal medicine and pediatrics had an increased ambulatory experience in which both generalists and subspecialists participated. The time spent in research by most generalist faculty members was modest at best.

Despite the changes in generalist education, the overall milieu of academic health centers was increasingly one of subspecialization.[29] It is not surprising that medical student interest in generalist disciplines gradually declined during the 1980s and reached its nadir in 1992, when only 14.5 percent of American medical school graduates indicated that they planned primary care careers on the graduate questionnaire of the Association of American Medical Colleges (AAMC).

The typical medical school family practice department consisted of six to ten family physicians and one or two behavioral scientists. Internal medicine and pediatrics generalist divisions were also small. In many departments, generalist faculty members were given responsibility for coordinating residency programs, and these residency programs increasingly provided half a day a week in a continuity practice, thereby providing some primary care experience.

The primary care residency tracks in medicine and pediatrics usually provided more time in continuity practice and more experience in the ambulatory setting and in other disciplines than the traditional categorical residency did. John Noble, a general internist at Boston University, and Barbara Starfield, a pediatrician at Johns Hopkins School of Public Health, demonstrated that higher percentages of the graduates of primary care tracks in internal medicine and pediatrics went on to become generalists than graduates of categorical programs in their specialties.[30,31] On the other hand, departments of internal medicine and pediatrics that did not develop primary care tracks perceived that the traditional track was excellent preparation both for those becoming generalists and for those becoming subspecialists.

Each of the generalist disciplines tried to develop substantial research programs, both because the research was needed and because research was the coin of the academic realm. The subspecialties had developed highly successful research programs with support from the National Institutes of Health. There were, however, only limited opportunities for funding research in primary care, which by its nature focused on common clinical ambulatory problems, clinical epidemiology, and health services research. Foundation support and funding from the National Center for Health Services Research, now the Agency for Healthcare Research and Quality (AHRQ), helped but has never approached levels comparable to the NIH budget. Research programs in general internal medicine at Seattle, San Francisco, and Boston; in pediatrics at Rochester and Boston; and in family practice at Seattle, Missouri, and Cleveland, as well as many others, were recognized for contributing to the generalist disciplines. These programs were small in scope, however, and clearly had less visible impact than the groundbreaking discoveries in basic sciences and subspecialties.

At Missouri, the 1980s were years of exuberance in family practice. We worked constantly to develop and enhance our educational, research, and patient care programs, with the aim of building a leading academic department of family medicine. We were fortunate to have a faculty consisting of family physicians, internists, epidemiologists, sociologists, psychologists, a nutritionist, and an educator. Our goal was to make our three practices true models of primary care delivery. The Robert Wood Johnson Family Practice Faculty Fellowship Program became the focus of intellectual activity within the department. Fellows completed a two-year program leading to a master of science degree with an emphasis in public health. Weekly research seminars supplemented clinical conferences. Jerry Perkoff's "Perk Reviews" of research papers and presentations by faculty members and fellows became legendary. Our fellows published consistently, and young faculty members began to get external grant support for their work. Gradually, we grew a second generation of faculty members.

Nevertheless, we struggled with financial realities. We had three sources of income: medical school support from the state, patient care income, and grant funding. Unlike family practice programs in most states, family practice at Missouri never received sustained direct support from the state. Our school provided modest support, which was fair when compared with that of other departments but small by national standards. We remained dependent on foundation support and federal training grant support from Title VII training grants. Efforts to obtain these grants constantly stimulated the creative juices of our faculty.

During the 1980s, we derived approximately a third of our support from the medical school, a third from grant funds, and a third from patient care. As is well known, the income of generalist physicians lies at the bottom of the ladder of physician reimbursement. In the academic setting, financial dilemmas are even greater. Income is reduced because of the service to indigent patients. Further, a significant proportion of the income of practicing generalists has been derived from electrocardiograms and laboratory and X-ray services, but in academic medical centers, this money goes to other departments. Overhead costs were also higher than those in private practice because of increased staffing in teaching settings, the increased costs of medical records, and higher institutional salary benefits for clinic employees. Thus, from the hospital's perspective and from the perspective of faculty members in other departments, our practice was a loser. Departments of medicine and pediatrics across the nation made similar observations about their primary care services.

Revenue shortfalls had to be met either by the hospital or by income earned by the more procedurally oriented specialties. Neither was enthusiastic about this prospect. We found that for each dollar billed by our family practice center, the hospital billed $4 and a consulting physician billed an additional $2. Getting across the concept that primary care services were a valuable loss leader was never easy. Still, the institution embraced and supported our practice. The financial instability of programs, however, was demonstrated by the decision by Duke University to close its family practice program. This outstanding residency was led by Harvey Estes, a former cardiologist and chair of the Institute of Medicine's 1978 Report on Primary Care. Estes felt compelled to resign his chairmanship in protest. The subsequent backlash by family physicians throughout the state and the threatened loss of referrals led Duke to reinstate the program.

In our medical school during this period, virtually all primary care was being provided by family practice. Despite this, derogatory comments in other departments about the quality of care provided by family practice faculty and residents remained a constant frustration. Most of this negative attitude seemed to come from our obstetrical residents and faculty members. While I knew that similar condescending statements were often made by internists about surgeons and by cardiologists about general internists, these continuing potshots made the milieu in which we worked more difficult. In reality, we were proud of the obstetrical services that we provided, and even today, after averaging more than two hundred deliveries a year for more than twenty-five years, our outcomes have been excellent, and we have never had an obstetrical malpractice case. During these years, for obvious reasons, our research focused on developing evidence-based obstetrical care—the most notable of which was the Radius trial, a randomized controlled trial evaluating the value of the routine use of obstetric ultrasound in pregnancy, led by Bernard Ewigman and Michael Le Fevre of our faculty.[32]

During the 1980s, the subspecialties continued to grow in departments of internal medicine and pediatrics. In internal medicine, inpatient hospital services were increasingly oriented along subspecialty lines. For the subspecialty faculty members, this made a lot of sense. On specialty services, they could care for patients with specialty-specific problems more efficiently. Faculty members were also more comfortable with clinical problems in their own disciplinary area. Coronary care units increasingly became the domain of the cardiologist, and intensive care units in internal medicine and pediatrics belonged to intensivists and neonatologists. These movements in academic medical centers were having a negative impact on the generalist vision of providing continuing care of patients in all settings. The scope of practice was narrowing.

The decade of the 1980s also was the time of the malpractice crisis. We seemed to be becoming a more litigious society in which the consumer was increasingly aware that the physician was not infallible. Malpractice insurance costs were skyrocketing. Many family physicians found that insurance costs exceeded their income from routine obstetrics and stopped performing obstetrics. While many of these doctors worried that the number of children in their practices would decline as a result, most of them also seemed relieved to get rid of the time demands of obstetrical practice.

# THE 1990s

The 1990s will forever be known as the decade of the most dramatic changes in health care delivery in the twentieth century. The nation entered the 1990s with health care expenditures continuing to rise at double-digit rates. Despite economic abundance, the number of medically uninsured people was increasing. Employers rebelled at the increasing costs of employee health care, and rising expenditures were depleting Medicare trust funds. Bill Clinton was elected president in 1992, promising health care reform. Washington and the nation as a whole seemed to believe that the key to controlling costs lay with managed competing systems of care.

At the time, there was a groundswell of concern that the supply of generalist physicians would be inadequate for a health care system rapidly moving toward managed care. Studies of group and staff model health maintenance organizations had demonstrated that perhaps half of their physicians were generalists.[33,34] However, the ratio of generalist physicians to population had remained unchanged from the 1960s, and interest in generalist careers among medical school graduates, declining throughout the 1980s, reached its nadir in

1992, when only 14.6 percent of medical school graduates planned careers in primary care.

In 1992, the Council on Graduate Medical Education reported that the nation had a continuing shortage of generalists and an increasing surplus of specialists.[33] The council recommended that the total number of physicians completing residency be reduced to 10 percent above the number of American graduates and that half of this reduced number of residents be generalists.[35] The call for increasing numbers of generalists was echoed by numerous foundations and medical organizations.[36-39] In the early 1990s, eleven state legislatures passed laws mandating that their medical schools increase the number of generalists graduating.[40]

In this setting, Steven A. Schroeder, the president of The Robert Wood Johnson Foundation, called me in 1992 and offered me a job that he said "I could not afford to turn down." He proposed that I assume the directorship of the Foundation's Generalist Physician Initiative (GPI), which was intended to help medical schools increase the number of their graduates who became generalists. Over the next nine years, Jerry Perkoff and Robin Blake, as associate directors, and I visited the fifteen GPI grant recipient medical schools annually. This opportunity provided us with insights into the education of generalists in each of the three specialties.[41]

When President Clinton's "managed competition" health reform failed, unmanaged competition ensued. Medical schools suddenly found themselves competing in a marketplace that was unwilling to pay for the higher costs of care in academic tertiary care centers. Hospitals and physician groups found that they had to compete in order to maintain "market share"—a new and distasteful term for most physicians. Managed care companies limited medical services and progressively ratcheted down payments for all providers. They sought contracts with integrated delivery systems, which could offer the full range of primary, secondary, and tertiary care. The game was to capture patient populations. Academic medical centers were handicapped not only by their high costs but also by their very limited primary care resources. How could they compete for the care of populations of patients without having a base of primary care providers? Almost overnight, primary care, which always had been low among the priorities of most academic medical centers, assumed major importance.

At Missouri, Dean Lester Bryant met with our faculty to tell us that we were developing an HMO, which would initially be for university employees and would then be expanded. He indicated that his highest anxiety was over the availability of primary care services and said he wasn't sure that our department was "up to the task." If that were the case, he would form another department of family medicine to meet the service needs.

From that day forward, our department was changed! Three months later, eight thousand additional patients entered our practice. The realities of the marketplace were fully upon us. We rapidly expanded the number of faculty members and provided them with appointments as clinician-teachers, with the vast majority of their effort spent in patient care. In addition, the institution recruited a network of family practices from throughout central Missouri to be its own primary care network.

Over the next few months, faculty members in other departments congratulated us for our success in meeting the needs of these patients. At the same time, the changes were to have a profound impact on the milieu of the department. All faculty members added clinic time, and they started evening clinics. All faculty members felt stressed by the increased patient loads. The primary focus of the practice moved slowly away from residency education to patient care. The maxim was "The patient comes first!" The new clinical challenge led several of our faculty members away from research careers toward practice and administration in the new system. The large increase in faculty members and the general feeling of overwork reduced the opportunity for reflective time. Consequently, research effort, which had been steadily rising, leveled and then dipped for several years.

A similar scenario was being followed at virtually every medical center across the country. Most academic medical centers sought to establish delivery systems and emphasized development of primary care. Each of them wanted to become the dominant provider in the region. The historical collegiality among practitioners declined in this competitive environment, and town-gown issues, always smoldering, flared almost everywhere. Academic physicians, like all other physicians, were increasingly frustrated by the control that insurers exerted over their day-to-day practice. For teaching physicians, these frustrations were compounded by the imposition of Medicare's teaching physician regulations. These defined the patient care services that attending physicians must personally provide when working with residents in order to bill for a service. Many faculty members felt that the required documentation took away time needed for the direct supervision of patient care and for teaching residents.

Despite the frustrations, the 1990s were also years of great opportunity for the academic primary care disciplines. The primary care imperative, stimulated by managed care, had a remarkable impact not only on patient care but also on the development of primary care educational programs. At Missouri, our departmental faculty provided leadership in replacing a traditional basic science curriculum with a problem-based curriculum for first-year and second-year students and then created a two-month family practice clerkship, replacing the earlier one-month primary care clerkship. One month of the clerkship was based in the teaching practices of the department, and the other was based in the offices of practicing physicians throughout the state. Interest among our medical students in primary care careers rose. A combined medicine-pediatrics residency was established. Faculty members ceased expressing concern about a shortage of residency applicants.

It was during this period that we began annual visits to each of the fifteen medical schools participating in the Generalist Physicians Initiative.[41] At each GPI school, the generalist faculty members were little short of exuberant as they accepted leadership roles and participated in curriculum reform. They cooperatively adopted programs emphasizing education in primary care in the first and second year, and they also involved physicians practicing in the community. Each school developed required family practice or primary care clerkships. Faculty members in the specialties, anticipating an underemployment of specialists because of a specialist glut, seemed to encourage students toward generalist careers for the first time. The changes that we observed at GPI schools were also occurring in medical schools nationally, and interest in the generalist specialties soared among medical school graduates.

In 2001, James Cultice, of the National Center for Health Workforce Analysis at the Health Resources and Services Administration (HRSA), and I completed studies indicating that between 1993 and 2000, the number of allopathic and osteopathic residency graduates entering practice in family practice increased 55 percent, to 3,885 graduates annually. Those entering general medicine practice increased 63 percent, to 3,701, and those entering general pediatrics practice increased 15 percent, to 1,716. At the same time, the number of first-year fellows in internal medicine had fallen 21 percent, and the percentage planning to enter a pediatric subspeciality dropped from 30 percent to 20 percent in 1997–98. After three decades in which the generalist physician-to-population ratio had remained steady at about 60 per 100,000, it appeared that the generalist shortage might be a thing of the past.[42]

Despite the increased numbers of generalist graduates, overt changes in residency curricula to enhance primary care skills were modest at best. Program directors for the GPI reported that the failure to change residency curricula was a major disappointment. The heavy demands of the inpatient services in medicine and pediatrics limited their ability to increase the emphasis on primary care. Further, the majority of people in both disciplines seemed to continue to believe that the best site for education is the acute inpatient service of the teaching hospital, believing that this setting fosters a more scholarly approach to understanding the pathogenesis and the management of disease. In their minds, the inpatient area is where the real action is. Nevertheless, influenced by new residency review requirements, all internal medicine and pediatrics residency programs now provided half a day a week in continuity practice and have also increased overall ambulatory experiences. A few even have two half-days weekly in continuity practice. None of the GPI schools have sought to initiate or expand primary care tracks in internal medicine or pediatrics. Nationally, the number of positions in primary care tracks in internal medicine offered in the

National Residency Matching Program (NRMP) fell from 514 in 1995 to 339 in 2001. Pediatrics had only 110 primary care track positions in 2002. So most residencies in medicine and pediatrics continued to emphasize acute hospital care and provided little education in common ambulatory problems outside their specialties.

In the late 1990s, a backlash against managed care began to appear, fueled by consumers and frustrated physicians and catalyzed by the press. Physician groups uniformly complained about regulations, precertification requirements, denial of tests and procedures, and other things that intruded into their care of patients. The public also articulated a desire for direct access to specialists and advocated a "patients' bill of rights." Concerns about restrictions on hospital stay, access to specialists, and the requirement that patients see their "gatekeeper" all led to highly negative publicity for HMOs. Vocal patient advocacy groups pointed to the inherent conflict of interest that many gatekeeping physicians faced. While their overriding responsibility was to their patients, gatekeeping physicians in some plans received incentive payments when they limited services such as hospitalizations, referrals, and diagnostic procedures.

After double-digit increases in HMO enrollment, the rate of increase slowed, and increasing numbers of patients entered point-of-service managed care plans, which guarantee access to the specialist for a price. Indeed, some insurers, such as United Health Care and Humana, began offering plans without a gatekeeper requirement. Enrollment in preferred provider organizations and point-of-service plans, however, continued to increase, while the old tried-and-true indemnity insurance, which had been the basis of employer-sponsored health insurance in earlier decades, seemed to be moribund.

In association with these changes, the number of medical school graduates entering generalist careers peaked in 1997 and then began to fall. The number of American medical school graduates in family practice residencies declined 19 percent between 1997 and 2002. Numbers entering primary care tracks in medicine, pediatrics, and joint internal medicine-pediatrics residencies have also declined, while the traditional categorical programs in internal medicine and pediatrics have held steady. More medical school graduates began to select residencies in radiology and in anesthesiology. The percentage of first-time takers of the pediatric certification exam who planned to become generalists fell from 73 percent in 1998 to 68 percent in 2000; the number of first-year fellows in internal medicine in 1999–2000 showed an increase for the first time since 1992–93.

In the early 1990s, many of us felt that medical students were sheltered from market forces in health care and that their choice of specialty was primarily influenced by the milieu for primary care within their own medical schools. Many studies had demonstrated the influence of the medical school on the selection of generalist careers.[43] The 1990s, with their dramatic shifts in students' specialty choices, clearly showed the pervasive power of the market-place.

# TODAY: OUR ACCOMPLISHMENTS

When the accomplishments of the generalist movement are viewed from the perspective of the last thirty-five years, they seem extraordinary. In 1966, the nation was crying for a new type of personal physician. The general practitioner was rapidly disappearing, and graduates of internal medicine and pediatrics residencies were increasingly entering subspecialties. Generalist faculty members were nonexistent in the nation's medical schools, and most institutions saw no role for generalists on their full-time academic faculty. Those internists and pediatricians who did not subspecialize typically became generalists, but their residency programs, like mine, had been hospital-based and provided limited training opportunities for providing primary care.

We may now be on the verge of solving the generalist shortage. The generalist movement blossomed during the 1970s, plateaued during the 1980s, and expanded explosively in the 1990s—reaching a peak in 1997. Jim Cultice from HRSA and I estimate that the number of generalists entering practice in 2000 was 9,579—a 50 percent increase from 1993. These included 3,885 family physicians, 3,701 general internists, and 1,716 general pediatricians. The Council on Graduate Medical Education (COGME) recommended that the nation reduce the number of first-year residency positions to 110 percent of United States medical school graduates and that half of this number become generalists. If this had occurred, the number of first-year residency positions would have fallen to 19,000, and 9,500 of those would have become generalists. So the number of generalist graduates in 2000 was at the level recommended by COGME. If this number of generalist graduates continues, and if past retirement rates from practice continue, we project that the number of practicing generalist physicians will increase to 83 per 100,000 population by 2020. This figure is slightly above the range of 60 to 80 specialists per 100,000 recommended by COGME. For the first time in a century, the United States has an increasing supply of generalist physicians. However, if the number of graduates were to return to 1993 levels, the number of generalists would fall to 66 per 100,000.[42]

The increases of the 1990s could not have happened without the development of academic programs in generalist medicine in the nation's medical schools. Today, 132 medical schools have departments of family medicine, and two have divisions. Only 10 have no educational programs in family medicine. Virtually all medical school departments of internal medicine and pediatrics have divisions of general internal medicine and general pediatrics. In many cases, these divisions are the largest divisions within their parent departments.

A typical department of family medicine will have more than thirty faculty members. Divisions of general internal medicine are of similar size, and a typical division of general pediatrics has more than fifteen faculty members.

The generalist faculty members have assumed a central role in undergraduate medical education. While visiting medical schools participating in The Robert Wood Johnson Foundation's Generalist Physician Initiative, we observed an increasing orientation of the curriculum toward primary care and generalist medicine. First- and second-year students are introduced to practicing community-based generalist physicians in their offices. Generalist faculty members provide leadership in enhancing courses that provide the introductory skills in clinical medicine. These courses now usually include clinical correlation with basic sciences, clinical epidemiology, evidence-based medicine, community medicine, medical ethics, and an emphasis on the biopsychosocial model of illness. Most schools developed third-year required clerkships in family practice. Many clerkships in internal medicine and pediatrics began to have more ambulatory experience. While family medicine took the lead in providing community-based education, some departments of pediatrics provided an even greater population-oriented focus and helped students understand broader issues of the community's health. Most important, generalist faculty members now serve as role models for students and residents.

Primary care services are now a central part of the delivery system at most academic medical centers. Although primary care is a financial loss leader, the institutions recognize that referrals from primary care contribute to the revenue-generating capacity of the institution. Generalist faculty members are also making major contributions to medical centers in their role as hospitalists. Finally, as a result of the breadth of their interests, generalist faculty members have increasingly assumed administrative leadership in the dean's office, in physician practice plans, and in other areas. In so doing, these faculty members are modifying the culture of our academic health sciences centers. They have helped expand the horizons of the medical center programs beyond traditional tertiary care services and have begun to bring educational programs out of the academic health center and into the community.

Our program at Missouri is one example. In 1964, we had only one generalist faculty member. Today at Missouri, our Department of Family and Community Medicine consists of approximately fifty faculty, including thirty-four physicians, four nurse practitioners, one sociologist, two psychologists, four health services researchers, a Ph.D. epidemiologist, a librarian, and nine M.D. fellows. The residency has produced 276 family practice graduates over the years. Twenty percent of this group is in academic medicine, and seven of these individuals head academic departments of family medicine. Two-thirds of the remaining 80 percent have entered practice in nonmetropolitan areas. The two-year fellowship program has fifty-six graduates, the vast majority of whom are in academic medicine. Faculty members provide more teaching time in the problem-based curriculum of the first two years than any other department in the school and also provide a two-month family practice clerkship in the third year. Eight of the faculty members are heavily involved in research, and five have funded grants. Several have major institutional leadership roles. Our practices have eighty thousand visits annually, and our inpatient services average sixteen hundred admissions and more than two hundred deliveries annually—even in this world of managed care. Faculty members feel that they are accomplishing their mission of primary care, rural health care, and academic family medicine.

## VISIONS NOT YET ACHIEVED

The growth of generalism in the 1990s was due in part to a national expectation that managed care would reshape the health care delivery system, with generalist physicians providing the majority of care and coordinating consultative care. There was a widespread belief that the nation needed more generalists and fewer specialists—a message trumpeted to the public and heard by all academic medical centers during the 1990s. As a result, highly efficient market forces increased the number of generalists. But these times appear to be changing.

Today we hear about the impending death of managed care.[44] Despite earlier expectations, most managed care plans never succeeded in developing cohesive systems to enhance the overall quality and efficiency of care for populations of patients. Despite major efforts, they were neither able to ensure that needed services were provided or that excessive services were reduced. In fact, most managed care companies did not succeed in managing care but did succeed in limiting expenditures. For several years during the 1990s, health care expenditures were held at or below the rate of growth of our economy. These efforts, however, fostered a tremendous backlash both by consumers and providers. Basic distrust of the profit motives of profit-driven HMOs added to this backlash.

Now, as HMOs loosen restrictions, health care expenditures are increasing at more than twice the rate of increase in the gross domestic product. Researchers at the Centers for Medicare and Medicaid Services project that medical expenditures will increase from 13 percent of GDP in 2000 to 16.8 percent in 2010.[45] Typical health insurance premiums are increasing at 20 percent a year. Our medical capabilities are approaching a point where they exceed payers' willingness to pay. Inevitably, government and employers will limit their contributions, but the public still expects to reap the rewards of new technologies. There is little evidence that the nation is willing to face this issue other than by linking services to the ability of the individual to pay.[46] Most experts expect employers to transfer increasing costs to patients through increasing deductibles and copayments. Many anticipate a three-tiered health care system based on the individual's ability to pay.[47]

Another fundamental issue is the growing number of medically uninsured individuals. No compassionate physician can ignore the fact that more than forty million Americans lack health insurance and another forty million are underinsured. Today, during the economic downturn of the early 2000s, millions of additional individuals are becoming uninsured.

Against this backdrop, a high percentage of physicians are distraught in their practices—frustrated by bureaucratic controls and above all by a sense of loss of autonomy. Prior authorization requirements, unfathomable fee schedules, rejected claims, chart audits, and higher overhead costs lead many to consider early retirement. Physicians feel that they must work longer hours and see more patients just to maintain their income. Some data, however, suggest that primary care physicians actually spend more time with patients than they did in the past.[48]

Although these issues affect all medical practitioners, generalist physicians have their own concerns. The vision of a health care delivery system built around competing integrated systems has become blurred. The demand for generalists seems to have leveled off, and anecdotal evidence suggests a newly increasing demand for specialists. The gatekeeper role of primary care physicians, with its potential for conflict of interest, is being challenged by consumers in their revolution against managed care, as well as by generalists themselves, who do not want to interfere with their patients' desire for access to specialists. Many fear that open-access insurance plans without a mandated gatekeeper will reduce the demand for generalists. In this competitive market, some are concerned that increasing numbers of nurse practitioners and physician assistants will limit practice opportunities for generalist physicians. Even though U.S. physicians continue to be highly paid, generalist physicians' incomes remain at the bottom of all specialties. But this has always been the case—and will continue to be the case as long as a fee-for-service system values technological services more than cognitive services. For many academics, the declining interest in generalist careers among the graduates of American medical schools is symbolic of a declining priority for generalist medicine nationally as well as in academic settings. Some feel that the modest primary care research programs weaken their identity as academicians. Each of these issues, while real, must be placed in perspective.

We must be deeply concerned about the declining interest in generalist careers among American medical school graduates. Interest by senior U.S. medical students in generalist careers fell from 35.6 percent of U.S. seniors to 24.5 percent between 1999 and 2001. These data from the AAMC Graduate Questionnaire revealed that interest in family practice fell 26 percent, general internal medicine fell 45 percent, and general pediatrics declined 25 percent. The number of United

States graduates seeking generalist careers has returned to 1992 levels. An adequate output of generalist graduates is being maintained by recruiting osteopathic and international graduates to our residency programs.

Over the years, the pendulum of interest among U.S. students in the various specialties has swung back and forth, depending on student perceptions of the medical marketplace.[49] The increased interest in generalist specialties during the 1990s occurred in association with a perceived glut of specialists, but now demand for specialists appears to be rising. Within a given national market, student views of generalist careers are also greatly influenced by the milieu for primary care in their medical schools. Schools with high orientations to primary care produce greater numbers of generalist physicians. Medical schools must continue to place high priority on education for primary care.[43] I anticipate that as history demonstrates, the pendulum will swing back.

Though many faculty in generalist disciplines perceive a decline in the priority for generalist medicine at academic medical centers, the reality is that generalist faculty members live in a world different from the one that they inhabited two decades ago. They are far more numerous; they are central to undergraduate and graduate medical education; they provide essential primary care services; and they provide leadership in their institutions. However, generalist faculty members continue to constitute only a small percentage of medical school faculties. The overall milieu continues to be oriented to tertiary care rather than primary care and continues to focus on the biomedical rather than the biopsychosocial. The emphasis continues to be on acute and episodic curative medicine rather than on prevention, chronic care, and the alleviation of symptoms. The medical student will continue to have far more contact with the tertiary care specialist than with the generalist. These are the realities of today and probably of tomorrow. These observations are less true for community-based medical schools and for schools that are less oriented to tertiary care and to biomedical research. It is not surprising that community-based schools continue to produce the highest percentage of generalists. The challenge for generalist faculty members will be to continue fostering and expanding education outside the tertiary care center. This movement will be expedited in many institutions as their clinical services increasingly focus on quaternary care and as educational experiences for students and residents in caring for routine problems become ever more limited.

In light of today's backlash against managed care, some observers may question the future of primary care. It is hard for me to conceive of a rational system of care that is not grounded in primary care provided by knowledgeable generalist physicians. Barbara Starfield, using international data, has demonstrated that the level of primary care orientation in a health care system is associated with lower costs, less use of medication, and better health levels.[50] A variety of researchers have shown that access to primary care is associated with lower mortality[51–54] and lower health care expenditures.[55] Access to specialty care does not have these associations. Whereas many suggest that specialists provide substantial primary care services, Roger Rosenblatt and colleagues' data show that specialists' practices include only modest primary care services.[56] Larry Green and colleagues have recently repeated Kerr White's classical study on the ecology of medical care and again has demonstrated the small proportion of human illness that finds its way to the academic health center.[57] The essential role for the generalist is as real today as it was at the time of the 1966 Millis Commission Report in 1966.

Despite the backlash against managed care, the vast majority of patients enrolled in gatekeeper plans are satisfied with their primary physician and seem to prefer seeing this physician initially for most problems, including severe problems.[58] Enrollment is increasing in the point-of-service (POS) plans, which give patients the option of having direct access to specialists and other generalists. However, a recent study of three POS plans suggests that patients enroll more to have the option of seeing other physicians than to use that option.[59] As an example, the University of Missouri in 2001 offered a new POS plan for university employees for $20 a month per family more than the university's gated-group type of HMO, which was based at University Hospital. This ungated POS plan permits both direct access to specialists and the option to seek care outside the network—options not available in the HMO. Only 6 percent of the employees switched to the new plan. Further, many who switched continue to use the university plan for primary care and specialty services.

Ethical issues exist when the physician gatekeeper benefits monetarily by limiting the use of resources. The solution to the gatekeeper dilemma is to eliminate individual financial incentives for physicians to limit services. Incentives for the patient and the generalist should be parallel. Ideally, the physicians should receive incentives based on quality as well as on consumer satisfaction, and the patient should have financial incentives to continue to use the primary care physician. In this way, the generalist becomes the coordinator of care rather than the gatekeeper to care.[60]

The nurse practitioner (NP) and physician assistant (PA) movements are now more than thirty years old. Both types of professionals play major roles in primary care. Studies by Richard Cooper and colleagues suggest large increases in numbers of nurse practitioners and physician assistants in the future.[61] Nursing has sought the right to independent practice for NPs. NPs as well as PAs now have the authority to prescribe medication in most states.[62] Mary Mundinger, dean of Columbia University's School of Nursing, and her colleagues completed a randomized trial of care by nurse practitioners for a relatively healthy immigrant population in New York City. The results of that study with this population suggest that the quality of care and costs of care are similar to services provided by physicians at a comparable clinic.[63] Many are concerned that a NP and PA surplus will reduce demand for generalist physicians.

It appears, however, that the role of NPs and PAs in office-based primary care practice is more modest than many have thought. Hooker and McCaig, using data from the National Ambulatory Medical Care Survey (NAMCS), found that NPs or PAs were involved in only 3 percent of 462 million visits to office-based primary care physicians annually between 1995 and 1999.[64] Their data indicated that approximately 25 percent of practicing generalist physicians work with an NP or a PA, but only 10 percent of total patient visits in these practices were provided by NPs or PAs. (NAMCS data may understate actual NP and PA visits because physician practices were sampled and some may not have provided data on NP and PA visits.) Hooker and McCaig, using data drawn from the NAMCS, found that that NPs and PAs actually had more visits in hospital-based clinics and emergency rooms than in the offices of primary care physicians. The role of the NP in independent practice also appears to be small. Ed Fryer of the AAFP's Graham Center provided me with data from the 1998 Medical Expenditure Panel Survey (MEPS) indicating that eight million visits were made to nurses (LPN, RN, NP) at locations where a physician does not work. Less than half of these visits were for diagnosis and treatment, services an NP might provide. The NP and the PA provide important services in many settings, but the bulk of this appears neither to be in physicians' practices nor in independent practice.

The nurse practitioner and physician assistant movements were initiated in the 1960s, when the nation faced a national shortage of primary care physicians and a major shortage of rural physicians. We do not know what the role of the NP will be in a setting where there is an adequate supply of generalist physicians. My feeling is that most people prefer to see a physician when they have a medical problem and that most nurse practitioners have little desire for independent medical practice, preferring rather to apply their advanced nursing expertise as members of primary care teams. After more than thirty years, there are relatively few examples of independent nursing practice. Some people in nursing now advocate Ph.D. nurses to provide greater competence in primary care. Even if such programs were established, it would be a generation before they could have a substantial impact on the delivery of primary care.

The future holds great promise for nurse practitioners and physician assistants in collaborative practice with generalists and specialists in a wide variety of settings. I believe that their services will continue to complement physician services but will not often replace them. There is an additional and relatively untapped market for NP and PA services in nursing homes, health departments, and schools that will expand as our health care system evolves.

Another concern of academic generalist faculty members is that their research contributions have been modest. This is a fair critique. Most successful researchers define a narrow research area and spend a career becoming a true expert in that area. Most generalists seem to desire a broader focus. Their gratification may come more from day-to-day comprehensive care of human beings with diverse problems than from focused inquiry. Internal medicine and pediatrics graduates have benefited from the fact that their residencies are based within academic health centers, in a setting where the intellectual milieu and the prestige of inquiry tend to be high. In family practice, the majority of the residencies are in community hospital settings, tend to be small, and have relatively few full-time faculty members and little research expertise. These settings provide patient care of high quality and outstanding teaching but do not usually provide a research-oriented milieu.

Nevertheless, generalists in each discipline are making significant research contributions. For them, the laboratory is the patient, the clinic, the community, and the larger delivery system. They are contributing to the understanding and management of common ambulatory problems, defining guidelines for preventive services, researching quality of care, and studying access to care. They have been among the leaders in the development of evidence-based medicine, clinical guidelines, and clinical decision analysis—areas that will help define the future practice of medicine. Their basic sciences are clinical epidemiology, statistics, and the behavioral sciences.

A challenge for all three disciplines is to develop a group of faculty members who are enthusiastic about research. Unfortunately, relatively small numbers of generalists apply either to The Robert Wood Johnson Foundation's Clinical Scholars Program or to its Generalist Faculty Fellows Program. The majority of those who do apply are internists, and the graduates of these programs are leaders in generalist medicine. At one point in the mid-1990s, more than fifty division heads in general internal medicine had been Clinical Scholars.

Research funding for common clinical problems and for health services research, which is central to primary care research, has been limited at best. However, current expansion of NIH funding into the primary care arena and increased funding of the Agency for Healthcare Research and Quality offer potential for future expansion of primary care research. Though contributions of generalist physicians to research have been modest, they are increasing and will continue to do so.

In summary, we live in a dynamic and changing environment. Over the past thirty years, the accomplishments of generalist medicine have been extraordinary. Although we appear to be on our way to solving the generalist shortage, we must still be deeply concerned about the declining proportion of American graduates among the trainees. The role of generalist medicine in the health care delivery system is evolving. As an academic discipline, generalist medicine is in its adolescence and still requires substantial development, but at this time it is well prepared for future challenges.

# THE PRACTICE OF TOMORROW'S GENERALISTS

Medicine and its delivery systems have been changing throughout my lifetime and will no doubt continue to change. Management of specific diseases constantly changes as new knowledge becomes available. As a resident, I had required rotations at a tuberculosis sanatorium and on an iron lung ward for polio patients. Fortunately, these are distant memories today. As residents, we were told that pregnant women should gain no more than twenty pounds during pregnancy out of concern that additional weight gain would increase the probability of preeclampsia. Then researchers found that rigid weight limitation during pregnancy increased the frequency of fetal growth retardation. We kept patients with myocardial infarction on complete bed rest for five weeks to allow maximum fibrosis of the damaged muscle but subsequently found increased mortality from thromboembolism. Chloramphenicol was our most commonly used antibiotic until we found that it occasionally caused agranulocytosis—loss of white blood cells. Now we find that giving postmenopausal estrogens and progesterone actually increases the risk of cardiovascular disease. I tell our residents, "Today's dogma may be tomorrow's malpractice."

Our systems of health care delivery have also changed. When I graduated from medical school in 1957, I expected universal access to medical care to be a reality within a few years. Congress did pass Medicare and Medicaid in 1965—a major step forward for a large segment of our population. With a few exceptions, the practice of medicine was fee-for-service and was organized around solo or small group practice. The corporatization of medicine was in its early infancy, and managed care existed in only a few group-model HMOs, which were demonized by organized medicine. We practiced medicine without thinking about cost. Patients with insurance were admitted to the hospital for thirty-day "rest cures." On the other hand, at indigent care hospitals, money was always a problem. During times of tight budget, we had weekly quotas on the number of lab tests we could order at the King County Hospital in Seattle.

Tomorrow's generalist will live in a brave new world of genomics and proteomics. We expect a new age of designer drugs that will be engineered to target specific receptors. Some observers suggest that the knowledge obtained from unlocking the human genome will require increasing specialization,[65] and a new specialty has been established in genetics. Others caution that gene therapy for most common diseases remains only a distant hope. They point out that most common diseases have multiple genetic loci. Consequently, genetic approaches may be less effective for these diseases than such well-recognized approaches as lifestyle and environmental modifications.[66] Thus the impact on day-to-day medical practice may be less than some people expect. In other areas, biomedical engineering promises great technological advances in specialties such as cardiology and physical medicine, and newer imaging techniques are revolutionizing the practice of radiologists.

For the generalist, the technology of the future is informatics. Information technology is already changing the lives of many generalists. Our residents maintain up-to-date information about their patients on handheld computers, which also provide immediate access to drug information, clinical guidelines, and other data. A major research focus in our department is to create a process whereby immediate online answers to clinical questions are available for physicians as they see patients in day-to-day practice. The movement toward electronic paperless records, which has been a promise for so long, is now being adopted in practices and medical centers across the nation. We are experiencing the greatest revolution in medical record keeping in half a century. These technological changes will increase the efficiency of the generalist, increase the comprehensiveness of care, reduce errors, and markedly expand access to medical knowledge right in the examining room.

Many observers expect the consumer, enabled by increasing medical information obtained from the Internet, to take a larger role in his or her care. But the consumer has always made decisions about care. As physicians grounded in hospital care, we have viewed ourselves as providers of care and have been frustrated when our patients have not complied with our directions. In reality, the patient—not the physician—is the provider of care in the ambulatory setting. The physician serves as one of many consultants for the patient, who makes decisions using the physician, members of the family, and information derived from other sources. Tomorrow's primary care physicians must recognize that they are consultants to their patients. These patients, though much more knowledgeable than in the past, will still need assistance in making rational decisions about their care.

In looking to the future, we must keep in mind the changing demographics of our society. We are becoming an increasingly mature society. The most rapidly growing segment of the population is the group above eighty-five years of age. By 2030, the number of people above age sixty-five will double and will constitute more than 20 percent of the population. Even today, with only 13 percent of the population older than sixty-five, this group accounts for 38 percent of health care expenditures in the United States.[67] As a result of advances in medicine, today's elderly are living longer and have decreased disability. Nevertheless, the burden of chronic disease can only increase as the population ages. Gerald Anderson, at the Johns Hopkins School of Public Health, points out that more than 40 percent of our population has one or more chronic illnesses and that this burden is responsible for 75 percent of today's health care spending. Tomorrow's generalists face an extraordinary challenge!

As my own patients have aged and have developed multiple chronic illnesses, I have come to realize that their care requires different skills and different orientations. I must now think less about curing and more about controlling symptoms, reducing disability, and maintaining quality of life. The task of providing continuing care for most of these patients is logically mine rather than that of the subspecialist. The chronic illnesses that these patients have are manageable. In my role as a primary provider, I confer with the various consultants and work with an interdisciplinary team to meet patient needs. The seemingly unresolvable problem, however, is that current fee-for-service reimbursement does not effectively pay for team care.

For many in medicine, gratification comes from curing rather than caring. Hospital-based education focuses on the acute and the emergent. The attitudes, competencies, and skills necessary for tomorrow's generalists can come only from generalists as team members providing longitudinal care for the chronically ill in the ambulatory setting.

Another universal trend in medical practice is a narrowing of the scope of physicians' practices. Even in ophthalmology, physicians are limiting their practices to narrow areas such as glaucoma or diseases of the cornea or retina. Orthopedists and other surgeons with whom I talk lament the fact that their practices have narrowed to performing only a few procedures. Some academic radiologists even limit their practices to MRIs of the knees.

By nature, generalists have felt that breadth of practice is essential for career gratification. Nevertheless, the scope of practice in the generalist disciplines has been narrowing. With the development of family practice as a new specialty, the general practitioner gave up most operative procedures. Subsequently, many family physicians gave up obstetrical practices in the malpractice crisis. In many settings today, general internists and general pediatricians are giving way to the cardiologist, the intensivist, and the hospitalist in the care of hospitalized patients. Increasingly, pediatricians devote 100 percent of their practice to ambulatory care.

These trends have been anathema for those of us who fear an increasing fragmentation of care. They may also lead some graduating students to relish the opportunity for "acute care" away from generalist specialties. Nevertheless, most family physicians did not grieve when they gave up obstetrics because of escalating malpractice premiums. Many in general internal medicine and family practice have vigorously opposed the hospitalist, but in reality many already prefer ambulatory practice because of the increased office efficiency. I was amazed to find that a third of our Missouri family practice residency graduates currently have no hospital practice. At the same time, 60 percent have intensive care privileges, usually in rural practice locations, and more than a third of them continue to care for obstetrical patients.

Current trends suggest that the practice of the general internist and the family physician will increasingly be based in the office, the nursing home, and the home. The pediatrician will be in the office, the home, and the school. Physicians in each generalist discipline will see their roles as being responsible for the health of defined populations. These generalists of the future should perhaps more appropriately be called "primary care physicians." They must be scholars and outstanding clinicians, well versed in the breadth of chronic disease and common ambulatory problems and knowledgeable in clinical epidemiology and behavioral science. Daniel Bryant of the Maine Medical Center suggests that these physicians, whom he calls "officists," will replace the education previously derived from hospital contacts with educational programs developed in the office.[68] In some ways, the example of a group of British GPs in a community-based practice, serving a defined population and working with an interdisciplinary group of providers, offers a model of what we might see in our own integrated delivery systems in the United States. The rural physician will continue to provide a breadth of services typically not offered by the urban physician, while acute hospital services for rural residents will increasingly be provided in an urban setting. Consequently, many family practice residencies should continue to provide rural training tracks, which ideally are located in rural settings.

We need to be developing tomorrow's models of primary care today. The beginnings are already present in primary care settings across the nation and are perhaps best developed in group- and staff-model HMOs.[69,70] Small interdisciplinary primary care teams will provide personalized care for defined populations utilizing evidence-based clinical guidelines. Programs of patient management will be integrated into these practices. In our practices at Missouri, small primary care teams consist of family physicians, nurse practitioners, and psychologists, with on-site psychiatric and dietary support. Northern California Kaiser Permanente has added a physical therapist to its primary care team. Our team, which includes residents, serves patients in the office, the nursing home, and the hospital and has links with home care agencies. As part of an academic group practice, we work closely with physicians in each clinical specialty. Communication between physicians, always a problem, has improved markedly with e-mail and our developing electronic medical record system.

Even though our team is in place and provides personalized care for a population of patients, key factors are absent. Consequently, the practice remains focused on the "numerator" patient and places inadequate emphasis on the "denominator," the population we serve. Information systems are not yet online to develop preventive reminder services for the healthy as well as for monitoring care for individuals with chronic illnesses. These information systems are essential for monitoring the quality of care. The predominance of fee-for-service reimbursement forces the practice to focus on the office visit rather than to make maximal use of the telephone and e-mail for efficiency and patient satisfaction. Little or no reimbursement is available for these services. A nurse practitioner maintains constant phone contact with our frail elderly, providing great support and assistance for them and, it is hoped, recognizing early warning signs in these individuals. But we have no means of reimbursement for these services! So even though fee-for-service has many strengths, it limits our potential to provide innovative and more efficient care. It is not surprising that much of the innovation in the delivery of primary care has occurred in group- and staff-model HMOs, which have clearly defined patient populations and are reimbursed by capitation.

The major questions now are "How will future insurance systems be organized?" and "Will these systems foster or impede the development of future-oriented primary care models?" During the 1990s, managed care became the enemy of the consumer and of the provider as it sought to control health care expenditures by limiting services. In the years ahead, new technologies, an aging population, insatiable consumer demand, and a more than adequate supply of physicians and hospital beds can only result in increasing utilization of services and increasing health care costs.[71] Managed care companies are passing increasing costs on to the payers. Government and industry are expected to transfer these increasing costs to consumers in an effort to make them more cost-conscious. The informed consumer will select from a menu of health plans based on coverage, quality, and costs. Consumers are expected to become more cost-conscious and to select insurance coverage from multiple options with varying coverage, deductibles, and coinsurance. One would expect the healthiest and those with lowest incomes to select the lower-cost, more tightly managed plans and plans with the least coverage. Those who have significant health problems and those who are more affluent are likely to select more comprehensive and more flexible plans. Adverse selection of these plans by those most ill may prohibitively increase the costs of these plans. Against this backdrop, the probability of a single-payer system increases.

The challenge for clinicians will be to provide the greatest value while meeting consumer needs for personalized care. Our services must be managed for both efficiency and quality. Most providers and delivery systems have not truly managed medical care, and our current delivery systems are plagued by extraordinary inefficiency, errors, redundancy, and fragmentation.[72] Tremendous geographic differences occur in services rendered, and much service is probably unnecessary.[54] We use the most expensive people to carry out the simplest of procedures. In this day, when colon cancer is second only to lung cancer in cancer mortality and colonoscopy seems to be the best screening test, can we afford to have gastroenterologists perform screening colonoscopy for the entire population at risk? Obviously, trained technicians under supervision of a gastroenterologist could markedly expand current capabilities and reduce costs in the event that alternative screening strategies do not become available.

The degree to which future models of primary care can be used will depend on the financial incentives within the system. Ideally, incentives should encourage the patient to use primary care, primary care physicians to provide comprehensive services, and consultants to be parsimonious in the use of their services.

## THE EDUCATION OF TOMORROW'S GENERALISTS

Education in the generalist disciplines faces major challenges. Often I feel we attempt to educate tomorrow's physicians in today's system while maintaining yesterday's beliefs. Perhaps my bias is showing, but I believe that the family practice educational model comes closest to meeting today's needs for primary care physicians. The categorical internal medicine residency is ideally suited to prepare today's hospitalists and subspecialists. However, physicians' roles will be different tomorrow and will require modified educational programs.

The boundaries of our disciplines are broadening in some areas as we provide more comprehensive care for the chronically ill and are narrowing in others. The orientations, skills, and attitudes for tomorrow's primary care physician can be developed only by immersion in models of tomorrow's primary care, where the resident develops skills in working with interdisciplinary teams and learns the gratification of providing complex longitudinal primary care services that meet patients' needs. Resident physicians must become integral members of these primary care practices. One half-day a week does not meet patient needs either for access or continuity, nor does it foster the knowledge and the orientation needed for tomorrow's primary care physicians. Our past focus on hospital-based education has fostered an orientation toward acute care and cure. Emphasizing tomorrow's models of primary care will foster an orientation focused on prevention, continuity, maintaining function, and assuming longitudinal responsibility for populations of patients.

Residency programs in primary care should be based in future-oriented primary care settings complemented by hospital inpatient rotations. Today most programs are driven by inpatient rotations supplemented by primary care experiences. Primary care residents in family practice and internal medicine would benefit from more emphasis on prevention, population medicine, evidence-based medicine, principles of rehabilitation, and end-of-life care. The resident in primary care internal medicine should also have additional experience in women's health, behavioral medicine, and musculoskeletal medicine. The pediatrics resident needs more developmental pediatrics, adolescent medicine, and school health. Each of the disciplines could accomplish these goals by reducing inpatient experiences.

In 1973, Joel Alpert and Evan Charney, in their monograph *The Education of Physicians for Primary Care,* pointed out that internal medicine and pediatrics had a dilemma as they attempted to educate physicians to be both primary care physicians and consulting specialists for those most ill.[10] Could they really educate physicians for both roles? Now, almost thirty years later, the issue is still unresolved. Larry Young and Ed Pellegrino, whose writings I discussed earlier, addressed these problems with remarkable insight in 1974 in *Controversy in Internal Medicine.*[73,74] Pellegrino believed the major manpower contribution of departments of medicine to be "the production of organ system specialists."[73] He also saw the need for a generalist in internal medicine who would be based in secondary and tertiary care, and would coordinate the care of hospitalized patients. He suggested that the coordination of inpatient care be provided by faculty members in general internal medicine who would also serve as role models for trainees in general internal medicine. The family physician would be a primary care physician with tasks specifically directed to "primary, preventive and general care of the common ills of mankind—the 85% of human disabilities that rarely enter the hospital." He went on, "The generally trained internist who wishes to become a bona fide family practitioner will find it necessary to acquire knowledge and skills beyond those he is apt to attain in the usual medical residency. His background in internal medicine is an excellent but far from sufficient preparation." Larry Young, on the other hand, emphasized that both the internist and the pediatrician must provide primary care in order to meet the need for personal physicians. He argued that educational programs in internal medicine and pediatrics had to be modified to provide competency in primary care, and he personally developed the primary care residency track in internal medicine at Rochester.[74]

It appears to me that internal medicine and pediatrics have three potential ways to resolve these long-standing dilemmas. First, each discipline could define itself as a secondary and tertiary care discipline and educate hospitalists and subspecialists, as suggested by Pellegrino almost thirty years ago. There is logic to this; it has precedence in other countries such as Canada and the United Kingdom and requires little change in educational programs. However, internal medicine's image of itself includes primary care, hospital care, and consulting care.[75,76] The same can be said for pediatrics. If Pellegrino's proposal were implemented, family practice, as the only primary care discipline, would have to more than double its residencies—not a very likely solution at this time. A second alternative would be to prepare all internists and pediatricians as primary care physicians as I have outlined. Those entering a subspecialty would enter that subspecialty as capable primary care physicians. I would view such an approach as highly desirable preparation both for those entering primary care and for those entering a subspecialty. This would meet the needs of the majority who enter primary care and would provide subspecialists with both the knowledge and the orientations required in primary care. The service demands of the inpatient services provide logistical dilemmas. The third option is to reinvent primary care tracks and make them available for graduates entering primary care. Those becoming hospitalists and those entering subspecialties would complete inpatient-oriented categorical programs, but the majority would enter primary care tracks. This seemed to be the direction that both primary care medicine and pediatrics were taking in the 1970s, but now these primary care tracks are dwindling. Either the second or the third option would provide a true primary care–oriented education for primary care graduates in internal medicine and pediatrics in which priorities are in the ambulatory settings and inpatient education complements ambulatory experiences.

I frequently ask myself whether the current organization of the three primary care disciplines in academic medical centers is optimally aligned with the future educational, service, and research objectives of the institutions. Each generalist discipline exists within its own disciplinary silo. In most institutions, there is little communication or cooperation among the three, except in the preclinical education of medical students. In fact, each frequently sees itself as competitive with the others. Many people in general internal medicine and general pediatrics feel dwarfed in subspecialty-dominated departments and feel that they have little ability in that setting to create needed generalist training programs. They recognize that their goals, aspirations, and functions have more in common with faculty members in the generalist disciplines than with those in the subspecialties. At the same time, primary care service and primary care education tend to be fragmented and uncoordinated, and primary care research programs lack the critical mass of investigators to initiate substantial projects. Some academic health centers have brought clinical primary care services together administratively as a "primary care service line," but the educational and research efforts have remained in their respective academic departments.

Logic would suggest that we bring the three generalist disciplines together in a new department of primary care. Such a department would have divisions of family practice, primary care internal medicine, and primary care pediatrics. The department would be responsible for primary care services, just as the department of surgery is responsible for surgical services. It would provide future-oriented primary care and would form the foundation of the institution's integrated delivery system. It would provide predoctoral educational programs in primary care across the four years of medical school and would offer primary care residency programs in each of the three disciplines. Categorical residency programs in internal medicine and pediatrics would remain within departments of specialty internal medicine and specialty pediatrics. Resident physicians in the primary care specialties might have a common first year and then differentiate to become board-eligible in the primary care specialty of their choice. The new department would bring together a group of researchers and would create the necessary critical mass. It would also promote interdisciplinary cooperation in primary care, and the walls between the three disciplines would begin to be torn down. Who knows, perhaps one day there will be one primary care discipline with various areas of emphasis.[77-81] Such an approach would have a tremendous impact on health care delivery in the United States.

Each of the three primary care disciplines has come from a unique heritage: the family physician from the general practitioner of old, the internist from the internist-diagnostician, and the pediatrician from the commitment to child health. They are three different but complementary cultures, and they have more in common with one another than with their own subspecialties. Our experience at Missouri with the multidisciplinary Department of Family and Community Medicine has demonstrated that each of the disciplines contributes to the overall mission. I believe that having both internists and family physicians in the department has strengthened our patient care, educational, and research efforts. From an institutional perspective, the logic of a department of primary care is irrefutable. Nevertheless, I was disappointed when none of the applicants for the Generalist Physician Initiative made such a proposal. Ties to the parent disciplines are not easily modified, but I hope that some institutions will explore the potential gains offered by a Department of Primary Care.

In conclusion, we seem to have come from what appeared to be the demise of the generalist to a place where today it appears that the nation may have an adequate future supply of generalists. Our health care system is still evolving, and all physicians live in a world of change. The challenges for primary care are great. The potential is perhaps even greater. The gratification that comes from caring for patients has always been there and will continue to be there. Those of us in academic medicine face the challenge of preparing practitioners for tomorrow's health care system. The opportunity and the excitement never end.

## Notes

1. Hertzler AE. *The Horse and Buggy Doctor.* New York: Harper; 1939.

2. Davis MM. The supply of doctors. *Med Care.* 1942;2:314–321.

3. The dangers of excessive specialization. *JAMA.* 1900;34:1420.

4. Ludmerer KM. *Time to Heal: American Medical Education from the Turn of the Century to the Era of Managed Care.* New York: Oxford University Press; 1999.

5. Flexner A. *Medical Education in the United States and Canada: A Report to the Carnegie Foundation for the Advancement of Teaching.* New York: Carnegie Foundation for the Advancement of Teaching; 1910.

6. Overpeck MD. Physicians in family practice, 1931–67. *Public Health Rep.* 1970; 85:485–494.

7. Stevens R. *American Medicine and the Public Interest.* Berkeley: University of California Press; 1998.

8. Engel GL, Green WL Jr, Reichsman F, Schmale A, Ashenburg N. A graduate and undergraduate teaching program on the psychological aspects of medicine. *J Med Educ.* 1957;32:859–871.

9. Engel GL. The need for a new medical model: a challenge for biomedicine. *Science.* 1977;196:129–136.

10. Alpert JJ, Charney E. *The Education of Physicians for Primary Care.* Rockville, Md: U.S. Department of Health, Education, and Welfare, Public Health Service, Health Resources Administration, Bureau of Health Services Research; 1973.

11. Young LE. Education and roles of personal physicians in medical practice. *JAMA.* 1964;187:927–933.

12. Perkoff GT. Teaching clinical medicine in the ambulatory setting: an idea whose time may have finally come. *N Engl J Med.* 1986;314:27–31.

13. White KL, Williams TF, Greenberg BG. The ecology of medical care. *N Engl J Med.* 1961;265:885–892.

14. Haggerty RJ. Community pediatrics. *N Engl J Med.* 1968;278:15–21.

15. Haggerty RJ. The university and primary medical care. *N Engl J Med.* 1969;281:416–422.

16. American Academy of Family Physicians. *Family Practice: Creation of a Specialty.* Kansas City, Mo.: American Academy of Family Physicians; 1980.

17. Citizens' Commission on Graduate Medical Education. *The Graduate Education of Physicians: The Report of the Citizens' Commission on Graduate Medical Education: Commissioned by the American Medical Association.* Chicago: Council on Medical Education, American Medical Association; 1966.

18. Ad Hoc Committee on Education for Family Practice of the American Medical Association. *Meeting the Challenge of Family Practice: The Report of the Ad Hoc Committee on Education for Family Practice of the Council of Medical Education of the American Medical Association.* Chicago: American Medical Association; 1966.

19. National Commission on Community Health Services. *Health Is a Community Affair: Report of the National Commission on Community Health Services.* Cambridge, Mass.: Harvard University Press; 1966.

20. Goroll AH, Stoeckle JD, Goldfinger SE, et al. Residency training in primary care internal medicine: report of an operational program. *Ann Intern Med.* 1975;83:872–877.

21. Alpert JJ, Bauchner H, Pelton SI, et al. Career choice in one general pediatric Title VII–supported residency. *Arch Pediatr Adolesc Med.* 1995;149:1019–1021.

22. Young LE. Changes in the postdoctoral education of internists? *Ann Intern Med.* 1975;83:728–730.

23. Pellegrino ED. The generalist function in medicine. *JAMA*. 1966;198:541–545.

24. Magraw RM. *Ferment in Medicine: A Study of the Essence of Medical Practice and of Its New Dilemmas*. Philadelphia: Saunders; 1966.

25. Magraw RM. Trends in medical education and health services: their implications for a career in family medicine. *N Engl J Med*. 1971;285:1407–1413.

26. McWhinney IR. *A Textbook of Family Medicine*. New York: Oxford University Press; 1989.

27. MacWhinney IR. Family medicine in perspective. *N Engl J Med*. 1975;293:176–181.

28. Stephens GG. *The Intellectual Basis of Family Practice*. Tucson, Ariz.: Winter; 1982.

29. Schroeder SA. The making of a medical generalist. *Health Aff*. 1985;4:22–46.

30. Noble J, Friedman RH, Starfield B, Ash A, Black C. Career differences between primary care and traditional trainees in internal medicine and pediatrics. *Ann Intern Med*. 1992;116:482–487.

31. Witzburg RA, Noble J. Career development among residents completing primary care and traditional residencies in medicine at the Boston City Hospital, 1974–1983. *J Gen Intern Med*. 1988;3:48–53.

32. Ewigman BG, Crane JP, Frigoletto FD, et al. Effect of prenatal ultrasound screening on perinatal outcome: RADIUS Study Group. *N Engl J Med*. 1993;329:821–827.

33. Council on Graduate Medical Education. *Third Report: Improving Access to Health Care Through Physician Workforce Reform: Directions for the 21st Century*. Rockville, Md: U.S. Department of Health and Human Services, Public Health Service, Health Resources and Services Administration; 1992.

34. Weiner JP. Forecasting the effects of health reform on U.S. physician workforce requirement: evidence from HMO staffing patterns. *JAMA*. 1994;272:222–230.

35. Council on Graduate Medical Education. *Fourth Report: Recommendations to Improve Access to Health Care Through Physician Workforce Reform*. Rockville, Md: U.S. Department of Health and Human Services, Public Health Service, Health Resources and Services Administration; 1994.

36. American Association of Colleges of Osteopathic Medicine, American Medical Association, American Osteopathic Association, Association of Academic Health Centers, Association of American Medical Colleges, and National Medical Association. Consensus statement on the physician workforce. Jan 1997.

37. Cohen JJ, Whitcomb ME. Are the recommendations of the AAMC's task force on the generalist physician still valid? *Acad Med*. 1997;72:13–16.

38. American Academy of Family Physicians. *Family Physician Workforce Reform: Recommendations of the American Academy of Family Physicians*. Kansas City, Mo.: American Academy of Family Physicians; 1995.

39. Institute of Medicine, Division of Health Care Services, Committee on the U.S. Physician Supply. *The Nation's Physician Workforce: Options for Balancing Supply and Requirements*. Lohr KN, Vanselow NA, Detmer DE, eds. Washington, DC: National Academy Press; 1996.

40. Weissert CS, Silberman SL. Sending a policy signal: state legislatures, medical schools, and primary care mandates. *J Health Polit Policy Law.* 1998;23:743–770.

41. Colwill JM, Perkoff GT, Blake RLJ, Paden C, Beachler M. Modifying the culture of medical education: the first three years of the RWJ Generalist Physician Initiative. *Acad Med.* 1997;72:745–753.

42. Colwill JM, Cultice J. The generalist physician supply: yesterday, today, and tomorrow. A Report to the COGME, HRSA, May 2002.

43. Colwill JM. Where have all the primary care applicants gone? *N Engl J Med.* 1992;326:387–393.

44. Robinson JC. The end of managed care. *JAMA.* 2001;285:2622–2628.

45. Heffler S, Smith S, Won G, et al. Health spending projections for 2001–2011: the latest outlook. *Health Aff.* 2002;21:207–218.

46. Aaron H, Schwartz WB. Rationing health care: the choice before us. *Science.* 1990;247:418–422.

47. Schroder SA. Primary care at crossroads. *Acad Med.* 2002;77:767–773.

48. Mechanic D, McAlpine DD, Rosenthal M. Are patients' office visits with physicians getting shorter? *N Engl J Med.* 2001;344:198–204.

49. Funkenstein DH. *Medical Students, Medical Schools, and Society During Five Eras: Factors Affecting the Career Choices of Physicians, 1958–1976.* Cambridge, Mass.: Ballinger; 1978.

50. Starfield B. Primary care and health: a cross-national comparison. *JAMA.* 1991;266:2268–2271.

51. Shea S, Misra D, Ehrlich MH, Field L, Francis CK. Predisposing factors for severe, uncontrolled hypertension in an inner-city minority population. *N Engl J Med.* 1992;327:776–781.

52. Ferrante JM, Gonzalez EC, Pal N, Roetzheim RG. Effects of physician supply on early detection of breast cancer. *J Am Board Fam Pract.* 2000;13:408–414.

53. Shi L, Starfield B, Kennedy B, Kawachi I. Income inequality, primary care, and health indicators. *J Fam Pract.* 1999;48:275–284.

54. Welch WP, Miller ME, Welch HG, Fisher ES, Wennberg JE. Geographic variation in expenditures for physicians' services in the United States. *N Engl J Med.* 1993;328:621–627.

55. Dartmouth Medical School, Center for the Evaluative Clinical Sciences. *The Dartmouth Atlas of Health Care in the United States.* Wennberg JE, Cooper MM, eds. Hanover, NH: Dartmouth Medical School, Center for the Evaluative Clinical Sciences; 1996.

56. Rosenblatt RA, Hart LG, Baldwin LM, Chan L, Schneeweiss R. The generalist role of specialty physicians: is there a hidden system of primary care? *JAMA.* 1998;279:1364–1370.

57. Green LA, Fryer GEJ, Yawn BP, Lanier D, Dovey SM. The ecology of medical care revisited. *N Engl J Med.* 2001;344:2021–2025.

58. Grumbach K, Selby JV, Damberg C, et al. Resolving the gatekeeper conundrum:

what patients value in primary care and referrals to specialists. *JAMA.* 1999;282:261–266.

59. Forrest CB, Weiner JP, Fowles J, et al. Self-referral in point-of-service health plans. *JAMA.* 2001;285:2223–2231.

60. Bodenheimer T, Lo B, Casalino L. Primary care physicians should be coordinators, not gatekeepers. *JAMA.* 1999;281:2045–2049.

61. Cooper RA, Laud P, Dietrich CL. Current and projected workforce of nonphysician clinicians. *JAMA.* 1998; 280:788–794.

62. Sox HC. Independent primary care practice by nurse practitioners. *JAMA.* 2000;283:106–108.

63. Mundinger MO, Kane RL, Lenz ER, et al. Primary care outcomes in patients treated by nurse practitioners or physicians: a randomized trial. *JAMA.* 2000; 283:59–68.

64. Hooker RS, McCaig LF. Use of physician assistants and nurse practitioners in primary care, 1995–1999. *Health Aff.* 2001;20:231–238.

65. Nathan DG, Fontanarosa PB, Wilson JD. Opportunities for medical research in the 21st century. *JAMA.* 2001;285:533–534.

66. Holtzman NA, Marteau TM. Will genetics revolutionize medicine? *N Engl J Med.* 2000;343:141–144.

67. Anderson GF, Hussey PS. *Health and Population Aging: A Multinational Comparison.* New York: Commonwealth Fund; 1999.

68. Bryant DC. Hospitalists and "officists" preparing for the future of general internal medicine. *J Gen Intern Med.* 1999;14:182–185.

69. Bodenheimer T, Wagner EH, Grumbach K. Improving primary care for patients with chronic illness. *JAMA.* 2002;288:1775–1779.

70. Bodenheimer T, Wagner EH, Grumbach K. Improving primary care for patients with chronic illness: the chronic care model, part 2. *JAMA.* 2002;288:1909–1914.

71. Schroeder SA, Sandy LG. Specialty distribution of U.S. physicians: the invisible driver of health care costs. *N Engl J Med.* 1993;328:961–963.

72. Institute of Medicine, Committee on Quality of Health Care in America. *Crossing the Quality Chasm: A New Health System for the 21st Century.* Washington, DC: National Academy Press; 2001.

73. Pellegrino ED. The identity crisis of an ideal. In: Ingelfinger FJ, Relman AS, Finland M, eds. *Controversy in Internal Medicine.* Philadelphia: Saunders; 1974:41–50.

74. Young LE. The broadly based internist as the backbone of medical practice. In: Ingelfinger FJ, Relman AS, Finland M, eds. *Controversy in Internal Medicine.* Philadelphia: Saunders; 1974:51–63.

75. American College of Physicians. The role of the future general internist defined. *Ann Intern Med.* 1994;121:616–622.

76. Ende J, Kelley M, Sox H. The federated council of internal medicines resource guide for residency education: an instrument for curricular change. *Ann Intern Med.* 1997;127:454–457.

77. Geyman JP, Bliss E. What does family practice need to do next? A cross-generational view. *Fam Med.* 2001;33:259–267.

78. Geyman JP. Training primary care physicians for the 21st century: alternative scenarios for competitive vs generic approaches. *JAMA.* 1986;255:2631–2635.

79. Perkoff GT. General internal medicine, family practice or something better? *N Engl J Med.* 1978;299:654–657.

80. Perkoff GT. Should there be a merger to a single primary care specialty for the 21st century? An affirmative view. *J Fam Pract.* 1989;29:185–188.

81. Colwill JM. Education of the primary physician: a time for reconsideration? *JAMA.* 1986;255:2643–2644.

# Reconstructing Primary Care for the Twenty-First Century

Kevin Grumbach, M.D.; Thomas Bodenheimer, M.D., M.P.H.
2003

Primary care in the United States faces many challenges in living up to the ideal set for it by the Institute of Medicine in 1996. The IOM defined primary care as "the provision of integrated, accessible health care services by clinicians who are accountable for addressing a large majority of personal health care needs, developing a sustained partnership with patients, and practicing in the context of family and community."[1] Abundant research has documented the importance of primary care to our health care system, yet that system has not traditionally valued and rewarded primary care and has offered relatively little support and few incentives to accomplish the monumental tasks of primary care.[2] For its part, primary care has shown a reluctance to adapt and respond to the changing context of medical practice in the twenty-first century.

Primary care now confronts a number of critical issues, and how they are resolved may determine whether or not it can emerge as a rejuvenated and energized sector of American health care. These issues include the following:

1. Can primary care deliver on the promises of the Institute of Medicine definition:[1] integrated care, accessible care, care for a large majority of health needs, a sustained partnership with patients, and an orientation toward the entire community?

2. Who should provide primary care, and who is available to provide it? What will happen if an adequate number and proper combination of clinicians needed to deliver primary care does not exist?

3. What is the meaning of primary care's changing face, with many more women entering the primary care workforce? Does this changing face include underrepresented minorities?

4. Primary care's promise of accessible care is meant to include all geographic regions of the country. But does primary care adequately serve inner cities and rural America?

5. Will primary care join the electronic revolution, which has left many medical institutions far behind? Will the new "e-health" technology solve primary care's problems, or will it compound them?

## THE ORGANIZATIONAL CONTEXT OF PRIMARY CARE

Health care systems are organized into primary, secondary, and tertiary levels. Primary care is the foundation of this structure and manages the prevalent health problems and needs of the majority of the people. Secondary care, provided by specialists and general hospitals, involves the management of more complex problems. Tertiary care, generally delivered in teaching institutions, handles rare and complicated illnesses. Primary care clinicians play a role in coordinating secondary and tertiary care through referrals and the integration of specialty care provided in non–primary care settings.[3]

In some countries—the United Kingdom and Scandinavia are examples— health care systems are highly structured, requiring patients to consult with a primary care provider for all except emergency health problems; difficult problems are referred to secondary or tertiary levels of the system after an initial evaluation by the primary care gatekeeper.

Historically, most care in the United States has taken place within a more dispersed model, allowing patients access to the secondary and tertiary levels without their first seeing their primary care clinician. In the mid-1960s, 45 percent of the population had no regular physician. By the 1970s, it became evident that our specialist-centered system encouraged the overuse of diagnostic procedures, surgeries, and prescription drugs, contributing to the rising costs of health care.[4] In the 1960s, the community medicine movement questioned this model and advocated a more central role for primary care. A number of commissions and reports in this era promoted primary care reforms, culminating in the establishment of the family medicine specialty in 1969. In the 1980s, the rapid growth of managed care transformed much of our health care into a system based on primary care, with many of the eighty million patients enrolled in health maintenance organizations required to gain permission from their primary care physician to get to secondary and tertiary destinations. At the dawn of the twenty-first century, however, the declining influence of managed care may spell a return to a more dispersed health care structure.

Over the past two decades, research has demonstrated that a more structured system with a strong primary care base has advantages over a dispersed system that emphasizes specialist care over generalist care. Continuity of care and the coordination of care are more likely to exist when care is given by primary care providers rather than specialists,[5] and primary care is associated with a greater use of preventive services,[6] reductions in hospitalization,[7] and reductions in overall health care costs.[8] Nations with strong primary care–based systems tend to have better outcomes on such measures as infant mortality and life expectancy.[9] The quality of care for a variety of common conditions such as low back pain, diabetes, and hypertension is similar between generalists and specialists.[10-12] Compared with specialists, however, generalists have been found to practice a less expensive style of medicine,[13] and health care costs are higher in regions with higher specialist-to-generalist ratios.[5,14]

In this first decade of the twenty-first century, the United States faces a major choice: renewed support for primary care or reversion to the dispersed model of care. As primary care–based managed care recedes in importance, the health care pendulum may swing back toward the dispersed and specialty-centered model of care, even though research shows that a primary care–based system is preferable and that the American public wants primary care. A recent survey showed that 94 percent of the patients enrolled in California physician groups valued having a primary care physician who knew about all their medical problems. A great majority preferred to seek initial care from their primary care physician rather than a specialist in the event of coughing and wheezing (91 percent), arthritis in the knee (75 percent), and blood in the stool (75 percent). And 89 percent wanted their primary care physician to participate in the process of specialty referral.[15]

The waning of managed care has given rise to fears that the recently arrived primary care–centered system will wither despite its proven advantages and remarkable popularity. To better understand the future prospects of primary care, it is necessary to appreciate the forces that inhibit its flourishing.

## CHALLENGES PAST AND FUTURE FOR PRIMARY CARE

Although specialty care has been responsible for remarkable medical achievements and advances, the United States has gone overboard in creating a cult of specialization. This cult has been shaped by four interrelated forces.[3] First, the public's acceptance of the biomedical model—the idea that there is a pill or a surgical procedure for every human difficulty—heightens the value of specialty care and undervalues primary care's contributions of preventive services, management of the 80 to 90 percent of medical visits that involve common and not immediately life-threatening problems, and integration of care in a patient-centered or family-centered manner. Second, the financial structure of physician reimbursement pays most specialists far more than primary care physicians for their time and their expertise. As a result, the average surgeon earns almost twice the income of the average family physician or pediatrician.[16] And these income disparities are not shrinking.[17] Third, specialist physicians wield sufficient professional power to control the flow of resources into the health care sector; for example, as physicians often centered in hospitals, they received a free workplace from the federally funded Hill-Burton hospital construction program while primary care physicians had to finance their own medical practices. Finally, unlike most nations, where regulations—administered by governmental or quasi-governmental health planning agencies—codify the central role of primary care through policies affecting physician payment, physician supply, and rules for obtaining specialty referrals, the United States lacks a formal publicly sanctioned role for primary care.[18]

Despite a not entirely propitious climate during the latter half of the twentieth century, primary care attracted a cadre of dedicated physicians drawn by the rewards of generalist practice: relationships with patients, families, and communities that endure over time, the intellectual breadth of comprehensive care, and the satisfaction of addressing fundamental human and clinical needs. Although the majority of medical school graduates pursued training in specialty fields, a solid foundation of primary care clinicians remained an essential piece of the system.

The advent of managed care created expectations of a golden age of primary care, with primary care gatekeepers playing a commanding role in patient care and with managed care organizations demanding their services. For health policy futurists of the mid-1990s, the triumph of managed care was a virtual certainty. The supply of specialists was designated as excessive for a health system soon to be dominated by managed care plans, with one prominent 1994 article predicting that the United States would have 165,000 specialists too many by 2000.[19] Medical students responded by briefly forsaking specialty careers and entering primary care in larger numbers.

Yet reality was not so lustrous. Primary care physicians were inundated with more patients than ever before, were expected to do far more for their patients than previously,[20] were given new administrative tasks that consumed their time and increased overhead expenses, and saw little if any additional money to pay for these growing tasks. In California, a state with many patients enrolled in managed care plans, primary care physician satisfaction dropped from 48 percent in 1991 to 36 percent in 1996.[21] As managed care plans pressured primary care physicians to limit specialty and ancillary services, some patients became disgruntled with their primary care gatekeepers.

While managed care transformed much of our system into a primary care–based structure, it also created enormous expectations of primary caregivers and often placed intolerable stresses on them. Today, even as managed care declines, the public's high expectations of primary care continue. The gatekeeper role is abating, but the stresses are not. Most worrisome, at the same time that the large and demanding baby boomer generation ages, medical school graduates are less inclined to enter primary care.

As managed care faltered, specialty opportunities and incomes blossomed. Medical students began to flock back into coveted specialty residencies. The number of medical students choosing generalist careers fell from 40 percent in 1997 to 32 percent in 2000 and may continue to drop to the 20 percent levels of the early 1990s.[22] Although graduates of foreign medical schools are entering primary care residency programs, in part offsetting the lower enrollment by Americans, the trends are still troubling.

At the very time that U.S. medical school graduates are showing diminishing interest in primary care careers, the aging of the population guarantees that the demand for primary services will increase. In the year 2010, the first wave of baby boomers—Americans born between 1946 and 1964—will reach age sixty-five. The sixty-five-and-over population will swell from thirty-five million in 2000 to thirty-nine million in 2010 and will then take off as the baby boomer population bulge fills the ranks of the elderly. Some fifty-three million in 2020 and seventy million in 2030 will have reached or surpassed age sixty-five, when chronic illness becomes common and begins to take its toll. From 2010 to 2030, the number of Americans eighty-five years and older will jump from six million to nine million.

What are the prospects that primary care will overcome the obstacles to having a more empowered and satisfying position in health care? They depend, to a large extent, on the responses to the five questions raised at the beginning of the chapter.

## CAN PRIMARY CARE DELIVER ON ITS PROMISES?

Primary care is supposed to be the first point of entry into the health system, and so must be accessible. It should handle most health care needs; that is, it should be comprehensive. As a sustained partnership with patients, primary care should provide continuity over time. In its coordinating role, primary care must interact easily with the secondary and tertiary rungs of the health system. And with an orientation toward the community, primary care practices should be held accountable to the entire population they serve rather than merely to individual patients.

Has primary care risen to these challenges? Thus far, not entirely—in part because of the many political and economic forces that inhibit primary care and in part because of primary care's own reluctance to innovate and to change. Primary care faces major new tensions in achieving each of its cardinal tasks.

## Continuity

In its ideal form, continuity of care means that a patient can always see his or her personal physician. The difficulty with this concept is that it would require physicians to be available to their patients twenty-four hours a day, seven days a week, every day of the year. It is remarkable that in the past, general practitioners were able to provide such care year in and year out. Today, even if a sufficient number of physicians were willing to make this total commitment, the cell phones and pagers would make it punishingly difficult.

In one study, patients consistently saw their own primary care physician only 36 percent of the time.[23] We need a new concept of continuity based on primary care teams; a single practitioner is not able to provide continuity all day every day.

## Accessibility

Many patients have difficulty obtaining timely appointments with any clinician in their primary care practice. In a 1999 national survey of insured adults under age sixty-five, 27 percent of people with health problems had difficulty gaining timely access to a clinician.[24] Forty percent of visits to emergency rooms are not urgent, and many of these occur because the patient is unable to obtain a prompt primary care appointment.[25]

## Comprehensiveness

Over the past two decades, the management of many illnesses has become far more complicated, placing a great strain on primary care's ability to handle most health care needs. The scope of care provided in primary care without referral to specialists has increased, with one-quarter of primary care physicians feeling that they are doing more than they are comfortable doing.[19] Preventive care has expanded from DPT and polio immunization, Pap smears, and breast exams to multiple periodic screenings for cancers, lipids, and coronary heart disease; treating numerous childhood and adult infections; and providing advice on healthy lifestyles. Primary care tasks in chronic illness management have multiplied geometrically.

The difficulty in providing comprehensive care is best demonstrated by studies of chronic illness performance. Only 35 percent of eligible patients with atrial fibrillation receive the blood thinner warfarin;[26] 54 percent of diabetics are not optimally controlled as measured by hemoglobin A1c levels above 7.0;[27] only

27 percent of hypertensives are adequately treated;[28] just 14 percent of patients with coronary heart disease reached levels of low-density lipoprotein cholesterol recommended by national standards,[29] and only half of tobacco users are counseled about smoking cessation by their clinician.[30]

## Coordination

Modern health care creates complex coordination problems for primary care. Primary care physicians must interact with a growing array of organizations and personnel involved in the care of many patients, such as home health agencies, public health nurses, mental health professionals, pharmacists, and physical therapists. These collaborating organizations and professionals generate more requests to primary care physicians for authorization of services and orders and additional information to incorporate into treatment plans.

## Accountability to the Community

Primary care physicians may have their clinical practice under constant surveillance—and at times made public through report cards and the Internet—by employers, Medicare, health plans, physician groups, and hospitals. This level of accountability requires primary care to concern itself not only with patients who make appointments to be seen but also with those who do not; the latter's care and outcomes—whether the hemoglobin A1c for diabetics or the use of beta-blockers for cardiac patients—may depress a physician's score by any measure of quality. The new population-based medicine requirement that primary care physicians be concerned with every patient on their panel—every patient for whom they are responsible—is not simply a burden created by quality measurement; it also means better care. In the past, the concept of a panel did not even exist.

In summary, given the current design of primary care practice, it has become increasingly difficult to convert the definition of primary care into daily reality. Many primary care physicians are stressed out and overwhelmed with crammed schedules, inefficient work environments, and unrewarding administrative tasks. A December 2000 editorial in the *British Medical Journal* noted, "Across the globe doctors are miserable because they feel like hamsters on a treadmill. They must run faster just to stand still. . . . The result of the wheel going faster is not only a reduction in the quality of care but also a reduction in professional satisfaction and an increase in burnout among doctors."[31]

Primary care visits last an average of sixteen to eighteen minutes and include a median of three patient problems, requiring the physician to make an average of 2.75 decisions per visit. At least half of these decisions are relatively complex.[32] A 1997 survey of young physicians in major metropolitan areas nationwide found only 32 percent reporting adequate time with their patients.[33]

Another survey found that the average family practitioner or general internist handled managed care hassles that wasted forty to fifty minutes every day.[34]

## Primary Care Innovations

Can primary care be redesigned to relieve the time stresses on physicians, reconceptualize the meaning of continuity of care, enable acute patients to be seen in a timely fashion, and provide optimal management to the entire panel of chronic patients? Fortunately, a number of medical innovators are initiating redesign projects in all four of these areas.

One concept underlying the redesign efforts is the primary care team.[35] At some primary care sites, a team of caregivers is being developed to relieve time pressures on the physician, to become the vehicle for continuity of care, and to allow a complementary division of labor. However, the literature on primary care teams is sparse, so it's still difficult to compare team versus nonteam care.

One model of a primary care team might bring together two family physicians, two nurse practitioners, a health educator, two medical assistants, and a receptionist. The physicians might directly care for eight to ten (rather than twenty-five to thirty) patients a day, spending thirty to forty-five minutes with more complex patients, thereby making the encounters more meaningful to both patient and physician. The physician would spend considerable time consulting with other team members and arranging referrals. More routine visits would be handled by nonphysician clinicians. Medical assistants would be trained to perform routine tasks associated with preventive health care and chronic illness, thereby relieving the physician of time-consuming work that is easily handled by caregivers with far less training.

The issue of continuity of care in a team-based system is more complicated. Patients expecting to see their own doctor would need to be willing to be seen by their team instead. Given how often patients currently see clinicians other than their own primary care physician, they may find it an improvement to be guaranteed access to a stable team.

Such access would be enhanced by guaranteeing that patients could see the appropriate caregiver on the primary care team the same day that they call for an appointment. Some medical practices have already redesigned their scheduling systems along these lines. For example, the scheduling innovation known as open access emphasizes providing same-day appointments for all patients, irrespective of whether they have routine or urgent needs.[36,37]

Improved management of chronic illness may be achievable through a set of innovations known as the chronic care model.[38] Components of this model, some of which have been adopted at a number of primary care sites, include the creation of disease registries to allow for population-based care of chronic illnesses; reminder systems and performance feedback for physicians; intensive case management of challenging patients; and planned chronic care visits with groups of patients.[39–41]

Chronically ill patients may also benefit from a new model of providing health care variously called provider-patient partnerships, patient empowerment, and collaborative care.[42,43] The essence of collaborative care is that the caregiver and the patient agree on a written plan to improve the patient's health. Collaborative care, which may be more effective than having physicians tell patients what they are supposed to do, takes more time than traditional paternalistic care, but physicians do not need to do all the work involved; other team members can be trained to work with patients on their action plans.[44]

The vision of ideal primary care is timeless: continuity, access, comprehensiveness, coordination, and accountability. But how to best accomplish these objectives is not a static process. The specific approaches that may have worked in the twentieth century—the solo primary care clinician single-handedly trying to perform each and every primary care task—may not be the model that will assure a vibrant and successful future for primary care.

The twenty-first-century model of primary care will have a number of objectives:

- To redesign the delivery of primary care through innovations in practice
- To create team care as the foundation for all redesign innovations
- To improve the care of chronic disease through multimodal innovations, including a division of labor so that urgent care does not always crowd out the management of chronic conditions
- To implement new appointment paradigms that will allow patients prompt access to primary care

Which innovations will help resolve primary care's dilemmas and which will prove to be worthless cannot be reliably predicted, but failing to experiment could result in an outmoded primary care system that no longer works for either patients or clinicians.

## WHO SHOULD AND WHO WILL PROVIDE PRIMARY CARE?

In addition to the question of what primary care physicians should be doing is the question of who should be the primary care clinicians. In most European countries, the answer to the question "Which physicians are primary care providers?" is straightforward: general practitioners. These countries have devised national health systems that give the general practitioner dominion over primary care.

The answer to the question "Who is the primary care provider?" is vastly more complicated in the United States, where no single physician specialty has a monopoly on primary care. General practitioners are virtually an extinct species, crowded out by the proliferation of specialists over the past century. The GP was reincarnated in the United States as the family physician with the advent of the board-certified specialty of family practice in 1969. But by then the ecological niche of primary care was already partly occupied by physicians in general internal medicine and general pediatrics. Currently, there are approximately equal numbers of family physicians, general internists, and general pediatricians. Collectively, these three generalist specialties account for one-third of all American physicians. All three specialties fulfill the essential primary care functions, although many observers consider family medicine the quintessential primary care specialty in the United States. Unlike physicians in internal medicine and pediatrics, those in family medicine care for patients irrespective of age and often perform services—obstetrical care, surgery—outside the scope of practice of the two other generalist specialties.

As if having three primary care specialties instead of one did not make for a confusing enough situation, the dispersed health care model further complicated matters by allowing other specialties to lay claim to portions of the primary care turf. For example, many women consider their obstetrician-gynecologist to be their primary care doctor. Studies have shown that neither in practice nor in training do specialties other than family medicine, general internal medicine, and general pediatrics fulfill the essential core functions of primary care.[45] Obstetrician-gynecologists, for example, can provide first contact and continuity of care, but they do not provide truly comprehensive care, given their focus on reproductive-health-related problems.

The permeable boundaries between primary, secondary, and tertiary care levels in the traditional health system have not only allowed specialists to perform some primary care functions but have also forced primary care physicians into more of a secondary care role compared with their counterparts in other nations. Whereas GPs in most nations work only in ambulatory care settings, family physicians in the United States have traditionally served as the inpatient attending physician, thereby allowing better continuity of care. Inpatient practice has had important political and financial benefits for primary care physicians; insurance plans pay much higher fees for inpatient than ambulatory visits, and the acute hospital setting has conferred professional prestige in the specialty-oriented world of American medicine.

Recent trends are forcing a reconsideration of the role of primary care physicians in inpatient medicine. Many health care organizations now have a dedicated staff of physicians who handle all general inpatient services. Primary care physicians voluntarily, or in some cases compulsorily, hand over care of their inpatients to a dedicated staff of "hospitalists" who handle all general inpatient services. Although the term *hospitalist* is an American invention,[46] the hospitalist arrangement is a long-standing one in most European nations. The role of general internists and general pediatricians in these nations is in fact largely that of hospitalists. Although hospitalists are well accepted in these nations, their advent in the United States is causing controversy. Many primary care physicians, particularly those in general internal medicine, are reluctant to relinquish hospital practice. On the other hand, research has indicated that many primary care physicians may welcome a reduced role in the hospital.[47] The demands of inpatient service often detract from the ability of generalist physicians to concentrate their efforts on the most critical dimension of primary care—ambulatory care.

In addition to the hospitalist movement, primary care physicians in the United States face a major development that has implications for their future: The nation is in the midst of an explosion in the supply of nonphysician primary care clinicians. These clinicians—nurse practitioners and physician assistants—have considerable overlap in functions with those of primary care physicians, and research has demonstrated that they can perform most of the tasks usually undertaken by primary care physicians with comparable quality of care.[48]

The professions of nurse practitioner and physician assistant developed in the 1970s in response to a shortage of primary care physicians. The number of nurse practitioners and physician assistants accelerated in the 1990s as the number of training positions abruptly increased. Current projections hold that between 1990 and 2015, the number of clinically active nurse practitioners in the United States will increase from 30,000 to 150,000 and the number of physician assistants from 20,000 to 80,000.[49] By 2015, there will be nearly as many nurse practitioners and physician assistants as generalist physicians in the United States. Although some nurse practitioners and physician assistants work in specialty areas, most are in primary care.

The rapid growth in the supply of nurse practitioners and physician assistants raises the question of whether such clinicians will function mainly as complements to primary care physicians or as competitors.[50] One complementary role would be as physician substitutes in settings, particularly at rural and inner city sites, where physicians are in short supply. Another would be as members of teams composed of primary care physicians and other health professionals, with different team members having roles that build on their particular strengths. For example, nurse practitioners could play a key role in health promotion and health education while physicians focus more of their effort on managing patients with multiple or complex medical problems.

As for competition, nurse practitioners and physician assistants could substitute for physicians not only where physicians are scarce but also even in settings with an abundance of physicians. Nonphysician clinicians might have a competitive advantage because of lower cost and, some advocates have argued, might even offer better patient satisfaction.[48] According to one group of economic theorists, all professions have a natural tendency to become more specialized over time. In this view, physicians will gravitate toward more specialized and technology-focused roles, ceding the field of primary care to nonphysician clinicians.

The twenty-first-century model of primary care in the United States will need to do two things to succeed. First, we will need to create a more unified primary care specialty for physicians. This model might take on more of the character of the European general practitioner, integrating the fields of family medicine, general internal medicine, and general pediatrics into a generalist specialty with a greater ambulatory care focus. Common generalist physician training could still allow for diversification through added qualifications—training for the full-spectrum American family physician role, including inpatient and obstetrical practice, which might remain well suited to remote rural communities. Each of the traditional primary care specialties would sacrifice something in the process— the internists their hospital practice, the pediatricians their exclusive focus on children, the family physicians their claim as the one specialty that can do it all. The question facing these disciplines is whether such sacrifices would ultimately result in a stronger, more focused primary care specialty for the United States.

Second, we will need to develop integrated primary care teams that build on the complementary strengths of physicians and nonphysicians in primary care fields.[51] Although nonphysician clinicians would continue to be physician substitutes in some settings, such as regions without enough doctors, most primary care physicians and nonphysician clinicians will be working in the same communities and will need to weigh the unique value that each discipline brings to primary care. For physicians, this may mean relinquishing some of the tasks they have traditionally performed as first-contact providers to take on more responsibility for managing integrated clinician teams.

# THE CHANGING FACE OF THE
# PRIMARY CARE PHYSICIAN WORKFORCE

The who of primary care involves more than simply deciding which professional groups should lay claim to the primary care turf. The changing role of women and the growing racial and ethnic diversity of the nation also demand a response from the primary care system.

## Women in Primary Care

The number of women entering medical school in the United States has increased dramatically since the 1970s. Before that time, many American medical schools had quotas on the number of female students who could enter.[52] In 1970, 11 percent of the students entering medical schools were women; by 1997, the number had increased to 43 percent. During this period, the percentage of women in all professional schools in the United States grew similarly, from 9 percent of enrollment in professional schools in 1970 to 42 percent in 1996.

Because more women are entering medical school, obviously there are more female physicians in the United States, from 7 percent of practicing physicians in 1970 to 20 percent in 1996. By the year 2010, 30 percent of the practicing physicians in this country will be women. Women now constitute 36 percent of the physicians under age thirty-five but only 11 percent of those in the fifty-five-to-sixty-four age group.[52,53]

Female physicians are much more likely to choose primary care specialties, obstetrics and gynecology, and psychiatry than their male counterparts. Almost 15 percent of the female residents in the United States are in pediatric training programs, compared with less than 5 percent of the male residents. So although 36 percent of the physicians in residency training overall are women, 63 percent of the residents in obstetrics-gynecology are women, 64 percent in pediatrics, and 45 percent in family medicine, but only 7 percent of the residents in orthopedic surgery and 15 percent in cardiology. Some observers have suggested that female physicians often choose these specialties because they involve fewer years of training and possibly allow for more flexibility in work once the residency training is finished. And of course, female medical students may face discrimination and related obstacles to specialty careers.[53]

Four times as many female physicians as male physicians are classified as inactive during their midcareer years, possibly because women reduce their professional activities for childbearing and child rearing. Female physicians who remain professionally active are also more likely than male physicians to work part time. One recent study of primary care physician staffing at a large HMO found that 58 percent of the female physicians worked less than full time, compared with only 12 percent of the male physicians.[54] Such patterns have raised questions about whether projections of the future physician supply should be adjusted downward—and if so, by how much—to account for the potentially lower productivity of female physicians. Because women do choose primary care specialties, these productivity differences will have a disproportionate effect on projections of the supply of primary care physicians.

Female physicians tend to have a different style of practice than male physicians and to attract more female patients. Female patients are more likely than male patients to value spending more time and receiving more explanations from their physicians.[55] Several studies have shown that female primary care physicians deliver more preventive services than male physicians, especially for their female patients.[56] Many studies also have found that female physicians spend more time with their patients than male physicians do.[55,57]

Female physicians also appear to communicate differently with their patients, being more likely to discuss lifestyle and social concerns and to give more information and explanations during a visit.[55] These differences in patterns of communication have been observed among pediatricians interacting with children and their parents,[57] as well as among internists and other primary care physicians caring for adults. A recent study demonstrated that female physicians are more likely to involve patients in medical decision making than male physicians are.[58]

The growing presence of women in medicine may be changing the way in which primary care is practiced. Female primary care physicians appear to have a more prevention-oriented, communicative approach to clinical practice. The demand for female physicians is high, especially among female patients. However, female physicians may experience work stress from the collision of heightened patient expectations and the constraints of their practice. Patients may expect that a female physician will be more communicative and patient-centered than a male physician, and yet pressures for increased physician productivity may mean that female physicians and male physicians alike face the same limitations on the amount of time that they can spend with patients in a typical office visit.

The twenty-first-century model of primary care will need to focus on two areas. First, it will have to openly confront the practice stresses, sexual inequities in family and household responsibilities, and experiences of sexism in training and practice that may increase stress and lead to professional and personal burnout among female physicians. This will require the development of more flexible primary care training and practice models that permit greater opportunities for part-time work and an accommodation of shared work and family responsibilities. Second, the model will also need to question its conventions and modify expectations about career roles for both men and women—potentially to the benefit of all physicians.

## Physician Race and Ethnicity

Many racial and ethnic minority groups are profoundly underrepresented in medicine. Although diversity in medical school classes has increased somewhat compared to that of the overall pool of practicing physicians, African Americans and Latinos remain markedly underrepresented relative to their share of the nation's population (see Tables 2.1 and 2.2).

Table 2.1. Medical School Enrollment by Student Race or Ethnicity, 1996–97.

| Racial/Ethnic Group | U.S. Population, 1996 | Allopathic Medicine | Osteopathic Medicine |
|---|---|---|---|
| Non-Hispanic white | 72.3% | 65.8% | 79.8% |
| Non-Hispanic black | 12.5% | 8.0% | 4.1% |
| Hispanic | 10.6% | 6.6% | 3.8% |
| Native American | 0.9% | 0.8% | 0.9% |
| Asian | 3.7% | 17.6% | 11.4% |

*Source:* U.S. Health Workforce Personnel Factbook, U.S. Department of Health and Human Services, 1998.

The population of the United States is now more diverse than at any time in the nation's history. Latinos make up as large a percentage of the population as African Americans. The number of Asian Americans has also increased dramatically. The three racial or ethnic groups traditionally underrepresented in the health professions—African Americans, Latinos, and Native Americans—now account for 25 percent of residents of the United States.[59]

This underrepresentation is a matter of concern for several reasons. The situation may be viewed as an indication of social injustice and inequity, but there is also an increasing recognition that the lack of greater racial and ethnic diversity in the medical professions is a public health concern. Minority communities experience poorer health and access to health care compared with communities populated primarily by non-Latino whites. Minority communities are less likely to have enough practicing physicians.[60] Minority primary care physicians are more likely to practice in underserved minority communities and to treat disadvantaged patients, such as the uninsured and those insured by Medicaid.[60–62] Minority individuals often prefer to receive care from physicians of the same race or ethnicity and are more satisfied with care provided by physicians of similar race or ethnicity.[58,63,64] Thus the underrepresentation of minorities is not simply a matter of fairness of opportunity for individuals desiring careers in the health professions. It is also an issue that has important ramifications for addressing inequities in access to care and health outcomes for the growing proportion of minorities.

Leaders in academic medicine have recognized the need to increase the number of underrepresented minorities entering medicine, and some progress has been achieved in this area. For example, the Association of American Medical Colleges (AAMC) implemented the "3000 by 2000" program in 1991 to increase the number of underrepresented minorities matriculating in American medical schools. This program consisted of efforts to create partnerships between aca-

Table 2.2.  Practicing Physicians by Race or Ethnicity, 1998.

| Racial/Ethnic Group | U.S. Population, 1996 | Physicians |
|---|---|---|
| Non-Hispanic white | 72.3% | 79.3% |
| Non-Hispanic black | 12.5% | 2.9% |
| Hispanic | 10.6% | 4.7% |
| Native American | 0.9% | 0.1% |
| Asian | 3.7% | 2.6% |
| Other | — | 2.6% |

*Source:* Pasko T et al. *Physician Characteristics and Distribution in the U.S.* 2000–2001 ed. Chicago: American Medical Association; 2000.

demic medical centers and K–12 schools and colleges to better prepare minority students for careers in medicine.[65] The AAMC's commitment to enhancing racial and ethnic diversity in medical schools initially appeared to yield benefits as reflected in an increase in underrepresented minority medical school matriculates from 1,470 in 1990 to 2,014 in 1994. However, a political movement opposed to affirmative action coincided with a downturn in underrepresented minority enrollment in American medical schools in the late 1990s. The number of underrepresented minority matriculates overall decreased from 2,014 in 1994 to 1,770 in 1997.[65] Almost half of the decrease between 1995 and 1997 was accounted for by drops in California, Texas, Louisiana, and Mississippi—states affected by the initial wave of anti–affirmative action legislation and court decisions. For example, underrepresented minority admissions and enrollment in California medical schools declined by 30 percent and 32 percent, respectively, in the late 1990s after a decision by the University of California Regents in 1995 to prohibit race-based admissions policies and the passage of Proposition 209 in 1996 repealing affirmative action in state agencies.[66]

Medical schools and training institutions are now trying to promote diversity in an era of growing legislative and judicial restrictions on affirmative action. Advocates on both sides of the debate agree on the need to enhance the quality of schooling for disadvantaged populations in the precollege and college years, to allow these individuals to become competitive for professional school admission.

The twenty-first-century model of primary care will need to change in two important ways. First, it must develop a primary care workforce that more closely resembles the racial and ethnic diversity of the nation's population. This will require major efforts to increase educational opportunities and success at all levels of schooling among students from underrepresented groups and to reconsider recent policies that inhibit flexibility in admissions decisions by medical schools.

Second, it must assist physicians from all cultural backgrounds to more effectively communicate with and care for the nation's ethnically diverse patient populations. The core skills of cross-cultural medicine include many of the skills basic to primary care practice: negotiating common ground in patient and clinician values and beliefs about health and illness, building trust and respect between clinician and patient, and promoting an honest exchange of information.

## PRIMARY CARE RESOURCES: HOW ARE THEY DISTRIBUTED?

Beyond the who and the what of primary care, there remains the question of where. Tremendous geographic variation exists in the supply of primary care physicians. Physicians have tended to locate their practices in urban areas and within cities have gravitated toward more affluent neighborhoods. About 2,500 communities in the United States qualify for federal designation as Primary Care Health Profession Shortage Areas (HPSAs).[67] One of the major criteria for receiving such a designation is having fewer than one primary care physician for every 3,500 residents. Despite the increase in the number of physicians, the number of HPSAs increased by 25 percent between 1980 and 2000.

Rural regions have fewer physicians than urban areas do. Whereas 20 percent of the population resides in rural areas, only 9 percent of the nation's physicians have offices there.[67] Metropolitan counties have over five times as many physicians per capita as small rural counties. Although it is to be expected that many specialists will locate their practices in urban areas near tertiary care hospitals, primary care physicians are also disproportionately concentrated in urban areas. Two-thirds of all HPSAs are in rural regions. In many sparsely populated regions, even individuals with the best health insurance coverage often find their access to care compromised by an absence of physicians within a convenient distance.

Rural communities face many challenges in recruiting and retaining primary care physicians. Some of these challenges stem from community characteristics that are difficult to modify, such as a lack of job opportunities for spouses of physicians; limited choices of schools; lack of cultural, recreation, and shopping opportunities; and an inhospitable climate. Other obstacles are related to the nature of primary care practice in rural areas. The higher rate of poverty in rural communities limits the number of persons with commercial health insurance coverage, making it difficult to financially sustain private primary care practices. The distance from specialists and hospitals poses obstacles to referrals and consultations and may compel primary care practitioners to provide a broader scope of care than they would in an urban setting. The lack of a critical mass of colleagues requires primary care practitioners to be on call more frequently and makes it difficult to leave town for professional conferences or vacation.

Although the geographic maldistribution of physicians is most acute in rural areas, such maldistribution also exists in metropolitan areas. Neighborhoods with a high proportion of minority residents are most likely to have a low supply of primary care physicians and to be designated as HPSAs.[60] The relationship between the supply of physicians and access to care is probably less clear cut in urban neighborhoods than in rural counties; most urban neighborhoods with few physicians are surrounded by communities with an abundant supply of physicians. However, inadequate public transportation and related factors may make it difficult for low-income people to avail themselves of health services outside of their neighborhood, and such difficulty argues for the importance of local primary care.

Federal and state agencies have developed policies to improve the geographic distribution of physicians. One of the most prominent programs is the National Health Service Corps and Loan Repayment Program, administered by the federal Bureau of Primary Health Care. This program provides scholarships to medical students and loan repayment to recent residency graduates in exchange for medical service in HPSAs. Several states operate similar loan repayment programs. The federal government also provides grants to community health centers in underserved communities, as well as augmenting Medicare fees for physicians practicing in HPSAs. Other federal and state programs have awarded grants to medical schools and residency training programs to encourage training opportunities that emphasize service to needy populations. Perhaps most influential in determining whether physicians will practice in underserved areas are the characteristics that physicians bring to their profession in the first place. Physicians who grew up in rural communities are much more likely than other physicians to locate their practice in rural communities when they complete their residency training. Similarly, physicians from minority racial and ethnic groups are much more likely to practice in underserved urban neighborhoods. A recent study demonstrated that four factors are highly predictive of which physicians care for underserved populations: being a member of a minority group, participating in the National Health Service Corps, having a strong interest before medical school in practicing in an underserved area, and growing up in an underserved area.[68] Eighty-six percent of the physicians with all four characteristics worked in shortage areas or cared for substantial numbers of underserved patients, compared with only 22 percent with none of these characteristics.

No discussion of access to primary care should fail to mention the single most critical barrier to health access in the United States: the lack of health insurance. The most corrosive element in our primary care system is the inability of the nation to agree on some form of universal coverage so that all people can have the benefits of health care, including primary care.

The twenty-first-century model of primary care will need to increase the racial and ethnic diversity of medical students and the number of students from rural backgrounds in order to improve the ultimate geographic distribution of physicians; expand community service in training programs and augment incentives to practice in underserved communities, such as the National Health Service Corps and Loan Repayment programs; and advocate the enactment of a national health insurance program that will guarantee all people access to comprehensive care.

# CAN THE ELECTRONIC REVOLUTION SOLVE PRIMARY CARE'S PROBLEMS?

Any discussion of redesigning primary care practice must consider the most powerful recent transformation of contemporary society: the computer revolution. The computer and the Internet are having a major impact on how primary care is delivered. Electronic health care—"e-health"—has the potential to facilitate several functions within primary care practice: access to information for physicians and patients, provider-patient communication, provider-provider communication, medical records, and quality improvement. The e-health revolution also raises new questions for primary care. Does the new medium increase or reduce the work of primary care physicians? Can the new technology supply easy connections among the insurers, specialists, ancillary providers, and pharmacies with which most primary care practices, in their coordinating function, must interact? Will the public's unfettered access to health information through the Internet improve or weaken the patient-physician relationship? And does e-health improve quality?

Studies of electronic medical records (EMRs) and other ways of computerizing primary care have demonstrated that these approaches can enhance the quality of care, though studies also find that this enhancement comes at the cost of greater demands on physician time. A review of eighty-nine studies evaluating primary care computing from 1980 to 1997 showed that in five out of six studies, primary care physicians spent slightly more time working with an EMR than with paper charts. Electronic protocols improved care for diabetes and hypertension but increased the length of consultations. A pediatric computer algorithm increased compliance with management plans, but doctors found it "too tedious to use during routine care." Computerized prescribing reduced physician and staff time, increased the use of generic drugs, and reduced costs. Many doctors said that the time commitment involved in learning and using computers was too great, resulting in additional stress.[69]

A review of sixty-eight controlled trials assessing the effects of computer-based clinical decision support systems on physician performance and patient outcomes found improved physician performance in forty-three of sixty-five studies, and six of fourteen studies assessing patient outcomes found a benefit.[70] Computerized reminder systems improve clinical processes for diabetes care, immunization, blood pressure screening, and Pap smears, though the improvements often fade if the reminders are stopped.[71] Sophisticated diagnostic software programs have been developed, but studies of their ability to improve quality show mixed results.[70] Computerized feedback systems in primary care appear to be effective in the treatment of diabetes. A review of thirty-seven studies found that the feedback of performance data to physicians had some effect in improving both process and outcome measures in diabetes.[72]

A controlled trial involving thirteen thousand adult diabetic patients examined primary care physicians with access to computerized practice guidelines, diabetes registries for proactive population-based interventions, and performance feedback. Physicians who used the system were more likely to order lipid studies and eye exams but not hemoglobin A1c tests. The message of the study was that most physicians did not use the computerized systems available to them because they were too busy.[73]

Electronic prescribing is an e-health application that has had some of the most consistently positive outcomes on quality. One common approach to electronic prescribing in primary care is the use of a personal digital assistant (PDA), with software that provides proper dosages, flags drug interactions, determines whether the prescribed drug is on the patient's insurance formulary, and sends the prescription to the patient's pharmacy. In the hospital setting, computerized physician prescribing can reduce medication errors by 55 percent.[74] With the number of medication errors growing, it is likely that e-prescribing can have salutary effects on patient safety.[75]

Can e-health seamlessly connect primary physicians with specialists, hospitals, ancillary providers, and pharmacies? Currently, the ever-changing array of vendors and software packages makes connecting a problem. In all likelihood, some form of standardization will eventually allow easy connections throughout the health care system; this would ease the work involved in coordinating the care of patients.

More than fifty million American adults use the Internet to get health information. Although 53 percent of the adults are distrustful of the information they find on the Internet, more than 70 percent report that the information has influenced a health care decision.[76] Seven percent of patients bring online search results into their doctors' offices, expecting the doctors to interpret the information.[77] Health information Web sites can be divided into those sponsored by respected institutions with data of good quality and those created by individuals and commercial interests (often pharmaceutical companies) with data of variable quality. Studies of Internet health information suggest that most Web sites have inaccuracies or other problems in the information posted.[78] On the one hand, Web-based information offers patients the opportunity to become better-informed partners with their primary care clinicians; on the other hand, the need for physicians to address the inaccuracies in many Internet sites may add to the work of primary care.[79]

In summary, research thus far suggests that one particular e-health innovation—electronic prescribing—is a win-win technology, improving quality while saving time. Other e-health innovations still pose trade-offs between quality improvement and work effort.

The twenty-first-century model of primary care will need to do three things successfully. First, it will have to capitalize on advances in technology, such as voice recognition software for electronic medical records, and seamless provider-to-provider communication that can combine improved patient outcomes with greater practice efficiency. Second, it will have to develop more coordinated regional planning to use electronic media that permit an exchange of information among organizations, such as the transfer of electronic medical records between doctors' offices and hospitals and the transfer of prescriptions between offices and pharmacies. And third, it will have to develop means to finance the acquisition and the operating costs of EMRs and other computer applications.

# CONCLUSION

Reconstructing primary care for the twenty-first century is a formidable task but one that can be accomplished. It is a task that requires honoring the noble traditions of primary care while being open to fresh ideas about how to best reconcile these traditions with the changing context of health care.[80] It is a task that carries both the risks of experimentation and the excitement of invigorated practices and practitioners. It is a task that calls for reflection about the identity of primary care—whether defined by medical specialty, health profession, or the sex and race or ethnicity of the people working in primary care—and action to weave the multifaceted strands of the primary care workforce into a whole cloth. Whatever the future holds for health care, that care will not be delivered effectively and efficiently without a vibrant primary care system at its core.

## Notes

1. Institute of Medicine. *Primary Care: America's Health in a New Era.* Washington, DC: National Academy Press; 1996.

2. Grumbach K, Bodenheimer T. A primary care home for Americans: putting the house in order. *JAMA.* 2002;288:889–893.

3. Bodenheimer T, Grumbach K. *Understanding Health Policy.* 3rd ed. New York: McGraw-Hill; 2002.

4. Bodenheimer T, Lo B, Casalino L. Primary care physicians should be coordinators, not gatekeepers. *JAMA.* 1999;281:2045–2049.

5. Starfield B. *Primary Care.* New York: Oxford University Press; 1998.

6. Benson P, Gabriel A, Katz H, et al. Preventive care and overall use of services: are they related? *Am J Dis Child.* 1984;134:74–78.

7. Wasson JH, Sauvigne AE, Mogielnicki RP, et al. Continuity of outpatient medical care in elderly men: a randomized trial. *JAMA.* 1984;252:2413–2417.

8. Weiss LJ, Blustein J. Faithful patients: the effects of long-term physician-patient relationships on the costs and use of health care by older Americans. *Am J Public Health.* 1996;86:1742–1747.

9. Starfield B. Primary care: is it essential? *Lancet.* 1994;344:1129–1133.

10. Carey TS, Garrett J, Jackman A, et al. The outcomes and costs of care for acute low back pain among patients seen by primary care practitioners, chiropractors, and orthopedic surgeons. *N Engl J Med.* 1995;339:913–917.

11. Greenfield S, Rogers W, Mangotich M, Carney MF, Tarlov AR. Outcomes of patients with hypertension and non-insulin-dependent diabetes mellitus treated by different systems and specialties. *JAMA.* 1995;274:1436–1444.

12. Harrold LR, Field TS, Gurwitz JH. Knowledge, patterns of care, and outcomes of care for generalists and specialists. *J Gen Intern Med.* 1999;14:499–511.

13. Greenfield S, Nelson EC, Zubkoff M, et al. Variations in resource utilization among medical specialties and systems of care. *JAMA.* 1992;267:1624–1630.

14. Welch WP, Miller ME, Welch HG, Fisher ES, Wennberg JE. Geographic variation in expenditures for physicians' services in the United States. *N Engl J Med.* 1993;328:621–627.

15. Grumbach K, Selby JV, Damberg C, et al. Resolving the gatekeeper conundrum: what patients value in primary care and referrals to specialists. *JAMA.* 1999;282:261–266.

16. Wassenaar JD, Thrar SL. *Physician Socioeconomic Statistics.* Chicago: American Medical Association; 2001.

17. American Medical Group Association. *2002 Medical Group Compensation and Productivity Survey.* Alexandria, Va.: American Medical Group Association; 2002.

18. Stevens R. The Americanization of family medicine: contradictions, challenges, and change, 1969–2000. *Fam Med.* 2001;33:232–243.

19. Weiner JP. Forecasting the effects of health care reform on U.S. physician workforce requirements: evidence from HMO staffing patterns. *JAMA.* 1994;272:222–230.

20. St Peter RF, Reed MC, Kemper P, Blumenthal D. Changes in the scope of care provided by primary care physicians. *N Engl J Med.* 1999;341:1980–1985.

21. Burdi MD, Baker LC. Physicians' perceptions of autonomy and satisfaction in California. *Health Aff.* 1999;18:134–145.

22. Sandy L, Schroeder S. Primary care in a new era: disillusion and dissolution? *Ann Intern Med.* 2003; 138(3), 262–267.

23. Speigel JS, Rubenstein LV, Scott B, Brook RH. Who is the primary physician? *N Engl J Med.* 1983;308:1208–1212.

24. Kaiser Family Foundation. *National Survey of Consumer Experiences with Health Plans.* Menlo Park, Calif: Kaiser Family Foundation; 2000.

25. Cunningham PJ, Clancy CM, Cohen JW, Wilets M. The use of hospital emergency departments for nonurgent health problems. *Med Care Res Rev.* 1995;52:453–474.

26. Samsa GP, Matchar DB, Goldstein LB, et al. Quality of anticoagulation management among patients with atrial fibrillation. *Arch Int Med.* 2000;160:967–973.

27. Clark CM, Fradkin JE, Hiss RG, et al. Promoting early diagnosis and treatment of Type 2 diabetes. *JAMA.* 2000;284:363–365.

28. Joint National Committee on Prevention, Detection, Evaluation, and Treatment of High Blood Pressure. Sixth report. *Arch Int Med.* 1997;157:2413–2446.

29. McBride P, Schrott HG, Plane MB, Underbakke G, Brown RL. Primary care practice adherence to National Cholesterol Education Program guidelines for patients with coronary heart disease. *Arch Intern Med.* 1998;158:1238–1244.

30. Perez-Stable EJ, Fuentes-Afflick E. Role of clinicians in cigarette smoking prevention. *West J Med.* 1998;169:23–29.

31. Morrison I, Smith R. Hamster health care. Time to stop running faster and redesign health care. *Br Med J.* 2000;321:1541–1542.

32. Braddock CH. Informed decision making in outpatient practice. *JAMA.* 1999;282:2313–2320.

33. Hadley J, Mitchell JM, Sulmasy DP, Bloche MG. Perceived financial incentives, HMO market penetration, and physicians' practice styles and satisfaction. *Health Serv Res.* 1999;34:307–321.

34. Sommers LS, Hacker TW, Schneider DM, Pugno PA, Garrett JB. A descriptive study of managed care hassles in 26 practices. *West J Med.* 2001;174:175–179.

35. Wagner EH. The role of patient care teams in chronic disease management. *Br Med J.* 2000;320:569–572.

36. Murray M, Tantau C. Redefining open access to primary care. *Managed Care Q.* 1999;7(3):49–59.

37. Grandinetti DA. You mean I can see the doctor today? *Med Econ.* 2000;77(6):102–114.

38. Wagner EH. Chronic disease management: what will it take to improve care for chronic illness? *Effect Clin Prac.* 1998;1:2–4.

39. Bodenheimer T, Wagner EH, Grumbach K. Improving primary care for patients with chronic illness: the chronic care model. *JAMA.* 2002;288:1775–1779.

40. Beck A, Scott J, Williams P, et al. A randomized trial of group outpatient visits for chronically ill older HMO members. *J Am Geriatr Soc.* 1997;45:543–549.

41. Sadur CN, Moline N, Costa M, et al. Diabetes management in a health maintenance organization: efficacy of care management using cluster visits. *Diabetes Care* 1999;22:2011–2017.

42. Lorig KR, Sobel DS, Stewart AL, et al. Evidence suggesting that a chronic disease self-management program can improve health status while reducing hospitalization. *Med Care.* 1999;37:5–14.

43. Holman H, Lorig KR. Patients as partners in managing chronic disease. *Br Med J.* 2000;320:526–527.

44. Bodenheimer T, Lorig KR, Holman H, Grumbach K. Patient self-management of chronic disease in primary care. *JAMA.* 2002;288:2469–2475.

45. Rivo ML, Saultz JW, Wartman SA, De Witt TG. Defining the generalist physician's training. *JAMA.* 1994;271:1499–1504.

46. Wachter RM, Goldman L. The emerging role of "hospitalists" in the American health care system. *N Engl J Med.* 1996;335:514–517.

47. Fernandez A, Grumbach K, Goitein L, et al. Friend or foe? How primary care physicians perceive hospitalists. *Arch Intern Med.* 2000;160:2902–2908.

48. Mundinger MO, Kane RL, Lenz ER, et al. Primary care outcomes in patients treated by nurse practitioners or physicians: a randomized trial. *JAMA.* 2000;283:59–68.

49. Cooper RA, Laud P, Dietrich CL. Current and projected workforce of nonphysician clinicians. *JAMA.* 1998;280:788–794.

50. Grumbach K, Coffman J. Physicians and nonphysicians clinicians: complements or competitors? *JAMA.* 1998;280:825–826.

51. Geyman JP, Bliss E. What does family practice need to do next? A cross-generational view. *Fam Med.* 2001;33:259–267.

52. Council on Graduate Medical Education. *Fifth Report: Women and Medicine.* Rockville, Md: Council on Graduate Medical Education; 1995.

53. Pasko T et al. *Physician Characteristics and Distribution in the U.S.* 2000–2001 ed. Chicago: American Medical Association; 2000.

54. Schmittdiel JA, Grumbach K, Selby JV, Quesenberry CP Jr. Effect of physician and patient gender concordance on patient satisfaction and preventive care practices. *J Gen Intern Med.* 2000;15:761–769.

55. Elderkin-Thompson B, Waitzkin H. Differences in clinical communication by gender. *J Gen Intern Med.* 1999;14:112–121.

56. Lurie N, Slater J, McGovern P, et al. Preventive care for women: does the sex of the physician matter? *N Engl J Med.* 1993;329:478–482.

57. Bernzweig J, Takayama JI, Phibbs C, Lewis C, Pantell RH. Gender differences in physician-patient communications. *Arch Pediatr Adolesc Med.* 1997;151:586–591.

58. Cooper-Patrick L, Gallo JJ, Gonzales JJ, et al. Race, gender and partnership in the patient-physician relationship. *JAMA.* 1999;282:583–589.

59. U.S. Census Bureau; 2001.

60. Komaromy M, Grumbach K, Drake M, et al. The role of black and Hispanic physicians in providing health care for underserved populations. *N Engl J Med.* 1996;334:1305–1310.

61. Cantor JC, Miles EJ, Baker LC, Barker DC. Physician service to the underserved: implications for affirmative action in medical education. *Inquiry.* 1996;33:167–180.

62. Moy E, Bartman BA. Physician race and care of minority and medically indigent patients. *JAMA.* 1995;273:1515–1520.

63. Saha S, Komaromy M, Koepsell TD, Bindman AB. Patient-physician racial concordance and the perceived quality and use of health care. *Arch Intern Med.* 1999;159:997–1004.

64. Saha S, Taggart SH, Komaromy M, Bindman AB. Do patients choose physicians of their own race? *Health Aff.* 2000;19(4):76–83.

65. Cohen J. Finishing the bridge to diversity. *Acad Med.* 1997;72:103–109.

66. Grumbach K, Mertz E, Coffman J. *Underrepresented Minorities and Medical Education in California: Recent Trends in Declining Admissions.* San Francisco: Center for California Health Workforce Studies; 1999.

67. Council on Graduate Medical Education. *Tenth Report: Physician Distribution and Health Care Challenges in Rural and Inner-City Areas.* Rockville, Md: Council on Graduate Medical Education; 1998.

68. Rabinowitz HK, Diamond JJ, Veloski JJ, Gayle JA. The impact of multiple predictors on generalist physicians' care of underserved populations. *Am J Public Health.* 2000;90:1225–1228.

69. Mitchell E, Sullivan F. A descriptive feast but an evaluative famine: systematic review of published articles on primary care computing during 1980–97. *Br Med J.* 2001;322:279–282.

70. Hunt DL, Haynes RB, Hanna SE, Smith K. Effects of computer-based clinical decision support systems on physician performance and patient outcomes: a systematic review. *JAMA.* 1998;280:1339–1346.

71. Demakis JG, Beauchamp C, Cull WL, et al. Improving residents' compliance with standards of ambulatory care. *JAMA.* 2000;284:1411–1416.

72. Thomson O'Brien MA, Oxman AD, Davis DA, et al. Audit and feedback: effects on professional practice and health care outcomes. *Cochrane Database of Systematic Reviews.* 1998;2:CD000259.

73. Baker AM, Lafata JE, Ward RE, Whitehouse F, Divine G. A Web-based diabetes care management support system. *Jt Comm J Qual Improv.* 2001;27:179–190.

74. Bates DW, Leape LL, Cullen DJ, et al. Effect of computerized physician order entry and a team intervention on prevention of serious medication errors. *JAMA.* 1998;280:1311–1316.

75. Phillips DP, Christenfeld N, Glynn LM. Increase in U.S. medication-error deaths between 1983 and 1993. *Lancet.* 1998;351:643–644.

76. Brodie M, Flournoy RE, Altman DE, et al. Health information, the Internet, and the digital divide. *Health Aff.* 2000;19:255–265.

77. Bard M, Farris J. Keeping customers through care. *Pharmaceutical Executive.* March 2002. Available at:

http://www.cyberdialogue.com/library/pdfs/pharma_exec.pdf. Accessed on November 5, 2003.

78. Eysenbach G, Powell J, Kuss O, Sa ER. Empirical studies assessing the quality of health information for consumers on the World Wide Web: a systematic review. *JAMA*. 2002;287:2691–2700.

79. Kleinke JD. Vaporware.com: the failed promise of the health care Internet. *Health Aff.* 2000;19(6):57–71.

80. Mullan F. *Big Doctoring in America: Profiles in Primary Care.* Berkeley: University of California Press; 2002.

# PRIMARY CARE AND THE ROLE OF GENERALIST PHYSICIANS

# Editors' Introduction to Section Two

This section begins with two reprints that explore the conceptual bases for a model of medical practice based on primary care. Chapter Three is a classic study published in 1961 in which Kerr White and his colleagues found that even though medical training is focused on high-tech hospital care, less than 1 percent of the adult population needs to be hospitalized in any given month, and few of these individuals require the sophisticated care offered by academic medical centers. They concluded that the practice and teaching of medicine is inappropriate and that it should be reoriented to focus on the primary care problems that affect the vast majority of patients. (Lawrence Green and his colleagues brought the study up to date forty years later and found that the conclusions were still valid; their article is abstracted in the Abstracts in this section.) In the article reprinted in Chapter Four, published in 1977, George Engel made a related argument: that the dominant model of treating disease is biomedical, leaving little room for the more important social, psychological, and behavioral dimensions of illness.

With these two chapters setting the conceptual stage, Chapter Five illuminates the content of primary care and the need for general practitioners to provide it. The 1966 Willard Committee Report, named after its chairperson, William Willard (the formal name is "Meeting the Challenge of Family Practice: The Report of the Ad Hoc Committee on Education for Family Practice of the Council on Medical Education of the American Medical Association"), is one of the most influential reports to appear on the topic of primary care and generalist physicians. It makes the argument for developing a field of family practitioners.

The succeeding reprints offer old and new perspectives on internal medicine and family practice, the two disciplines providing primary care to adults. (The third discipline providing primary care is pediatrics.) Chapter Six, by Edmund Pellegrino, written in 1966, explains why general internists are needed, what it is they should do, and how they should be trained. In Chapter Seven, published in 2001, Eric Larson explores one of the major challenges facing general internal medicine today: the need to care for an increasingly aging population with an array of chronic illnesses. Reports such as The Willard Committee Report and The Millis Commission Report (reprinted in Section Four) ultimately led to family practice's becoming a formal specialty in 1969. More than thirty years later, in 2001, John Geyman and Erika Bliss reviewed the development of family practice and made some projections about its future; their article is reprinted in Chapter Eight. These two perspectives are followed in Chapter Nine by a reprint of a 1989 article by Gerald Perkoff in which he suggests that combining the primary care functions of internal medicine, pediatrics, and family practice into a single medical specialty would result in better and more efficient patient care.

A much-debated issue is whether specialists provide primary care to their patients. The Mendenhall Report, written in 1979, found that subspecialists provided a substantial amount of primary care for their patients (an abstract of the report can be found in the Abstracts section). In 1998, Roger Rosenblatt and his colleagues conducted further research on the topic. They found, in an article reprinted as Chapter Ten, that while certain specialists such as pulmonologists, gynecologists, and rheumatologists do provide a substantial amount of primary care, on the whole specialists rarely provide substantial amounts of care beyond the boundaries of their own specialty.

The final two chapters in this section offer a wide-ranging view of primary care and generalist physicians. In Chapter Eleven, originally published in 1991, Barbara Starfield compares primary care in ten industrialized Western nations and finds the United States ranking low in primary care services, levels of health indicators, and patient satisfaction; she notes that the three are associated, so that countries ranking low in primary care services also ranked low in health indicators and patient satisfaction. In Chapter Twelve, published in 2002, Lewis Sandy and Steven Schroeder offer an innovative view of the future of primary care, suggesting that primary care physicians will offer markedly different kinds of services, depending on whether they are serving an upper, middle, or lower tier of patients.

Abstracts of relevant articles, books, and reports appear next.

The Robert Wood Johnson Foundation has funded programs to improve the health care workforce—in particular, to promote and improve primary care—

since the 1970s. The reprint in Chapter Thirteen of the article by Stephen Isaacs, Lewis Sandy, and Steven Schroeder from *To Improve Health and Health Care, 1997: The Robert Wood Johnson Foundation Anthology,* examines these programs. The section concludes with summaries of reports, written by the Foundation's Grant Results Reporting Unit, of projects dealing with primary care funded by The Robert Wood Johnson Foundation.

CHAPTER THREE

# The Ecology of Medical Care

Kerr L. White, M.D.; T. Franklin Williams, M.D.; Bernard G. Greenberg, Ph.D.

1961

Current discussions about medical care appear largely concerned with two questions: Is the burgeoning harvest of new knowledge fostered by immense public investment in medical research being delivered effectively to the consumers? Is the available quantity, quality and distribution of contemporary medical care optimum in the opinion of the consumers? In addition, it may be asked: Whose responsibility is it to examine these questions and provide data upon which sound judgments and effective programs can be based?

The traditional indexes of the public's health, such as mortality and morbidity rates, are useful for defining patterns of ill-health and demographic characteristics of populations who experience specific diseases. They are of limited value in describing actions taken by individual patients and physicians about disease and other unclassified manifestations of ill-health. It is the collective impact of these actions that largely determines the demand for and utilization of medical-care resources. To assess the adequacy of the resources, it may be as important to ask questions about medical-care decisions, and to relate the data to clearly defined populations and health facilities, as it is to ask questions about mortality and morbidity for other purposes. In the context of medical care the patient may be a more relevant primary unit of observation than the disease,

Supported in part by a research grant (W-74) from the Division of Hospital and Medical Facilities, United States Public Health Service.

the visit or the admission. The natural history of the patient's medical care may be a more appropriate concern than the natural history of his disease. Similarly, data for short periods (weeks or months) may be more useful than data for longer periods (a year or more) for relating potential needs and demands to medical-care resources.

Little is known about the process by which persons, perceiving some disturbance in their sense of well-being or health, decide to seek help. Nor is much known about their sources of help,[1] or about the second and third stages of decision making at which patients and their health advisors, whether physicians, pharmacists or faith healers, seek or advise help and consultations from other medical-care resources. The available data suggest that patients control the decision-making process with respect not only to seeking but also to accepting and using medical care to a substantial extent.[2,3] Each practitioner or administrator sees a biased sample of medical-care problems presented to him; rarely has any individual, specialty or institution a broad appreciation of the ecology of medical care that enables unique and frequently isolated contributions to be seen in relation to those of others and to the over-all needs of the community.[4]

The dimensions of these relations may be described quantitatively by estimation of the proportions of defined populations who, within the relatively short period of one month, are "sick," consult a physician, are referred by him to another physician, are hospitalized or are sent to a university medical center. Such information could be a helpful prelude to further studies of the processes by which patients move from level to level up and down the hierarchy of medical-care resources, and of the best ways in which to relate these resources to one another.

## AVAILABLE DATA

Reliable data that can be related to defined groups are available from several sources; although not strictly comparable, because of differences in time, place and criteria, they appear adequate for the present purpose and may reflect, not too inaccurately, the dimensions of certain medical-care problems. Only adults sixteen years of age and over (fifteen and over, for certain data) will be considered, first because the data lend themselves most readily to consideration of the adult population, and second because most decisions about children's medical care are customarily made by their parents or guardians. A month has been taken as the unit of time, since it is probably a more realistic period than a year for evaluating decisions affecting the prompt and adequate delivery of medical care. This short time has the additional advantage that surveys asking respondents to recall experiences during the previous month or two are apt to be less influenced by memory than those based on longer recall periods.

In a population of 1000 adults (sixteen years of age and over) with an age distribution comparable to those found currently in the United States and England, it would be important to know the number who consider themselves to have been "sick" or "ill" during a month. For the present purpose, *The Survey of Sickness*[5] reports useful data for a continuing representative population sample of England and Wales over a ten-year period. The "sickness rate," as defined in this survey, is "the number of people (sixteen years of age and over) per 100 interviewed reporting some illness or injury in a month regardless of when they began to be ill"; uncomplicated pregnancies are excluded, and the rate cannot exceed 100. It does not reflect the number of illnesses, injuries or diagnoses during a month, the extent of disability or incapacity or the patient's position on the gradient from "perfect" health to terminal illness. It is a monthly "sick-person" prevalence rate. It does reflect individual, subjective perception and definition of ill-health, the initial responses that lead to decisions affecting the qualitative and quantitative demand for and utilization of medical-care resources. Since potential "patients" themselves usually define this primary unit of illness for purposes of medical care, the findings from such a survey will differ from those based on screening procedures or medical examinations. Physicians, depending upon their education, experiences, interests, facilities and the cultures in which they work, may define "illness" differently from their patients or from those who never consult physicians. In a medical sense, there is probably under-reporting in the English sickness survey of occult congenital anomalies, of asymptomatic sequelae of chronic diseases and of latent, incipient or minimal illnesses of many kinds, particularly mental illness.

Data from this survey for a four-year period (1946–47 to 1949–50) show variations in the mean monthly sickness rates with age, sex and season between extremes of 51 and 89 per 100 adults (sixteen years of age and over), as shown in Table 3.1. The annual mean monthly rates are rather constant at about 68, suggesting that in a broad-based population survey, 68 adults out of every 100, in an average month, will experience at least one episode of ill-health or injury that they can recall at the end of that month.

This rate may be compared with those calculated from the reports of the Committee on the Costs of Medical Care.[6] In this study, based on a broad, representative sample of the white population of the United States in 1928–31, an illness is defined more rigidly than in the English survey, as "any symptom, disorder, or affection which persisted for one or more days or for which medical service was received or medicine purchased," and it includes "the results of both disease and injury." The data are influenced by the informant's (usually the housewife's) concept of illness and her memory over periods of two to four months between the interviewer's visits. Annual rates for adults ill or injured one or more times per year vary between 41 and 65 per 100 adults (fifteen years of age and over). Mean monthly sickness rates would probably be lower than the over-all annual rate of 49 (see Table 3.2), but use of criteria for defining

Table 3.1. Mean Monthly Sickness Rates (Persons Sick per Month), According to Sex, Age and Quarter, per 100 Adults (Sixteen Years of Age and Over) Interviewed July 1946 to June 1950.

| Yr. and Quarter (1946–1950) | 16–44 Yr. of Age | | 45–64 Yr. of Age | | 65 Yr. of Age & Over | | All Ages (16 & Over) | | Monthly Sickness Rates for All Persons (Annual Means) |
|---|---|---|---|---|---|---|---|---|---|
| | Monthly Sickness Rates for Men | Monthly Sickness Rates for Women | Monthly Sickness Rates for Men | Monthly Sickness Rates for Women | Monthly Sickness Rates for Men | Monthly Sickness Rates for Women | Monthly Sickness Rates for Men | Monthly Sickness Rates for Women | |
| 1946 July–Sept. | 54 | 64 | 65 | 80 | 76 | 85 | 60 | 72 | |
| Oct.–Dec. | 61 | 71 | 72 | 81 | 81 | 88 | 67 | 76 | 68 |
| 1947 Jan.–Mar. | 60 | 68 | 68 | 78 | 79 | 86 | 65 | 73 | |
| Apr.–June | 52 | 61 | 61 | 76 | 76 | 86 | 58 | 69 | |
| July–Sept. | 51 | 59 | 62 | 74 | 73 | 84 | 57 | 67 | |
| Oct.–Dec. | 59 | 69 | 67 | 78 | 79 | 88 | 64 | 74 | 66 |
| 1948 Jan.–Mar. | 55 | 65 | 67 | 75 | 79 | 85 | 62 | 71 | |
| Apr.–June | 52 | 62 | 61 | 74 | 73 | 83 | 58 | 69 | |
| July–Sept. | 51 | 62 | 62 | 76 | 75 | 84 | 58 | 70 | |
| Oct.–Dec. | 60 | 70 | 70 | 81 | 79 | 88 | 66 | 76 | 69 |
| 1949 Jan.–Mar. | 62 | 73 | 70 | 81 | 82 | 89 | 67 | 78 | |
| Apr.–June | 56 | 67 | 66 | 79 | 78 | 87 | 62 | 73 | |
| July–Sept. | 51 | 63 | 64 | 76 | 74 | 85 | 58 | 71 | |
| Oct.–Dec. | 61 | 70 | 68 | 80 | 76 | 87 | 65 | 76 | 68 |
| 1950 Jan.–Mar. | 60 | 69 | 70 | 79 | 79 | 88 | 66 | 75 | |
| Apr.–June | 55 | 66 | 66 | 77 | 80 | 88 | 62 | 73 | |
| Mean monthly rates | 56 | 66 | 66 | 78 | 77 | 81 | 62 | 73 | 68 |

Source: Logan WPD, Brooke EM. The Survey of Sickness, 1943–1952. London: Her Majesty's Stationery Office, 1957; tables. 2 and 3.

**Table 3.2. Annual Sickness Rates (Persons Sick One or More Times per Year) from All Causes, According to Sex and Age, per 100 Adults (Fifteen Years of Age and Over) Among 8,758 Canvassed White Families (22,561 Adults) in Eighteen States During Twelve Consecutive Months, 1928–31.**

| 15–44 Yr. of Age | | 45–64 Yr. of Age | | 65 Yr. of Age & Over | | All Ages (15 & Over) | | |
|---|---|---|---|---|---|---|---|---|
| Annual Sickness Rates for Men | Annual Sickness Rates for Women | Annual Sickness Rates for Men | Annual Sickness Rates for Women | Annual Sickness Rates for Men | Annual Sickness Rates for Women | Annual Sickness Rates for Men | Annual Sickness Rates for Women | Annual Sickness Rates for All Persons |
| 41 | 55 | 44 | 57 | 55 | 65 | 42 | 56 | 49 |

*Source:* Collins SD. Cases and days of illness among males and females, with special reference to confinement to bed, based on 9,000 families visited periodically for 12 months, 1928–31. *Public Health Rep.* 1940;55:47–93, table 4.

"sickness" comparable to those employed in the English survey would probably increase the rates materially.

From these two surveys, it seems reasonable to conclude that the mean monthly sickness rate is unlikely to be as low as 50 or to be more than 75 per 100 adults. During an average month, in a population of 1000 adults (sixteen years of age and over), bearing in mind contemporary preoccupation with health, one may estimate that as many as 750 will experience what they recognize as injuries or illnesses.

From this population that experiences "sickness" in the course of a month, a proportion will consult physicians; a few who are not ill will do the same. The rate at which sick persons in the community consult physicians also is available from "The Survey of Sickness" in England and Wales.[7] Table 3.3 shows the mean numbers and rates of medical consultations per month in 1947 per 100 adults (sixteen years of age and over) who were "sick" as defined above. Only 23 per cent of all adults reporting at least one illness or injury during a month consulted a physician at least once; there are no differences in sex and slight differences in age. Expressed in relation to the base population of 100 adults, the mean monthly medical-consultation rate becomes $23/100 \times 75$, or 17 per 100 adults (sixteen years of age and over).

Data from the current United States National Health Survey[8] are also helpful in this regard, although the sampling period for the relevant published data covers only three months (July to September 1957) in contrast to the English sickness survey, which covers one year and therefore reflects seasonal fluctuations. Monthly Medical-Consultation Rates calculated from the published data vary from 13 to 26, with an over-all monthly rate of 19 adult patients (fifteen years of age and over) consulting at least once per 100 adults (see Table 3.4). In the English sickness survey,[5] the July–September quarter has lower mean monthly medical-consultation rates than the other quarters. In the United States National Health Survey data,[9] the physician visit rates per person during a two-year period tend to be lower in the July–September quarters than in the other three quarters for less than half the adult age-sex classifications reported.

The circumstances under which the English data were collected tend to diminish the under-reporting of persons consulting a physician each month, but the United States National Health Survey data could be more substantially biased in this respect. A preliminary study, comparing data from records of the Health Insurance Plan of Greater New York with those from the National Health Survey household interviews, suggests that the latter could under-report the number of persons consulting a physician during a two-week period by as much as a third.[10]

Considering the available data, as well as possible sources of bias, it seems reasonable to estimate the mean monthly medical-consultation rate at about 25 patients per 100 adult population. In an average month, in a population of

Table 3.3. Mean Monthly Medical Consultation Rates (Persons Consulting a Physician), According to Sex and Age, per 100 "Sick" Adults (Sixteen Years of Age and Over) Who Suffered from Any Illness or Injury, 1947.

| Mean No. of Medical Consultations/Mo. | 16–64 Yr. of Age | | 65 Yr. of Age & Over | | All Ages (16 & Over) |
|---|---|---|---|---|---|
| | Monthly Medical Consultation Rates for Men | Monthly Medical Consultation Rates for Women | Monthly Medical Consultation Rates for Men | Monthly Medical Consultation Rates for Women | Monthly Medical Consultation Rates for All Persons |
| 0 | 77 | 78 | 72 | 73 | 77 |
| 1 | 9 | 9 | 12 | 12 | 10 |
| 2 | 5 | 5 | 7 | 6 | 5 |
| 3 | 3 | 2 | 2 | 2 | 2 |
| 4 | 3 | 3 | 5 | 4 | 3 |
| 5–9 | 2 | 2 | 1 | 2 | 2 |
| 10 or more | 1 | 1 | 1 | 1 | 1 |
| Mean | 23 | 22 | 28 | 27 | 23 |

*Source:* Adapted from Stocks P. *Sickness in the Population of England and Wales in 1944–1947.* London: His Majesty's Stationery Office; 1949. (General Register Office, *Studies on Medical and Population Subjects,* No. 2.)

1000 adults (sixteen years of age and over) it may be expected that about 250 adults will consult a physician at least once. It is this population that is at risk of hospitalization, referral to another physician or referral to a university medical center.

The United States National Health Survey[11] has published annual rates based on household interviews for patients discharged from short-stay hospitals (including those with obstetric beds)—that is, those in which most patients stay for less than thirty days. From these annual rates, corrected both for under-reporting by respondents and to reflect patients hospitalized, rather than episodes of hospitalization, rates per 100 adults (fifteen years of age and over) may be estimated[12] (see Table 3.5). Rates by age and sex groups vary between 0.35 and 1.06, with an over-all rate of 0.61. Younger women admitted for delivery or related problems are reflected in the 1.06 rate; there are no differences in the rates for men and women in the other broad age groups.

More accurate mean monthly rates can be calculated from data developed by Forsyth and Logan[13] for a defined population served by the Barrow and Furness Group of Hospitals in England, a group that includes among its 9 hospitals, 2

Table 3.4. Monthly Medical Consultation Rates (Persons Consulting a Physician), According to Sex and Age, per 100 Adults (Fifteen Years of Age and Over) Who Had Visited a Physician in the Month Before Interview, July–September, 1957.

| 15–44 Yr. of Age | | 45–64 Yr. of Age | | 65 Yr. of Age & Over | | All Ages (15 & Over) | | |
|---|---|---|---|---|---|---|---|---|
| Monthly Medical Consultation Rates for Men | Monthly Medical Consultation Rates for Women | Monthly Medical Consultation Rates for Men | Monthly Medical Consultation Rates for Women | Monthly Medical Consultation Rates for Men | Monthly Medical Consultation Rates for Women | Monthly Medical Consultation Rates for Men | Monthly Medical Consultation Rates for Women | Monthly Medical Consultation Rates for All Persons |
| 13 | 26 | 14 | 21 | 21 | 26 | 14 | 23 | 19 |

*Source:* Adapted from Public Health Service: *United States National Health Survey: Preliminary Report on Volume of Physician Visits, United States, July–Sept. 1957.* Washington, DC: Public Health Service; 1958, table 17.

**Table 3.5. Monthly Hospitalization Rates (Patients Reporting Hospitalization), According to Sex and Age, per 100 Adults (Fifteen Years of Age and Over) in "Short-Stay" Hospitals, 1957–58 and 1959.**

| Age Group | Annual Episodes of Hospitalization[a] | Correction Factor for Under-Reporting & to Reduce Episodes to Persons Hospitalized[b] | Persons Hospitalized /Year[c] | Persons Hospitalized /Month[d] | Base Population[a] | Monthly Hospitalization Rates[e] |
|---|---|---|---|---|---|---|
| 15–44 years of age: | | | | | | |
| Men | 2,018 | 0.34 | 1,332 | 111 | 31,686 | 0.35 |
| Women | 6,751 | 0.34 | 4,456 | 371 | 35,064 | 1.06 |
| 45–64 yr. of age: | | | | | | |
| Men | 1,670 | 0.43 | 952 | 79 | 16,739 | 0.47 |
| Women | 1,743 | 0.43 | 993 | 83 | 17,731 | 0.47 |
| 65 yr. of age & over: | | | | | | |
| Men | 810 | 0.55 | 365 | 31 | 6,642 | 0.47 |
| Women | 944 | 0.54 | 435 | 36 | 7,871 | 0.46 |
| All ages (15 & over): | | | | | | |
| Men | 4,498 | 0.41 | 2,649 | 221 | 55,067 | 0.40 |
| Women | 9,438 | 0.38 | 5,884 | 490 | 60,666 | 0.81 |
| All persons | 13,936 | 0.39 | 8,533 | 711 | 115,733 | 0.61 |

[a]Adapted from Public Health Service. *Hospitalization: Patients Discharged from Short-Stay Hospitals, United States, July 1957–June 1958.* Washington, DC: Public Health Service; 1958, table 1.

[b]Based on Public Health Service. *Reporting of Hospitalization in the Health Interview Study: Methodological Study of Several Factors Affecting Reporting of Hospital Episodes.* Washington, DC: Public Health Service; 1961, tables 1 and 3.

[c]Annual episodes—correction factor × annual episodes.

[d]Persons hospitalized/yr. ÷ 12.

[e]Persons hospitalized/mo. ÷ base population × 100.

for the "chronic sick" and 4 with obstetric beds. The monthly hospitalization rates for adults (sixteen years of age and over) during a period of twelve months vary between 0.59 and 0.77 per 100 adults, with a mean monthly hospitalization rate based on the twelve-month period of 0.70 (see Table 3.6).

Further data are available from three samples of New York City residents.[14] The "eight-week" hospitalization rate for all ages varies between 1.4 and 1.7 per 100 persons, and it can be estimated that the monthly rate would be about 0.80 or less per 100 adults (see Table 3.7).

Rates derived from the three studies cited are remarkably similar (0.61, 0.70 and 0.80), and allowing for possible under-reporting[10] in connection with the New York study, it appears that the mean monthly hospitalization rate is unlikely to exceed a level of about 0.90 per 100 adults (sixteen years of age and over). In a population of 1000 adults (sixteen years of age and over) it may be estimated that, in an average month, about 9 will be hospitalized.

Table 3.6. Monthly Hospitalization Rates (Patients Recommended for Admission) per 100 Adults (Sixteen Years of Age and Over) in the Barrow and Furness Group of Hospitals, 1957.

| | Patients 16 Years of Age and Over Recommended for Hospitalization[a] | |
| --- | --- | --- |
| Month | Number | Rate |
| Jan. | 595 | 0.66 |
| Feb. | 656 | 0.73 |
| Mar. | 656 | 0.73 |
| Apr. | 690 | 0.77 |
| May | 677 | 0.75 |
| June | 586 | 0.65 |
| July | 602 | 0.67 |
| Aug. | 567 | 0.63 |
| Sept. | 659 | 0.73 |
| Oct. | 675 | 0.75 |
| Nov. | 534 | 0.59 |
| Dec. | 646 | 0.72 |
| Means | 628 | 0.70 |

*Source:* Adapted from Forsyth G, Logan RFL. *The Demand for Medical Care: A Study of the Case-Load in the Barrow and Furness Group of Hospitals.* London: Oxford University Press; 1960, p. 79 and Appendix 3.

[a]Populaton at risk (16 yr. of age & over) in the area served by Barrow & Furness Group of Hospitals (1951 census), 89,400.

Table 3.7. Hospitalization Rates (Persons Hospitalized) per 100 Persons
(All Ages) for New York City, 1952.

| Bases of Study | 8 Week Hospitalization Rates | Monthly Hospitalization Rates[a] |
|---|---|---|
| Health Insurance Plan enrollees | 1.4 | 0.70 |
| New York City sample: | | |
| Total | 1.6 | 0.80 |
| Insured | 1.7 | 0.85 |
| Uninsured | 1.6 | 0.80 |

*Source:* Adapted from a Report by the Committee for the Special Research Project in the Health Insurance Plan of Greater New York. *Health and Medical Care in New York City.* Cambridge, Mass: Commonwealth Fund, Harvard University; 1957.
[a]8-wk. rates ÷ 2.

Monthly prevalence rates for referral of patients from one physician to another are even more difficult to obtain. Many patients in the United States receive primary, continuing medical care from a specialist; some may visit several specialists concurrently. Frequently, patients "refer" themselves, and in general, patients appear to control the referral process about half the time.[3] In a stratified random sample of North Carolina general practitioners, 91 physicians (97 per cent return rate) recorded their patient visits for one week; these one-week samples were spread over the period July 1953 to June 1954.[15] The 91 general practitioners reported 11,765 visits of adult patients (sixteen years of age and over), or a mean of 129 adult patient visits per one-week sample. Since patient visits over a period of one week are likely to approximate closely patients seen, a mean of 250 adult patients seen per two-week period seems a reasonable estimate. In a second stratified random sample of the same population of North Carolina general practitioners, 93 physicians (87 per cent return rate) reported 460 adult patients (sixteen years of age and over) referred to other physicians (excluding university medical centers) during two-week sampling periods spread from August 1957 to February 1959.[16,17] The mean number of adult patients referred was 4.94, or about 5 patients referred per two-week period. The mean monthly patient-referral rate to other physicians for North Carolina general practitioners may be estimated as follows: 5/250 × 100, or 2 patients, are referred per 100 adult patients seen, and since other estimates suggest that, on the average, 250 adults per 1000 consult a physician at least once a month, approximately 5 adult patients are referred per 1000 adult population (sixteen years of age and over) per month.

Other published referral data[18-22] do not permit calculation of rates for short periods (such as a month) for patients referred, in contrast to rates for numbers of referrals. The risks of a given patient being referred to either another physician or a university medical center increase the longer he is under the care of a given physician. Annual patient-referral rates, like annual patient-hospitalization rates, will be higher than monthly rates, but the latter probably more accurately reflect the decision-making process as it affects current utilization of medical-care resources.

The final court of appeal, both for investigation of obscure medical problems and for specialized treatments, and one of the central sources of new medical knowledge and personnel, is the university medical center or teaching hospital. The composition of the patient population seen in each medical center will depend on the ecology of medical care in the region in which it is located, the demographic characteristics of the community it serves, and its own acceptance and admission policies. There may be wide differences between adjacent medical centers, between regions and between countries, but since in theory, and frequently in practice, such centers constitute the apices of referral hierarchies, it should be helpful to estimate the over-all proportion of sick persons in the community referred to them by physicians. Where primary, continuing medical care (in contrast to episodic or consultant care) is provided by university hospitals to groups of patients, or where a large proportion of self-referred patients are accepted, the compositions of the patient populations seen may differ materially from those seen at centers accepting predominantly physician-referred patients.

From the two North Carolina studies, it is possible to estimate the referral rate of general practitioners to the three university medical centers serving that state and its population of over 4,000,000 persons. The 93 North Carolina general practitioners surveyed,[16,17] as discussed above, referred 96 adult patients (sixteen years of age and over) to the three university medical centers during two-week sampling periods in 1957–59, with a mean of about 1 patient per two-week period. The mean monthly university medical-center patient-referral rate of North Carolina general practitioners may be estimated as follows: $1/250 \times 100$, or 0.4 patients, are referred per 100 adult patients seen, and since other estimates suggest that, on the average, 250 adults consult a physician at least once a month, approximately 1 adult patient is referred to a university medical center per 1000 adult population (sixteen years of age and over) per month.

"Hard" data on the "natural history of medical care" are in short supply. Studies such as those described only suggest the broad dimensions of relative utilization for several important medical-care resources. In summary, it appears that within an average month in Great Britain or the United States, for every 1000 adults (sixteen years of age and over) in the population, about 750 will experience what they recognize and recall as an episode of illness or injury. Two hundred and fifty of the 750 will consult a physician at least once during that month. Nine of the 250 will be hospitalized, 5 will be referred to another physician, and 1 will be sent to a university medical center within that month. Expressed in other terms, 0.75 of the adult population experience sickness each month, 0.25 consult a physician, 0.009 are hospitalized, 0.005 are referred to another physician, and 0.001 are referred to a university medical center. In an average month, 0.009/0.75, or 0.012 of the "sick" adults in the community, are seen on hospital wards, and 0.001/0.75, or 0.004, are seen at university medical centers. These relations are shown in Figure 3.1.

# DISCUSSION

The relations reflected in the data presented are subject to wide variations. All the surveys referred to were conducted carefully, but the rates are only approximate. Precise sampling methods were used in all the studies, but sampling fluctuations should be considered before any confidence limits can be placed around these estimates. Sampling errors are probably small in comparison to other sources of discrepancy, and although these are discussed in connection with the original studies, no effort has been made to deal with them here. The characteristics of the populations at risk, the health resources available and the decisions made about health problems by individuals, physicians and community leaders all affect both the way in which health facilities and manpower are deployed and the characteristics, quality and quantity of medical care available to a particular society, but the broad relations and the orders of magnitude of the differences depicted in Figure 3.1 probably reflect the patterns of medical care in the United States and Great Britain with reasonable accuracy.

Appreciation of these relations helps to bring the contributions made by advances in the medical sciences into better perspective in the over-all view of society's health. Medical science does not make its contributions in a vacuum, and the absolute value of these to society may be substantially modified by other factors that have received relatively little attention as yet and may impose critical limitations to the attainment of better health.

Medical-care research is concerned with the problems of assessing needs and of delivering medical care; more specifically, it is concerned with problems of implementing the advances achieved by medical science. Its concerns are not the characteristics, prevalence and mechanisms of disease, but the social, psychologic, cultural, economic, informational, administrative and organizational factors that inhibit and facilitate access to and delivery of the best contemporary health care to individuals and communities. It is concerned with the identification and measurement of medical-care needs, demands and resources, and the evaluation of the qualitative and quantitative aspects of programs, person-

**Figure 3.1.** Monthly Prevalence Estimates of Illness in the Community and the Roles of Physicians, Hospitals and University Medical Centers in the Provision of Medical Care (Adults Sixteen Years of Age and Over).

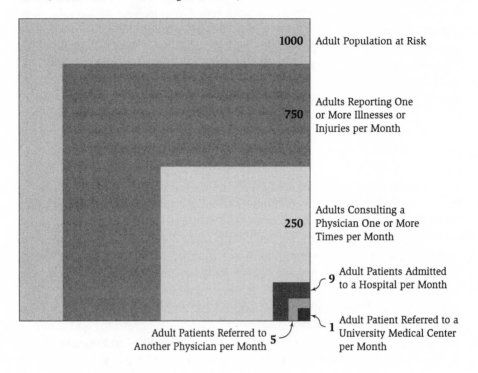

1000 Adult Population at Risk

750 Adults Reporting One or More Illnesses or Injuries per Month

250 Adults Consulting a Physician One or More Times per Month

9 Adult Patients Admitted to a Hospital per Month

1 Adult Patient Referred to a University Medical Center per Month

Adult Patients Referred to Another Physician per Month 5

nel, services and facilities, and their utilization in the provision of preventive, diagnostic and therapeutic care and rehabilitation. It is as concerned with the health of those who do not use medical-care resources as with the health of those who do. In essence, it is concerned with medicine as a social institution.

Much more needs to be known about patients' thresholds for perceiving, acknowledging and describing their own disordered function and behavior. What factors govern the patients' assumption or rejection of the "sick" role, or the "patient" role? More needs to be known about patients' sources of help in understanding and coping with their health problems. How do patients select their physicians, and physicians their patients? Under what circumstances do physicians refer patients to other physicians and to medical centers? What kinds of patients, problems and diseases are seen at different health facilities? Do the "right" patients get to the "right" facilities at the "right" time? More specifically, do the 500 "sick" people per month who do not consult physicians enjoy better health than those who do? Are the 5 patients per 1000 referred each month those most in need of consultation? What factors determine which person in every thousand adults will be referred to a university medical center each month? Are these processes in the best interests of all patients? Are they best for medical education?

For many years, it was an unchallenged assumption that physicians always knew what was best for the people's health. Whatever the origins of this authoritarian assumption, it presumably was transmitted by the medical schools as part of the "image" of the physician. Serious questions can be raised about the nature of the average medical student's experience, and perhaps that of some of his clinical teachers, with the substantive problems of health and disease in the community. In general, this experience must be both limited and unusually biased if, in a month, only 0.0013 of the "sick" adults (or even ten times this figure), or 0.004 of the patients (or even ten times this), in a community are referred to university medical centers. The size of the sample is of much less importance than the fact that, on the average, it is preselected twice. Under such circumstances, it would be difficult, if not impossible, for those at medical centers, without special efforts, to obtain valid impressions of the overall health problems of the community. Medical, nursing and other students of the health professions cannot fail to receive unrealistic impressions of medicine's task in contemporary Western society, to say nothing of its task in developing countries.

The present arrangements for *delivering* medical care to the consumers in the United States (or any other Western country for that matter) owe relatively little to data, ideas or proposals developed in university medical centers. Over the years, individual physicians and groups have concerned themselves with the profession's social responsibilities, but with rare exceptions the substantive problems of medical care have not been a continuing concern of either schools of medicine or schools of public health. It is one of the purposes of this communication to suggest that it is now time for schools of medicine, schools of public health and teaching hospitals to address themselves to the urgent need for medical-care research and education. It is now time for the health professions, and particularly for faculty members with clinical interests, to join their colleagues from the other disciplines, and to accord to medical-care research and teaching the same priority they have accorded research in the fundamental mechanisms of pathologic process. Investigation and teaching directed at improved understanding of the ecology of medical care and ways of favorably modifying it eventually should reduce the time lag between developments in the laboratory and delivery to the consumers of new knowledge accruing from the vast sums of money that the latter are currently paying for disease-oriented research.

# SUMMARY AND CONCLUSIONS

Data from medical-care studies in the United States and Great Britain suggest that in a population of 1000 adults (sixteen years of age and over), in an average month 750 will experience an episode of illness, 250 of these will consult a physician, 9 will be hospitalized, 5 will be referred to another physician, and 1 will be referred to a university medical center. The latter sees biased samples of 0.0013 of the "sick" adults and 0.004 of the patients in the community, from which students of the health professions must get an unrealistic concept of medicine's task in both Western and developing countries.

Medical-care research is defined, and the need for according it equal priority with research on disease mechanisms is discussed. Recognizing medicine as a social institution, in addition to disease as a cellular aberration, the objective of medical-care research is reduction of the time lag between advances in the laboratory and measurable improvement in the health of a society's members.

## Notes

1. Koos EL. *The Health of Regionville: What the People Thought and Did About It.* New York: Columbia University Press; 1954.

2. Freidson, E. Organization of medical practice and patient behavior. *Am J Public Health.* 1961;51:43–52.

3. Williams TF et al. Patient referral to university clinic: patterns in rural state. *Am J Public Health.* 1960;50:1493–1507.

4. Horder J, Horder E. Illness in general practice. *Practitioner.* 1954;173:177–187.

5. Logan WPD, Brooke EM. *The Survey of Sickness, 1943–1952.* London: Her Majesty's Stationery Office; 1957. (General Register Office, *Studies on Medical and Population Subjects,* No. 12.)

6. Collins SD. Cases and days of illness among males and females, with special reference to confinement to bed, based on 9,000 families visited periodically for 12 months, 1928–31. *Public Health Rep.* 1940;55:47–93.

7. Stocks P. *Sickness in the Population of England and Wales in 1944–1947.* London: His Majesty's Stationery Office; 1949. (General Register Office, *Studies on Medical and Population Subjects,* No. 2.)

8. Public Health Service: *United States National Health Survey: Preliminary Report on Volume of Physician Visits, United States, July–Sept. 1957.* Washington, DC: Public Health Service; 1958.

9. Public Health Service. *Volume of Physician Visits, United States, July 1957–June 1959: Statistics on Volume of Physician Visits by Place of Visit, Type of Service, Age, Sex, Residence, Region, Race, Income and Education: Based on Data Collected in*

*Household Interviews During July 1957–June 1959.* Washington, DC: Public Health Service; 1960.

10. Public Health Service. *Health Interview Responses Compared with Medical Records: Study of Illness and Hospitalization Experience Among Health Plan Enrollees as Reported in Household Interviews, in Comparison with Information Recorded by Physicians and Hospitals.* Washington, DC: Public Health Service; 1961.

11. Public Health Service. *Hospitalization: Patients Discharged from Short-Stay Hospitals, United States, July 1957–June 1958.* Washington, DC: Public Health Service; 1958.

12. Public Health Service. *Reporting of Hospitalization in the Health Interview Study: Methodological Study of Several Factors Affecting Reporting of Hospital Episodes.* Washington, DC: Public Health Service; 1961.

13. Forsyth G, Logan RFL. *The Demand for Medical Care: A Study of the Case-Load in the Barrow and Furness Group of Hospitals.* London: Oxford University Press; 1960.

14. Committee for the Special Research Project in the Health Insurance Plan of Greater New York. *Health and Medical Care in New York City.* Cambridge, Mass: Commonwealth Fund, Harvard University; 1957.

15. Peterson AL, Andrews LP, Spain RS, Greenberg BG. Analytical study of North Carolina general practice, 1953–1954. *J Med Educ.* 1956;31(12):1–165, pt 2.

16. Andrews LP et al. Study of patterns of patient referral to medical clinic in rural state: methodology. *Am J Public Health.* 1959;49:634–643.

17. Williams TF, White KL, Fleming WL, Greenberg BG. Referral process in medical care and university clinic's role. *J Med Educ.* 1961;36:899–907.

18. Fry J. Why patients go to hospitals: study of usage. *Br Med J.* 1959;2:1322–1327.

19. Hopkins P. Referrals in general practice. *Br Med J.* 1956;2:873–877.

20. General Register Office. *General Practitioners' Records: An Analysis of the Clinical Records of Some General Practices During the Period April 1952 to March 1954.* London: Her Majesty's Stationery Office; 1955. (General Register Office, *Studies on Population and Medical Subjects,* No. 9.)

21. Logan WPD. *General Practitioners' Records: An Analysis of Clinical Records of Eight Practices During the Period April 1951 to March 1952.* London: Her Majesty's Stationery Office; 1953. (General Register Office, *Studies on Medical and Population Subjects,* No. 7.)

22. Taubenhaus LJ. Study of one rural practice, 1953. *GP.* 1955;12:97–102.

# CHAPTER FOUR

# The Need for a New Medical Model

## A Challenge for Biomedicine

George L. Engel, M.D.
1977

A t a recent conference on psychiatric education, many psychiatrists seemed to be saying to medicine, "Please take us back and we will never again deviate from the 'medical model.'" For as one critical psychiatrist put it, "Psychiatry has become a hodgepodge of unscientific opinions, assorted philosophies and 'schools of thought,' mixed metaphors, role diffusion, propaganda, and politicking for 'mental health' and other esoteric goals."[1] In contrast, the rest of medicine appears neat and tidy. It has a firm base in the biological sciences, enormous technologic resources at its command, and a record of astonishing achievement in elucidating mechanisms of disease and devising new treatments. It would seem that psychiatry would do well to emulate its sister medical disciplines by finally embracing once and for all the medical model of disease.

But I do not accept such a premise. Rather, I contend that all medicine is in crisis and, further, that medicine's crisis derives from the same basic fault as

This article was adapted from material presented as the Loren Stephens Memorial Lecture, University of Southern California Medical Center, 1976; the Griffith McKerracher Memorial Lecture at the University of Saskatchewan, 1976; and the Annual Hutchings Society Lecture, State University of New York-Upstate Medical Center, Syracuse, 1976. It was also presented during 1975–76 at the University of Maryland School of Medicine, University of California–San Diego School of Medicine, University of California–Los Angeles School of Medicine, Massachusetts Mental Health Center, and the 21st annual meeting of Midwest Professors of Psychiatry, Philadelphia. The author is a career research awardee in the U.S. Public Health Service.

psychiatry's, namely, adherence to a model of disease no longer adequate for the scientific tasks and social responsibilities of either medicine or psychiatry. The importance of how physicians conceptualize disease derives from how such concepts determine what are considered the proper boundaries of professional responsibility and how they influence attitudes toward and behavior with patients. Psychiatry's crisis revolves around the question of whether the categories of human distress with which it is concerned are properly considered "disease" as currently conceptualized and whether exercise of the traditional authority of the physician is appropriate for their helping functions. Medicine's crisis stems from the logical inference that since "disease" is defined in terms of somatic parameters, physicians need not be concerned with psychosocial issues which lie outside medicine's responsibility and authority. At a recent Rockefeller Foundation seminar on the concept of health, one authority urged that medicine "concentrate on the 'real' diseases and not get lost in the psychosociological underbrush. The physician should not be saddled with problems that have arisen from the abdication of the theologian and the philosopher." Another participant called for "a disentanglement of the organic elements of disease from the psychosocial elements of human malfunction," arguing that medicine should deal with the former only.[2]

## THE TWO POSITIONS

Psychiatrists have responded to their crisis by embracing two ostensibly opposite positions. One would simply exclude psychiatry from the field of medicine, while the other would adhere strictly to the "medical model" and limit psychiatry's field to behavioral disorders consequent to brain dysfunction. The first is exemplified in the writings of Szasz and others who advance the position that "mental illness is a myth" since it does not conform with the accepted concept of disease.[3] Supporters of this position advocate the removal of the functions now performed by psychiatry from the conceptual and professional jurisdiction of medicine and their reallocation to a new discipline based on behavioral science. Henceforth medicine would be responsible for the treatment and cure of disease, while the new discipline would be concerned with the reeducation of people with "problems of living." Implicit in this argument is the premise that while the medical model constitutes a sound framework within which to understand and treat disease, it is not relevant to the behavioral and psychological problems classically deemed the domain of psychiatry. Disorders directly ascribable to brain disorder would be taken care of by neurologists, while psychiatry as such would disappear as a medical discipline.

The contrasting posture of strict adherence to the medical model is caricatured in Ludwig's view of the psychiatrist as physician.[1] According to Ludwig, the medical model premises "that sufficient deviation from normal represents *disease,* that disease is due to known or unknown natural causes, and that elimination of these causes will result in cure or improvement in individual patients" (Ludwig's italics). While acknowledging that most psychiatric diagnoses have a lower level of confirmation than most medical diagnoses, he adds that they are not "qualitatively different provided that mental disease is assumed to arise largely from 'natural' rather than metapsychological, interpersonal or societal causes." "Natural" is defined as "biological brain dysfunctions, either biochemical or neurophysiological in nature." On the other hand, "disorders such as problems of living, social adjustment reactions, character disorders, dependency syndromes, existential depressions, and various social deviancy conditions [would] be excluded from the concept of mental illness since these disorders arise in individuals with presumably intact neurophysiological functioning and are produced primarily by psychosocial variables." Such "nonpsychiatric disorders" are not properly the concern of the physician-psychiatrist and are more appropriately handled by nonmedical professionals.

In sum, psychiatry struggles to clarify its status within the mainstream of medicine, if indeed it belongs in medicine at all. The criterion by which this question is supposed to be resolved rests on the degree to which the field of activity of psychiatry is deemed congruent with the existing medical model of disease. But crucial to this problem is another, that of whether the contemporary model is, in fact, any longer adequate for medicine, much less for psychiatry. For if it is not, then perhaps the crisis of psychiatry is part and parcel of a larger crisis that has its roots in the model itself. Should that be the case, then it would be imprudent for psychiatry prematurely to abandon its models in favor of one that may also be flawed.

## THE BIOMEDICAL MODEL

The dominant model of disease today is biomedical, with molecular biology its basic scientific discipline. It assumes disease to be fully accounted for by deviations from the norm of measurable biological (somatic) variables. It leaves no room within its framework for the social, psychological, and behavioral dimensions of illness. The biomedical model not only requires that disease be dealt with as an entity independent of social behavior, it also demands that behavioral aberrations be explained on the basis of disordered somatic (biochemical or neurophysiological) processes. Thus the biomedical model embraces both reductionism, the philosophic view that complex phenomena are ultimately derived from a single primary principle, and mind-body dualism, the doctrine that separates the mental from the somatic. Here the reductionistic primary principle is physicalistic; that is, it assumes that the language of chemistry and physics will ultimately suffice to explain biological phenomena. From the reductionist viewpoint, the only conceptual tools available to characterize and experimental tools to study biological systems are physical in nature.[4]

The biomedical model was devised by medical scientists for the study of disease. As such it was a scientific model; that is, it involved a shared set of assumptions and rules of conduct based on the scientific method and constituted a blueprint for research. Not all models are scientific. Indeed, broadly defined, a model is nothing more than a belief system utilized to explain natural phenomena, to make sense out of what is puzzling or disturbing. The more socially disruptive or individually upsetting the phenomenon, the more pressing the need of humans to devise explanatory systems. Such efforts at explanation constitute devices for social adaptation. Disease par excellence exemplifies a category of natural phenomena urgently demanding explanation.[5] As Fabrega has pointed out, "disease" in its generic sense is a linguistic term used to refer to a certain class of phenomena that members of all social groups, at all times in the history of man, have been exposed to. "When people of various intellectual and cultural persuasions use terms analogous to 'disease,' they have in mind, among other things, that the phenomena in question involve a person-centered, harmful, and undesirable deviation of discontinuity . . . associated with impairment or discomfort." Since the condition is not desired it gives rise to a need for corrective actions. The latter involve beliefs and explanations about disease as well as rules of conduct to rationalize treatment actions. These constitute socially adaptive devices to resolve, for the individual as well as for the society in which the sick person lives, the crises and uncertainties surrounding disease.[6]

Such culturally derived belief systems about disease also constitute models, but they are not scientific models. These may be referred to as popular or folk models. As efforts at social adaptation, they contrast with scientific models, which are primarily designed to promote scientific investigation. The historical fact we have to face is that in modern Western society biomedicine not only has provided a basis for the scientific study of disease, it has also become our own culturally specific perspective about disease, that is, our folk model. Indeed the biomedical model is now the dominant folk model of disease in the Western world.[5,6]

In our culture the attitudes and belief systems of physicians are molded by this model long before they embark on their professional education, which in turn reinforces it without necessarily clarifying how its use for social adaptation contrasts with its use for scientific research. The biomedical model has thus become a cultural imperative, its limitations easily overlooked. In brief, it has now acquired the status of *dogma*. In science, a model is revised or abandoned when it fails to account adequately for all the data. A dogma, on the other hand, requires that discrepant data be forced to fit the model or be excluded. Biomedical dogma requires that all disease, including "mental" disease, be conceptualized in terms of derangement of underlying physical mechanisms. This permits only two alternatives whereby behavior and disease can be reconciled: the *reductionist*, which says that all behavioral phenomena of disease must be conceptualized in terms of physicochemical principles; and the *exclusionist*, which says that whatever is not capable of being so explained must be excluded from the category of disease. The reductionists concede that some disturbances in behavior belong in the spectrum of disease. They categorize these as mental diseases and designate psychiatry as the relevant medical discipline. The exclusionists regard mental illness as a myth and would eliminate psychiatry from medicine. Among physicians and psychiatrists today the reductionists are the true believers, the exclusionists are the apostates, while both condemn as heretics those who dare to question the ultimate truth of the biomedical model and advocate a more useful model.

# HISTORICAL ORIGINS OF THE REDUCTIONISTIC BIOMEDICAL MODEL

In considering the requirements for a more inclusive scientific medical model for the study of disease, an ethnomedical perspective is helpful.[6] In all societies, ancient and modern, preliterate and literate, the major criteria for identification of disease have always been behavioral, psychological, and social in nature. Classically, the onset of disease is marked by changes in physical appearance that frighten, puzzle, or awe, and by alterations in functioning, in feelings, in performance, in behavior, or in relationships that are experienced or perceived as threatening, harmful, unpleasant, deviant, undesirable, or unwanted. Reported verbally or demonstrated by the sufferer or by a witness, these constitute the primary data upon which are based first-order judgments as to whether or not a person is sick.[7] To such disturbing behavior and reports all societies typically respond by designating individuals and evolving social institutions whose primary function is to evaluate, interpret, and provide corrective measures.[5,6] Medicine as an institution and as a discipline, and physicians as professionals, evolved as one form of response to such social needs. In the course of history, medicine became scientific as physicians and other scientists developed a taxonomy and applied scientific methods to the understanding, treatment, and prevention of disturbances which the public first had designated as "disease" or "sickness."

Why did the reductionistic, dualistic biomedical model evolve in the West? Rasmussen identifies one source in the concession of established Christian orthodoxy to permit dissection of the human body some five centuries ago.[8]

Such a concession was in keeping with the Christian view of the body as a weak and imperfect vessel for the transfer of the soul from this world to the next. Not surprisingly, the Church's mission to study the human body included a tacit interdiction against corresponding scientific investigation of man's mind and behavior. For in the eyes of the Church these had more to do with religion and the soul and hence properly remained its domain. This compact may be considered largely responsible for the anatomical and structural base upon which scientific Western medicine eventually was to be built. For at the same time, the basic principle of the science of the day, as enunciated by Galileo, Newton, and Descartes, was analytical, meaning that entities to be investigated be resolved into isolable causal chains or units, from which it was assumed that the whole could be understood, both materially and conceptually, by reconstituting the parts. With mind-body dualism firmly established under the imprimatur of the Church, classical science readily fostered the notion of the body as a machine, of disease as the consequence of breakdown of the machine, and of the doctor's task as repair of the machine. Thus, the scientific approach to disease began by focusing in a fractional-analytic way on biological (somatic) processes and ignoring the behavioral and psychosocial. This was so even though in practice many physicians, at least until the beginning of the 20th century, regarded emotions as important for the development and course of disease. Actually, such arbitrary exclusion is an acceptable strategy in scientific research, especially when concepts and methods appropriate for the excluded areas are not yet available. But it becomes counterproductive when such strategy becomes policy and the area originally put aside for practical reasons is permanently excluded, if not forgotten altogether. The greater the success of the narrow approach the more likely is this to happen. The biomedical approach to disease has been successful beyond all expectations, but at a cost. For in serving as guideline and justification for medical care policy, biomedicine has also contributed to a host of problems, which I shall consider later.

## LIMITATIONS OF THE BIOMEDICAL MODEL

We are now faced with the necessity and the challenge to broaden the approach to disease to include the psychosocial without sacrificing the enormous advantages of the biomedical approach. On the importance of the latter all agree, the reductionist, the exclusionist, and the heretic. In a recent critique of the exclusionist position, Kety put the contrast between the two in such a way as to help define the issues.[9] "According to the medical model, a human illness does not become a specific disease all at once and is not equivalent to it. The medical model of an illness is a process that moves from the recognition and palliation of symptoms to the characterization of a specific disease in which the etiology and pathogenesis are known and treatment is rational and specific." Thus taxonomy progresses from symptoms, to clusters of symptoms, to syndromes, and finally to diseases with specific pathogenesis and pathology. This sequence accurately describes the successful application of the scientific method to the elucidation and the classification into discrete entities of disease in its generic sense.[5,6] The merit of such an approach needs no argument. What do require scrutiny are the distortions introduced by the reductionistic tendency to regard the specific disease as adequately, if not best, characterized in terms of the smallest isolable component having causal implications, for example, the biochemical; or even more critical, is the contention that the designation "disease" does not apply in the absence of perturbations at the biochemical level.

Kety approaches this problem by comparing diabetes mellitus and schizophrenia as paradigms of somatic and mental diseases, pointing out the appropriateness of the medical model for both. "Both are symptom clusters or syndromes, one described by somatic and biochemical abnormalities, the other by psychological. Each may have many etiologies and shows a range of intensity from severe and debilitating to latent or borderline. There is also evidence that genetic and environmental influences operate in the development of both."[9] In this description, at least in reductionistic terms, the scientific characterization of diabetes is the more advanced in that it has progressed from the behavioral framework of symptoms to that of biochemical abnormalities. Ultimately, the reductionists assume schizophrenia will achieve a similar degree of resolution. In developing his position, Kety makes clear that he does not regard the genetic factors and biological processes in schizophrenia as are now known to exist (or may be discovered in the future) as the only important influences in its etiology. He insists that equally important is elucidation of "how experiential factors and their interactions with biological vulnerability make possible or prevent the development of schizophrenia." But whether such a caveat will suffice to counteract basic reductionism is far from certain.

## THE REQUIREMENTS OF A NEW MEDICAL MODEL

To explore the requirements of a medical model that would account for the reality of diabetes and schizophrenia as human experiences as well as disease abstractions, let us expand Kety's analogy by making the assumption that a specific biochemical abnormality capable of being influenced pharmacologically exists in schizophrenia as well as in diabetes, certainly a plausible possibility. By obliging ourselves to think of patients with diabetes, a "somatic disease," and with schizophrenia, a "mental disease," in exactly the same terms, we will see more clearly how inclusion of somatic and psychosocial factors is indispensable for both; or more pointedly, how concentration on the biomedical and exclusion of the psychosocial distorts perspectives and even interferes with patient care.

1. In the biomedical model, demonstration of the specific biochemical deviation is generally regarded as a specific diagnostic criterion for the disease. Yet in terms of the human experience of illness, laboratory documentation may only indicate disease potential, not the actuality of the disease at the time. The abnormality may be present, yet the patient not be ill. Thus the presence of the biochemical defect of diabetes or schizophrenia at best defines a necessary but not a sufficient condition for the occurrence of the human experience of the disease, the illness. More accurately, the biochemical defect constitutes but one factor among many, the complex interaction of which ultimately may culminate in active disease or manifest illness.[10] Nor can the biochemical defect be made to account for all of the illness, for full understanding requires additional concepts and frames of reference. Thus, while the diagnosis of diabetes is first suggested by certain core clinical manifestations, for example, polyuria, polydipsia, polyphagia, and weight loss, and is then confirmed by laboratory documentation of relative insulin deficiency, how these are experienced and how they are reported by any one individual, and how they affect him, all require consideration of psychological, social, and cultural factors, not to mention other concurrent or complicating biological factors. Variability in the clinical expression of diabetes as well as of schizophrenia, and in the individual experience and expression of these illnesses, reflects as much these other elements as it does quantitative variations in the specific biochemical defect.

2. Establishing a relationship between particular biochemical processes and the clinical data of illness requires a scientifically rational approach to behavioral and psychosocial data, for these are the terms in which most clinical phenomena are reported by patients. Without such, the reliability of observations and the validity of correlations will be flawed. It serves little to be able to specify a biochemical defect in schizophrenia if one does not know how to relate this to particular psychological and behavioral expressions of the disorder. The biomedical model gives insufficient heed to this requirement. Instead it encourages bypassing the patient's verbal account by placing greater reliance on technical procedures and laboratory measurements. In actuality the task is appreciably more complex than the biomedical model encourages one to believe. An examination of the correlations between clinical and laboratory data requires not only reliable methods of clinical data collection, specifically highlevel interviewing skills, but also basic understanding of the psychological, social, and cultural determinants of how patients communicate symptoms of disease. For example, many verbal expressions derive from bodily experiences early in life, resulting in a significant degree of ambiguity in the language patients use to report symptoms. Hence the same words may serve to express

primary psychological as well as bodily disturbances, both of which may coexist and overlap in complex ways. Thus, virtually each of the symptoms classically associated with diabetes may also be expressions of or reactions to psychological distress, just as ketoacidosis and hypoglycemia may induce psychiatric manifestations, including some considered characteristics of schizophrenia. The most essential skills of the physician involve the ability to elicit accurately and then analyze correctly the patient's verbal account of his illness experience. The biomedical model ignores both the rigor required to achieve reliability in the interview process and the necessity to analyze the meaning of the patient's report in psychological, social, and cultural as well as in anatomical, physiological, or biochemical terms.[7]

3. Diabetes and schizophrenia have in common the fact that conditions of life and living constitute significant variables influencing the time of reported onset of the manifest disease as well as of variations in its course. In both conditions this results from the fact that psychophysiologic responses to life change may interact with existing somatic factors to alter susceptibility and thereby influence the time of onset, the severity, and the course of a disease. Experimental studies in animals amply document the role of early, previous, and current life experience in altering susceptibility to a wide variety of diseases even in the presence of a genetic predisposition.[11] Cassel's demonstration of higher rates of ill health among populations exposed to incongruity between the demands of the social system in which they are living and working and the culture they bring with them provides another illustration among humans of the role of psychosocial variables in disease causation.[12]

4. Psychological and social factors are also crucial in determining whether and when patients with the biochemical abnormality of diabetes or of schizophrenia come to view themselves or be viewed by others as sick. Still other factors of a similar nature influence whether or not and when any individual enters a health care system and becomes a patient. Thus, the biochemical defect may determine certain characteristics of the disease, but not necessarily the point in time when the person falls ill or accepts the sick role or the status of a patient.

5. "Rational treatment" (Kety's term) directed only at the biochemical abnormality does not necessarily restore the patient to health even in the face of documented correction or major alleviation of the abnormality. This is no less true for diabetes than it will be for schizophrenia when a biochemical defect is established. Other factors may combine to sustain patienthood even in the face of biochemical recovery. Conspicuously responsible for such discrepancies between correction of biological abnormalities and treatment outcome are psychological and social variables.

6. Even with the application of rational therapies, the behavior of the physician and the relationship between patient and physician powerfully influence therapeutic outcome for better or for worse. These constitute psychological

effects which may directly modify the illness experience or indirectly affect underlying biochemical processes, the latter by virtue of interactions between psychophysiological reactions and biochemical processes implicated in the disease.[11] Thus, insulin requirements of a diabetic patient may fluctuate significantly depending on how the patient perceives his relationship with his doctor. Furthermore, the successful application of rational therapies is limited by the physician's ability to influence and modify the patient's behavior in directions concordant with health needs. Contrary to what the exclusionists would have us believe, the physician's role is, and always has been, very much that of educator and psychotherapist. To know how to induce peace of mind in the patient and enhance his faith in the healing powers of his physician requires psychological knowledge and skills, not merely charisma. These too are outside the biomedical framework.

## THE ADVANTAGES OF A BIOPSYCHOSOCIAL MODEL

This list surely is not complete but it should suffice to document that diabetes mellitus and schizophrenia as paradigms of "somatic" and "mental" disorders are entirely analogous and, as Kety argues, are appropriately conceptualized within the framework of a medical model of disease. But the existing biomedical model does not suffice. To provide a basis for understanding the determinants of disease and arriving at rational treatments and patterns of health care, a medical model must also take into account the patient, the social context in which he lives, and the complementary system devised by society to deal with the disruptive effects of illness, that is, the physician role and the health care system. This requires a biopsychosocial model. Its scope is determined by the historic function of the physician to establish whether the person soliciting help is "sick" or "well"; and if sick, why sick and in which ways sick; and then to develop a rational program to treat the illness and restore and maintain health.

The boundaries between health and disease, between well and sick, are far from clear and never will be clear, for they are diffused by cultural, social, and psychological considerations. The traditional biomedical view, that biological indices are the ultimate criteria defining disease, leads to the present paradox that some people with positive laboratory findings are told that they are in need of treatment when in fact they are feeling quite well, while others feeling sick are assured that they are well, that is, they have no "disease."[5,6] A biopsychosocial model which includes the patient as well as the illness would encompass both circumstances. The doctor's task is to account for the dysphoria and the dysfunction which lead individuals to seek medical help, adopt the sick role, and accept the status of patienthood. He must weight the relative contributions of social and psychological as well as of biological factors implicated in the patient's dysphoria and dysfunction as well as in his decision to accept or not accept patienthood and with it the responsibility to cooperate in his own health care.

By evaluating all the factors contributing to both illness and patienthood, rather than giving primacy to biological factors alone, a biopsychosocial model would make it possible to explain why some individuals experience as "illness" conditions which others regard merely as "problems of living," be they emotional reactions to life circumstances or somatic symptoms. For from the individual's point of view his decision between whether he has a "problem of living" or is "sick" has basically to do with whether or not he accepts the sick role and seeks entry into the health care system, not with what, in fact, is responsible for his distress. Indeed, some people deny the unwelcome reality of illness by dismissing as "a problem of living" symptoms which may in actuality be indicative of a serious organic process. It is the doctor's, not the patient's, responsibility to establish the nature of the problem and to decide whether or not it is best handled in a medical framework. Clearly the dichotomy between "disease" and "problems of living" is by no means a sharp one, either for patient or for doctor.

# WHEN IS GRIEF A DISEASE?

To enhance our understanding of how it is that "problems of living" are experienced as illness by some and not by others, it might be helpful to consider grief as a paradigm of such a borderline condition. For while grief has never been considered in a medical framework, a significant number of grieving people do consult doctors because of disturbing symptoms, which they do not necessarily relate to grief. Fifteen years ago I addressed this question in a paper entitled "Is Grief a Disease? A Challenge for Medical Research."[13] Its aim too was to raise questions about the adequacy of the biomedical model. A better title might have been, "When Is Grief a Disease?"—just as one might ask when schizophrenia or when diabetes is a disease. For while there are some obvious analogies between grief and disease, there are also some important differences. But these very contradictions help to clarify the psychosocial dimensions of the biopsychosocial model.

Grief clearly exemplifies a situation in which psychological factors are primary; no preexisting chemical or physiological defects or agents need be invoked. Yet as with classic diseases, ordinary grief constitutes a discrete syndrome with a relatively predictable symptomatology which includes, incidentally, both bodily and psychological disturbances. It displays the autonomy typical of disease; that is, it runs its course despite the sufferer's efforts or wish to bring it to a close. A consistent etiologic factor can be identified, namely, a significant loss. On the other hand, neither the sufferer nor society has ever dealt with ordinary grief as an illness even though such expressions as "sick with grief" would indicate some connection in people's minds. And while every culture makes provisions for the mourner, these have generally been regarded more as the responsibility of religion than of medicine.

On the face of it, the arguments against including grief in a medical model would seem to be the more persuasive. In the 1961 paper I countered these by comparing grief to a wound. Both are natural responses to environmental trauma, one psychological, the other physical. But even at the time I felt a vague uneasiness that this analogy did not quite make the case. Now 15 years later a better grasp of the cultural origins of disease concepts and medical care systems clarifies the apparent inconsistency. The critical factor underlying man's need to develop folk models of disease, and to develop social adaptations to deal with the individual and group disruptions brought about by disease, has always been the victim's ignorance of what is responsible for his dysphoric or disturbing experience.[5,6] Neither grief nor a wound fits fully into that category. In both, the reasons for the pain, suffering, and disability are only too clear. Wounds or fractures incurred in battle or by accident by and large were self-treated or ministered to with folk remedies or by individuals who had acquired certain technical skills in such matters. Surgery developed out of the need for treatment of wounds and injuries and has different historical roots than medicine, which was always closer in origin to magic and religion. Only later in Western history did surgery and medicine merge as healing arts. But even from earliest times there were people who behaved as though grief-stricken, yet seemed not to have suffered any loss; and others who developed what for all the world looked like wounds or fractures, yet had not been subjected to any known trauma. And there were people who suffered losses whose grief deviated in one way or another from what the culture had come to accept as the normal course; and others whose wounds failed to heal or festered or who became ill even though the wound had apparently healed. Then, as now, two elements were crucial in defining the role of patient and physician and hence in determining what should be regarded as disease. For the patient it has been his not knowing why he felt or functioned badly or what to do about it, coupled with the belief or knowledge that the healer or physician did know and could provide relief. For the physician in turn it has been his commitment to his professional role as healer. From these have evolved sets of expectations which are reinforced by the culture, though these are not necessarily the same for patient as for physician.

A biopsychosocial model would take all of these factors into account. It would acknowledge the fundamental fact that the patient comes to the physician because either he does not know what is wrong or, if he does, he feels incapable of helping himself. The psychobiological unity of man requires that the physician accept the responsibility to evaluate whatever problems the patient presents and recommend a course of action, including referral to other helping professions. Hence the physician's basic professional knowledge and skills must span the social, psychological, and biological, for his decisions and actions on the patient's behalf involve all three. Is the patient suffering normal grief or melancholia? Are the fatigue and weakness of the woman who recently lost her husband conversion symptoms, psychophysiological reactions, manifestations of a somatic disorder, or a combination of these? The patient soliciting the aid of a physician must have confidence that the M.D. degree has indeed rendered that physician competent to make such differentiations.

# A CHALLENGE FOR BOTH MEDICINE AND PSYCHIATRY

The development of a biopsychosocial medical model is posed as a challenge for both medicine and psychiatry. For despite the enormous gains which have accrued from biomedical research, there is a growing uneasiness among the public as well as among physicians, and especially among the younger generation, that health needs are not being met and that biomedical research is not having a sufficient impact in human terms. This is usually ascribed to the all too obvious inadequacies of existing health care delivery systems. But this certainly is not a complete explanation, for many who do have adequate access to health care also complain that physicians are lacking in interest and understanding, are preoccupied with procedures, and are insensitive to the personal problems of patients and their families. Medical institutions are seen as cold and impersonal; the more prestigious they are as centers for biomedical research, the more common such complaints.[14] Medicine's unrest derives from a growing awareness among many physicians of the contradiction between the excellence of their biomedical background on the one hand and the weakness of their qualifications in certain attributes essential for good patient care on the other.[7] Many recognize that these cannot be improved by working within the biomedical model alone.

The present upsurge of interest in primary care and family medicine clearly reflects disenchantment among some physicians with an approach to disease that neglects the patient. They are now more ready for a medical model which would take psychosocial issues into account. Even from within academic circles are coming some sharp challenges to biomedical dogmatism.[8,15] Thus Holman ascribes directly to biomedical reductionism and to the professional dominance of its adherents over the health care system such undesirable practices as unnecessary hospitalization, overuse of drugs, excessive surgery, and inappropriate utilization of diagnostic tests. He writes, "While reductionism is a powerful tool for understanding, it also creates profound misunderstanding when unwisely applied. Reductionism is particularly harmful when it neglects the impact of nonbiological circumstances upon biologic processes." And, "Some medical outcomes are inadequate not because appropriate technical interventions are lacking but because our conceptual thinking is inadequate."[15] How ironic it would be were psychiatry to insist on subscribing to a medical model which some leaders in medicine already are beginning to question.

Psychiatrists, unconsciously committed to the biomedical model and split into the warring camps of reductionists and exclusionists, are today so preoccupied with their own professional identity and status in relation to medicine that many are failing to appreciate that psychiatry now is the only clinical discipline within medicine concerned primarily with the study of man and the human condition. While the behavioral sciences have made some limited incursions into medical school teaching programs, it is mainly upon psychiatrists, and to a lesser extent clinical psychologists, that the responsibility falls to develop approaches to the understanding of health and disease and patient care not readily accomplished within the more narrow framework and with the specialized techniques of traditional biomedicine. Indeed, the fact is that the major formulations of more integrated and holistic concepts of health and disease proposed in the past 30 years have come not from within the biomedical establishment but from physicians who have drawn upon concepts and methods which originated within psychiatry, notably the psychodynamic approach of Sigmund Freud and psychoanalysis and the reaction-to-life-stress approach of Adolf Meyer and psychobiology.[16] Actually, one of the more lasting contributions of both Freud and Meyer has been to provide frames of reference whereby psychological processes could be included in a concept of disease. Psychosomatic medicine—the term itself a vestige of dualism—became the medium whereby the gap between the two parallel but independent ideologies of medicine, the biological and the psychosocial, was to be bridged. Its progress has been slow and halting, not only because of the extreme complexities intrinsic to the field itself, but also because of unremitting pressures, from within as well as from without, to conform to scientific methodologies basically mechanistic and reductionistic in conception and inappropriate for many of the problems under study. Nonetheless, by now a sizable body of knowledge, based on clinical and experimental studies of man and animals has accumulated. Most, however, remains unknown to the general medical public and to the biomedical community and is largely ignored in the education of physicians. The recent solemn pronouncement by an eminent biomedical leader[2] that "the emotional content of organic medicine [has been] exaggerated" and "psychosomatic medicine is on the way out" can only be ascribed to the blinding effects of dogmatism.

The fact is that medical schools have constituted unreceptive if not hostile environments for those interested in psychosomatic research and teaching, and medical journals have all too often followed a double standard in accepting papers dealing with psychosomatic relationships.[17] Further, much of the work documenting experimentally in animals the significance of life circumstances or change in altering susceptibility to disease has been done by experimental psychologists and appears in psychology journals rarely read by physicians or basic biomedical scientists.[11]

## GENERAL SYSTEMS THEORY PERSPECTIVE

The struggle to reconcile the psychosocial and the biological in medicine has had its parallel in biology, also dominated by the reductionistic approach of molecular biology. Among biologists too have emerged advocates of the need to develop holistic as well as reductionistic explanations of life processes, to answer the "why?" and the "what for?" as well as the "how?"[18,19] Von Bertalanffy, arguing the need for a more fundamental reorientation in scientific perspectives in order to open the way to holistic approaches more amenable to scientific inquiry and conceptualization, developed general systems theory.[19,20] This approach, by treating sets of related events collectively as systems manifesting functions and properties on the specific level of the whole, has made possible recognition of isomorphies across different levels of organization, as molecules, cells, organs, the organism, the person, the family, the society, or the biosphere. From such isomorphies can be developed fundamental laws and principles that operate commonly at all levels of organization, as compared to those which are unique for each. Since systems theory holds that all levels of organization are linked to each other in a hierarchical relationship so that change in one affects change in the others, its adoption as a scientific approach should do much to mitigate the holist-reductionist dichotomy and improve communication across scientific disciplines. For medicine, systems theory provides a conceptual approach suitable not only for the proposed biopsychosocial concept of disease but also for studying disease and medical care as interrelated processes.[10,21] If and when a general-systems approach becomes part of the basic scientific and philosophic education of future physicians and medical scientists, a greater readiness to encompass a biopsychosocial perspective of disease may be anticipated.

## BIOMEDICINE AS SCIENCE AND AS DOGMA

In the meantime, what is being and can be done to neutralize the dogmatism of biomedicine and all the undesirable social and scientific consequences that flow therefrom? How can a proper balance be established between the fractional-analytic and the natural history approaches, both so integral for the work of the physician and the medical scientist?[22] How can the clinician be helped to understand the extent to which his scientific approach to patients represents a distinctly "human science," one in which "reliance is on the integrative powers of the observer of a complex nonreplicable event and on the experiments that are provided by history and by animals living in particular ecological settings," as Margaret Mead puts it?[23] The history of the rise and fall of scientific dogmas throughout history may give some clues. Certainly mere emergence of new findings and theories rarely suffices to overthrow well-entrenched dogmas. The power of vested interests, social, political, and economic, are formidable deterrents to any effective assault on biomedical dogmatism. The delivery of health care is a major industry, considering that more than 8 percent of our national economic product is devoted to health.[2] The enormous existing and planned investment in diagnostic and therapeutic technology alone strongly favors approaches to clinical study and care of patients that emphasize the impersonal and the mechanical.[24] For example, from 1967 to 1972 there was an increase of 33 percent in the number of laboratory tests conducted per hospital admission.[25] Planning for systems of medical care and their financing is excessively influenced by the availability and promise of technology, the application and effectiveness of which are often used as the criteria by which decisions are made as to what constitutes illness and who qualifies for medical care. The frustration of those who find what they believe to be their legitimate health needs inadequately met by too technologically oriented physicians is generally misinterpreted by the biomedical establishment as indicating "unrealistic expectations" on the part of the public rather than being recognized as reflecting a genuine discrepancy between illness as actually experienced by the patient and as it is conceptualized in the biomedical mode.[26] The professionalization of biomedicine constitutes still another formidable barrier.[8,15] Professionalization has engendered a caste system among health care personnel and a peck order concerning what constitute appropriate areas for medical concern and care, with the most esoteric disorders at the top of the list. Professional dominance "has perpetuated prevailing practices, deflected criticisms, and insulated the profession from alternate views and social relations that would illuminate and improve health care."[15(p21)] Holman argues, not unconvincingly, that "the medical establishment is not primarily engaged in the disinterested pursuit of knowledge and the translation of that knowledge into medical practice; rather in significant part it is engaged in special interest advocacy, pursuing and preserving social power."[15]

Under such conditions it is difficult to see how reforms can be brought about. Certainly contributing another critical essay is hardly likely to bring about any major changes in attitude. The problem is hardly new, for the first efforts to introduce a more holistic approach into the undergraduate medical curriculum actually date back to Adolph Meyer's program at Johns Hopkins, which was initiated before 1920.[27] At Rochester, a program directed to medical students and to physicians during and after their residency training, and designed to inculcate psychosocial knowledge and skills appropriate for their future work as clinicians or teachers, has been in existence for 30 years.[28] While difficult to measure outcome objectively, its impact, as indicated by a questionnaire on how students and graduates view the issues involved in illness and patient care, appears to have been appreciable.[29] In other schools, especially in the immediate post–World War II period, similar efforts were launched, and while some flourished briefly, most soon faded away under the competition of more glamorous and acceptable biomedical careers. Today, within many medical schools there is again a revival of interest among some faculty, but they are few in number and lack the influence, prestige, power, and access to funding from peer review groups that goes with conformity to the prevailing biomedical structure.

Yet today, interest among students and young physicians is high, and where learning opportunities exist they quickly overwhelm the available meager resources. It would appear that given the opportunity, the younger generation is very ready to accept the importance of learning more about the psychosocial dimensions of illness and health care and the need for such education to be soundly based on scientific principles. Once exposed to such an approach, most recognize how ephemeral and insubstantial are appeals to humanism and compassion when not based on rational principles. They reject as simplistic the notion that in past generations doctors understood their patients better, a myth that has persisted for centuries.[30] Clearly, the gap to be closed is between teachers ready to teach and students eager to learn. But nothing will change unless or until those who control resources have the wisdom to venture off the beaten path of exclusive reliance on biomedicine as the only approach to health care. The proposed biopsychosocial model provides a blueprint for research, a framework for teaching, and a design for action in the real world of health care. Whether it is useful or not remains to be seen. But the answer will not be forthcoming if conditions are not provided to do so. In a free society, outcome will depend upon those who have the courage to try new paths and the wisdom to provide the necessary support.

# SUMMARY

The dominant model of disease today is biomedical, and it leaves no room within its framework for the social, psychological, and behavioral dimensions of illness. A biopsychosocial model is proposed that provides a blueprint for research, a framework for teaching, and a design for action in the real world of health care.

# Notes

1. A. M. Ludwig, *JAMA*, 234, 603 (1975).

2. *RF Illustrated*, 3, 5 (1976).

3. T. S. Szasz, *The Myth of Mental Illness* (Harper & Row, New York, 1961); E. F. Torrey, *The Death of Psychiatry* (Chilton, Radnor, Pa., 1974).

4. R. Rosen, in *The Relevance of General Systems Theory*, E. Laszlo, Ed. (Braziller, New York, 1972), p. 45.

5. H. Fabrega, *Arch Gen Psychiatry*, 32, 1501 (1972).

6. H. Fabrega, *Science*, 189, 969 (1975).

7. G. L. Engel, *Ann Intern Med*, 78, 587 (1973).

8. H. Rasmussen, *Pharos* 38, 53 (1975).

9. S. Kety, *Am J Psychiatry*, 131, 957 (1974).

10. G. L. Engel, *Perspect Biol Med*, 3, 459 (1960).

11. R. Ader, in *Ethology and Development*, S. A. Barnett, Ed. (Heinemann, London, 1973), p. 37; G. L. Engel, *Gastroenterology*, 67, 1085 (1974).

12. J. Cassel, *Am J Public Health*, 54, 1482 (1964).

13. G. L. Engel, *Psychosom Med*, 23, 18 (1961).

14. R. S. Duff and A. B. Hollingshead, *Sickness and Society* (Harper & Row, New York, 1968).

15. H. R. Holman, *Hosp Pract*, 11, 11 (1976).

16. K. Menninger, *Ann Intern Med*, 29, 318 (1948); J. Romano, *JAMA*, 143, 409 (1950); G. L. Engel, *Midcentury Psychiatry*, R. Grinker, Ed. (Thomas, Springfield, Ill., 1953), p. 33; H. G. Wolff, Ed., *An Outline of Man's Knowledge* (Doubleday, New York, 1960), p. 41; G. L. Engel, *Psychological Development in Health and Disease* (Saunders, Philadelphia, 1962).

17. G. L. Engel and S. Salzman, *N Engl J Med*, 288, 44 (1973).

18. R. Dubos, *Mirage of Health* (Harper & Row, New York, 1959); *Reason Awake* (Columbia Univ. Press, New York, 1970); E. Mayr, in *Behavior and Evolution*, A. Roe and G. G. Simpson, Eds. (Yale Univ. Press, New Haven, Conn., 1958), p. 341; *Science*, 134, 1501 (1961); *Am Sci*, 62, 650 (1974); J. T. Bonner, *On Development. The Biology of Form* (Harvard Univ. Press, Cambridge, Mass., 1974); G. G. Simpson, *Science*, 139, 81 (1963).

19. R. Dubos, *Man Adapting* (Yale Univ. Press, New Haven, Conn., 1965).

20. L. von Bertalanffy, *Problems of Life* (Wiley, New York, 1952); *General Systems Theory* (Braziller, New York, 1968). See also E. Laszlo, *The Relevance of General Systems Theory* (Braziller, New York, 1972); *The Systems View of the World* (Braziller, New York, 1972).

21. K. Menninger, *The Vital Balance* (Viking, New York, 1963); A. Sheldon, in *Systems*

*and Medical Care,* A. Sheldon, F. Baker, and C. P. McLaughlin, Eds. (MIT Press, Cambridge, Mass., 1970), p. 84; H. Brody, *Perspect Biol Med,* 16, 71 (1973).

22. G. L. Engel, in *Physiology, Emotion, and Psychosomatic Illness,* R. Porter and J. Knight, Eds. (Elsevier-Excerpta Medica, Amsterdam, 1972), p. 384.

23. M. Mead, *Science,* 191, 903 (1976).

24. G. L. Engel, *JAMA,* 236, 861 (1976).

25. J. M. McGinnis, *J Med Educ,* 51, 602 (176).

26. H. Fabrega and P. R. Manning, *Psychosom Med,* 35, 223 (1973).

27. A. Meyer, *JAMA,* 69, 861 (1917).

28. A. H. Schmale, W. A. Greene, F. Reichsman, M. Kehoe, and G. L. Engel, *Adv Psychosom Me,* 4, 4 (1964); G. L. Engel, *J Psychosom Res,* 11, 77 (1967); L. Young, *Ann Intern Med,* 83, 728 (1975).

29. G. L. Engel, *J Nerv Ment Dis,* 154, 159 (1972); *Univ Rochester Med Rev* (Winter 1971–1972), p. 10.

30. G. L. Engel, *Pharos,* 39, 127 (1976).

# CHAPTER FIVE

# Meeting the Challenge of Family Practice (The Willard Committee Report)

## *Introduction*

Ad Hoc Committee on Education for Family Practice of the
Council on Medical Education of the American Medical Association
1996

M*eeting the Challenge of Family Practice: The Report of the Ad Hoc Committee on Education for Family Practice of the Council on Medical Education of the American Medical Association (1996) is commonly referred to as "The Willard Committee Report" after William Willard, the chair of the committee. The Introduction is reprinted here.*

## Introduction

### THE CHARGE TO THE COMMITTEE

The Ad Hoc Committee on Education for Family Practice was appointed in September 1964 by the Council on Medical Education of the American Medical Association with the concurrence of the AMA Board of Trustees, with the following charge:

1. To review present AMA policy regarding the future of family and/or general practice and determine whether the goals of such policy are being achieved.

2. To recommend the educational approach by which present goals may be achieved if they are not being achieved now.

---

This chapter originally appeared as Ad Hoc Committee on Education for Family Practice of the Council on Medical Education. *Meeting the Challenge of Family Practice/The Willard Committee Report,* 1966; used by the permission of the American Medical Association.

3. To define and recommend policies by which these goals may be achieved.

The Committee understood that it was free to pursue its explorations without restrictions and accordingly has done so. However, the charge given by the Board of Trustees overlapped to some extent that of the Citizens' Commission on Graduate Medical Education.[1] The Ad Hoc Committee therefore established liaison with the Commission and calls attention to the fact that many of the recommendations of the two bodies are consistent and reinforcing.

The Committee has also been aware of the activities of the National Commission on Community Health Services, established in 1962 by the National Health Council and the American Public Health Association, whose report entitled *Health Is a Community Affair*[2] was published earlier this year. Six task forces contributed to the total effort of NCCHS and each published an independent report. One of these was the Task Force on Comprehensive Personal Health Service, and its report was entitled "Comprehensive Health Care, a Challenge to American Communities."[3] One chapter of the full NCCHS report deals with the subject "Comprehensive Personal Health Services" and contains an extensive section on "The Changing Role of the Personal Physician" which was derived from the Task Force report. The recommendations of that portion of the NCCHS report and of the Ad Hoc Committee are quite similar in philosophy and detail.

Although there are similarities between this report and the expressions of other bodies, the Ad Hoc Committee has conducted its studies and deliberations separately and independently, and has reached its own conclusions and recommendations.

# REASON FOR THE APPOINTMENT OF THE COMMITTEE

Previous actions of the AMA House of Delegates have affirmed the opinion of the House that family practice is important for optimum health care. The House believes, however, that the number and percentage of family practitioners in the United States are declining, and that positive action is necessary to reverse that trend. A Committee on Preparation for Family Practice was appointed in 1957 and issued a report[4] in 1959 which led to the establishment of new residency programs in family practice. Neither that report and the resultant training programs, nor other actions to date, most of which have been aimed at the area of graduate medical education, have yet been productive. The present Committee was therefore appointed to reexamine the problem and its causes and to suggest solutions which might be effective in increasing the supply of family physicians.

# GENERAL CONSIDERATIONS

There are few valid data for a determination of trends about family practice. There are, however, some data concerning the number of general practitioners and it is these data which are usually cited as evidence of a trend in the decline of family practitioners. While general practice and family practice are not necessarily the same, it is believed that the decline in the number of general practitioners is indicative of a decline in the number of physicians interested in family practice.

In 1931 there were 112,000 physicians who classified themselves as general practitioners on AMA's annual directory cards. In 1960, the number had declined to 75,000 and in 1965, to 66,000.

Data from the Weiskotten studies[5] indicate that the percentage of young physicians in "pure" general practice (i.e., those who begin in general practice and stay in general practice) has remained relatively constant, at 15%-25%. However, in previous years many physicians started out in general practice and later became specialists by limiting their practice to a particular field; the modern trend is to enter specialty practice directly, through training in specialty internships and residencies. The earlier group was classified in general practice, while the modern group is obviously listed in the specialist class, but many physicians in both groups undoubtedly have carried on family practice. Therefore, the decline in numbers of general practitioners does not necessarily mean a decline in family practice.

Valid data do not exist on the number of recognized specialists who are in fact engaged in family practice, regardless of the nature of their past training. This number may be quite large, and hence the number of physicians who classify themselves as general practitioners, and are so recorded in the AMA records department, probably understates considerably the number engaged in family practice. It has been reported that about 75% of the membership of the American College of Physicians serve as family practitioners for many of their patients. An editorial in the Bulletin of the College has stated, in fact, that "the College thinks a man certified by the American Board of Internal Medicine is the ideally trained man for adult family practice as currently defined."[6]

While this information may indicate that the declining number of recognized general practitioners should not be translated directly into a conclusion that there is a declining number of family physicians, the fact remains that virtually no physicians are being trained specifically for careers in family practice. Since many physicians trained specifically for other specialty practice are instead or in addition engaging in family practice, it is reasonable to assume that this is done in response to public demand and need and reflects their interest in carrying on this kind of practice. In spite of this apparent demand and need, training programs in the currently recognized specialties continue to attract more and more medical graduates. But none of the currently recognized specialty programs known to the Ad Hoc Committee would satisfy the criteria which it considers essential for the proper preparation of the family practitioner.

The question is often raised whether the American people really need and want family practitioners today. Most persons who raise the question appear to be equating the family physician with the old-time general practitioner, the "horse-and-buggy" doctor of an earlier generation. The Ad Hoc Committee in no sense advocates a return to that era.

The Committee believes, however, that there is need for a new kind of specialist in family medicine, educated to provide comprehensive personal health care, because of the complexity of modern medicine and the health care system. The Committee feels that the American public does want and need a large number of well-qualified family physicians, as defined in Chapter II of this Report, and that the preparation of a large number of family physicians is essential if the people are to receive the maximal benefits from American medicine.

The Committee's opinion is based upon several items:

- The indirect evidence mentioned above that many specialists are called upon by their patients to practice family medicine even though their education has not prepared them to do so

- Expressions of concern from many specialists that they are asked by their patients to recommend family physicians but are unable to identify any who are available

- Studies carried out by the American Academy of General Practice[7] suggesting that most people would like to have a family practitioner

- The findings of the Task Force on Comprehensive Personal Health Services of the National Commission on Community Health Services[3]

- The deliberations and conclusions of the Citizens' Commission on Graduate Medical Education[1]

- Evidence from AMA's Placement Service that a large majority of requests from communities for physicians are for family practitioners

- The results of personal discussions with many individuals, in and out of the medical profession

It is not possible now to determine what proportion of practicing physicians should be family physicians, or indeed what the total number of physicians should be. Physician-population studies show that the number of physicians in the United States is increasing proportionately more rapidly than the total population[8]—primarily because of the large numbers of new foreign medical graduates—but that the proportion of physicians in the private practice of medicine is declining. This is largely a reflection of the number and variety of new career opportunities now open to physicians.

There is a school of thought which states that all of the public needs for family practitioners would be met if there were simply enough physicians and that the solution to the problem is therefore a massive increase in the number and size of medical schools. While this might encourage many more graduates to engage in family practice for economic reasons, it would not solve the problem of their adequate preparation for such practice. The Ad Hoc Committee has concluded that the medical profession should augment its efforts to increase the total number of physicians but that it should also strive to increase the number and proportion of physicians educated specifically to enter the field of family practice.

# DEFINITION AND FUNCTIONS OF THE FAMILY PHYSICIAN

In defining the family physician and describing his functions, the Ad Hoc Committee is referring for the most part to a physician of the future who will be educated in accordance with programs described in Section IV. Many of today's physicians are called upon to function in this manner, but few have had the educational preparation to do so.

## Definition of the Family Physician

The family physician is one who (1) serves as the physician of first contact with the patient and provides a means of entry into the health care system; (2) evaluates the patient's total health needs, provides personal medical care within one or more fields of medicine, and refers the patient when indicated to appropriate sources of care while preserving the continuity of his care; (3) assumes responsibility for the patient's comprehensive and continuous health care and acts as leader or coordinator of the team that provides health services; and (4) accepts responsibility for the patient's total health care within the context of his environment, including the community and the family or comparable social unit.

The family physician is a personal physician, oriented to the whole patient, who practices both scientific and humanistic medicine. He may provide care for only one member of the family, but more often does so for several or all members. Usually he himself provides medical care in more than one of the traditional specialty fields of medicine, and he coordinates the care obtained by referral to or consultation with other physicians and allied health personnel. He assumes responsibility for the patient's comprehensive and continuing health care and in effect serves as captain of the health team.

Comprehensive health care includes preventive, diagnostic, therapeutic, rehabilitative and health-maintenance services, and requires appropriate referral of patients for selected specialized and supporting services. This implies and requires effective coordination among physicians within the various specialties and with personnel in the allied health fields. It also requires adequate interpretation to the patient and his family of the nature and progress of the patient's illness and the services being recommended and provides in the context of the patient's expectations.

In today's society, it is estimated that 20% of the population changes residence every year, while the average family moves about every 7 years.[2] Under these conditions, and with the highly complex health resources now available, continuity of patient care through one physician is not always possible. However, even for the mobile patient, a measure of continuity can be provided by appropriate organization of medical practice and medical records.

In some instances, continuity may be provided by several physicians working together in formal or informal association, with each member having access to the patient's records. Continuity may also be facilitated by the appropriate use of nurses and other allied health personnel under proper supervision, in situations where continuing attention by the same physician is not possible.

However, the Committee believes that the best medical care is provided if the patient has continuing relationship with a family physician. Even where a group of physicians provides the total medical care, one physician in the group should assume responsibility for the comprehensive and continuous nature of the care for each patient. This will not necessarily be the same physician for all patients seen by the group, although usually the family practitioner role will fall naturally to a specific physician or physicians who have interest, talent and training to serve this function.

## Functions of the Family Physician

The functions of the family physician must be clearly understood, because they determine the nature of the required educational programs. The functions may be viewed from three perspectives: the first relates to the services which the family physician provides for his patients, the second to his administrative role in the health team, and the third to his role of community leadership.

**Patient Care Functions.** *The family physician is the first medical contact for patients, facilitating their access to medical care and to the whole health care system.* Because of his intimate personal relationships with the patient and his family, which grow with time, it is easy for the patient to contact him, and to obtain medical care. The family physician insures the ready availability of medical services, twenty-four hours a day and seven days a week, services that he either gives personally or arranges.

He takes positive action to see that his patients' medical care needs are met. He helps to remove barriers—barriers of all kinds—economic, emotional, social and occupational, and he minimizes as much as possible the disruption in the patients' way of life caused by illness. In appropriate instances the physician seeks out individual patients and advises them of their need for medical care (e.g., cancer patients who need periodic check-ups).

The family physician, himself, provides a major portion of medical care. Without referral he cares for a high percentage of his patients' problems, in those fields in which he is adequately trained and interested. He identifies the emergency or urgent problems of his patients and takes the necessary steps to solve them. As the primary physician, he is in excellent position to detect the earliest onset of disease or functional abnormality.

As he acquires a continuing and stable relationship with his patients, he becomes highly effective in dealing with their frequent emotional problems and with the social dimensions of their illnesses. He also becomes more selective in the use of diagnostic procedures and applies them more easily in proper sequence. Because of his prior and continuing knowledge of his patients' problems, there is less need to carry out or repeat many diagnostic procedures. As a result, treatment will often be less complicated but even more effective. There may be less need to hospitalize patients, and competent medical care will frequently be less costly in time and money.

*The family physician is the key to the referral process for problems beyond his scope of practice and competence.* Because he can not provide definitive care himself for all types of problems, he must know and respect his limitations and obtain help either by consultation or by referral of the patient to appropriate sources. To refer properly, he must know all the health resources in his geographic area and how to use them when indicated. Ideally, patients should gain access to all of their specialty care through the family physician.

Furthermore, the family physician is in the key position to follow up the findings and results to insure that the patient receives maximum benefit from the referral. For this to happen, referral must be recognized as a two-way process, with the patient being returned to the family physician in accordance with appropriate arrangements made at the time of referral.

Effective referrals and the use of consultation services require skill which the family physician must acquire through training and practice. This is a much more difficult and important function than serving as a triage officer.

*The family physician is the integrator of health services received by his patient.* He also interprets them to the patient, explaining the nature of the illness, the implications of the treatment and the effect of both upon his way of life. This function has increased in importance as medicine has become more highly specialized and complex and as patients have become more medically sophisticated and better able to participate actively in their own care. The process of achieving integration is often difficult and requires skill, energy and commitment on the part of the physician.

*The family physician insures continuity and comprehensiveness of medical care. This is one of his most important functions.*

**Coordinating Functions.** The family physician provides leadership for the many allied personnel who offer services for his patients. Whether he works within a formal group or as a solo practitioner, there will be many occasions on which his patients will need the professional services of a physical therapist, a public health nurse, a social worker or some other health worker. The family physician helps to mobilize these resources to provide whatever services his patients may need. To do this effectively, he must understand the training and skills of other professional and technical personnel and must know how persons in the allied health fields can best contribute to the care of his patients.

There are several advantages to be realized if the family physician plays his coordinating role properly:

a. The health team functions more effectively if it has a leader who can coordinate and monitor the activities of the other personnel. However, the family physician can not assume this position of leader simply by right of his medical degree, but must justify his leadership by demonstration of his understanding of the total health care picture.

b. By proper use of the skills of allied health personnel, the time and energy of the physician may be conserved for those functions which only he can perform. This, in effect, increases the supply of physicians and is one practical way of helping to meet escalating demands for medical care.

c. Special professional and technical skills of which the patient may not be aware are available in modern medical care through allied health personnel. The family physician can advise the patient in their use and direct him to the proper source to obtain these services.

The family physician must, of course, appreciate and value the contributions of the allied health personnel. He must have training in the medical school and hospital under conditions in which the health team approach to patient care is demonstrated effectively. While still a medical student, he must learn to understand the role of the registered nurse, the occupational therapist, the dietitian, and all other health personnel. In addition, he should understand the various kinds of problems and approaches to their solution, which interfere with effective teamwork.

**Community Functions.** The family physician is concerned with the other resources available in his community and region, (e.g., rehabilitation and mental health facilities) in order to insure that his patients will receive the best available in comprehensive medical care. He evaluates the adequacy of available services and facilities, and is aware of the unmet needs and of what might be done to resolve them. Where the community and region are lacking in certain important resources, he is knowledgeable about the mechanisms for transport and referral of patients to other regions. He exerts leadership to improve the quantity and quality of resources and services available in the area in accordance with demonstrated needs.

## Relation of the Terms "Family Physician" and "General Practitioner"

The terms "family physician" or "family practitioner" and "general practitioner" have often been used interchangeably. However, in the opinion of the Ad Hoc Committee, there are conceptual differences which should be understood to avoid semantic problems and confusion.

A family physician provides medical care within one or more, usually more than one, specialty disciplines of medicine. He assumes responsibility for providing a continuous and comprehensive care for the individual patient within the family contexture, supplying portions of the care himself when appropriate and coordinating portions obtained by referral or consultation with other physicians and allied health personnel. He provides access to appropriate community resources for his patients as needed.

A general practitioner provides medical care involving two or more specialty disciplines of medicine—usually from several disciplines. Whether he functions as a family physician rather than as a general practitioner depends upon whether he assumes responsibility for comprehensive, continuous health care for his patients within the context of their family groups. Most general practitioners function as family physicians, but many others do not.

Family practice refers to the *function* of the practitioner, while general practice refers to the *content* of his practice.

A family physician may limit his own practice to one or two fields of medicine, but he assumes responsibility for seeing that the patient receives the comprehensive continuing care that is required, and he coordinates this care for the benefit of the patient and his family. A specialist who limits his practice to a single field of medicine may therefore, function as a family physician.

A group of physicians, assembled in formal or informal association, may be able to provide all of the medical services needed by a patient. However, if such a group proposes to assume the responsibilities of a family physician, one physician within the group must serve as the first contact physician and be responsible for the continuing, comprehensive care of each patient and for seeing that all of his health care needs are met. In this instance the one physician who assumes this responsibility functions as the family physician for that patient.

Presently in group practice an internist or a general practitioner most often serves as family physician. However, a surgeon or obstetrician could also assume responsibility for the continuing comprehensive care of the patient and thus be the family physician for that patient, even though he has not been specifically educated for that role.

## Relation of the Term "Family Physician" to the Terms "Personal Physician" and "Primary Physician"

There are striking similarities among the descriptions of the family physician as given here, the "personal physician" as given in the Report of the National Commission on Community Health Services, and the "primary physician" of the Citizens' Commission on Graduate Medical Education. The following paragraphs are from the Report of NCCHS:[2]

> Every individual should have a personal physician who is the central point for integration and continuity of all medical and medically related services to his patient. Such a physician will emphasize the practice of preventive medicine, both through his own efforts and in partnership with the health and social resources of the community.
>
> He will be aware of the many and varied social, emotional and environmental factors that influence the health of his patient and his patient's family. He will either render, or direct the patient to, whatever services best suit his needs. His concern will be for the patient as a whole and his relationship with the patient must be a continuing one. In order to carry out his coordinating role, it is essential that all pertinent health information be channeled through him regardless of what institution, agency, or individual renders the service. He will have knowledge of and access to all the health resources of the community—social, preventive, diagnostic, therapeutic, and rehabilitative—and will mobilize them for the patient.

Remarkably similar are these segments of the Report of the Citizens' Commission on Graduate Medical Education:[1]

> Many leaders of medical thought have proclaimed the desirability of training physicians who are able and willing to offer comprehensive medical care of a quality far higher than that provided by the typical general practitioner of the past. The physician they conceive of is knowledgeable—as are other physicians—about organs, systems, and techniques, but he never forgets that organs and systems are parts of a whole man, that the whole man lives in a complex social setting, and that diagnosis or treatment of a part, as if it existed in isolation, often overlooks major causative factors and therapeutic opportunities.
>
> One of the qualifications of the physician who renders comprehensive care is thorough knowledge of and access to the whole range of medical services of the community. Thus he can readily call upon the special skills of others when they can help his patient. If the full range of medical competence is to be made effec-

tively and efficiently available, it is mandatory that means be found to increase the supply of physicians who are properly trained and willing to serve in this comprehensive role.

What is wanted is comprehensive and continuing health care, including not only the diagnosis and treatment of illness but also its prevention and the supportive and rehabilitative care that helps a person to maintain or to return to, as high a level of physical and mental health and well being as he can attain. Neither the hospital nor any of the existing specialists is willing, equipped, or able to assume this comprehensive and continuing responsibility; and too few of the present general practitioners are qualified to do so. A different kind of physician is called for.

We suggest that he be called a *primary physician.* He should usually be primary in the first-contact sense. He will serve as the primary medical resource and counselor to an individual or a family. When a patient needs hospitalization, the services of other medical specialists, or other medical or paramedical assistance, the primary physician will see that the necessary arrangements are made, giving such responsibility to others as is appropriate, and retaining his own continuing and comprehensive responsibility.

While the term used is different in each case, it seems clear that the same physician is being described by each of these three bodies.

## Notes

1. *The Graduate Education of the Physician: Report of the Citizens' Commission on Graduate Medical Education,* American Medical Association, September 1966.

2. *Health Is a Community Affair: Report of the National Commission on Community Health Services,* May 1966.

3. *Comprehensive Health Care: A Challenge to American Communities: Report of the Task Force on Comprehensive Personal Health Service of the National Commission on Community Health Services,* May 1966.

4. *Final Report on Preparation for Family Practice: Report of the Committee on Preparation for General Practice,* American Medical Association, June 1959.

5. Weiskotten, H. G., Wiggins, W. S., Altenderfer, M. G., and Tipner, A., Trends in medical practice, *J Med Educ* 35:1071–1095, (Dec.) 1960.

6. Executive director's page, *Bull Am Coll Phys* 6:218 (July–Aug.) 1965.

7. Cahal, M. F., What the public thinks of the family doctor—folklore or fact, *GP* 25:146–157 (Feb.) 1962.

8. Ruhe, C.H.W., Present projections of physician production, *JAMA* 198:1094–1100, (Dec.) 1966.

# CHAPTER SIX

# The Generalist Function in Medicine

Edmund D. Pellegrino, M.D.
1966

I am sincerely grateful for the privilege of presenting the first annual American Academy of General Practice (AAGP) lecture and of expressing my convictions on the matter of general medicine—a matter of increasing moment for profession and public alike.

I am of the firm conviction that the generalist function is an urgent need of present and future society. I am genuinely concerned about its gradual attenuation even in such broad fields as medicine and pediatrics, and I am convinced that for its refurbishment it must be firmly based in the medical school and the university. We have here one of a growing number of issues in which medical schools and practitioners must confront a public need cooperatively, if they are to meet current social responsibilities.

There is much public anxiety that the maximum of new knowledge is not now easily available to all in their own communities. This anxiety will transform the current evolution in medical education and practice into a revolution and the current ferment into a crisis. Questions which a few short years ago were the special province of the educator and the profession are now questions of the widest public interest. A high value has been placed upon health in our society and we are entering an era in which the public will determine more directly how to apportion its resources. The initiative for the design of patterns of medical care no longer lies exclusively with the profession.

This public interest is not to be deprecated, nor can it be wished away. It is most appropriate in a democracy. The health professions must prepare for an era of cooperative effort with the community in defining the goals of medical

This chapter originally appeared as Pellegrino ED. The generalist function in medicine. *JAMA.* 1966;198(5):127–131. Copyright © 1966, American Medical Association. Reprinted with permission.

care, selecting the means to attain them, and providing the scientific basis for the choice of alternatives. In this, the role of the professional is a critical one, if unrealistic programs initiated on insecure scientific footings are to be avoided. The physician's focal contribution is to dissect out of the scientific and social forces transforming our lives those which enhance, those which impede, and those which redefine the essential social and individual purposes of medicine.

# PRESENT AND FUTURE NEEDS

It is within the context of what is at the heart of medical care that I wish to consider the first of my questions. Is there a present and future need for the generalist in optimal patient care? There are few subjects more inducive to cosmic certitude on the part of public, practitioner, and educator. The stigma of heresy and anathema is nowhere more freely applied nor is the display of visceral reactions anywhere so varied and intense. This occurs because the question is at the very root of medicine for both the patient and the physician—that personal confrontation of one human in distress by another who presumes to help with special knowledge.

This confrontation will remain despite every convolution which may beset the science and organization of patient care. The sick person wants to know what is wrong, how he got that way, what will happen to him, whether he can be helped and how, and what it will cost in discomfort, money, and personal dignity. In getting the answers the patient wants to be understood as a person in distress and he wants to be treated compassionately. It has always been the job of medical practice to answer these questions as competently as the science and resources of the day allow and always the job of the educator to prepare students with the requisite intellectual equipment.

The satisfaction of these specific needs of patients is an unchanging imperative for medicine and the benchmark against which all practitioners must measure themselves. The central question is whether these needs can be competently met by specialists alone or whether they require in addition someone specifically trained as a generalist. It is my contention that they cannot be satisfied competently for the bulk of human ills without specific attention to a redefinition of the generalist function—a redefinition urgently needed and one which the educator cannot ignore.

# REDEFINITION OF THE GENERALIST FUNCTION

There are an increasing number who would categorically oppose this contention. They say that family and general medicine are anachronisms without a recognizable body of knowledge and impossible of attainment in a world in which medical knowledge doubles every ten years. They insist that if there were a real demand for the generalist his numbers and his rewards would be increasing and not dwindling as they now are. Still others are certain that a new species of technical assistants will assume all the functions now performed by the general physician.

The proponents of these views assume, of course, that they know the definition of general medicine, that it will remain static, and that it can be supplied adequately by some combination of specialists or technicians. Let us examine these assumptions.

Anyone who has seriously pursued a life in clinical medicine is aware that human illness does not come in neatly labeled categories. Nor are humans so accommodating as to herald clearly what organ system is ailing; nor do they develop disease in one organ system at a time. Among students and practicing physicians, specialists and subspecialists, the ability deteriorating most rapidly at all levels is the ability to meet the patient with an unbiased and unselected set of problems, assess the template of that patient's needs, and establish a logical plan for meeting those needs. While specialization is an unquestioned benefit in every phase of clinical medicine, it greatly sharpens the need for a parallel development of the synthesizing and integrative functions required to understand and treat humans and their diseases. Concentration on an organ system or technique too often produces an insensitivity to distress signals elsewhere in the body or in the person.

The abilities which define this generalist function more specifically are the following: (1) to assume responsibility for primary assessment of the health care needs of *unselected* patients—their diagnostic, personal, social, and family needs; (2) to make a judicious decision about which of these can be met by the generalist himself and which must be referred to a specialist, a social agency, or allied health professional; (3) to design and coordinate the plan of management; (4) to provide continuing care and support for the large number of patients for whom definitive care is not available but who need relief, comfort, and understanding. All this implies an ability to handle the majority of common ills as they occur in the community, a sensitive consideration and personal involvement in their psychosocial determinants, and an interest in patient education and health maintenance. It also necessarily implies the use of the health team and medical institution and agencies.

It is not the content of this type of medicine, however, which is unique. Its disciplines and techniques are those of internal medicine, pediatrics, psychiatry, and community medicine. The critical factor is an attitude of mind—rare in most professions today—"the power of viewing many things as one whole, referring them severally to their true place . . . , understanding their respective values, and determining their mutual dependence."[1(p136)] This is nothing less than the attitude of the liberal mind exercised on the data of medical practice.

It should be clear that this generalist function is a respectable intellectual activity not to be reserved for the inept or those who cannot pursue specialization. It should be clear, too, that no simple addition of specialties can equal the generalist function. To build a wall one needs more than the aimless piling up of bricks; one needs an architect. Every operation which analyzes some part of the human mechanism requires to be balanced by another which synthesizes and coordinates.

## GENERAL MEDICINE TODAY

If the need for the generalist arises out of an important need of patients, why is the state of general medicine as precarious as it is today? First, the need is still with us but it is now parceled out among a variety of people and institutions. Family practitioners of the traditional type, though diminishing in numbers, are still providing the first contact function. In addition, internists perform the generalist function for the adult and pediatricians for infants and children. Hospital emergency rooms and outpatient departments are performing the first-contact function for an ever widening range of social and economic groups. Even the more restricted specialists see nonreferred patients and act as assessors and coordinators of care. We can add to varying degrees industrial and school physicians, pharmacists, and others.

A more important reason for deterioration of the generalist is the failure to redefine general medicine in terms consistent with today's expanded knowledge and health resources. The patient has a right to expect access to the maximum of knowledge in the solution of his health problem. General practice as conceived in the past cannot meet the standards of competence required in today's scientific medicine. But, if it can be recast as the discipline which concentrates on the generalist function specifically, and if it emphasizes first contact assessment, coordination, continuity of care and prevention, then it can reemerge as a most necessary and satisfying role for the majority of physicians. At present, few of the many people who fill the vacuum left by the attenuation of general medicine are specifically trained for this function. Each specialist must, of course, cover thoroughly the small spectrum of illness he has selected. But, only the generalist has the comprehensive approach as a prime contribution.

## THE GENERALIST FUNCTION TOMORROW

Will the generalist function survive in future patterns of medical care? If so, will it be changed? How? To answer these questions, we need to look at only the very immediate future. Medical competence today has an ever-expanding definition. It implies the capacity to bring all pertinent information techniques, organizations, and people to bear on a patient's problem. Indeed, the patient has the right to this information and his right should not be restricted by his own physician's limitations. Therefore, we must expand the capabilities of each physician. Four mechanisms now in use are sure to be extended further in an attempt to make maximum use of the physician's one nonexpandable asset—time. I will only mention these mechanisms: (1) the further increase of specialization, (2) the use of computers in almost every phase of patient care, (3) the better use of the health care team in and out of the hospital, and (4) regionalization of medical facilities, equipment, and personnel. The question is not whether we shall use these mechanisms—they are already with us. Rather, it is to learn to use them without choking off the prime purposes of medicine, the satisfaction of certain needs of the sick person.

Devices like specialization, the team, regionalization and the computer will only deepen further the need for a new type of generalist. They all tend to fragmentation and depersonalization as the patient is dissected into parts and problems each attended by a separate specialist, technician, or process. The more steps we interpose in the patient care process—whether machines, men, or institutions—the more we enhance the possibilities for error and misunderstanding. Simple tasks can become enormously complicated. More energy must be spent in communicating with others. Responsibility becomes diffused and difficult to fix with certainty.

If these newer mechanisms in medical care are not to be self-defeating, it is essential that we resuscitate the generalist function, define it in new terms and prepare our students specifically for it. The future generalist will have several critical roles. He will in many places continue to function as the first-contact physician, as previously defined, for individuals and families. But his task will be both easier and harder. He will have more at his command, but a more complex system to handle. He will experience a closer institutional identification than is now the case.

In some places he will be prime assessor of care; in others he will be prime assessor, once removed—that is, he will supervise a series of clinical assistants who provide the first contact function for certain prescribed clinical situations (minor medical illnesses, minor surgical emergencies, well-baby care, and antepartum and postpartum care). He will be required to define and limit what these assistants do and establish the programs and standards under which they operate. He will be essential, in and out of the hospital, as the coordinator of the health care team and responsible for the design of the plan of care, its synthesis, execution, and follow-up. He will devote more of his time to the noncategorizable problem and to the patient with emotional and personal problems.

These are functions different from those now readily assumed by the generalist. They imply less emphasis on manipulative functions and direct care and more emphasis on supervision, coordination, interpretation, and diagnosis of total needs. Though a little unsettling in their prospect some combination of these functions seems essential if we are to keep pace with the demands of a growing population and make maximal use of the physician's time and education.

None of the present specialties—even the broader ones like pediatrics and internal medicine—as now constituted, can satisfy the requirements of this generalist function. Though they exercise an integrative function over a wide spectrum of disorders, both internal medicine and pediatrics are restricted by the age of the patients they serve. Each emphasizes a different aspect of medical care. The pediatrician is more sensitive to the growth and development process, to the family setting of illness, and to ambulant medicine. The internist lays greater stress on the complexities of the diagnostic process and on complicated diseases of long duration. Neither places sufficient emphasis on the social and community determinants of illness. Psychiatry and community medicine which fill the latter needs do not have a strong enough base in everyday clinical medicine.

On the other hand, it has been evident for some time that neither pediatrician nor internist can function adequately as consultants in all the branches of their own fields. Thus, the pediatrician finds that he is needed for the intercurrent illness, the baby who is well, the behavioral problem, and not for the complicated diagnostic problem. The general internist finds he is needed for a general evaluation of the patient and for long-term care. The difficult categorizable problems go directly to the subspecialists in both fields and will do so increasingly.

Pediatricians and internists are being drawn into caring for other members of the family and thus into the role of family physician. Meanwhile, the general practitioner is gradually foregoing surgery and even obstetrics in an attempt to meet the needs of his patient for first-contact services. As the general pediatricians and internists broaden themselves and the general practitioners constrict their field, the distinctions between them seem certain to be obliterated. The resultant fusion will provide a valuable base of family practice upon which can be engrafted the newer and less traditional functions of the generalist required by future patterns of medical care.

# CHALLENGE TO MEDICAL INSTITUTIONS

Preparation of young people for the redefined roles of family medicine and generalist is a community need to which our universities and medical centers are just beginning to respond. Programs of training at the undergraduate and postgraduate levels are emerging as new and old medical centers awaken to the somewhat insistent demands of the public they must ultimately serve.

The new roles will require attitudes of mind and skills for which we do not specifically prepare students at this time. If he is to be ultimately captain of the health care team, the student must learn something of group dynamics and psychology and how to coordinate disparate disciplines to a common end. He will need more of the language of the behavioral scientist, ecologist, and epidemiologist than he now has if he is to take proper cognizance of the community dimensions of illness. If, and it appears reasonably certain, the computer becomes a part of his daily clinical life, the student must know how they operate, how they can be made into extensions of his brain, and what new intellectual demands will be made of him when the computer takes over the manipulative aspects of thinking.

Obviously more of the student's education before, during, and after medical school must emphasize thought processes—finding information, putting it in order, selecting out the essential from the trivial, generating new hypotheses and making value judgments—in short, those functions in which his brain surpasses the machine. Stuffing the mind with evanescent data will no longer be as essential as before and more time will be available hopefully for the design of a rational plan of management, coordinating it, and making it manifest to the patient.

The challenge to medical faculties is to discern which of these intellectual attitudes to teach, to recruit the requisite faculty skilled in these approaches, and they are few, and to do so by a discriminating choice of the objectives of medical education.

If these and other intellectual skills are to have any meaning the student must have some experience in their use. He should have clinical experience as a member of a well-run health care team; he should understand the computer and use it in the solution of clinical problems; he should have a community experience wherein he can study the family and social determinants of illness in their local setting.

There are many roles in medicine and many minds attracted to it. Among them are individuals suited by intellect and temperament for the generalist function. They should be identified and their interests developed early. Multiple and alternate pathways to the MD degree are needed. The MD with a designated major is a possible solution. The quintessential core of the MD degree is the interest in health and disease from the point of view of any of the disciplines which can contribute. All recipients of this degree need exposure to the language of cellular and human biology and clinical experience in the basic arts and skills of the clinician. After this, their pathways could diverge. One could envision four routes: (1) the medical sciences; (2) a clinical specialty; (3) general and family medicine; and (4) an undifferentiated route for those who wish to keep the alternatives open.

In such a plan, students interested in the generalist function could receive more training specifically designed to provide the intellectual skills their roles will require. The postgraduate years would then provide depth of experience in the major field. Perhaps, the student could even be available earlier to take his place in society.

Education for family practice and the generalist function is both a postgraduate and an undergraduate endeavor just as it is for the specialties. Certain experiences and opportunities must be provided in medical school to encourage and stimulate those students motivated to a life in family medicine. Exposure to the behavioral sciences, emphasis on the comprehensive approach in clinical medicine, a community medicine experience, as provided at the University of Kentucky, and elective opportunities with selected family physicians can all help to prepare the way.

If the generalist function is really needed and if it is to be resuscitated, every clinical department will need to direct some of its energies to this important end. The major responsibility, however, lies with departments of medicine which have thus far interpreted their responsibilities too narrowly. They themselves are in urgent need of redefining general medicine—a traditional concern much endangered by the growth of subspecialization.

# PROGRAM IN OPERATION

We have found it most useful in our own department at the University of Kentucky to appoint two academically-oriented general practitioners to our faculty. They are full-time members of the faculty of the Department of Medicine at the University of Kentucky. They are charged with the coordination of the graduate program in family practice. Even more importantly, they advise and counsel students who express an interest in family medicine even as early as the first year. These men, in addition, take the regular teaching assignments of any member of the department—on the wards, in the outpatient department, and in physical diagnosis. It is essential, we feel, that students see family physicians accepted as members of our Department of Medicine and appreciate that academic stature can be realized by excellence in this field as in any other.

The graduate program in family medicine at the University of Kentucky, which begins this year, is based in the Department of Medicine, but is interdisciplinary in organization involving the departments of pediatrics, psychiatry, community medicine, and obstetrics. The first year is devoted to basic medicine and pediatrics in the hospital; the second year, to internal medicine, pediatrics, and psychiatry with emphasis on the ambulant patient; and the last year, to a period in community medicine as well as to experience in a model family practice outside the medical school. This last year of experience is supervised by full-time general practitioners who are members of the faculty. In the last two years seminars have been arranged on a wide variety of topics by contributors from appropriate departments devoted to basic studies and issues pertinent to the family, e.g., developmental biology, behavioral science, law, theology, and economics. Obstetrics, except for antenatal and postpartum physiology, is elective for those who will practice in areas without adequate coverage in these fields. Throughout, emphasis is on the same academic quality which permeates good residency programs in the specialties. The last year is structured as a fellowship similar to the clinical fellowships now available in the subspecialties of medicine and pediatrics.

At the same time that he was asserting the importance of the university as an influence on contemporary life, Flexner felt constrained to warn: "A University seeking to be modern, seeking to evolve theory, seeking to solve problems, may thus readily find itself complicating its task and dissipating energy and funds by doing a host of inconsequential things."[2(p25)]

A concern for family practice illustrates the dilemmas faculties of medicine must face as they try to respond to social pressures and remain true to their mission as "students of problems and trainers of men."[2(p16)] The natural fear of the academician is that scientific medicine, basic research, and intellectual rigor must necessarily be sacrificed if we concern ourselves with how best to deliver medical care as intensively as we do with the content of that care.

General family practice, however, needs just those qualities of research-mindedness and critical inquiry which an academic department imparts. Nor is the existence of a program of family practice without its benefits to today's academic clinical departments. The scarcest commodity in these departments is often the physician willing and competent to evaluate the problems of the noncategorized patient. Students, house staff, and faculty all need a constant reminder of the importance of the general as well as the special needs of the sick.

Certainly, without a strong academic footing family medicine cannot compete successfully for students and house staff. Too many young people with an instinct for the kind of medicine we are describing are disaffected in medical school when they see that the academic coin of the realm lies elsewhere. Surely, if students are not to detect a certain note of hypocrisy, when family practice is recommended, they must be exposed to its actual practice and to a model of what their institution conceives as the best way to provide such care.

A genuine concern with the provision of general physicians is a legitimate and compelling responsibility of today's university and medical school as they enter the era of increasing involvement in the community around them. The nature of human illness is such that the integrative functions of the general clinician will always be necessary. The coming fusion of internal medicine, pediatrics, and general practice promises to be a synergistic one which will yield a family physician and a generalist who will meet certain specific needs for adults, children, and, hopefully, the family unit. The intellectual development of this field and its ability to engage the young is dependent on a firm academic base in the medical centers where intellectual rigor, research, and a model of practice can be provided simultaneously.

## Notes

1. Newman JH. *Idea of a University.* New York: Doubleday; 1954.
2. Flexner A. *Universities: American, English, German.* New York: Oxford University Press; 1930.

CHAPTER SEVEN

# General Internal Medicine at the Crossroads of Prosperity and Despair

## *Caring for Patients with Chronic Diseases in an Aging Society*

Eric B. Larson, M.D., M.P.H.
2001

During the past quarter century, general internal medicine in the United States has emerged as a vital discipline in the pantheon of academic internal medicine and as an important provider of general care for adults.[1] At the start of the 1970s, academic general internal medicine was almost nonexistent and the number of general internal medicine practitioners was dwindling.[2] Since then, the field has revitalized, as evidenced by increases in numbers of practitioners, trainees, and a well-established cadre of clinical researchers. However, as the field has seemingly flourished, many worry about general internal medicine's future and that of all primary care specialists.[3] We hear of demoralized practitioners selling practices, changing practices, leaving practices for other opportunities, or abandoning medicine altogether. Prosperity and despair seem to coexist side-by-side in general internal medicine.

General internal medicine arguably could be the specialty most highly valued by the segment of the population that requires the most care—the geriatric population. However, the instability of today's medical marketplace makes the future of general internal medicine uncertain. To thrive, general internal medicine must build on its strengths within the medical marketplace, seize the opportunities offered by demographic changes, and take a primary role in serving the needs of older patients with chronic diseases.

---

This chapter is based on a presentation given at a Hartford Foundation–sponsored geriatric educational retreat for general internal medicine in August 1999.

# PATIENT CARE

The need for a cadre of competent generalists to meet patient care needs was the driving force behind the resurgence of general internal medicine that began in the 1970s.[4] The preeminence of the randomized trial and the increasing acceptance of more robust clinical epidemiologic methods have expanded the ways in which all practitioners can meet patients' needs. But general internal medicine has always been, and continues to be, the integrating discipline par excellence, maintaining the broad perspective on each patient's medical situation and keeping that care from being fragmented. Today's generalists are thus faced with the challenge of integrating advances of dizzying speed and complexity across a wide range of areas of internal medicine (a not atypical example is managing anticoagulant therapy for thromboembolic disease in a patient with type 2 diabetes mellitus, coronary artery disease, and asthma).

Ironically, as practice becomes more effective and the challenges of weaving together these complex elements of care increase, practitioners have more difficulty earning a living from practice. Increasingly, physicians are no longer self-employed. In the early 1990s, hospitals and delivery systems acquired practices in anticipation of health care reform based on managed competition. These practices and their practitioners now cannot cover their owners' expenses. In some markets, these acquired practices do not have the strategic value that their owners anticipated, and many have been abandoned.

Employers (and the economics of practice) pressure physicians to work harder and faster. Cognitive services are still relatively undervalued compared with procedural and diagnostic services. Fee schedules do not account for the increasing complexity found in many internal medicine patients. Time pressure probably limits the translation of clinical research results into patient care and challenges adherence to practice guidelines.

Pressures to be more time-efficient have also forced many practitioners to abandon the traditional combination of office- and hospital-based practice. In many communities, hospitalists and subspecialists now fill this breach. There is an increasing tendency for patients to change insurance coverage (a recent report stated that one in six patients changes insurance every year).[5] Thus, many forces combine to undermine continuity of care, which has long been seen as important for the effectiveness of primary care, especially in older persons with chronic disease.[6,7]

The commitment to excellent patient care has been the strength of general internal medicine. This idealism and commitment could suffer terminal "burnout" from overwhelming market forces. Physician burnout has gone from a theoretical concern to a well-recognized threat. A comparison survey[8] of California physicians in 1991 and 1996 demonstrated that the proportion of primary care physicians willing to go to medical school again had decreased steeply, from 79% in 1991 to 61% in 1996, whereas the proportions for specialists changed very little (68% vs. 63%).

# RESEARCH

Research in general internal medicine, as well as support for that research, was virtually nonexistent in 1975. General internal medicine research is now robust, a leader in many departments of medicine and a source of departmental prestige. Further, the results of general internal medicine research have truly changed practice. For example, contrast the relatively nihilistic message of a 1977 article,[9] which argued that health services and medical care research "didn't make a difference," to today, when research has prompted beneficial changes in practice that are literally too numerous to count. Examples range from research-based strategies defining more effective use of common diagnostic tests for patients with sore throat[10] and other common problems[11] and more precise use of everyday treatments for common conditions (such as bed rest for low back pain[12]) to the more dramatic changes in how we care for patients hospitalized with acute myocardial infarction[13] and patients with venous thrombosis and other thromboembolic diseases.[14-16] The care of both outpatients and inpatients at the millennium is almost unrecognizable compared with the treatments we offered 25 years ago. Most important, it is not only the process of care but also the outcomes that are better.

Despite these successes, overall research funding for general internists is still relatively modest, especially compared with funding for biomedical and traditional subspecialty research. General medicine research often involves studying chronic disease, and these types of studies often require years. "Programmatic" research, a paradigm described by Sackett[17] for researchers interested in chronic diseases, depends on collaborations with bridging disciplines, often including biostatistics and social sciences, and requires a substantial infrastructure to support a collaborative group. Building such infrastructures is challenging and expensive.

Another threat to research in divisions of general internal medicine is the practice of hiring only clinicians or clinician-teachers in departments of medicine. An increasing, almost unquenchable need to recruit young clinicians to staff growing clinical empires in academic medical centers will increase the total size of academic departments. However, the absence in the ranks of young, entry-level general internist researchers threatens to erase the gains of the past 25 years. This threat to clinical research is hardly unique to academic general internal medicine, but the existence of strong general medicine research programs is a relatively recent phenomenon, making these programs more vulnerable than programs in the subspecialties of internal medicine.

# EDUCATION

The teaching ability of general internal medicine faculty has emerged as one of their greatest assets. They are highly visible to students and residents since they provide a disproportionate share of clinically related teaching in many, if not most, schools. They are highly visible and attractive to learners both as inpatient attendings and, increasingly, as role models in the clinic. As clinician-teachers, general internists lead by example in their commitment to evidence-based patient care.

However, while education in general internal medicine has improved, weaknesses persist in the broader teaching enterprise. Many teaching programs fail to emphasize the "bedside" (or "deskside") skills most important for clinical practice, despite persuasive narratives[18] and research[19] pointing out deficiencies in traditional training. Technical skills tend to be overemphasized.[20] Faculty find it easier to rely on ready-made "chalk talks" that are suited to faculty interests rather than based on the patient's problems or the learner's needs.[19] Case-based iterative teaching[21] and bedside teaching are used less than they should be.[22]

Skills training for managing a successful practice is generally not offered, reflecting internal medicine's traditional obsession with mastery of medical knowledge to the exclusion of more pragmatic, everyday practice concerns. By contrast, leaders in family medicine have placed more emphasis on successful practice management. Moreover, even with increases in ambulatory clinic experience, most residency programs find it difficult to provide experiential opportunities for their trainees to learn chronic disease management both over time and across several sites. The opportunity to continuously follow single patients with chronic disease is further complicated by the continued emergence of sub-specialties within general internal medicine—now including emergency medical specialists, hospitalists, and possibly "officists"—which further threatens the traditional primary care emphasis on continuity.

Internal medicine residency programs have recently had difficulties adapting to the changing nature of inpatient care in major teaching hospitals. Thus, they offer residents an experience with inpatient general medicine that can be dispiriting and discouraging. Patients admitted to all inpatient teaching services are increasingly ill, and many, particularly on general medical services, have several complex problems or near-terminal conditions. Financial incentives have dramatically reduced the duration of hospitalization, leading to rapid turnover as many patients are transferred as soon as possible to alternative, less expensive sites of care. House staff are stressed by intense service demands and the lack of opportunities to care for patients over time.

Perhaps the greatest threat to the continued vigor of general internal medicine education, however, is the persistence of unattractive practice conditions out in the "real world." This persistence, along with overly stressful residency programs, threatens to decrease the size and quality of the pool of applicants to internal medicine training programs, in the long run threatening the very existence of general internal medicine.

# OPPORTUNITIES

The greatest opportunities for general internal medicine relate to its strength as an integrating, cognitive specialty. Adult medical care is predominantly care of patients with common chronic diseases plus some acute care diagnosis and prevention, precisely the knowledge base and domain of general internal medicine. The best care of patients with common chronic diseases, especially geriatric patients (who often have several chronic diseases), will be deeply knowledge-based and will involve skills in managing complexity. I believe that the best place to invest time and effort in general internal medicine is in the knowledge base of practice, including systems thinking and quality improvement. This investment can occur either as individuals pursue traditional self-improvement or as innovators look for unique ways to provide both knowledge and care to patients and groups of patients. A growing market for that knowledge base is and will continue to be in geriatrics.

As more services are delivered to an increasingly aging population, clinical research in geriatrics will, and should, be in high demand and should be attractive to internists interested in chronic diseases. Natural experiments, as a result of rapid changes, provide opportunities to observe the effects of system changes[23] on process and outcome of care. The most vulnerable populations, including the elderly, are those most likely to experience the effects of such natural experiments.

Training of general internists could appropriately be based primarily in the growing geriatric population. Skill development in geriatrics should be a high priority and, in addition to allowing trainees to experience the joys of geriatrics (and there are many), could become a focus for education in general internal medicine.

# SUMMARY

General internal medicine in the United States has emerged as a robust specialty. In the past 20 to 25 years, general internists have developed a successful research enterprise with a "clinical" research focus. General internal medicine faculty are committed, enthusiastic, and idealistic. Today's marketplace, however, finds internist practitioners beleaguered, disheartened, and under intense pressures to "produce." What is most disheartening to internist practitioners, particularly experienced practitioners with aging practices, is a lack of any evident solution to the practice crisis, especially at a time when they have so much to offer their patients.

Yet, despite the many forces assailing it, the strengths of general internal medicine and the opportunities for it to succeed are considerable. The professional organizations representing general internists can join forces with public groups that advocate for older persons (such as the American Association of Retired Persons and the Hartford Foundation). Both professional and lay groups must make more concerted and serious efforts to address the threats to practice experienced by generalist practitioners and their patients. Finding alternatives to payment systems that devalue such a commodity as knowledge, which is difficult to measure, will be a real challenge. Developing revenue in exchange for application of knowledge to improve patient care will be no less challenging. However, it is time that leaders in medicine, along with an informed public sector, confront the reality that brief visits and rapid cycling of patients through physicians' offices, sites of care, and insurance plans are probably damaging to patients and could also destroy the viability of a specialty with much to offer aging patients, especially those with chronic diseases. At the very least, payment coding for evaluation and management services needs to allow practitioners and their patients more flexibility. Finally, internists need to work with patient advocacy groups and insurers, including government payers, to create a stabler practice environment—one that will reward practitioners for applying the remarkable knowledge base of internal medicine, especially to ongoing care of patients over time.

## Notes

1. Roberg N. Internal medicine in the 1930s. *JAMA*. 1988;260:3645–3646. [PMID: 0003057255]

2. Roback G, Mason HK. *Physician Distribution and Licensure in the U.S., 1975.* Chicago: American Medical Association; 1977.

3. Grumbach K. Primary care in the United States—the best of times, the worst of times [Editorial]. *N Engl J Med.* 1999;341:2008–2010. [PMID: 0010607821]

4. Massachusetts Department of Public Health. The outpatient department—ambulatory care at the hospital. *N Engl J Med.* 1975;293:775. [PMID: 0001160958]

5. Cunningham PJ, Kohn L. Health plan switching: choice or circumstance? *Health Aff.* 2000;19:158–164. [PMID: 0010812794]

6. Wasson JH, Sauvigne AE, Mogielnicki RP, et al. Continuity of outpatient medical care in elderly men: a randomized trial. *JAMA*. 1984;252:2413–2417. [PMID: 0006481927]

7. Campion EW. Continuity counts [Editorial]. *JAMA*. 1984;252:2459. [PMID: 0006481937]

8. Burdi MD, Baker LC. Physicians' perceptions of autonomy and satisfaction in California. *Health Aff.* 1999;18:134–145. [PMID: 0010425851]

9. Lewis C. Health-services research and innovations in health-care delivery: does research make a difference? *N Engl J Med.* 1977;297:423–427. [PMID: 0000882112]

10. Komaroff AL, Pass TM, Aronson MD, et al. The prediction of streptococcal pharyngitis in adults. *J Gen Intern Med.* 1986;1:1–7. [PMID: 0003534166]

11. Panzer RJ, Black ER, Griner PF, eds. *Diagnostic Strategies for Common Medical Problems.* Philadelphia: American College of Physicians; 1991.

12. Malmivaara A, Häkkinen U, Aro T, et al. The treatment of acute low back pain—bed rest, exercises, or ordinary activity? *N Engl J Med.* 1995;332:351–355. [PMID: 0007823996]

13. Every NR, Parsons LS, Hlatky M, Martin JS, Weaver WD. A comparison of thrombolytic therapy with primary coronary angioplasty for acute myocardial infarction: Myocardial Infarction Triage and Intervention Investigators. *N Engl J Med.* 1996;335:1253–1260. [PMID: 0008857004]

14. Levine M, Gent M, Hirsh J, et al. A comparison of low-molecular-weight heparin administered primarily at home with unfractionated heparin administered in the hospital for proximal deep-vein thrombosis. *N Engl J Med.* 1996;334:677–681. [PMID: 0008594425]

15. Koopman MM, Prandoni P, Piovella F, et al. Treatment of venous thrombosis with intravenous unfractionated heparin administered in the hospital as compared with subcutaneous low-molecular-weight heparin administered at home: the Tasman Study Group. *N Engl J Med.* 1996;334:682–687. [PMID: 0008594426]

16. Schulman S, Rhedin AS, Lindmarker P, et al. A comparison of six weeks with six months of oral anticoagulant therapy after a first episode of venous thromboembolism: Duration of Anticoagulation Trial Study Group. *N Engl J Med.* 1995;332:1661–1665. [PMID: 0007760866]

17. Sackett DL. Zlinkoff honor lecture: basic research, clinical research, clinical epidemiology, and general internal medicine. *J Gen Intern Med.* 1987;2:40–47. [PMID: 0003806269]

18. Eichna LW. Medical-school education, 1975–1979: a student's perspective. *N Engl J Med.* 1980;303:727–734. [PMID: 0007402270]

19. Kern DC, Parrino TA, Korst DR. The lasting value of clinical skills. *JAMA.* 1985;254:70–76. [PMID: 0003999353]

20. La Combe MA. On bedside teaching. *Ann Intern Med.* 1997;126:217–220. [PMID: 0009027273]

21. Kassirer JP. Teaching clinical medicine by iterative hypothesis testing: let's preach what we practice. *N Engl J Med.* 1983;309:921–923. [PMID: 0006888486]

22. Fitzgerald FT. Physical diagnosis versus modern technology: a review. *West J Med.* 1990;152:377–382. [PMID: 0002190412]

23. Lowrie EG, Hampers CL. The success of Medicare's end-stage renal-disease program: the case for profits and the private marketplace. *N Engl J Med.* 1981;305:434–438. [PMID: 0007019710]

# CHAPTER EIGHT

# What Does Family Practice Need to Do Next?

## *A Cross-Generational View*

John P. Geyman, M.D.; Erika Bliss, M.D.
2001

It is an honor and privilege to contribute to this Keystone III conference on the future of family practice. We have chosen to take a 60-year view of the discipline—30 years back and 30 years forward. Our perspectives are those of two family physicians of different generations, one (JPG) graduating from medical school in 1960, the other (EB) graduating in 2000. We challenged ourselves first to independently distill our respective views about the next steps for family practice and then collated them into this cross-generational perspective. We have tried to be as objective and evidence based as possible, which at times leads to potentially provocative or politically incorrect recommendations.

The purpose of this paper is four-fold: (1) to compare the major hopes for family practice at its genesis in 1969 to the realities of the year 2000, (2) to summarize some of the major lessons learned by the discipline over the last 30 years, (3) to briefly mention some of the most important changes affecting the health care system over the last 30 years, and (4) to present our vision for future primary care, together with our recommendations on the next steps for family practice in the areas of patient care, education, research, and organizational development.

## FAMILY PRACTICE: 1969 AND 2000

Table 8.1 lists some of the major hopes that many individuals had for family practice when it became the 20th specialty in American medicine in 1969.

This chapter originally appeared as Geyman JP, Bliss E. What does family practice need to do next? A cross-generational view. *Fam Med.* 2001;33:259–267. Copyright © 2001, Society of Teachers of Family Medicine, www.stfm.org. Reprinted with permission.

Table 8.1. Family Practice: 1969 Versus 2000.

| Hopes in 1969 | Reality in 2000 |
| --- | --- |
| Family practice would become the main primary care discipline. | Family practice is only one of three or four primary care disciplines, with general internal medicine being the largest. |
| Family physicians would increase as a proportion of all U.S. physicians. | Family physicians represent only 12% of U.S. physicians, down from 18% in 1969. |
| Family practice would have a well-accepted, central role in medical schools. | Family practice is rarely central and often is marginal. |
| Family practice residency positions would represent 25% of all U.S. residency positions. | Family practice residency positions represent less than 15% of residency positions. |
| There would be a family physician for every family in the United States. | Way short. |
| Family practice would integrate the biopsychosocial approach into practice. | Mixed record. |

Despite its many successes, it is apparent that the hopes held in 1969 for the future of family practice fell far short of the mark by 2000.

## Lessons from the Last 30 Years

We believe five overall lessons can be learned from the first 30 years' evolution of family practice.

*Lesson 1: We didn't reform medical education, medical practice, or the health care system.*

Despite some interdisciplinary initiatives in medical education, such as the Association of American Medical Colleges' General Professional Education of the Physician (GPEP) report and its aftermath, to which family medicine made important contributions, medical education and clinical practice remain largely specialist dominated and rely heavily on the biomedical model.

*Lesson 2: Because of family practice's limited numbers, family physicians remain only one of several options for primary care.*

Although the evolution of family practice so far has been remarkable in many respects, particularly in education, the number of family physicians remains far too limited to provide the major source of primary care for the U.S. population.

*Lesson 3: Since 1970, the generalist-specialist ratio in the United Sates has shifted farther to specialists and shows no signs of shifting back toward generalists.*

The numbers of family physicians, general internists, and general pediatricians grew by only 13% between 1965 and 1992 (to 88 per 100,000 population), while the number of specialists increased by 121% (to 124 per 100,000).[1] By 1994, the proportion of primary care physicians (by the federal definition) had dropped to only 32% of active physicians in the United States.[2] Moreover, there is no evidence that this trend will reverse over the next 30 years. In fact, according to recent data from the National Resident Matching Program (NRMP), the proportion of graduating U.S. seniors entering generalist residency positions dropped from about 30% in recent years to 28.4% in the 2000 Match.

Rivo and Kindig have made projections to the year 2040 for the generalist-specialist mix, based on different assumptions for the entry levels of medical graduates to generalist residency training. At the 30% entry level, there will be no significant increase in the number of primary care physicians between now and 2040.[1]

*Lesson 4: The United States remains unique among Western industrialized nations in having multiple generalist specialties.*

In the arena of primary care, the United States continues to see competition among three generalist specialties (four if obstetrics-gynecology is included), as well as a "hidden" system of primary care provided by physicians in the more limited specialties. By comparison, general practice is the unambiguous foundation of primary care in other Western industrialized countries, representing 70% of active physicians in the United Kingdom and 50% in Canada.[3]

*Lesson 5: The three primary care disciplines remain distinct tribes on parallel but separate courses.* Though they have much in common with family practice in terms of clinical skills, function, and values as they relate to the care of their respective patients, general internal medicine and general pediatrics still have largely separate educational programs, read different literature, and are organizationally more separated than collaborative—from each other and from family medicine. This divide is ironic, as general internal medicine, perhaps partly due to the influence of family medicine, has shown more interest in the biopsychosocial model and has added to its own residency training in such areas as office gynecology and dermatology. Further, practice patterns of general internists have become quite similar to those of family physicians, 75% of whom do not provide obstetric care and thereby have fewer and fewer children in their practices.

# CHANGES IN THE HEALTH CARE SYSTEM AND NEEDS FOR HEALTH CARE

To set the stage for a consideration of a future course for family practice, we must first recognize how the health care system, as well as needs for health care, have changed since 1969. The extent of change is remarkable, as reflected by eight aspects mentioned here.

## The Advent of Managed Care

Although managed care traces its origins to the populist movement of the 1940s (e.g., Kaiser Permanente, Group Health Cooperative of Puget Sound), the term *managed care* has taken center stage today because of factors relating to cost containment. As it has evolved over the last 2 decades, managed care now more often involves managed *reimbursement* than managed *care*. In this new landscape, there has been intense economic competition among health maintenance organizations (HMOs), preferred-provider organizations (PPOs) and point-of-service programs. The essential elements of managed reimbursement have led to growing frustration on the part of physicians and patients alike.

Currently, some form of managed care has virtually replaced cost-based reimbursement to hospitals and fee-for-service medicine, both for people covered by employer-based insurance and for those on federally funded assistance programs. In fact, some kind of managed reimbursement now covers 75% of the U.S. population[4] (R. Black, Health Care Financing Administration, Office of Managed Care, personal communication to M. H. Bailit, February 28, 1997). About 50% of primary care physicians receive part of their reimbursement through capitation, and almost 50% are employed by a health care organization.[4,5]

## Increased Burden of Chronic Illness

Aging of the U.S. population has major implications for the kind of health care needed by the population. The proportion of Americans over age 65 will double (to almost 70 million) between 1995 and 2030.[6] As the population ages and medical technology provides more effective and efficient care of acute illnesses, the predominant burden of disease is shifting to chronic conditions. These chronic diseases are often multifactorial, coexist with other chronic diseases, and require care beyond the biomedical model. Of growing importance are such approaches as disease management, palliative care, and application of the biopsychosocial model through shared decision making with well-informed patients.

## Deemphasis of Hospital Care

Although the acute care hospital has been the base of the U.S. health care system for most of the last 100 years, its role is rapidly diminishing as more care is provided in outpatient settings. Hospitals are becoming the site of care only for patients with serious illnesses that often require intensive care. The length of hospital stays has shortened, and patients discharged from hospitals frequently need considerable medical and nursing care after discharge. The escalating costs of hospitalization are partly responsible for this shift from hospital care to ambulatory and other sectors of care, but containment of hospital costs has still not been achieved.[7]

As inpatient care has become more intensive, ambulatory care has become more demanding. The pressures of outpatient care have made it more difficult and less efficient for primary care physicians to remain involved with inpatient care. Twenty years ago, many primary care physicians cared for up to 10 inpatients on any given day, but that number has dropped to one or two today.[8]

Hospital care is now increasingly being provided by dedicated hospital physicians—i.e., "hospitalists." The hospitalist movement is gaining momentum rapidly; it most involves general internists but also some family physicians. Hospitalists, by definition, spend at least 25% of their time on inpatient care and typically care for 10 to 15 inpatients at any one time.[9] There are some preliminary data that suggest that hospitalist care may reduce lengths of stay and costs of hospitalization without compromising quality of care.[10–12]

## Proliferation of Health Care Professionals Involved in Primary Care

The primary care marketplace has become more competitive than ever as physicians in other specialties and many nonphysician professionals assert their claims to one aspect or another of primary care. As Edward O'Neill, internist at the University of California, San Francisco, has observed: "There are 150,000 'born again' primary care providers out there."[13]

Managed care plans, and even state legislatures, have increasingly responded to public pressure by enabling point-of-service access to specialists. In 1997, for example, the Georgia legislature passed a law requiring managed care plans to offer direct access to dermatologists without referral, while Indiana has mandated the opportunity for direct access to anesthesiologists, dermatologists, mental health professionals, and others.[14]

The number of nonphysician clinicians (NPC) doubled between 1992 and 1997,[15] with 63,000 nurse practitioners and 29,000 physician assistants in the country's NPC workforce by 1997.[16] Although less than 15% of nurse practitioners are in independent practice, 25 states and the District of Columbia have passed legislation removing requirements for nurse practitioners to have physician supervision and/or mandatory collaboration with physicians.[17]

Other health professions are also vying for a piece of primary care, including clinical pharmacists[18] and some alternative care providers. Of 18 major managed care organizations (including Aetna, Kaiser Permanente, and Medicare), 14 now offer at least 11 of 34 complementary and alternative medicine therapies, while Blue Cross Blue Shield now permits its HMO enrollees to select chiropractors as their primary care provider, even though they lack prescriptive authority.[19]

## Shared Decision Making with Empowered Patients

There has been a big change in recent decades in public expectations of health care and in empowerment of patients. Many factors have contributed to this change, including the Great Society programs of the 1960s, increased expectations of the Baby Boom generation for a voice in their health care, and recent advances in information technology (now patients can be instant experts on their problems after 20 minutes on the Internet). Many of these changes are for the better, but the physician-patient relationship has often suffered in this process. Radowski notes the effect on the physician-patient relationship in these terms:

> Patients are better informed, less submissive, and more open. They still seek a captain to lead them against fate but do not sign on as readily and usually wish to know where they are headed. To the extent that science has replaced magic, the doctor-patient relationship has been weakened. The relationship is more fragmented among specialists, in health maintenance organizations (where the organization may be the physician), and in hospitals, because of the house staff. The requirement for second opinions has also changed the relationship, along with the critical view of medical care expressed in magazines, books, newspapers, and on television. Malpractice suits may partly be a consequence of a poorer doctor-patient relationship, but they probably contribute to it also, as must the larger number of people who re-locate, have two homes, or visit walk-in centers or emergency rooms for their care.[20]

## Advances in Information and Communication Technologies

A revolution in information and communication technologies has already transformed much of the nation's business community. Health care has not been in the forefront of these changes, but it will not be far behind. In its recently published book, *Health and Health Care 2010: the Forecast, the Challenge,* The Institute for the Future predicts that these information and communication technologies will affect health care in four principal areas: (1) process-management systems, (2) clinical information interfaces, (3) data analysis, and (4) telehealth and remote monitoring.[21]

New technologies are already bringing electronic clinical data systems to physicians by means of handheld computers, and electronic communication between patients, physicians, and consultants is transforming the process of care in ways unimagined only 10 years ago. Joe Scherger, MD, for example, has found that increased e-mail communication with patients has resulted in more continuous and less episodic communication with patients within a busy practice, while reducing unnecessary office visits, providing more service, and enhancing the physician-patient relationship.[22]

## Increased Emphasis on Cost-Effectiveness and Value

National expenditures for health care have more than quadrupled since 1980, while per capita expenditures have surged from just over $1,000 in 1988 to $4,000 in 1998.[23] This increase in the cost of health care has led to increasing cost containment measures by payers, both public and private. At the same time, questions of cost-effectiveness and value of health care services are being asked more seriously, especially by government, other payers, and managed care organizations. David Eddy has this to say about this new dynamic:

> That environment (in which medical decisions are made) is demanding something that seems impossible; we must simultaneously increase the quality of medical care while curtailing its costs. Indeed, the last quarter century has delivered two huge forces that are changing the way medicine is and will be practiced, forever. They both begin with the people who pay the bills—whether out of pocket, through insurance premiums or HMO dues, higher costs for goods and services (which pay for employee health benefits), or income taxes. The bill payers have said they will not continue to pay health care costs that rise twice as fast as the general inflation rate and incomes. Simultaneously, they have begun to ask about the quality of the product they are receiving for their money. The latter is not a pretty sight: wide variations in practice patterns without any obvious medical justification; studies indicating that, according to expert panels, from one fourth to one half of the indications for which some major procedures are done are inappropriate or equivocal; studies showing that the experts themselves might not know what they are talking about; and exposes that major diseases are being treated on the flimsiest of evidence. Clearly, we need to rethink what we are trying to do and how we are doing it.[24]

## Future Evolution of Managed Care

Managed care has become the latest "whipping boy" in U.S. health care. Despite its initial success in cost containment, a powerful backlash against managed care organizations has gathered momentum since the mid-1990s over such issues as "gag rules" for HMO physicians, denial of services, and "drive-through deliveries."[25] It is already clear that managed care will not continue without major changes. Many HMOs, for example, are acceding to enrollees' demands for point-of-service access to specialists, and less-effective cost containment appears inevitable.

It is important to recognize the distinction between managed care, described here, and managed reimbursement, which was mentioned earlier. Some managed care organizations, especially in the for-profit group, have focused on management of costs of care at the expense of quality of care, for the purpose of making profits for shareholders. Unfortunately, the many achievements toward cost-effective comprehensive care based on evidence-based outcomes, as exemplified by many non-profit managed care organizations, are being unfairly included in the backlash to managed care. Indeed, some HMOs have been committed for up to 50 years to health promotion, preventive medicine, and a population-based approach to optimizing health care outcomes. It is unclear to what extent these efforts will continue.

# WHERE TO GO NEXT IN FAMILY PRACTICE?

Based on the foregoing discussion, including what has been successful or less successful for family practice over its first 30 years, we now propose our cross-generational recommendations for significant course changes for family practice. These recommendations fall into four major categories: patient care, education, research, and organizational/political strategies.

## Patient Care

Our overriding recommendation is that the foundation of the health care system, for the entire U.S. population, must be a system of accessible, affordable, comprehensive, high-quality primary care. For this recommendation to be put into action, several enabling steps must occur.

**Embrace New Paradigms.** The first enabling step is the need for the health care system in general, and for family practice in particular, to embrace new paradigms of care. These paradigms include evidence-based medicine, population-based care, and chronic disease management.

1. *Evidence-Based Medicine.* With its roots in clinical epidemiology, evidence-based medicine can inform and guide clinical decision making for individual patients as well as populations.[26,27] The process of evidence-based medicine, augmented by information mastery as developed by Slawson et al.,[28] is becoming more widely accepted and applied in family practice. Evidence-based medicine, with an emphasis on positive outcomes that matter to patients, should underpin clinical practice and education in family practice.[29]

2. *Population-Based Care.* Although its application may vary somewhat from one health care organization to another, population-based care typically involves

a systematic structure for identifying patients under the health care organization's care that are at high risk for disease or have an established chronic disease, implementing clinical practice guidelines to deal with the patients' health care problems, and tracking health status, outcomes, and clinical performance. The concept is still somewhat controversial, but there are good examples of its effectiveness. For example, after implementing its population-based family practice model, Group Health Cooperative of Puget Sound has demonstrated a 32% decrease in late-stage breast cancer (1989 to 1990), as well as an increase from 4% to 48% in bicycle helmet use among children, with a concomitant 67% decrease in bicycle-related head injuries (1987 to 1992).[30] Some family physicians advocate that population-based approaches can be usefully applied in small group or even solo family practice,[31] while others caution against the possible erosion of continuity of personal care when focused on populations instead of individuals in large health care systems.[32]

3. *Chronic Disease Management.* As one of the main approaches to population-based care, chronic disease management broadens the goals of health care to include important areas often relatively neglected in our current biomedical paradigm. These include restoring functional capacity; care when cure is not possible; prevention of illness, injury, and untimely death; and health promotion.[21(p187)]

There is good evidence that disease management can lead to improved patient outcomes, as shown by a 1997 HMO Industry Report by Inter Study.[33] Moreover, research on the contribution of health-related quality of life (HRQOL) measures to patient satisfaction and health care decision making indicates that patients with chronic conditions value mental and social health interventions as much or more than they value specific disease treatments.[34] Since chronically ill patients frequently have associated mental and/or social impairments, there is an increasing need to reorient medical practice to address these needs more effectively.

**Modify Practice Style and Redesign Systems.** An enabling second step in family practice's role in transforming the health care system involves redesigning our practices and practice systems. We believe that several actions are necessary.

1. *Group Practices.* Because of the infrastructure required for effective family practice, we believe that solo practice is no longer a viable practice option. The trend will be toward larger groups and more integration of smaller groups into larger health care organizations. The minimum effective practice size is probably four physicians, even in rural areas.

2. *Electronic Medical Record.* Electronic medical records should be implemented in all practices, permitting physicians to take advantage of its full capabilities, including clinical decision support and reminder systems, quality

assurance monitoring, and monitoring of patient outcomes and clinical performance.

3. *Variable Patient Scheduling.* Family physicians should have more variable
patient scheduling, whereby e-mail communication with patients can obviate
the need for office visits for some minor problems, while extended office visits
can be scheduled for patients with more-complex medical problems, multisystem disease, or personal/family problems requiring more time.

4. *Seamless System of Personal Care.* It is essential to develop "seamless" systems of personal care, facilitated by electronic information systems, whereby
effective care can be rendered regardless of a patient's location—office, hospital, nursing home, at home, or elsewhere.

5. *Team Practice.* We recommend expanded team practice with other clinical disciplines, including nurse practitioners/physician assistants, clinical pharmacists, medical social workers, and clinical psychologists. Other team members
may be actively involved in such areas as care of minor illness, patient education and health promotion programs, disease management, and monitoring of
drug therapy and health status.

The family physician's roles in expanded team practice will include emergency care for patients of all ages, including skills in advanced cardiac and
trauma life support skills for adults and children. It will also include extended
office visits for new patients, including full personal and family history, physical examination, baseline laboratory tests, and assessment of health status; diagnosis, management, and follow-up of complex and multisystem disease;
person-centered care of biopsychosocial problems; shared decision making with
patients confronting alternative therapies for serious illness; and coordination
of care for the population being served by the group.

The future family physician will not need to see every patient cared for by
the team but will be in touch electronically with many others. Continuity of care
should continue into the hospital when family physicians' patients are hospitalized, most likely through colleagues within the group who have opted for
training with an emphasis on hospital practice.

6. *Public Health.* We should seek closer collaboration with public health officials. Local and state public health departments can help the personal care sector to extend needed health care services to defined populations, plus provide
community-based epidemiological surveillance and targeted public health interventions. Strategic alliances should be developed with public health agencies,
including electronic communication of clinical information for populations being
served (e.g., information on immunization rates).

**Embrace Increased Differentiation Within Family Practice.** In the 1960s,
there was a tendency among general practitioners who became board certified

in family practice to hold a "macho" view of what family practice should be—full-breadth practice including obstetrics and some surgery. Extent of surgical privileges was a key issue, much as intensive care privileges are an issue today. Given the increasing complexity of our evolving health care system and the progressive shift from acute care to the care of chronic conditions, family practice will need to lose its focus on full-scope practice for all family physicians and diversify more than it has to date. Some family physicians will become hospitalists for adults, with little or no role in ambulatory care or child care. Others will be office-based physicians without a hospital practice, even though their patients may be covered in the hospital by hospitalists from their group practice. Still others may work in a part-time or job-sharing arrangement. In short, it will no longer be possible to "do it all."

## Education

The overall goal of family medicine education at all levels should be the translation of best evidence into practice. Education will thus include emphasis on effective systems of practice, shared decision making with patients, team practice, quality assurance, and optimizing clinical outcomes for individual patients and populations being served. Enabling steps to reach this goal involve revision of our educational programs at all levels.

**Medical Student Education.** Medical student (predoctoral) teaching programs in many medical schools with departments of family medicine are already well established along appropriate lines, including involvement in preclinical courses such as Introduction to Clinical Medicine, plus clinical preceptorships and clerkships with family physicians. The main challenge to improve these programs will be to place medical students in exemplary family practice groups that also use a modern systems approach to family practice as described above. Medical students should also be introduced to the relationships of primary care to public health and a changing health care system, including important policy issues concerning access to care and quality and costs of health care.

**Residency Education.** The development of family practice residencies has been the real success story in family practice, but there is still room for improvement. A classic paper in 1978 by Stephen Abramson, medical educator for many years at the University of Southern California, called attention to diseases of the curriculum—"curriculosclerosis" (hardening of the categories) and "curriculum ossification" (an often epidemic casting of the curriculum in concrete).[35]

We have examples of both disorders in our family practice residencies, though it may be difficult to see them. For example, is our continuity-of-care requirement for the family practice center (1 half day, 2–4 half days, and 3–5 half-days in the first, second, and third years, respectively) still essential, or has it become so restrictive that it limits or prevents other essential training?

Rivo et al. have derived a useful set of 60 generalist training components from a number of national data sources for conditions encountered in primary care.[36] They recommended that generalist residency programs require training in at least 90% of these 60 components, together with a continuity-of-care experience for a panel of patients during at least 10% of the entire training period.

We propose that the following changes be seriously considered for graduate education in family practice: First, we should establish tracks for selected practice competencies, including rural practice, hospitalist practice, and perhaps others. Second, we should restructure required time in the family practice center, permitting more flexibility to allow family practice residents to prepare for special kinds of practice or for additional training in areas of special interest. Third, we should focus on areas that have not yet received sufficient emphasis, such as information and communication systems, cost-effectiveness of care, shared decision making, medical ethics, palliative care, and home and hospice care. Finally, we should model and provide training in aspects of improved systems of primary care, including team practice, quality assurance, leadership and management skills, linkage with public health, and promotion of scholarly projects related to patient outcomes and population-based health.

**Continuing Medical Education (CME).** Many of our CME programs still rely on the traditional paradigm of medical education—the global subjective judgment of "experts." As outcomes-based clinical research and electronic clinical databases continue to develop, we should transform our CME to make use of these evolving approaches to practice.

**Increased Emphasis on Fellowship Training.** We need to expand the number of family physicians with master of public health degrees and increase the participation of family physicians in faculty development programs. These include programs such as the Clinical Scholars Program of The Robert Wood Johnson Foundation and other career development awards.

## Research

The overall goal of family medicine research should be to study outcomes that matter to patients, such as investigate the quality and cost-effectiveness of primary care interventions for both individuals and defined populations in real-world practice settings. Enabling steps to achieve this goal will involve considerable development of family medicine's research infrastructure.

**Practice-Based Research.** To answer important clinical questions with sufficient generalizability and power, it will be necessary to use a networking approach that links the primary care information systems of multiple practices—so-called "practice-based research net-works."

**Electronic Databases.** For effective research in family medicine, we need to develop electronic databases that capture the data from practice. For physicians to use the information generated by family medicine research, they will need access to handheld computers or similar devices that provide them with the results of research in ways that are practical to use in everyday clinical practice.

## Organizational and Political Strategies

We must set a goal of having primary care clinicians assume their full potential as the foundation of the U.S. health care system. Enabling steps to achieve this goal involve organizational and political strategies.

**Organizational Strategies.** First, and most importantly, we should work to establish linkages among the current primary care specialties to accomplish development of a unified primary care generalist discipline by 2030. This will involve expanding the number of true generalist residency positions in primary care by reserving a larger proportion (perhaps 50%) of internal medicine positions for primary care. This could become possible as some medical schools close, resulting in contraction in the number of specialty residency positions. Within a unified primary care discipline, we should develop tracks for areas of emphasis for future practice (e.g., rural, adult, hospitalist).

A second enabling step is to assure the long-term viability of primary care clinical research journals. In family practice in particular, the environment of our clinical research journals remains fragile 30 years after the specialty was founded, mostly due to continued reductions of pharmaceutical advertising. The various family medicine organizations should consider how to stabilize this environment to assure the viability of at least one excellent clinical research journal that is not dependent on and vulnerable to changes in pharmaceutical advertising policies.

**Political Strategies.** It is essential that we advocate for changes in the structure of the U.S. health care system, not merely changes in reimbursement systems. We should educate the public about problems with our current health care system, as well as progress toward resolving them. We should be active in organizations such as the Physicians' Work Group on Universal Coverage. We should build bridges to public health and advocate for increased primary care emphasis in medical schools and residency training programs. Finally, we must increase our representation with government agencies involved in health care education, policy, and research.

# CONCLUSIONS

Our cross-generational perspectives have been remarkably congruent. We agree that much has been achieved. We agree that more needs to be done before family practice, or preferably a unified generalist physician specialty, can sufficiently expand its numbers and capability to serve as the primary care foundation for the entire health care system.

Today, family practice meets only a fraction of the nation's primary health care needs, which are also being addressed by other competing allopathic specialties (including a "hidden system" of non-primary care physicians), other health professionals (including allied health and alternative care providers), and osteopathic physicians. The health care system has already been restructured by powerful forces, including public demand, cost-containment efforts by large employers, health care insurers, and governmental and other payers. Medicine, for better or worse, is also no longer the sovereign profession it once was.

Medicine, and family practice within it, remains a service profession, so the question becomes how can it best serve the public interest in a new health care environment. This is not the time for family practice to rest on the laurels of its initial development. The field must look forward and outward and critically reassess where it is and where it is not. Family practice of the 1970s and 1980s is no longer the best model for the 21st century, but the accomplishments of the last 30 years provide excellent groundwork for what needs to be done next. Opportunities for family practice have never been greater, and there is no better time in history to be a family physician, but continuance of the status quo will assure that family practice is just one option for primary care in 2030, perhaps even a marginalized one at that.

Family medicine is but one part of the larger and rapidly changing health care system in this country, the future shape of which is still uncertain. We can be leaders in the effort to transform that system into one that is effective, efficient, and structured to meet the primary care needs of all Americans. In that spirit, we close with these observations:

> The underlying problems that led to turbulence in medicine—the earlier acceptance of the myth of unbridled resources and national capacity, the preoccupation with short-term rather than long-term thinking, the emphasis on immediate gratification, the difficulty of retaining purpose and values in a culture that champions greed and material excess, and the dilemma of providing for public goods and human needs through a private market system beholden only to owners and shareholders—were the same problems that jeopardized other aspects of the country's prosperity.

The key (to rebuilding the public trust in medicine) lies in restoring the tattered social contract between medicine and society. The medical profession must remember that it exists to serve. (*Kenneth Ludmerer,* 1999)[37]

and further:

We are the intersection between care and cure, between technology and trust, between economics and social equity. (*Bob Graham, executive vice president of American Academy of Family Physicians,* 1997)[38]

# Notes

1. Rivo MC, Kindig DA. A report card on the physician workforce in the United States. *N Engl J Med.* 1996;334:892–896.

2. Donaldson MS, Yordy KD, Vanselow NA. *Primary Care: America's Health in a New Era.* Washington, DC: National Academy Press; 1996:155.

3. Starfield B. Is primary care essential? *Lancet.* 1994;344:1129–1133.

4. Jensen GA, Morrisey MA, Gaffney S, Liston DK. The new dominance of managed care: insurance trends in the 1990s. *Health Aff.* 1997;16(1):125–136.

5. Simon C, Emmons DW. Physician earnings at risk: an examination of capitated contracts. *Health Aff.* 1997;16(3):120–126.

6. Institute for the Future. *Health and Health Care 2010: The Forecast,The Challenge.* San Francisco: Jossey-Bass; 2000:17–24.

7. Fisher ES. What is a hospital? *Effect Clin Pract.* 1999;2(3):138–140.

8. Chesanow N. When hospitalists take over—who wins? Who loses? *Med Econ.* 1998;December 28:107.

9. Lindenauer PK, Pantilat SZ, Katz PP, Wachter RM. Hospitalists and the practice of inpatient medicine: results of a survey of the National Association of Inpatient Physicians. *Ann Intern Med.* 1999;130(4, pt2):343–349.

10. Lurie JD, Wachter RM. Hospitalist staffing requirements. *Effect Clin Pract.* 1999;2(3):126–130.

11. Diamond HS, Goldberg E, Janosky JE. The effect of full-time faculty hospitalists on the efficiency of care at a community teaching hospital. *Ann Intern Med.* 1998;129:197–203.

12. Wachter RM, Katz P, Showstack J, Bindman AB, Goldman L. Reorganizing an academic medical service: impact on cost, quality, patient satisfaction, and education. *JAMA.* 1998;279:1560–1565.

13. Kane T. Too many primary care doctors? It could happen. *Med Econ.* 1997;July 14:119–145.

14. Applelsy C. Open access plans: will family physicians be left behind? *Fam Pract Manag.* 1997;March:58–67.

15. Cooper RA. The growing independence of nonphysician clinicians in clinical practice. *JAMA.* 1997;277:1092–1093.

16. Kostreski F. Mid-level provider debate divides FPs. *Fam Pract News.* 1997;September 1:93.

17. Flanagan L. Nurse practitioners: growing competition for family physicians? *Fam Pract Manag.* 1998;October:34–43.

18. Washington State Medical Association. Pharmacists want to shift from drug dispensing to managing drug therapy. *WSMA Reports.* 1999;October:1,3.

19. Jancin B. Rocky marriage: payers and alternative medicine. *Fam Pract News.* 2000;January 1:44.

20. Radovsky SS. U.S. medical practice before Medicare and now—differences and consequences. *N Engl J Med.* 1990;322:263–267.

21. Institute for the Future. *Health and Health Care 2010: The Forecast, The Challenge.* San Francisco: Jossey-Bass; 2000:109–122.

22. Scherger JE. E-mail enhanced relationships: getting back to basics. *Hippocrates.* 1999;November:7–8.

23. Levit K, Cowan C, Lazenby H, et al. Health spending in 1998: signals of change: the health accounts team. *Health Aff.* 2000;19(1):124–132.

24. Eddy DM. *Clinical Decision Making: From Theory to Practice.* Sudbury, Mass: Jones & Bartlett; 1996:xi.

25. Bailit MH. Ominous signs and portents: a purchaser's view of health care market trends. *Health Aff.* 1997;16(6):85–88.

26. Sackett DL, Richardson WS, Rosenberg W, Haynes RB. *Evidence-Based Medicine: How to Practice and Teach EBM.* New York: Churchill Livingstone,1997:2–16.

27. Evidence-Based Medicine Working Group. Evidence-based medicine: a new approach to teaching the practice of medicine. *JAMA.* 1992;268:2420–2425.

28. Slawson DC, Shaughnessy AF, Bennett JH. Becoming a medical information master: feeling good about not knowing everything. *J Fam Pract.* 1994;38:505–513.

29. Ebell M. Information at the point of care: answering clinical questions. *J Am Board Fam Pract.* 1999;12:225–235.

30. Thompson RS, Taplin SH, McAfee TA, Mandelson M, Smith AE. Primary and secondary prevention services in clinical practice: 20 years' experience in development, implementation, and evaluation. *JAMA.* 1995;273:1130–1135.

31. Rivo ML. It's time to start practicing population-based health care. *Fam Pract Manag.* 1998;June:44.

32. Scherger JE. Does the personal physician continue in managed care? *J Am Board Fam Pract.* 1996;9:67–68.

33. Inter Study. *The Inter Study Competitive Edge: HMO Industry Report 7.2.* Minneapolis: Inter Study; 1997.

34. Sherbourne CD, Sturm R, Wells KB. What outcomes matter to patients? *J Gen Intern Med.* 1999;14:357–366.

35. Abramson S. Diseases of the curriculum. *J Med Educ.* 1978;53:951–957.

36. Rivo ML, Saultz JW, Wartman SA, De Witt TG. Defining the generalist physician's training. *JAMA*. 1994;271:1499–1504.

37. Ludmerer KM. *Time to Heal: American Medical Education from the Turn of the Century to the Era of Managed Care.* New York: Oxford University Press; 1999:398–399.

38. Academy EVP defines specialty's challenges for next 25 years. *FP Report.* 1997;July:3.

# CHAPTER NINE

# Should There Be a Merger to a Single Primary Care Specialty for the Twenty-First Century?

## *An Affirmative View*

Gerald T. Perkoff, M.D.
1989

Debating whether there should be a single or multiple primary care specialties should be nothing more than an exercise in reasoning. Logically, a united front in primary care could be a much more important force in American medicine than the present warring groups ever could be. Again, logically, there are characteristics of each of the existing primary care disciplines that could strengthen the others if they were combined into a single discipline.

Family practice can take a good deal of the credit for the current understanding of primary care and for the definition of current strengths and weaknesses in primary care training and practice. We would not even have this question to debate had our discipline not developed and challenged the other primary care disciplines. Would it not now be logical to improve medical training and medical care by combining the positive aspects of the three disciplines—family practice, internal medicine, and pediatrics—strengthening primary care in the process? Not only could a single primary care specialty provide improved training for practice in general medicine, but it could also eliminate the continued competition for status, money, and patients that characterizes the current relationships among primary care specialties.

Let me first make an important initial disclaimer. Despite a large literature, there is no convincing evidence that supports any one primary care specialty over any other. The bulk of the evidence is that outcome of care provided by family physicians and the other primary care specialists is similar, with neither family practice nor any other specialty showing consistently superior results.[1-10]

---

This chapter is reprinted with permission from Perkoff GT. Should there be a merger into a single primary care specialty for the 21st century? An affirmative view. *J Fam Pract.* 1989;29(2):185–190. Copyright © 1989, Dowden Health Media.

# COMMON BACKGROUND

The generalist origins of the primary care disciplines suggest that there may be emotional and professional support for a single primary care specialty which could make such a development easier to bring about than many presently think.

We know that family practice developed in response to the steadily decreasing number of needed general practitioners.[11] Many forget, however, that at the time the stirrings began which led to family practice as a specialty—the late 1940s to early 1950s—internal medicine still was a general medical discipline. Physicians who trained in internal medicine as late as 1960 believed in continuity of care, often worked closely in their training with social workers and psychologists, emphasized the importance of family members in at least the management of illness, if not in its genesis, and saw themselves as the central managerial physician in a medical care system that even then was becoming complex. Chairmen of departments of medicine insisted that their trainees were general internists first and specialists only later. Understandably, the leaders of internal medicine viewed the developing specialty of family practice as a threat.

The success of family practice should not make us overlook the viability of the current programs in general internal medicine, which are considerably more successful than many in family practice realize. According to the American College of Physicians (in conversation, January 1989), there now are over 200 primary care internal medicine residency and fellowship training programs, and most departments of internal medicine have a formal division of general internal medicine. Some such departments have as many as 40 full-time general internists on their faculty participating actively in training and patient care. The problem of competition in primary care will not go away by our merely emphasizing family practice as the best primary care specialty, as some wish to do. Internal medicine in particular will remain a competitor for the minds of students, the business of patients, and the funds of the public.

Pediatrics, too, was committed to ambulatory care before family practice came into existence, and still considers itself the major primary care specialty for children. Indeed, it is only within the last decade that departments of pediatrics have come to be so subspecialized. The Society for Ambulatory Pediatrics, founded in 1960, now has almost 2000 members (B. Starfield, personal communication, June 1989). Practicing pediatricians, too, do mainly primary care. Thus, like general internal medicine, general and ambulatory pediatrics represents a significant force in American medicine. What we are talking about here, then, are three strong disciplines doing similar things competitively.

It is the positive aspects of each specialty that we would seek to combine, and in the current primary care specialties, positive aspects are not hard to find, both in the characteristics and features of each specialty's training programs and in their practices. In general, all of the primary care specialties espouse the importance of training to assure intellectual curiosity and competence. Family practice, in particular, endorses specific primary care training in the belief that specialty training does not prepare one to do family practice or any other kind of primary care. Likewise, competent specialty care requires special training. Thus pediatricians are trained to provide more detailed and often higher quality child care over a wider range of patient problems, especially for seriously ill children. Internal medicine training emphasizes meticulous inpatient care of patients with complex illnesses. That family physicians use internists for consultation for our more difficult medical patients emphasizes the usefulness and importance of this extra inpatient training. Both pediatrics and internal medicine stress the biological basis of medicine over the social and behavioral components of patient care. Family practice emphasizes strong training in ambulatory care of common patient problems with a special weight given to the social and behavioral aspects of medicine. A combination of the three specialties would give us a physician well trained in both the ambulatory and inpatient care of adults and children, and in both the biological and the social and behavioral aspects of illness.

## ADVANTAGES OF A MERGER

What would each discipline gain from combination? Some of the gains would be directly related to desirable improvements in training for medical practice. Others deal with political, fiscal, and organizational matters. Family practice would gain from consolidation by balancing its present important emphasis on ambulatory care with enhanced emphasis on the biological aspects of diagnosis and treatment and inpatient care of internal medicine and pediatrics.

The family practice resident's expected first allegiance to the ambulatory care patient makes his or her inpatient experience inefficient. Even the best of today's residents lack the sophistication in detailed physical examination, reasoning about diagnosis, and breadth of clinical acumen that characterized their earlier colleagues. Increased impatient and specialty clinic experiences could help correct this deficiency. Further, internal medicine and pediatric faculty supervisors in family practice would be more likely to probe the primary care resident's knowledge and reasoning in the biological aspects of the patients' illnesses more effectively than current faculty, while family practice faculty would be much more likely to be successful teachers of the social and behavioral aspects of patient care.

Anyone from family practice, an already predominantly ambulatory specialty, could fairly ask why these same goals could not be achieved in the ambulatory instead of the inpatient setting. Medical care already is moving in this direction, and Steven Schroeder and I have made just such a suggestion.[12,13] The sheer volume of patients required in a primary care practice to yield several patients with specific disorders that usually are treated in the hospital or in specialty clinics, however, suggests that such training can still be the most efficient for some purposes. The extent to which internal medicine and pediatrics modify their standard programs over the years to move toward ambulatory specialty care of seriously ill patients will help determine the actual sites and content of any increased training in those disciplines.

A common primary care specialty would be stronger politically as well as medically. The competition among current primary care specialties for patients, money, and academic status could not exist if there were only one primary care specialty. Further, combining presently divided scarce training dollars could help raise support for primary care training to more adequate levels, both by making more efficient use of a single sum of money and by improving the persuasiveness of the argument for primary care in the halls of Congress and of academe. Not only would a voluntary solution made within our profession be respected, but it would be clear that we, as primary care physicians, have the welfare of the public at heart if we stop destructive infighting and unite to prepare a better physician.

A common primary care specialty would fare well financially in other ways as well. A new resource-based relative value scale to determine pay for physicians' work has been developed by Hsiao and his co-workers.[14] Their analyses provide support for the long-held view that the nonsurgical work of family physicians, internists, and pediatricians has been compensated inadequately. Although new Medicare legislation will change reimbursement policies, the different primary care specialties can still be paid differently for similar services. A single specialty would not face this problem at all. In addition, a single primary care specialty would be a potent political force in maintaining these gains in the continuing discussions among the various specialties, which will lose income under the new system, and the federal government— discussions that are certain to follow initial implementation of the new payment system.

A common primary care specialty could also strengthen recruitment of future primary care physicians. Schroeder[15] and Colwill[16] have used recent data on entry level university and medical students, as well as analyses of the numbers of individuals entering primary care specialties over time, to document a leveling off and diminishing interest in primary care among current students. This serious problem deserves attention both from disciplinary and health policy points of view. Schroeder, in particular, has detailed the continuing imbalance between primary care and subspecialty physicians that characterizes our current medical educational and medical care systems. Even the success of family practice as a specialty and the resurgence of general internal medicine and pediatrics have not prevented this disparity from worsening.

The major influence medical school has upon career choice by medical students lies in the faculty role models students learn to emulate during their clinical clerkships.[15] Medical students are primarily exposed to specialty, inpatient-based faculty. Further, the academic stature of generalist physicians in medical schools is limited both by their relatively small number and by the entrenched biomedical science value structure of the majority of the faculty. Research emphasis in current medical schools is still strong, and even the growing research efforts of the primary care specialties are less well accepted by the majority of medical school faculty than is work in the biomedical sciences.

Having a single primary care specialty would result in increased effectiveness of primary care faculty in policy deliberations in each medical school even without increased numbers, as this faculty would all be working in a single discipline with concentrated exposure to students. In addition, a single primary care discipline would eliminate the competition that divides primary care faculty recruits into small, less-effective groups, and would represent a potent force for reorganization of medical education around primary care as a major clinical experience. The proportion of primary care faculty would increase, and subspecialty faculty would proportionately decrease. Students would see primary care role models in positions of authority in medical education and in patient care.

Finally, a single primary care specialty makes sense in light of recent changes in the organization of medical care. Primary care generalists are in demand as the central figures in physicians' medical service organizations. Unfortunately, particularly in staff-type health maintenance organizations, family physicians commonly are relegated either to an exclusively gatekeeper or combined gatekeeper-ambulatory care role, doing little or no inpatient care or obstetrics. Internists, on the other hand, have a greater generalist role in such organizations, both in the care of more complex patient problems in the ambulatory setting and in the hospital. A single primary care specialty would prepare physicians for a more complete role in medical care that could provide all the generalist functions needed in organized medical care systems, and provide it cost effectively.

# EFFECTING A MERGER

First, we would have to overcome present unreasoned fears. I already have described the threat presented by the successes of family practice to internal medicine, both in numbers and in the image internists have of themselves as generalists who go on to specialize. Another, even deeper fear is that voiced by family physicians, who feel that family practice would be absorbed into internal medicine and would be lost. If we can recognize and examine the degree to which internal medicine and pediatrics have changed their primary care residency programs to emulate those of family practice, we should be able to put those fears at rest.

The entry of primary care trainees into internal medicine and pediatrics has fallen off even more than it has into family practice. Family physicians surely spend more of their time actually doing primary care than do even general internists. If any discipline was going to "lose its identity," it would be general internal medicine and pediatrics, since the new specialty would resemble family practice more than either of them. And if such a specialty were to have the strong characteristics of each existing specialty, then all three would lose their current identities in a new and better identity.

Fear of loss of subspecialty trainees is one reason some chairmen of departments of internal medicine oppose a common primary care discipline. A successful residency that resulted in the combination of present general medicine, pediatrics, and family practice would perforce play a central role in resident training. At the present time, departments of pediatrics and internal medicine depend upon their traditional residencies and on their primary care–general medicine programs for recruits into all the subspecialties. An increasingly successful primary care residency that was central to hospitals and medical schools would gradually supplant these more traditional programs and become a major source of trainees for the specialties in addition to graduating the new primary care specialist. In time, the new primary care practitioner would also become a dominant generalist in medical practice.

From a practical point of view, several steps can be outlined that could lead in the directions proposed. First of all, a new residency program would have to be devised and approval obtained from all three existing specialty boards to sanction trainees from such programs. Second, several schools would have to be willing to experiment with the new training program, setting it up either alongside or instead of existing programs. Such training programs would include more inpatient care and at least as much ambulatory care as current family practice programs, and would have to be the initial training programs for some physicians who want to specialize as well as those who wished to enter primary care. These training programs might be somewhat longer than the current three years devoted to primary care residencies, as well as more flexible. Already some programs are in place that represent first steps in this direction.[17,18]

Further, some decisions would have to be made about obstetric aspects of primary care training. Most agree at the least that obstetrics is an essential part of rural family practice in addition to being a superb model of family care for trainees. Much remains to be decided here, and the place of obstetrics in family practice overall is undergoing changes. The outcomes of these changes cannot now be predicted, but they will have to be dealt with and plans made for rural obstetric care in any new specialty.

Creatively designed training programs for a new primary care specialty would be exciting and attract inquisitive trainees. Overall outcomes would have to be monitored according to previously determined guidelines that would define levels of competence of program graduates and would monitor the content and breadth of their medical training. Finally, the outcomes would have to be accepted by the specialty boards, which would then be expected to amalgamate. These new training programs and their faculty would bear the burden of leading the changes in medical education and practice that would necessarily follow upon these initial steps.

Amalgamation might not be as difficult as it may seem. Changes already made have led to more similarities in the existing specialties than we might expect to find. Internal medicine programs now must provide one fourth of all their experience in ambulatory care settings, behavioral as well as biomedical aspects of medicine must be emphasized, and experiences in otolaryngology, dermatology, orthopedics, and office gynecology are strongly suggested. These requirements are remarkably similar to the experiences required in family practice training, and in time will make the differences between us smaller in actuality than they are in our minds. Even Dr. John R. Ball, Executive Director of the American College of Physicians, suggests that the concept of a merger of family practice, internal medicine and pediatrics makes sense (personal communication, October 1988). It really is time to begin the spadework necessary to make this exciting and revolutionary development a reality.

## Notes

1. Eisenberg JM, Nicklin D. Use of diagnostic services by physicians in community practice. *Med Care.* 1981;19:297–309.

2. Singh BM, Holland MR, Thorn PA. Metabolic control of diabetes in general practice clinics: comparison with a hospital clinic. *Br Med J.* 1984;289:726–728.

3. Klein R, Klein BEK, Anderson S, Moss SE. Hypoglycemic therapy in patients diagnosed to have diabetes at 30 years of age or older. *J Chronic Dis.* 1984;37:159–165.

4. Franks P, Dickinson JC. Comparison of family physicians and internists: process and outcome in adult patients at a community hospital. *Med Care.* 1986;24:941–948.

5. Meyer BA. Audit of obstetrical care: comparison between family practitioners and obstetricians. *Fam Pract Res J.* 1981;1:20–27.

6. Caetano DF. The relationship of medical specialization (obstetricians and general practitioners) to complications in pregnancy and delivery, birth injury, and malformation. *Am J Obstet Gynecol.* 1975;123:221–227.

7. Ely JW, Ueland K, Gordon MJ. An audit of obstetric care in a university family medicine department and an obstetrics-gynecology department. *J Fam Pract.* 1976;3:397–401.

8. Phillips WR, Rice GA, Layton RH. Audit of obstetrical care and outcome in family medicine obstetrics and family practice. *J Fam Pract.* 1978;6:1209–1216.

9. Kriebel SH, Pitts JD. Obstetric outcomes in a rural family practice: an eight-year experience. *J Fam Pract.* 1988;27:377–384.

10. Roos NP. Who should do the surgery? Tonsillectomy-adenoidectomy in one Canadian province. *Inquiry.* 1979:83:73–83.

11. Overpeck M. Physicians in family practice, 1931–1967. *Public Health Rep.* 1970;85:485–494.

12. Schroeder SA, Showstack JA, Gerbert B. Residency training in internal medicine: time for a change? *Ann Intern Med.* 1986;104:555–561.

13. Perkoff GT. Teaching clinical medicine in ambulatory care settings: an idea whose time may have finally come. *N Eng J Med.* 1986;314:27–31.

14. Hsiao WC, Braun P, Dunn D, Baker ER. Resource-based relative values: an overview. *JAMA.* 1988;260:2347–2353.

15. Schroeder SA: The making of a medical generalist. *Health Aff.* 1985;4:23–46.

16. Colwill JM. Primary care education: a shortage of positions and applicants. *Fam Med.* 1988;20:250–254.

17. Strelnick AH, Bateman WB, Jones C, et al. Graduate primary care training: a collaborative alternative for family practice, internal medicine, and pediatrics. *Ann Intern Med.* 1988;109:324–334.

18. Christiansen RG, Johnson LP, Boyd GE, et al. A proposal for a combined family practice and internal medicine residency. *JAMA.* 1986;255:2628–2630.

# The Generalist Role of Specialty Physicians

## *Is There a Hidden System of Primary Care?*

Roger A. Rosenblatt, M.D., M.P.H.; L. Gary Hart, Ph.D.;
Laura-Mae Baldwin, M.D., M.P.H.; Leighton Chan, M.D.;
Ronald Schneeweiss, M.D.
1998

There have been persistent concerns that the predominance of specialty physicians in the United States reduces access for vulnerable populations and increases the total cost of medical care.[1-5] In response, a wide variety of programs have been initiated to increase the production of generalists,[6] but not without controversy.[7-9] Many specialists argue that they can discharge the responsibilities usually associated with primary care physicians—in particular the provision of accessible, continuous, coordinated, and comprehensive care.[10] This model has been called the hidden system of primary care.[11,12]

The debate as to which approach is preferable has taken on new importance as a result of the emergence of managed care systems.[13] Most structured systems use some variant of the gatekeeper model, restricting access to specialists by requiring that patients begin care with a designated generalist.[14] If specialists routinely provide a broad spectrum of care to their patients, the requirement that patients receive their basic medical care from generalists may be unnecessary or counterproductive.[15-17] This study addresses this issue by determining the extent to which medical and surgical specialists take on the generalist physician role in their care of elderly patients.

## METHODS

This study is based on the medical care utilization patterns of Washington State residents aged 65 years and older who were Medicare beneficiaries throughout the calendar years 1994 and 1995 and did not belong to a capitated health care

---

plan. The data come from the Health Care Financing Administration's National Claims History File, an administrative data set that captures diagnostic, therapeutic, and fiscal information about services rendered to Medicare Part B beneficiaries that were submitted to Medicare for payment.[18,19]

# DATA

## Encounters and Diagnoses

The Medicare Part B file contains a series of line items, each representing a discrete billable service provided to a Medicare beneficiary. We define a physician encounter as all the line items provided on an outpatient basis to an individual patient on a given date by a single physician.

Each physician encounter includes at least 1 line item with a valid *International Classification of Diseases, Ninth Revision, Clinical Modification (ICD-9-CM)* code. In encounters with multiple line items, we selected an index diagnosis from the line item containing the "Evaluation and Management" code. In cases without such a code, we selected the index diagnosis from the line item with the highest charge.

## Identifying Physicians

We used 3 sources to assign physician specialty: American Board of Medical Specialties certifications, the primary self-designated specialty captured in the American Medical Association Masterfile, and the specialty recorded by Health Care Financing Administration. We used American Board of Medical Specialties certification to determine specialty whenever possible. Where a physician had certificates in multiple specialties or no certificates, we assigned the American Medical Association specialty. When the American Medical Association specialty was missing, we assigned the Health Care Financing Administration specialty.

## Generalist Care

We measured 2 of the core attributes of primary care as defined by the Institute of Medicine: continuity and comprehensiveness.[20–24] We operationalized these concepts as follows:

**Continuity: The Majority-of-Care Relationship.** We used the existence of a majority-of-care relationship between patient and physician as a surrogate for continuity, an approach developed in earlier studies.[11,22,25,26] We defined a *majority-of-care relationship* as a single physician providing more than 50% of all ambulatory visits to 1 patient during the study period. If a patient split his or her visits equally between 2 physicians, the physician with the higher total charges was designated as the majority-of-care provider.

**Comprehensiveness.** Comprehensiveness is the ability of the physician to address a broad range of patient problems, whether or not the conditions are within the traditional domain of the specialty in which the physician is trained.[11,23,27] Most medical and surgical subspecialties tend to concentrate their efforts on a narrow range of diagnostic categories related to their specialty.[28] One sign that a specialist is providing comprehensive care is the inclusion of diagnoses outside the traditional domain of that specialty.

For each specialty in this study, we constructed a specialty domain based on the diagnostic rubrics assigned to the ambulatory visits made by Medicare patients. Using diagnosis clusters (DCs)—a method of aggregating *International Classification of Diseases, Ninth Revision (ICD-9)* rubrics into related medical conditions—we constructed a set of DCs and *ICD-9* rubrics that fell within the medical realm generally addressed by a specific specialty.[29] These domains were constructed by the study team and reviewed and revised by the Carrier Advisory Committee—specialists who advise the Medicare intermediary within Washington State. For example, the most common DCs within dermatology were skin keratoses, dermatitis and eczema, and skin cancers; diagnoses within these clusters were "in domain." By contrast, a dermatologist who provided care for hypertension would be considered to be providing "out-of-domain" care.

## Preventive Care: Influenza Immunization

Part of the primary care role is ensuring that patients receive such preventive interventions as annual influenza vaccinations, an injection that can be easily administered in the physician's office and is reimbursed separately by Medicare.[30,31] We defined an *immunization* as any line item that included the appropriate diagnostic or billing code for an influenza vaccination (*Current Procedural Terminology* 90724 or the Health Care Financing Administration Common Procedure Coding System G0008, and *ICD-9* V048); duplicates were eliminated. For each specialty, we computed the immunization rate for their majority-of-care patients and determined whether the patient received the immunization from the majority-of-care specialty or some other identifiable physician.

## Statistical Considerations

Because of the large number of patients in this study, confidence intervals for the figures in the tables that follow are relatively narrow. As an example, the 95% confidence interval for the vaccination rate of patients of neurologists—the group with the fewest majority-of-care patients—is 35.5 to 41.7, with a point estimate of 38.6; confidence intervals for all other specialties are narrower. The differences among groups (generalists vs. medical specialists vs. surgical specialists) are highly significant in all tables ($P < .001$).

# RESULTS

## Description of Washington State Medicare Patients and Physicians

During the study period, 373,505 Health Care Financing Administration beneficiaries from Washington State received all their medical care within Washington State, had at least 1 outpatient visit in both 1994 and 1995, and were alive at the end of the study period. In the aggregate, these patients made 5,590,687 ambulatory visits over the 2-year period, or an average of 7.48 outpatient visits per patient per year. A total of 9.6% of patients made visits only to generalists during the 2-year period, while 14.7% of patients made visits only to specialists.

General internists (GIMs) and family physicians (FPs) accounted for 40.4% of outpatient visits during the study period. The 13 largest medical and surgical specialties in the aggregate have roughly the same number of ambulatory visits as GIMs and FPs combined. The balance of ambulatory visits are to office- and hospital-based specialists, who in the aggregate account for 17.5% of all ambulatory visits (see Table 10.1).

Generalists and specialists have very different diagnostic repertoires. The GIMs and FPs have very similar diagnostic profiles and provide care for a broad and diverse spectrum of conditions. Medical and surgical specialists devote the majority of their visits to conditions primarily within the organ systems or pathological conditions around which the specialty is organized (see Figure 10.1).

## Continuity of Care: The Majority-of-Care Relationship

Specialties differed greatly in the extent to which they established majority-of-care relationships with patients. The GIMs and FPs spend roughly half of their outpatient practices with patients with whom they have a majority-of-care relationship: 49.8% of all their visits occur with the 32.8% of patients with whom they have a majority-of-care relationship. By contrast, medical specialists have roughly one quarter as many (7.8%) and surgical specialists have about one sixth as many (5.2%) majority-of-care patients (see Table 10.2).

Although specialists are much less likely to have such relationships, there are some notable exceptions. Oncology stands out in this respect, probably because oncologists become the dominant caregiver for patients being treated for cancer. Although only 18.9% of the patients of oncologists have a majority-of-care relationship with their physician, these patients account for almost half of all

**Table 10.1. Outpatient Visits by Washington State Medicare Beneficiaries to Selected Physician Specialties, 1994–1995.**

| Specialty | No. of Physicians | % of Physicians | Total Ambulatory Visits | % of Ambulatory Visits | Ambulatory Visits per Physician | Medicare Patients per Physician |
|---|---|---|---|---|---|---|
| Generalists | | | | | | |
| Family practice | 1682 | 18.4 | 1,129,106 | 20.2 | 671.3 | 105.5 |
| Internal medicine | 921 | 10.1 | 1,131,673 | 20.2 | 1228.7 | 191.6 |
| **All Generalists** | **2603** | **28.5** | **2,260,779** | **40.4** | **868.5** | **136.0** |
| Medical specialties | | | | | | |
| Cardiology | 232 | 2.5 | 300,203 | 5.4 | 1294.0 | 286.6 |
| Dermatology | 147 | 1.6 | 199,965 | 3.6 | 1360.3 | 527.7 |
| Gastroenterology | 146 | 1.6 | 119,829 | 2.1 | 820.7 | 296.6 |
| Neurology | 139 | 1.5 | 75,059 | 1.3 | 540.0 | 201.6 |
| Oncology | 125 | 1.4 | 124,079 | 2.2 | 992.6 | 131.7 |
| Pulmonology | 100 | 1.1 | 110,065 | 2.0 | 1100.7 | 222.0 |
| Rheumatology | 57 | 0.6 | 79,979 | 1.4 | 1403.1 | 268.1 |
| **All Medical Specialists** | **946** | **10.4** | **1,009,179** | **18.1** | **1066.8** | **284.7** |
| Surgical specialties | | | | | | |
| General surgery | 351 | 3.8 | 121,722 | 2.2 | 346.8 | 137.1 |
| Gynecology | 495 | 5.4 | 72,289 | 1.3 | 146.0 | 59.6 |
| Ophthalmology | 287 | 3.1 | 612,711 | 11.0 | 2134.9 | 689.0 |
| Orthopedic surgery | 416 | 4.6 | 214,248 | 3.8 | 515.0 | 177.0 |
| Otolaryngology | 180 | 2.0 | 121,801 | 2.2 | 676.7 | 305.7 |
| Urology | 158 | 1.7 | 200,266 | 3.6 | 1267.5 | 369.2 |
| **All Surgical Specialists** | **1887** | **20.7** | **1,343,037** | **24.0** | **711.7** | **245.0** |
| Other specialties[a] | 3682 | 40.4 | 977,692 | 17.5 | 265.5 | 110.8 |
| **Total** | **9118** | **100.0** | **5,590,687** | **100.0** | **613.1** | **163.8** |

[a]"Other" includes the following specialties with 10,000 or more patient encounters during the study period: allergy and immunology, anesthesia, colon and rectal surgery, emergency medicine, endocrinology, general preventive medicine, hand surgery, infectious disease, nephrology, neurosurgery, psychiatry, physiatry, plastic surgery, radiology, and vascular surgery; physicians whose specialties could not be determined accounted for 4.3% of all visits and are included in the "other" category.

**Figure 10.1.** Diagnosis Clusters Accounting for the Majority of Ambulatory Visits by Medicare Patients to Physicians in Selected Specialties.

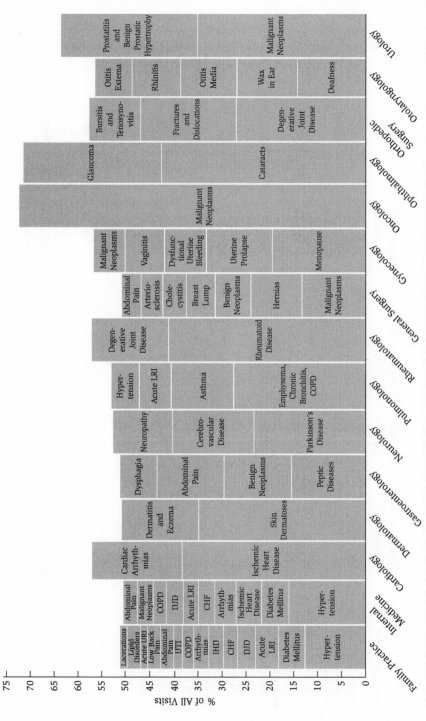

*Notes:* The list is truncated after diagnoses representing 50% of all outpatient visits for each discipline depicted. URI indicates upper respiratory tract infection; UTI, urinary tract infection; COPD, chronic obstructive pulmonary disease; IHD, ischemic heart disease; CHF, congestive heart failure; DJD, degenerative joint disease; and LRI, lower respiratory tract infection.

**Table 10.2. Majority-of-Care Relationships Between Washington State Medicare Patients and Selected Physician Specialties, 1994–1995.**

| | Patients | | | Outpatient Visits | | |
|---|---|---|---|---|---|---|
| | Majority-of-Care Patients | Total Patients | % Majority-of-Care Patients | Majority-of-Care Visits | Total Visits | % Majority-of-Care Visits |
| Specialty | | | | | | |
| Generalists | | | | | | |
| Family practice | 61,545 | 177,476 | 34.7 | 591,507 | 1,129,106 | 52.4 |
| General internal medicine | 54,589 | 176,460 | 30.9 | 533,438 | 1,131,673 | 47.1 |
| **All Generalists** | **116,134** | **353,936** | **32.8** | **1,124,945** | **2,260,779** | **49.8** |
| Medical specialties | | | | | | |
| Cardiology | 7060 | 66,501 | 10.6 | 62,785 | 300,203 | 20.9 |
| Dermatology | 3029 | 77,569 | 3.9 | 16,898 | 199,965 | 8.5 |
| Gastroenterology | 1553 | 43,304 | 3.6 | 11,285 | 119,829 | 9.4 |
| Neurology | 976 | 28,016 | 3.5 | 7,177 | 75,059 | 9.6 |
| Oncology | 3114 | 16,466 | 18.9 | 55,905 | 124,079 | 45.1 |
| Pulmonology | 3434 | 22,203 | 15.5 | 33,870 | 110,065 | 30.8 |
| Rheumatology | 1755 | 15,280 | 11.5 | 24,138 | 79,979 | 30.2 |
| **All Medical Specialists** | **20,921** | **269,339** | **7.8** | **212,058** | **1,009,179** | **21.0** |
| Surgical specialties | | | | | | |
| General surgery | 1705 | 48,105 | 3.5 | 14,928 | 121,722 | 12.3 |
| Gynecology | 1532 | 29,511 | 5.2 | 10,876 | 72,289 | 15.1 |
| Ophthalmology | 13,429 | 197,730 | 6.8 | 80,733 | 612,711 | 13.2 |
| Orthopedics | 2,466 | 73,638 | 3.4 | 14,309 | 214,248 | 6.7 |
| Otolaryngology | 1,222 | 55,032 | 2.2 | 7,164 | 121,801 | 5.9 |
| Urology | 3,729 | 58,329 | 6.4 | 29,268 | 200,266 | 14.6 |
| **All Surgical Specialists** | **24,083** | **462,345** | **5.2** | **157,278** | **1,343,037** | **11.7** |

the outpatient visits to oncologists in the 2-year study period. Pulmonologists and rheumatologists also devote an appreciable part of their practices to majority-of-care patients, 30.8% and 30.2%, respectively.

The pattern portrayed in Table 10.2 persists even for several important subsets of patients. Restricting the analysis only to patients without a major disease episode—those with no hospitalizations during the 2-year period—does not affect the results. In similar fashion, focusing only on patients with 5 or more visits per year—about 60% of the patient population—also does not change this measure of continuity of care. Patients who have more visits are slightly less likely to have a specific physician who provides the majority of visits, but the effect is slight. The specialty-specific patterns are remarkably stable.

Defining majority of care as 50% or more of all visits to a single physician may unfairly exclude patients with a nearly even distribution of visits among several physicians. We therefore reanalyzed the data, designating the physician who provided more visits than any other physician as the plurality-of-care physician; in the case of a tie, the physician with the higher total charges was considered to be the plurality physician. Generalists are the plurality-of-care physician for 53.0% of the patients and the rank order across specialties does not change, but several specialties stand out. Of the patients seen by oncologists, 35.9% have a plurality-of-care relationship with their oncologists, and these patients account for 71.6% of all ambulatory visits to oncologists over a 2-year period. Pulmonologists and rheumatologists also have the majority of their ambulatory visits with patients for whom they are the plurality-of-care physicians.

## Comprehensiveness of Care: Specialists Providing Out-of-Domain Care

The vast majority of ambulatory patient visits to specialists are for conditions that lie within that specialist's traditional domain of expertise. The medical specialty with the most comprehensive practice using this particular measure was pulmonology, with 36.0% of diagnoses out of domain. Other medical specialties had relatively few ambulatory visits for diagnoses that were not part of their traditional repertoire. The surgical specialists show a similar pattern. General surgeons—with 24.5% of visits for out-of-domain diagnoses—and gynecologists—with 27.8%—appear to have a much broader diagnostic scope than other surgical specialists (see Table 10.3).

If out-of-domain care is an accurate marker of the generalist role, physicians would be expected to provide more out-of-domain care to those patients with whom they have a majority-of-care relationship. Table 10.4 tests this supposition.

In general, specialists provide more out-of-domain care for patients with whom they have a majority-of-care relationship. The differences are substantial for several of the internal medicine subspecialties, such as gastroenterology

Table 10.3. Proportion of Diagnoses In and Out of Selected Specialty
Domains of Washington State Medicare Beneficiaries, 1994–1995.

| Specialty | % in Domain | % Out of Domain | Total Visits |
|---|---|---|---|
| Medical specialties | | | |
| Cardiology | 95.5 | 4.5 | 300,203 |
| Dermatology | 98.0 | 2.0 | 199,965 |
| Gastroenterology | 87.2 | 12.8 | 119,829 |
| Neurology | 84.3 | 15.7 | 75,059 |
| Oncology | 84.6 | 15.4 | 124,079 |
| Pulmonology | 64.0 | 36.0 | 110,065 |
| Rheumatology | 80.8 | 19.2 | 79,979 |
| **All Medical Specialties** | 88.2 | 11.8 | **1,009,179** |
| Surgical specialties | | | |
| General surgery | 75.5 | 24.5 | 121,722 |
| Gynecology | 72.2 | 27.8 | 72 ,89 |
| Ophthalmology | 97.7 | 2.3 | 612,711 |
| Orthopedics | 94.5 | 5.5 | 214,248 |
| Otolaryngology | 93.0 | 7.0 | 121,801 |
| Urology | 97.6 | 2.4 | 200,266 |
| **All Surgical Specialties** | 93.4 | 6.6 | **1,343,037** |

and neurology. And, the differences are dramatic for general surgery and gynecology.

Pulmonologists, oncologists, and gynecologists each have a substantial proportion of patients—26.7%, 20.9%, and 19.6%, respectively—for whom most of the services they provide are outside their specialty domain. This reinforces the impression that generalist care is something they provide to at least a segment of their patient populations.

Preventive care interventions—as measured by the rate at which physicians provide influenza vaccinations to their majority-of-care patients—tend to validate the other ways of examining the generalist role. As seen in Table 10.5, patients whose majority-of-care physicians are GIMs or FPs have significantly higher immunization rates than patients who have specialists as their dominant source of care: 55.4% of the majority-of-care patients of generalists receive an annual influenza immunization vs. 47.7% of the patients of medical specialists and 39.6% of the patients of surgical specialists.

Of equal interest is the source of the immunizations: generalists administer most of the immunizations that their patients receive in their offices, while patients of most specialists get immunizations either from GIMs and FPs who see them less frequently than do the specialists, or from undefined sources that probably represent public health facilities, hospital outpatient clinics, and

Table 10.4. Percentage of Out-of-Domain Visits Made by
Majority-of-Care and Minority-of-Care Patients to Selected Specialties, Washington State, 1994–1995.

| | % of Out-of-Domain Visits | |
| --- | --- | --- |
| | Majority-of-Care Relationship With Physician | Minority-of-Care Relationship With Physician |
| Medical specialties | | |
| Cardiology | 6.8 | 3.9 |
| Dermatology | 2.0 | 2.0 |
| Gastroenterology | 37.2 | 10.2 |
| Neurology | 31.4 | 14.0 |
| Oncology | 13.1 | 17.3 |
| Pulmonology | 40.8 | 33.8 |
| Rheumatology | 22.9 | 17.6 |
| All Medical Specialists | 17.8 | 10.2 |
| Surgical specialties | | |
| General surgery | 60.6 | 19.5 |
| Gynecology | 56.8 | 22.6 |
| Ophthalmology | 4.5 | 2.0 |
| Orthopedics | 20.5 | 4.5 |
| Otolaryngology | 6.8 | 7.0 |
| Urology | 2.1 | 2.5 |
| All Surgical Specialists | 14.6 | 5.6 |

similar settings. It is noteworthy that the 2 specialty groups that tend to administer influenza vaccinations in their own offices—pulmonologists and rheumatologists—are also the 2 specialties whose patients have the highest immunization rates.

# COMMENT

## Who Are the Generalists?

There are systematic differences between the 2 traditional adult generalist disciplines—general internal medicine and family practice—and many of the medical and surgical subspecialties examined in this study. The GIMs and FPs provide care for a broad range of diagnoses and devote a large proportion of

Table 10.5. Influenza Vaccination Rates for Washington State Medicare Beneficiaries by Specialty of Majority-of-Care Physician.

| Specialty | No. of Patients | No. (%) Vaccinated | Vaccine Administered by, % | | | |
|---|---|---|---|---|---|---|
| | | | Majority-of-Care Specialists | Nonmajority-of-Care Specialists | Nonmajority-of-Care Generalists | Other or Missing |
| Generalists | | | | | | |
| Family practice | 61,545 | 32,848 (53.4) | 73.4 | 1.3 | 1.3 | 23.9 |
| Internal medicine | 54,589 | 31,475 (57.7) | 73.8 | 1.6 | 4.5 | 20.1 |
| **All Generalists** | **116,134** | **64,323 (55.4)** | 73.6 | 1.5 | 2.9 | 22.1 |
| Medical specialties | | | | | | |
| Cardiology | 7,060 | 3,193 (45.2) | 26.4 | 5.8 | 28.6 | 39.2 |
| Dermatology | 3,029 | 1,136 (37.5) | 0.9 | 7.8 | 43.5 | 47.8 |
| Gastroenterology | 1,553 | 710 (45.7) | 36.9 | 4.2 | 23.9 | 34.9 |
| Neurology | 976 | 377 (38.6) | 26.3 | 7.2 | 25.5 | 41.1 |
| Oncology | 3,114 | 1,475 (47.4) | 44.5 | 5.8 | 24.5 | 25.1 |
| Pulmonology | 3,434 | 2,107 (61.4) | 71.8 | 1.5 | 8.5 | 18.2 |
| Rheumatology | 1,755 | 971 (55.3) | 51.8 | 5.0 | 21.4 | 21.7 |
| **All Medical Specialists** | **20,921** | **9,969 (47.7)** | 39.0 | 5.0 | 24.3 | 31.7 |
| Surgical specialties | | | | | | |
| General surgery | 1,705 | 670 (39.3) | 36.3 | 3.0 | 18.5 | 42.2 |
| Gynecology | 1,532 | 642 (41.9) | 25.4 | 5.6 | 21.8 | 47.2 |
| Ophthalmology | 13,429 | 5,327 (39.7) | 1.8 | 7.0 | 45.0 | 46.2 |
| Orthopedics | 2,466 | 858 (34.8) | 16.8 | 6.4 | 34.5 | 42.3 |
| Otolaryngology | 1,222 | 447 (36.6) | 0.9 | 8.3 | 45.2 | 45.6 |
| Urology | 3,729 | 1,583 (42.5) | 2.1 | 8.9 | 42.3 | 46.7 |
| **All Surgical Specialists** | **24,083** | **9,527 (39.6)** | 7.2 | 6.9 | 40.2 | 45.7 |

their efforts to patients with whom they have a continuous relationship.[32] By contrast, many of the medical and surgical specialties appear to function primarily as specialists. They form majority-of-care relationships with a much smaller proportion of their patients, render care for a focused group of diagnoses, and rarely stray outside the traditional domain of their specialty.

There are some notable exceptions to these generalizations.[33] Pulmonary specialists and rheumatologists have a relatively large proportion of majority-of-care patients and provide a substantial amount of out-of-domain care. Oncologists have more majority-of-care relationships than any of the other specialists, but most of their visits are for diagnoses related to cancer. Overall, there is probably a continuum in which some medical specialists also have a component of their practice devoted to general internal medicine. That component is large in pulmonary medicine, small in dermatology.

Surgical specialists—with the exception of general surgery and gynecology— rarely assume the generalist role. Although general surgeons and gynecologists do not have a greater proportion of majority-of-care patients than their counterparts, they provide large amounts of out-of-domain care to patients with whom they have such a tie and are much more likely to administer influenza immunizations in their offices. One would speculate that they are taking on the generalist role in their care of these patients.

## Limitations

Generalism and primary care are difficult to define and to measure, yet they remain useful constructs in our analysis of the health care system.[21,34] The strength of this study is its ability to examine the health care provided to an entire population; its weakness is the reliance on a secondary data set designed as an administrative and reimbursement tool. Our measures of generalism are, by necessity, based on quantitative proxies for generalist care rather than direct observation of the patient-physician relationship itself. Specific threats to the validity of our inferences are described below:

### Using Majority of Care as a Measure of Continuity

The selection of majority of care as a measure of continuity is arbitrary. Other investigators have used similar measures,[11,26,27] but there is no a priori reason to draw the line between continuity and a lack of continuity at 50% of all visits.[35] However, the findings in this study do not change if we restrict the analysis only to patients who are treated frequently (5 or more times per year) or to patients who have not had a hospitalization during the study period and whose care is probably not distorted by the occurrence of a major disease episode. Changing the threshold for determining continuity from the majority to the plurality of visits does not change the relationship across specialties, but underlines the fact that oncologists, pulmonologists, and rheumatologists devote most of their ambulatory care to patients whom they see more frequently than any other physician.

### Using Out-of-Domain Care as a Measure of Comprehensiveness

Determining whether a given visit to a specialist is within or outside that specialist's domain of care is problematic. We used a normative process in which—aided by a panel of specialists—we assigned every diagnosis within a specialty to within or outside the domain of that specialty. There was little disagreement among the panel and the advisory committee about the core diagnoses defining each specialty. Disagreement was common at the margin, but the prevalence of the disputed diagnoses was so low that including or excluding those in question had no meaningful impact on the results. We were conservative in assigning diagnoses to a specialty domain; when there was substantial disagreement, the diagnosis was considered out of domain.

Using this concept is not entirely satisfactory, but no externally validated criterion standard exists. We examined documents published by the respective specialty boards and residency review committees, but neither source provided adequate specificity.[36]

### Coding Bias

A possible source of error may be that specialists select a diagnosis within their domain for payment to ensure Medicare reimbursement. We examined secondary and tertiary diagnoses, but they rarely changed our determination as to whether a specific visit was within domain. However, if specialists systematically do not code for services that they provide that fall outside their customary domains, we will underestimate the comprehensiveness of their practices.

### Reliance on Outpatient Care

We restricted our examination to outpatient care because it represents the majority of interactions between patients and their physicians. We do not think our exclusion of inpatient care introduces systematic error. Instead, we feel that physicians are more likely to restrict themselves to their specialty area when providing hospital care.

## GENERALIZABILITY OF THESE RESULTS

First, this study is restricted to Washington State Medicare beneficiaries 65 years or older who are not members of capitated managed care programs. Younger patients may have a different relationship with their physicians than the elderly. However, since older patients are sicker and see their physicians more frequently, it seems they would be more likely to establish strong relationships with individual physicians.[37]

Second, this study excludes patients within capitated managed care systems, who constituted 15% of the Medicare elderly in Washington State in 1994. The results reported here cannot be extrapolated to health maintenance organizations. However, virtually all health maintenance organizations restrict access to specialists, and most in Washington State confer the gatekeeper role on an internist or family physician, making it unlikely that the results would be different in those settings.

Third, it is not clear that these results can be generalized to other parts of the country. Washington State is a middle-sized state with both rural and urban areas and a fairly typical mix and supply of physicians. However, there can be profound variations even within small regions, and specialists in areas where they are in greater surplus may be more predisposed to provide generalist care to their patients.

# IS THERE A HIDDEN SYSTEM OF PRIMARY CARE?

In their exploration of the contribution of specialists to the delivery of medical care, Aiken and colleagues[11] concluded that specialists are the "principal source of care to a substantial portion of their patients" and provide care for "a range of ailments not confined to the physician's area of specialization." They concluded that there is a "hidden system" of general medical care in which specialty physicians "spend considerable amounts of their time serving as providers of continuing care, irrespective of their patients' medical needs."

The picture that emerges from our study agrees in some ways with earlier work but suggests a different interpretation.[25] Specialists play an enormous role in providing ambulatory care to elderly patients; 14.7% of the patients saw only specialists during the entire 2-year period, and most ambulatory visits are with specialists. Whether or not these specialists were consciously adopting a principal-care role, they were the dominant physicians for a large number of patients. Aiken et al concluded that specialists "serve as primary physicians for almost one in every five Americans." Given that almost 1 of every 6 patients in this study saw only specialists during a 2-year period, there is no question that specialists are the principal physicians in the lives of a large number of patients.

However, the data also suggest that principal care means something quite different for most specialists than it does for most generalists. Specialists tend to focus on the interrelated diagnoses that define their specialty. Although they may be the principal—and in some cases only—physician for a subset of their patients, they probably only rarely provide substantial amounts of care beyond the boundaries of their specialty.

The advent of the age of managed care—and the growing surplus of specialists—has led many specialties to assert their ability to act as primary care physicians.[38] Although this may be true, this study suggests that this phenomenon is specialty-specific. Specialties such as pulmonary medicine, rheumatology, and gynecology already have a substantial number of patients for whom they provide primary care services, such as immunizations. To the extent that these specialties wish to modify training and practice, they might well take on generalist roles in managed care settings.[39] On the other hand, specialties such as dermatology or urology would have to fundamentally change the nature of their practices.

All this ignores the question as to whether it would be good for patients—or payers—to encourage this migration of specialists to generalism. The crucial issue is whether it makes a difference—both in cost and outcomes—if a patient has a generalist physician, and if that physician is a general internist or family physician or a specialist.[40,41] But these data show that, even in the relatively unstructured world of indemnity insurance, most specialists do not assume the generalist role.

# Notes

1. Moore GT. The case of the disappearing generalist: does it need to be solved? *Milbank Q.* 1992;70:361–379.

2. Schroeder SA. Training an appropriate mix of physicians to meet the nation's needs. *Acad Med.* 1993;68:118–122.

3. Millis JS. *The Graduate Education of Physicians: Report of the Citizens Commission on Graduate Medical Education.* Chicago: American Medical Association; 1966.

4. Schroeder SA, Sandy LG. Specialty distribution of U.S. physicians: the invisible driver of health care costs. *N Engl J Med.* 1993;328:961–963.

5. Mark DH, Gottlieb MS, Zellner BB, Chetty VK, Midtling JE. Medicare costs in urban areas and the supply of primary care physicians. *J Fam Pract.* 1996;43:33–39.

6. Kindig DA, Cultice JM, Mullan F. The elusive generalist physician: can we reach a 50% goal? *JAMA.* 1993;270:1069–1073.

7. Schwarz WB, Williams AP, Newhouse JP, Witsberger C. Are we training too many medical subspecialists? *JAMA.* 1988;259:233–239.

8. Meltzer D. Are generalists the answer for primary care? *JAMA.* 1993;269:1711–1714.

9. Rogers DE. Who should give primary care? the continuing debate. *N Engl J Med.* 1981;305:577–578.

10. Peterson ML. The Institute of Medicine report, "A Manpower Policy for Primary Health Care": a commentary from the American College of Physicians. *Ann Intern Med.* 1980;92:843–851.

11. Aiken LH, Lewis CE, Craig J, et al. The contribution of specialists to the delivery of primary care: a new perspective. *N Engl J Med.* 1979;300:1363–1370.

12. Barr DM. Primary and consultant care: can they be distinguished? *JAMA.* 1980;243:2510–2512.

13. Forrest CB, Starfield B. The effect of first-contact care with primary care clinicians on ambulatory health care expenditures. *J Fam Pract.* 1996;43:40–48.

14. Franks P, Clancy CM, Nutting PA. Gatekeeping revisited: protecting patients from overtreatment. *N Engl J Med.* 1992;327:424–429.

15. Grumbach K, Selby JV, Schmittdiel J, Quesenberry CP Jr. Quality of primary care practice in a large HMO according to physician specialty and physician sex. *Health Serv Res.* 1999;34:485–502.

16. Safran DG, Tarlov AR, Rogers WH. Primary care performance in fee-for-service and prepaid health care systems: results from the Medical Outcomes Study. *JAMA.* 1994;271:1579–1586.

17. Kravitz RL, Greenfield S, Rogers W, et al. Differences in the mix of patients among medical specialties and systems of care: results from the Medical Outcomes Study. *JAMA.* 1992;267:1617–1623.

18. Lave JR, Pashos CL, Anderson GF, et al. Costing medical care: using Medicare administrative data. *Med Care.* 1994;32:JS77–JS89.

19. Parente ST, Weiner JP, Garnick DW, et al. Developing a quality improvement database using health insurance data: a guided tour with application to Medicare's National Claims History File. *Am J Med Qual.* 1995;10:162–176.

20. Donaldson MS, Vanselow NA. The nature of primary care. *J Fam Pract.* 1996;42:113–116.

21. Institute of Medicine. *A Manpower Policy for Primary Health Care.* Washington, DC: National Academy Press; 1978.

22. Weiss LJ, Blustein J. Faithful patients: the effect of long-term physician-patient relationships on the costs and use of health care by older Americans. *Am J Public Health.* 1996;86:1742–1747.

23. Goldberg HI, Dietrich AJ. The continuity of care provided to primary care patients: a comparison of family physicians, general internists, and medical subspecialists. *Med Care.* 1985;23:63–73.

24. Wasson JH, Sauvigne AE, Mogielnicki RP, et al. Continuity of outpatient medical care in elderly men: a randomized trial. *JAMA.* 1984;252:2413–2417.

25. Spiegel JS, Rubenstein LV, Scott B, Brook RH. Who is the primary physician? *N Engl J Med.* 1983;308:1208–1212.

26. Dietrich AJ, Marton KI. Does continuous care from a physician make a difference? *J Fam Pract.* 1982;15:929–937.

27. Mendenhall RC, Tarlov AR, Girard RA, Michel JK, Radecki SE. A national study of internal medicine and its specialties, II: primary care in internal medicine. *Ann Intern Med.* 1979;91:275–287.

28. Rosenblatt RA, Cherkin DC, Schneeweiss R, Hart LG. The content of ambulatory medical care in the United States: an interspecialty comparison. *N Engl J Med.* 1983;309:892–897.

29. Schneeweiss R, Rosenblatt RA, Cherkin DC, Kirkwood CR, Hart LG. Diagnosis

clusters: a new tool for analyzing the content of ambulatory medical care. *Med Care.* 1983;21:105–122.

30. Morrissey JP, Harris RP, Kincade-Norburn J, et al. Medicare reimbursement for preventive care: changes in performance of services, quality of life, and health care costs. *Med Care.* 1995;33:315–331.

31. Ives DG, Lave JR, Traven ND, Kuller LH. Impact of Medicare reimbursement on influenza vaccination rates in the elderly. *Prev Med.* 1994;23:134–141.

32. Dietrich AJ, Goldberg H. Preventive content of adult primary care: do generalists and subspecialists differ? *Am J Public Health.* 1984;74:223–227.

33. Braunwald E. Subspecialists and internal medicine: a perspective. *Ann Intern Med.* 1991;114:76–78.

34. Institute of Medicine. *Primary Care: America's Health in a New Era.* Washington, DC: National Academy Press; 1996.

35. Lambrew JM, De Friese GH, Carey TS, Ricketts TC, Biddle AK. The effects of having a regular doctor on access to primary care. *Med Care.* 1996;34:138–151.

36. Accreditation Council for Graduate Medical Education. *Essentials and Information Items, 1993–1994.* Chicago: Accreditation Council for Graduate Medical Education; 1993.

37. Vladeck BC, King KM. Medicare at 30: preparing for the future. *JAMA.* 1995;274:259–262.

38. Lundberg GD, Lamm RD. Solving our primary care crisis by retraining specialists to gain specific primary care competencies. *JAMA.* 1993;270:380–381.

39. Eisenberg JM. The internist as gatekeeper: preparing the general internist for a new role. *Ann Intern Med.* 1985;102:537–543.

40. Rhee SO, Luke RD, Lyons TF, Payne BC. Domain of practice and the quality of physician performance. *Med Care.* 1981;19:14–23.

41. Payne BC, Lyons TF, Neuhaus E. Relationships of physician characteristics to performance quality and improvement. *Health Serv Res.* 1984;19:307–332.

# CHAPTER ELEVEN

# Primary Care and Health

## *A Cross-National Comparison*

Barbara Starfield, M.D., M.P.H.
1991

A persisting sense of crisis in the U.S. health service system is responsible for a new willingness to consider experiences from abroad. Debates focus on the relative advantages of various other systems, with the leading contenders for emulation emerging as the Canadian and West German models.[1,2]

Arguments for and against these and other national systems focus largely on their philosophical underpinnings, especially concerning the appropriate balance between the private sector and government and on the costs associated with the different systems. Little of the debate centers on the value of the systems as reflected by indicators of health that are amenable to medical care.

This article presents the results of an analysis of the characteristics of the systems of primary care in 10 Western industrialized nations and the relationship to the attitudes of the populations toward their health service systems and to levels of health as reflected by 12 indicators.

Since primary care is the place of entry (the "gatekeeper") into health services and the locus of continuing care for most of the health problems that occur in the population, it is an appropriate point of departure for an examination of the relationship between the health system and levels of health.

## METHODS

Ten Western industrialized nations that have comparable data on characteristics of their primary care health systems and health status indicators for the same years were chosen for comparison. Information concerning the characteristics of

This article was updated by Barbara Starfield and Leiyu Shi in June 2002 in Policy Relevant Determinants of Health: An International Perspective. *Health Policy.* 2002;60:201–218.

primary care in the 10 countries was obtained from six major sources.[3-8] Where particular items of information were lacking in these six sources, information was sought from individuals who were from the particular country and who either had access to published data in their country or were experts concerning their country's health services system. Information from the published sources was also confirmed by these individuals or updated where necessary.

Characteristics of primary care were of two types: those related to the overall system and those related to the mode of practice. The former category comprised five characteristics: the type of system (in particular the extent of regulation on place of practice of primary care practitioners); the type of physician who provides primary care (family physician, internist, pediatrician, or specialist); financial access to care (national health insurance sponsored by government, by nongovernmental agencies, or no national health insurance); percentage of active physicians who are specialists; and income of primary care physicians relative to that of specialists.

Six characteristics of primary care were considered to be related to the mode of practice: the extent to which the primary care physician acts as the point of entry into the system; the extent to which that physician provides continuous (longitudinal) care over time; the comprehensiveness of the care provided; the extent of coordination of services by the primary care physician; the extent to which the physician is "family-centered"; and the community orientation of the physician. All of these characteristics have been considered essential or, at least, important in primary care practice.[9-11]

Possible scores for each of the characteristics ranged from zero (where the level of achievement was not conducive to primary care) to two (where the level of achievement was most conducive to primary care). Intermediate levels of achievement were given a score of one. Table 11.1 describes the method of scoring. The core for each country was the average of these 11 scores.

A satisfaction-expense ratio was obtained from a study conducted by Blendon et al.[12] These investigators conducted a telephone survey of a random sample of individuals in 10 countries, seven of which are countries in this analysis. Three statements were posed to people who were asked to indicate which came closest to expressing their overall view of the health care system in their country: "On the whole, the health care system works pretty well, and only minor changes are necessary to make it work better"; "There are some good things in our health care system, but fundamental changes are needed to make it work better"; and "Our health care system has so much wrong with it that we need to completely rebuild it." Hellander and Wolfe[13] used the data from that study to calculate a ratio. The numerator of the ratio is the percentage of people who said that their system needed only minor changes divided by the percentage of people who said that the system needed to be completely rebuilt, and the denominator is the per capita cost of the health care system in thousands of dollars.

Table 11.1. Rating Criteria.

## Criteria for Rating of Health System
## Characteristics Related to Primary Care

1. **Type of System**
   Regulated primary care or public health centers are considered to be the highest commitment to primary care. Regulated primary care implies that national policies influence the location of physician practice so that they are distributed throughout the population rather than concentrated in certain geographic areas. Public health centers are also assumed to represent the equitable distribution of physician resources. Intermediate scores connote systems where incentives for equitable distribution are present and moderately effective.

2. **Type of Primary Care Practitioner**
   Generalists (family or general practitioners) are the prototypical primary care physicians because the nature of their training is exclusively devoted to primary care practice. General pediatricians and general internists are considered intermediate primary care practitioners because their training has a major subspecialty focus. Other specialists are not considered primary care physicians because their training is focused on subspecialty issues.

3. **Financial Access to Care**
   Universal government-sponsored national health insurance or a national health entitlement is considered most conducive to access to primary care services. National health insurance sponsored by nongovernmental agencies is considered intermediate because of the absence of uniform benefits. Absence of national health insurance is not considered conducive to access to primary care.

4. **Percentage of Active Physicians Who Are Specialists**
   A value below 50% is considered indicative of an orientation toward primary care. Values of 50% to 75% are considered intermediate, and values above 75% are considered to indicate a specialty-oriented system.

5. **Salary of Primary Care Physicians Relative to Specialists**
   A high ratio (0.9:1 or above) is considered an incentive toward a specialty-oriented system. Ratios between 0.8 and 0.9 are considered intermediate.

System characteristics not scored for primary care are where care is provided (since there is not evidence that one type of site is better than another), the type of reimbursement of generalists and of specialists (since the impact of type of reimbursement on incentives for primary care practice is unknown), whether or not generalists care for patients in hospitals (since there is little evidence on the impact of this feature of a health service system), and whether or not specialists are restricted to hospitals (since

*(continued)*

**Table 11.1. Rating Criteria** *(continued).*

consultations with primary care physicians might be enhanced by limited specialty practice in the community). Even though the assignment of primary care services to a defined geographic area is considered conducive to community orientation and hence potentially pursuant to high level primary care, no points are assigned since community orientation is assessed directly.

### Criteria for Rating Practice Characteristics Related to Primary Care

6. First Contact

   First contact implies that decisions about the need for specialty services are made after consulting the primary care physician. Requirements for access to specialists via referral from primary care are considered most consistent with the first-contact aspect of primary care. The ability of patients to self-refer to specialists is considered conducive to a specialty-oriented health system. Where there are incentives to reduce direct access to specialists but no requirement for a referral, an intermediate score is assigned.

7. Longitudinality

   Longitudinality connotes the extent of relationship with a practitioner or facility over time that is not based on the presence of specific types of diagnoses or health problems. Highest ratings are given where the relationship is based on enrollment with a source of primary care, with the intent that all nonreferred or nondelegated care will be provided by the practitioner. Lowest rates are given where there is not an implicit or explicit relationship over time and intermediate scores are assigned where this relationship exists by default rather than intent.

8. Comprehensiveness

   The extent to which a full range of services is either directly provided by the primary care physician or specifically arranged for elsewhere is the measure of comprehensiveness. Highest ratings are given to arrangements for the universal provision of extensive and uniform benefits and for preventive care. Intermediate ratings are given to arrangements for the provision of either extensive benefits or preventive care, or for concerted efforts to improve these for needy segments of the population. Low ratings are given when there is no policy regarding a minimum uniform set of benefits.

9. Coordination

   Care is considered coordinated where there are formal guidelines for the transfer of information between primary care physicians and specialists. Where this is present for only certain aspects of care (such as long-term care), intermediate ratings are given. Low ratings reflect the general absence of guidelines for the transfer of information about patients.

Table 11.1. Rating Criteria *(continued)*.

10. Family-Centeredness

High ratings are given to explicit assumption of responsibility for family-centered care. Only one point is assigned to this characteristic, however, since it is related (although not necessarily identical) to the type of primary care physician.

11. Community Orientation

High ratings are given where practitioners use community data in planning for services or for the identification of problems. Intermediate values are assigned where clinical data derived from analysis of data from the practice are used to identify priorities for care. Low ratings are given when there is little or no attempt to use data or organize services.

Twelve indicators of health obtained from reliable sources[14–17] were used to compare the countries: neonatal mortality, postneonatal mortality, total infant mortality, age-adjusted death rate, average life expectancy at age 1 year for males and females separately, average life expectancy at age 20 years for males and females separately, average life expectancy at age 65 years for males and females separately, years of potential life lost, and percentage of birth weights below 2500 g. All of these indicators are relatively standard indicators of health. The only one that may require special explanation is years of potential life lost, because it may not be widely known. It reflects that component of mortality occurring before age 65 years that is considered preventable.[16,17] All data on health indicators were from the mid-1980s except for average life expectancy at ages 1 year and 20 years (1980) and low birth weight (1983 or 1894). The data on each indicator were almost always from the same year for every country. Greater detail regarding each indicator is in Starfield.[18]

To summarize the findings for the health indicators, each country was categorized as being in the upper third, middle third, or lower third of the distribution for all 10 countries. Sometimes there were three countries and sometimes four in the bottom third, depending on whether the adjacent countries had very similar values. In the case of the top third, there were sometimes only two countries because they had values far better than the middle group, which had values very close together. For example, the rates of infant mortality ranged from 5.85 to 10.35 per 1000 live births. Finland and Sweden had values of 5.85 and 5.93 per 1000 live births, respectively, whereas the countries in the middle third had values of 7.76, 7.88, 8.19, 8.54, and 8.85 per 1000 live births. The countries in the bottom third had values of 9.55, 9.69 and 10.35 per 1000 live births.

All characteristics reflected the situation existing in the middle to late 1980s.

Additional details concerning the components of the items, the methods of scoring, and the raw data on the scoring of the primary care components and the levels of each of the health indicators can be found in Starfield[18] or obtained from the author.

# RESULTS

The primary care scores ranged from 0.2 in the United States to 1.7 in the United Kingdom. Scores for the other countries were as follows: West Germany, 0.5; Belgium, 0.8; Australia, 1.1; Canada and Sweden, 1.2; and the Netherlands, Denmark, and Finland, 1.5.

The satisfaction-expense index ranged from 0.2 in the United States to 9.0 in the Netherlands. Intermediate values were obtained for the United Kingdom and Australia, 2.1; West Germany, 2.9; Sweden, 4.3; and Canada, 7.6. These data were not available for Belgium, Denmark, and Finland.

Table 11.2 summarizes the position of each country with regard to the health indicators. The United States was in the top third of the distribution for only one indicator—life expectancy at age 65 years for men, in the bottom third for seven of the 12 indicators, and in the middle third for four—life expectancy at ages 1, 20, and 65 years for females and age-adjusted death rate.

West Germany was in the top third for one indicator (neonatal mortality rate), in the bottom third for seven indicators, and in the middle third for four indicator conditions (infant mortality, age-adjusted mortality, years of potential life lost, and the percentage of infants born at low birth weight).

Canada ranked in the top third for five indicators: age-adjusted death rate and life expectancy at ages 1, 20, and 65 years for females and at age 65 years for men. For the remainder of the seven indicators, Canada ranked in the middle third.

The Netherlands and Sweden ranked in the top third for all 12 indicators; only Australia, Canada, the Netherlands, and Sweden had no conditions for which they were in the bottom third of the distribution for the 10 countries.

The United Kingdom had no indicator conditions in the top third of the distribution and eight in the bottom third. The only conditions in the middle third of the distribution were neonatal mortality, life expectancy at age 1 year and 20 years for males, and years of potential life lost.

Figure 11.1 summarizes the relationship between the ranking for the primary care score, the satisfaction-expense index, and the health indicators for each of the seven countries for which all three were available. There is a general tendency for the three indicators to relate to each other. That is, where the primary care score is high, so are the satisfaction-expense index and the number of indicator conditions in the top third of the distribution, while the number of indicator conditions in the bottom third of the distribution is low. The major exception was the United Kingdom, which had the highest primary care score but a low

**Table 11.2. Health Indicator Status by Country.**

| | Health Indicators[a] | |
| Countries | Top Third | Bottom Third |
| --- | --- | --- |
| Australia | 3 | 0 |
| Belgium | 0 | 9 |
| Canada | 5 | 0 |
| Denmark | 0 | 3 |
| Finland | 5 | 6 |
| West Germany | 1 | 7 |
| Netherlands | 10 | 0 |
| Sweden | 10 | 0 |
| United Kingdom | 0 | 8 |
| United States | 1 | 7 |

[a]These columns present the number of indicators for which the country falls in the top (best) third of the distribution and the number for which it falls in the bottom (worst) third. Sometimes there were 3 and sometimes 4 countries in the bottom third, depending on whether or not the countries had very similar values on the indicator. In the case of the top third, there were sometimes only 2 countries because they had values far better than the middle group, which had values very close to each other. Although there were 31 indicators in all (including separate breakdowns by age and sex), comparable information was available for all countries for only 12 of the indicators (excluding death rates from injuries and natural causes by individual child age group, and immunization rates). Similar ratings are obtained, however, when the other indicators are added and used for comparisons among countries for which they were available.

satisfaction-expense index, no conditions in the top third of the distribution, and a large number of conditions in the lowest third of the distribution.

# COMMENT

There are several potential limitations of these analyses. The findings are from one point in time only, during the middle to late 1980s. The analyses are descriptive and, in part, based on judgments rather than precise measurements of primary care. The data concerning the health indicators assume accuracy of those indicators and the divisions of the indicators into thirds could only be roughly accomplished.

Nevertheless, the data stem from multiple independent sources which confirm each other. The ranking of the countries on those indicators for which more

**Figure 11.1.** Indicators of Health, Primary Care, and Satisfaction and Expense.

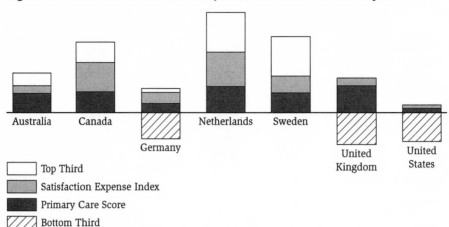

Notes: The top third and the bottom third of the distribution contain the number of indicators for which the country was in that third. The ratings for the primary care score were multiplied by 4 to make their ranges comparable with the other two indicators. The satisfaction-expense ratio for the United States was 0.2.

recent data are available (such as infant mortality) remain the same. The data on health indicators are from reliable published sources, such as the World Health Organization, the Organization for Economic Cooperation and Development, the National Center for Health Statistics, and the Centers for Disease Control.[14–17] The characterization of the countries as high, middle, or low for each of the health indicators was essentially the same when they were characterized by having clearly extreme values on the top or bottom of the distribution or when the countries were ranked and arbitrary cuts were made so that four countries were always in the top third and four in the bottom third of the distribution. That is, the United States, the United Kingdom, and West Germany were low in their standing, whereas the Netherlands, Sweden, and Canada were high in their standing.

The anomalous position of the United Kingdom, with its high primary care score and low ranking on the health indicators, bears comment. The United Kingdom has the lowest per capita spending on health of all of the countries studied. However, per capita spending does not guarantee high performance on the health indicators, as the United States has by far the highest level of spending of all of the countries. Another possible explanation derives from the observation that the United Kingdom and the United States are the only two countries of the 10 studied that are in the lowest third of the distribution both for the percentage of central government expenditures for housing, social security, and welfare, and for education.[19] Although the United Kingdom, the United States, and West Germany are in the top third of the distribution for the percentage of central governmental expenditures for health, there appears to be little relationship between this indicator and levels of health. Access to primary care services may have little impact on health when other social services are underdeveloped and where resources for public education are relatively inadequate.

The findings of this study have implications for the public debate on appropriate models for modifying the financing and organization of health services in the United States. The specialty orientation of the system and underdevelopment of the primary health care system in this country are well recognized.[20] Financial barriers to services in the absence of national health insurance and restrictions in coverage of many existing health insurance policies exacerbate the limitations on access to primary care.

Alternative explanations for the apparent relationship between the level of health indicators and the extent of development of the primary care sector are not readily evident. One commonly expressed view is that the heterogeneity of U.S. population is responsible for its relatively low health levels when compared with the more homogeneous populations of many other industrialized countries. Other analyses have shown that most of the other countries in this study also have substantial minority populations, including the Lapps in Finland, the native American population in Canada, and the foreign workers who have immigrated into many central and northern European countries.[21] At the very least, the findings of this study should indicate the need for consideration of both health levels and the adequacy of the primary care sector when competing systems are debated as possible models for this country.

## Notes

1. Letter from Senator John Heinz to the General Accounting Office; February 12, 1990.

2. U.S. Bipartisan Commission on Comprehensive Health Care (Pepper Commission). *A Call for Action.* Washington, DC: US Senate; September 1990.

3. Stephen WJ. *An Analysis of Primary Medical Care: An International Study.* New York: Cambridge University Press; 1979.

4. Swedish Health Services. *Primary Healthcare Today: Some International Comparisons.* Stockholm: Swedish Health Services; 1981. Publication HS90.

5. Schroeder SA. Western European responses to physician oversupply: lessons for the United States. *JAMA.* 1984;252:373–384.

6. Fry J, Hasler J. *Primary Health Care 2000.* New York: Churchill Livingstone; 1986.

7. Weiner J. Primary care delivery in the United States and four northwest European countries: comparing the "corporatized" with the "socialized." *Milbank Q.* 1987;65:426–461.

8. Iglehart, J. Germany's health care system. *N Engl J Med.* 1991;324:503–508.

9. Millis JS. *The Graduate Education of Physicians: Report of the Citizens Commission on Graduate Medical Education.* Chicago: American Medical Association; 1966:37.

10. Alpert J, Charney E. *The Education of Physicians for Primary Care.* Rockville, Md: Public Health Service, Health Resources Administration; 1974.

11. Institute of Medicine. *A Manpower Policy for Primary Health Care.* Washington, DC: National Academy Press; 1978.

12. Blendon R, Leitman R, Morrison I, Donelan K. Satisfaction with health systems in ten nations. *Health Aff.* 1990;9:185–192.

13. Hellander I, Wolfe S. Which countries are satisfied with their health care? *Health Lett.* 1990;6(8):9–10.

14. World Health Organization. *World Statistics Annual.* Geneva, Switzerland: World Health Organization; 1986.

15. Organization for Economic Cooperation and Development. *Living Conditions in OECD Countries.* Paris, France: Organization for Economic Cooperation and Development; 1986.

16. Centers for Disease Control. Premature mortality in the United States. *MMWR.* 1986;35:29–31.

17. Centers for Disease Control. Mortality in developed countries. *MMWR.* 1990;39:205–209.

18. Starfield B. *Primary Care: Concept, Evaluation, and Policy.* New York: Oxford University Press; 1992.

19. World Bank. *World Development Report, 1990.* New York: Oxford University Press; 1990.

20. Beeson P. Too many specialists, too few generalists. *Pharos.* 1991;54:2–6.

21. Williams B, Miller A. *Preventive Health Care for Young Children: Findings from a 10-Country Study and Directions for United States Policy.* Arlington, Va: National Center for Clinical Infant Programs; 1991.

CHAPTER TWELVE

# Primary Care in a New Era: Disillusion and Dissolution?

Lewis G. Sandy, M.D.; Steven A. Schroeder, M.D.

2003

For decades, health policy experts have bemoaned the beleaguered status of primary care. Rather than building our health care system based on "provision of integrated, accessible health care services by clinicians who are accountable for addressing a large majority of personal health care needs, developing sustained partnerships with patients, and practicing in the context of family and community,"[1] our health care system continues to emphasize technologically oriented specialty care.

While this contrast is unremarkable, given the long-standing pro-specialty biases in our medical payment and education systems,[2,3] what is perhaps more surprising is that primary care seems more precarious than ever, even as forces thought to promote it continue to strengthen. Managed care, with its emphasis on cost-effective care for populations, was envisioned by many as a major stimulus to promote primary care. Medical school curricula have evolved to place greater emphasis on early exposures to patients, longitudinal clinical experiences, and clinical clerkships with community-based physicians, all of which are thought to increase interest in primary care.

Yet primary care residency matches were down 3.8% in 2001, the fourth straight year of decline.[4] Graduating medical student interest in generalism declined from 40% in 1997 to 32% in 2000[5] (see Figure 12.1). Primary care

---

This chapter originally appeared as Sandy LG, Schroeder SA. Primary care in a new era: disillusion and dissolution? *Ann Intern Med.* 2003;138:262–267. Copyright © 2003, American College of Physicians–American Society of Internal Medicine. Reprinted with permission.

physicians feel beleaguered, and evidence of a primary care "backlash" is emerging among students and medical school faculty.

We suggest that the current dilemmas in primary care stem from the unintended consequences of forces thought to promote primary care, and the "disruptive technologies of care" that attack the very concept of primary care itself. These forces, in combination with "tiering" in the health insurance market, could cause the dissolution of primary care as a single concept, replaced by alignment of providers by economic niche, not role.

## THE ASSAULT ON PRIMARY CARE

Ironically, primary care is being assaulted by forces that had been thought to be friendly to it—managed care and medical education reform. The growth of managed care, particularly capitation, would, the theory went, create new incentives for primary care, by increasing income, status, and reputation and promoting comprehensive and cost-effective care. Under capitation, primary care providers would reap real financial rewards for providing continuous, comprehensive, high quality care by reducing unneeded procedures, hospitalizations, and specialty services. Medical education reform, with an emphasis on early patient care experiences and curriculum changes beyond biomedical science, would also promote primary care.

In reality, although managed care dominated the market, payment policy perpetuated a discounted fee-for-service financing system. Few physicians could

**Figure 12.1.** Interest in Generalist Specialities Among Graduating Medical Students, 1984–2000.

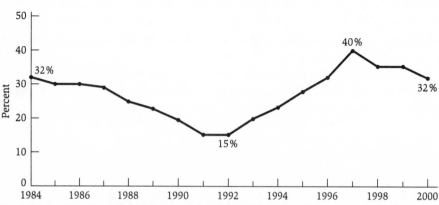

*Source:* Association of American Medical Colleges. *1996 AAMC Medical School Graduation Questionnaire.* Washington, DC: Association of American Medical Colleges; 1996.

actually manage care under capitation financing, and the managed care marketplace evolved such that most health maintenance organizations (HMOs) paid physicians discounted fee-for-service rates, as did preferred provider organizations (PPOs). As a result, in 1999 the average physician derived only 17% of revenues from capitation.[6] Thus, neither enhanced income nor incentives for cost-effective care came to pass as a result of managed care. The technology-intensive biases of fee-for-service payment continue to penalize physicians with less resort to technology (see Figure 12.2).

Nonetheless, consumer and provider anger over "gatekeeper" arrangements and highly publicized limitations on care in HMOs caused a managed care backlash in which primary care was swept up. Consumers equated "quality" with "choice" and began to frame primary care as a barrier to quality, not as an enhancer.

**Figure 12.2**. Mean Annual Physician Net Income After Expenses and Before Taxes, 1981–1998 (in real dollars).

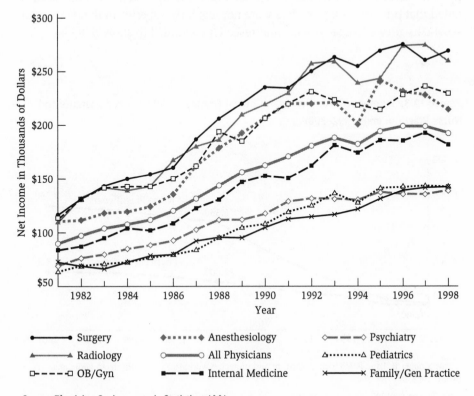

*Source:* Physician Socioeconomic Statistics, AMA.

Moreover, managed care promoted "disruptive technologies" in primary care, creating new challenges. As described by Christensen, Bohmer, and Kenagy in their widely cited *Harvard Business Review* paper "Will Disruptive Innovations Cure Health Care?"[7] "disruptive" innovation in a field occurs from below when less expensive approaches enable a product or service to be delivered faster, better, or cheaper. Managed care promoted the growth of nurse practitioner and physician assistant programs, both to enhance the productivity of physician practice and to offer a more cost-effective form of primary care itself. From 1992 to 1997, this group of health professionals doubled, and further growth is anticipated[8] (see Figure 12.3).

Managed care also created the need for hospitals and medical groups to become more efficient in inpatient care, giving rise to the hospitalist movement.[9,10] While the debate continues on the virtues of hospitalists, clearly the hospitalist movement created an "alternative pathway" for internists interested in a broad practice that crosses subspecialty boundaries. By 1999, 65% of internists had hospitalists in their community,[11] and the hospitalist movement is projected to grow significantly.[12,13]

Most devastatingly, the policy promise that primary care could increase quality and reduce health care costs was not supported by evidence. Some studies noted that primary care providers were not regularly superior in the delivery of secondary preventive services,[14] and research continued to show that—not sur-

**Figure 12.3.** Number of Nonphysician Clinical Graduates (Physician Assistants and Nurse Practitioners), 1992–2001.

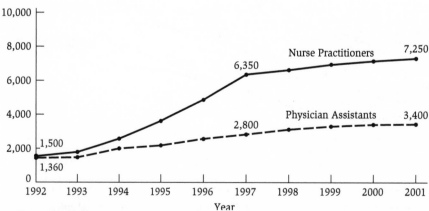

*Source:* Cooper R, Laud P, Dietrich C. Current and projected workforce of nonphysician clinicians. *JAMA.* 1998;280:788–794.

*Note:* Figures for 1998–2001 are estimates.

prisingly—specialists are more current in their practices than primary care physicians.[15] Managed care's use of discounts and the health insurance underwriting cycle succeeded in moderating health care costs in the mid- to late 1990s—an important object lesson suggesting that market forces independent of primary care can attack cost inflation.[16]

Primary care fared scarcely better within the walls of academe. Although many medical schools revised their overt curricula to achieve a better balance between generalism and specialism, the "hidden" curriculum that serves powerfully to socialize learners continued to promote subspecialty training and tertiary care. The population-based approaches of the best managed care organizations, some of which worked in partnership with academic health centers, were overshadowed by more aggressive health plans with limited interest in social mission.[17]

Finally, the 21st century began with some fundamental dynamics in place in the U.S. health care system: (1) "managed care" hasn't succeeding in improving the cost, quality, and access issues its advocates envisioned; (2) health care costs are bound to escalate in years ahead, driven by demographic forces and new technologies; (3) the public has a powerful appetite for health care that shows no signs of abating; and (4) public policy is adrift, with no coherent strategy in evidence.

## Primary Care Circa 2001: Excess Supply Meets Tiered Demand

These factors have combined with the unique dynamics among the health professions to create greater primary care supply than demand. The growth in the overall number of physicians has led the Council on Graduate Medical Education (COGME) and other policy bodies to the new view that no significant shortage of primary care providers currently exists.[18] For nonphysician primary care providers, the promise of prestige and access to reimbursement has resulted in dramatic growth in the supply of nurse practitioners and physician assistants providing primary care[19] (see Table 12.1). Nurses in particular may find the troubled landscape of primary care a relative nirvana when compared with the problems facing "regular" hospital nursing practice. Nursing leaders, consequently, have emphasized attainment of advanced credentials and training to increase nursing's prestige and scope.[20]

These nonphysician providers, in turn, are augmented by both a wide variety of other health professionals providing "alternative medicine" and by specialists delivering principal care to their patients with a single chronic condition.

While the majority of those with private health insurance are in "loose" managed care arrangements, such as open-network HMOs and PPOs, these arrangements offer little prospect of reining in costs over the long haul. Indeed, after several years of moderation in health care costs, both health insurance premiums and underlying costs increased at nearly double-digit rates in 2000.[21]

Table 12.1. Reimbursement of Nurse Practitioners and Physician Assistants, 1998

| | Medicaid Reimbursement | Private Insurance Mandates[a] | Medicare Reimbursement |
|---|---|---|---|
| Nurse Practitioners | 48 States | 29 States | Yes |
| Physician Assistants | 49 States | 3 States | Yes |

Source: McDonnell K et al. EBRI Databook on Employee Benefits. Washington, DC: Employee Benefit Research Institute; 1997:244.

[a]Shows the number of states that have enacted mandates that require private insurers to offer the services of various nonphysician clinician disciplines.

Most analysts believe that employees will gradually assume a greater burden of cost sharing over time and that should the economy go into prolonged recession, employees will face far greater cost sharing and will have to pay a significant premium for the open access to wide networks that many currently enjoy.[22]

Consequently, lower-income workers may increasingly "tier" into tightly managed HMOs, while higher-paid workers will prefer to pay for greater flexibility. Preliminary evidence suggests that this is already occurring. Gabel et al. found that workers in high-wage firms tend to enroll in PPOs and POS-type HMOs (which tend to cost more), while low-wage firms tend to offer traditional HMO coverage (which costs less).[23] Similarly, the percentage of Medicaid recipients in managed care has increased from 10% in 1991 to 56% in 2000.[24] This tiering, predicted some time ago by Reinhardt,[25] has become the common wisdom among health care futurists.[26]

As the system tightens for middle- and low-income groups, however, the affluent, particularly empowered aging baby boomers, will demand not only free choice of provider but also the highest level of customer service. Already, some practices offer a "medical concierge" service where physicians are only a cell phone away 24/7; others offer "integrative" medical practices, which combine traditional Western medicine with acupuncture, massage therapy, aromatherapy, and other adjunctive treatments.

In summary, the under-65-year-old health insurance and patient markets will in all likelihood begin to "tier" into three tiers. The top tier will be the affluent, with full coverage and/or the ability to pay out of pocket. The middle tier will be the middle-class or upper-middle-class employee, with some choice but significant cost-sharing; the bottom tier will include low-income workers, Medicaid patients, and the uninsured.

## Medicare: Tiering's "Wild Card"

Will Medicare tier like the private insurance market? Medicare managed care grew significantly in the mid-1990s, driven by consumer demand for coverage of prescription drugs. Recently, however, Medicare HMOs have begun to exit certain markets; enrollment in Medicare HMOs declined from a peak of 6.1 million enrollees in 1999 to 5.5 million as of December 2001.[27] To the extent that Medicare remains static, its nontiered, fee-for-service-oriented approach would provide a countervailing force against tiering.

It is unlikely, however, that Medicare will remain in its current form over the long haul. First, pressures exist to expand Medicare to include prescription drug coverage and cover the near-elderly uninsured. Second, both government and market-oriented policy experts believe that Medicare requires revamping to move from a structure modeled on 1960s health insurance benefits and financing to one that supports introduction of practices to improve quality and control costs.[28]

The most likely future direction of Medicare reform will be in the general direction outlined by the 1999 Bipartisan Commission on the Future of Medicare. The commission, although it did not make an official recommendation to Congress, had a majority in favor of a "premium support" model, in which the government would pay a fixed, risk-adjusted premium to plans, thereby exposing consumers to the cost impact of their choice of plans and providers.[29] The commission's views clearly indicate a consensus, first, to move Medicare toward greater use of competitive markets and, second, to create greater price sensitivity among consumers. Both of these forces, if actualized, would increase the likelihood of significant tiering in our health care system.

# PRIMARY CARE IN A TIERED MARKETPLACE

If the marketplace does evolve in this fashion, the function and approach of primary care could vary significantly by tier. In each tier, the epidemiology of disease and risk, the expectations of the provider, and the supporting financial incentives and drivers will vary. These variations will begin to splinter primary care itself, in terms of both what is done and who does it. As this occurs, the very notion of "primary care" as a unified field of practice, applied in varying circumstances, faces the prospect of dissolution, superseded by an orientation to economic niche.

## Upper-Tier Primary Care: The Full-Service Broker

Just as the affluent engage the services of their accountant, stockbroker, and personal trainer, they will engage health professionals in the same manner and expect the same level of service. Baby boomers will spend their earned and inherited wealth to bypass the usual hassles of medical care practice. They will expect to reach their physician quickly by cell phone, fax, e-mail, or the Internet. They will expect their provider to offer customized syntheses of information and to arrange their visits to a preferred subspecialist. The "medical concierge" will grow as a niche, most likely as an adjunct service to high-end single-specialty or multispecialty groups. Providers will begin to offer comprehensive "wellness" programs, building off current executive physical fitness programs and "lifestyle" programs such as Canyon Ranch, a luxury spa that now offers medical services.

These providers will be continually thinking about how to enhance both service quality and revenues. One could envision attempts to brand these programs or develop franchises—consider the current value of the brand of internationally know wellness gurus Andrew Weil or Deepak Chopra. Most likely, high-end specialty practices will begin to add primary care not because they believe in the basic concept but as a way to attract and retain patients—in marketing, this is known as a wraparound, loss-leader service.

## Middle-Tier Primary Care: Responsive Advocate or Diffident Bureaucrat?

This tier will most dramatically feel the tug between retaining classic concepts of professional autonomy and obligation to the patient versus accommodating to the bureaucratic reality of contemporary medical practice. These strains can already be observed in large multispecialty groups and in prepaid group practices. Providers will want to provide high-quality comprehensive care, coordination, and continuity. On the other hand, they will also attempt to maintain their income and preferred work style while continually struggling with demands placed on them by insurers, regulators, and patients. They will be asked by demanding patients to provide the same level of service as in the upper tier, without commensurate reimbursement. To adapt to these tensions, the more innovative will explore new team arrangements for care, group visits, or some forms of technology assistance. New services will spring up to help offload some of the burden on these providers. For example, providers can now buy a practice newsletter off-the-shelf, adding some customized information for their practice. Providers may "outsource" their e-mail and telephone queries from patients, utilizing existing nurse triage services, essentially buying round-the-clock "customer support." Physician Web site companies will offer a range of services, competing with vendors supplying electronic medical record systems and handheld prescription-writing devices.

On the other hand, as they practice from day to day and month to month, fighting with indifferent insurance companies and attempting to satisfy demanding patients, burnout and loss will be close to the surface for many physicians. Some will find renewal in new developments in their practice such as technology enhancements or in building communications skills. Others will become diffident bureaucrats, going through the motions, but seeking satisfaction in family and outside interests, viewing medicine more as a job than a calling.

### Lower-Tier Primary Care: The Community-Oriented Primary Care Advocate

As the second-tier physicians struggle to meet personal and professional goals, low-income patients will find access to care increasingly difficult. In most locales, low-income populations will become even more concentrated in safety-net hospitals and existing community health centers.

Primary care in these tiers will increasingly be thought of as a social mission. Physicians entering this tier will have no illusion as to their income possibilities and will be attracted to the possibility of community-oriented primary care or their role as social advocates. Providers in this tier will become less connected to primary care and more aligned with advocacy movements for social justice. They will join Health Care for All, not the ACP or the ASIM.

Further, these physicians will begin to bridge medicine and public health. Working with vulnerable populations, they will readily observe the impact that community, social, and economic factors play in the health of their patients and will work at the community level with public health advocates on issues of violence, substance abuse, lack of economic opportunity, and racism.

Clearly, these physicians will find the practice of primary care different from physicians in higher tiers. Their organizations will have far greater public than private financing, their personal incomes will be lower, and they may be happier. The teams needed to provide care in this tier will be broader in scope and function, including not only health professionals but also community health advocates, community organizers, and local community leaders.

# IMPLICATIONS FOR PRIMARY CARE

As the marketplace evolves, practitioners will increasingly begin to align with their economic niche, not their specialty domain. For example, an upper-tier wellness practice will have more in common with an upper-tier cardiology group that with a lower-tier practice. Thus, whatever current solidarity exists within and among primary care disciplines will begin to erode over time. Accelerating this will be greater income stratification within primary care, with the greatest income growth naturally occurring in the upper tier. This emergence of a "class" distinction in primary care will further erode solidarity.

Each of the primary care disciplines will face unique challenges. For family medicine, its orientation to families and communities will lead it to populate the middle and lower tiers, although a few will take their discipline's holistic approach to the upper-tier "wellness" market. For general pediatrics, those in the top tier niche will need to develop novel ways to provide the level of service expected while developing a sustainable "business model" for practice. For example, upper-tier pediatricians may begin to bill for phone consultation but also send nurses to the schools and soccer fields in affluent communities.

General internal medicine faces the most daunting challenges for the future. Though patients with complex and chronic illnesses will be concentrated in the middle and lower tiers, few internal medicine residencies have developed a training model for practice in either a bureaucratic organization or in a low-income community. Some upper-tier internists will develop and market their acumen around complex areas of medical decision making. Although the aging of the population will increase the population base for GIM, general internists will also be competing with specialists for these patients. Indeed, falling age-specific disability rates[30] suggest that "healthy aging" could be better for plastic surgeons than for internists. In order to survive and even thrive, general internists in the middle and lower tiers will need to develop competencies and practice styles much closer to family medicine, since family medicine's training model, which emphasizes family and community context and a biopsychosocial model of care, is more congruent with this tier's practice realities. Another niche for general internists will also be the management of multiple, complex, and chronic conditions, a practice that will blur the specialty boundary between GIM and geriatrics.

# IMPLICATIONS FOR THE FUTURE

If these predictions about the future organization and financing of care come to pass, clear implications for the immediate future exist. First, how managed care evolves will have a major impact on the future of primary care. If managed care returns to a tightly managed gatekeeping model and retains its bureaucratic, low-customer service ethos, primary care will continue to be tarred by its brush. Given this, we can expect medical student interest in primary care to drop to the 20% levels seen in the early 1990s.

On the other hand, if managed care principles and practices evolve into "kinder and gentler" forms, through consumer pressure, regulation, or changes in payment policy, the middle tier will look much more promising. Providers could see the opportunity to use advanced information technology to rationalize their practices and make better use of their time and energy.

Second, primary care policy should concern itself less with workforce issues and more with macro-level organization and financing. A new consortium might begin analyzing the impact that Medicare reform, Health Insurance Portability and Accountability Act (HIPAA) regulations, patient bill of rights, or HMO lawsuits will have on primary care.

For all primary care providers, however, we see five major challenges embodied in this forecast. First, current training in primary care does not provide the requisite skills for effective practice in any of the tiers we describe. Major training enhancements in communications skills, information technology, working in teams, prevention, and behavior change counseling will be needed.[31]

Second, for primary care to survive as a construct in a new era, greater attention is needed for the essential "core values" of primary care. Perhaps primary care's overarching focus should be on values and ethos, not solely on functions, since these functions will vary significantly in the future. Just as all of medicine has sought to unify the profession by focusing on core values of professionalism, primary care may need to do the same.

Third, this analysis suggests the need to consider primary care as a function that could be delivered by specialty physicians, not just the "generalist specialties." Perhaps a new organization such as the "Society for Primary Care Practice," open to any specialty, should be developed.

Fourth, general internal medicine, and its relationship to primary care and to internal medicine, requires further thought. Simply put, the underlying conceptual basis of GIM, wherein the parent discipline of internal medicine is applied to the primary care of adults, is not tracking with either the changing marketplace for medical care or the evolution of internal medicine and the rise of the hospitalist movement.

Finally, like most ideas, primary care is a concept that must continue to have demonstrated utility—to the public, to the health professions, and to health care. The future segmentation of the market suggests that unless fundamental changes in training, acculturation, and professional development of those who practice primary care occur, as a concept it will be swept away by economic, demographic, and social forces.

## Notes

1. Donaldson MS, Yordy KD, Lohr KN, Vanselow NA, eds. Primary Care: *America's Health in a New Era*. Washington, DC: National Academic Press; 1996.

2. Schroeder SA, Showstack JA. Financial incentives to perform medical procedures and laboratory tests: illustrative models of office practice. *Med Care*. 1978;16:289–298.

3. Showstack JA, Blumberg BD, Schwartz J, Schroeder SA. Fee-for-service physician payment: analysis of current methods and their development. *Inquiry*. 1979;16:230–246.

4. Greene J. Primary care matches down again; fourth year of decline worries some. *Am Med News* [serial online]. 2001;1(1)[5 screens]. Available from: American Medical News, http://www.ama-assn.org/sci-pubs/amnews/pick_01/prse0409.htm. Accessed April 9, 2001.

5. Association of American Medical Colleges. *1996 AAMC Medical School Graduation Questionnaire.* Washington, DC: Association of American Medical Colleges; 1996.

6. Center for Studying Health System Change. Community tracking study physician survey, 1998–1999: [United States] [Computer file]. Washington, DC: Center for Studying Health System Change [producer], 2001.

7. Christensen CM, Bohner R, Kenagy J. Will disruptive innovations cure health care? *Harvard Bus Rev.* 2000;78:102–112.

8. Cooper RA. Current and projected workforce of nonphysician clinicians. *JAMA.* 1998;28:788–794.

9. Schroeder SA, Schapiro R. The hospitalist: new boon for internal medicine or retreat from primary care? *Ann Intern Med.* 1999;130(4, pt 2):382–387.

10. Wachter RM, Goldman L. The emerging role of "hospitalists" in the American health care system. *N Engl J Med.* 1996;335:514–517.

11. Auerbach AD, Nelson EA, Lindenauer PK, et al. Physician attitudes toward and prevalence of the hospitalist model of care: results of a national survey. *Am J Med.* 2000;109:648–653.

12. Lurie JD, Miller DP, Lindenauer PK, Wachter RM, Sox HC. The potential size of the hospitalist workforce in the United States. *Am J Med.* 1999;106:441–445.

13. Wachter RM, Goldman L. The hospitalist movement 5 years later. *JAMA.* 2002;287:487–494.

14. Chen J. Care and outcomes of elderly patients with acute myocardial infarction by physician specialty: the effects of comorbidity and functional limitations. *Am J Med.* 2000;108:460–469.

15. Solomon DH, Bates DW, Panush RS, Katz JN. Costs, outcomes and patient satisfactions by provider type for patients with rheumatic and musculoskeletal conditions: a critical review of the literature and proposed methodologic standards. *Ann Intern Med.* 1997;127:52–60.

16. Ginsberg P. Tracking health care costs: long-predicted upturn appears. *Center for Studying Health System Change Issue Brief.* 1999;23:1–4.

17. Firshein J, Sandy LG. The changing approach to managed care. In: Isaacs SL, Knickman JR, eds. *To Improve Health and Health Care: The Robert Wood Johnson Foundation Anthology.* San Francisco: Jossey-Bass; 2001:77–100.

18. Council on Graduate Medical Education. Summary of fourteenth report:COGME physician workforce policies: recent developments and remaining challenges in meeting national goals. Available from: Council on Graduate Medical Education, http://www.cogme.gov/rpt14.htm. Accessed November 19, 2001.

19. Cooper RA. Current and projected workforce of nonphysician clinicians. *JAMA.* 1998;28:788–794.

20. Mundinger MO. Advanced-practice nursing: good medicine for physicians? *N Engl J Med.* 1994;330:211–214.

21. Hogan C, Ginsburg PB, Gabel JR. Tracking health care costs: inflation returns. *Health Aff.* 2000;19:217–223.

22. Council on the Economic Impact of Health System Change. Renewed health care spending growth: implications and policy options. Available from: Council on the Economic Impact of Health System Change, http://ihp.brandeis.edu/council/html/spendingsum.htm. Accessed November 19, 2001.

23. Gabel J, Hurst K, Whitmore H, Hoffman C. Class and benefits at the workplace. *Health Aff.*1999;18:144–150.

24. Centers for Medicare and Medicaid Services. Medicaid managed care enrollment report: summary statistics as of June 30, 1995–June 30, 2000. Available from: Centers for Medicare and Medicaid, http://www.hcfa.gov/medicaid/mcaidsad.htm. Accessed November 8, 2001.

25. Reinhardt UE. Rationing health care: what it is, what it is not, and why we cannot avoid it. *Baxter Health Policy Rev.* 1996;2:63–99.

26. Grosel C, Hamilton, M, Koyano, J, Eastwood, S, eds. *Health and Health Care, 2010: The Forecast, the Challenge.* San Francisco: Jossey-Bass; 2000.

27. Centers for Medicare and Medicaid Services. Medicare Managed Care Contract (MMCC) plans monthly summary report, December 2001. Available from: Centers for Medicare and Medicaid, http://www.hcfa.gov/stats/monthly.htm. Accessed February 4, 2002.

28. Reischauer RD, Butler S, Lave, JR, eds. *Medicare: Preparing for the Challenges of the 21st Century.* Washington, DC: Brookings Institution; 1998.

29. Oberlander J. Is premium support the right medicine for Medicare? *Health Aff.* 2000;19:84–99.

30. Manton KG, Gu X. Changes in the prevalence of chronic disability in the United States: black and nonblack population above age 65 from 1982 to 1999. *Proc Natl Acad Sci USA.* 2001;98:6354–6359.

31. Yedidia MJ, Gillespie CC, Moore GT. Specific clinical competencies for managing care: views of residency directors and managed care medical directors. *JAMA.* 2000;284:1093–1098.

# Abstracts from the Literature

*Primary Care and the Role of Generalist Physicians*

## BOOKS AND REPORTS

Institute of Medicine. *Role of the Primary Care Physician in Occupational and Environmental Medicine.* Washington, DC: National Academy Press; 1988.

Institute of Medicine. *Primary Care: America's Health in a New Era.* Donaldson MS, Yordy KD, Lohr KN, Vanselow NA, eds. Washington, DC: National Academy Press; 1996. In early 1994, the Institute of Medicine appointed a study committee to consider the future of primary care chaired by Neal A. Vanselow, MD. This book presents the findings and recommendations of that committee which include a definition of primary care; an examination of the value, scope and nature of primary care; an analysis of primary care workforce trends and supply projections and the education and training of primary care practitioners, and suggestions for primary care research.

Pew Health Professions Commission. *Critical Challenges: Revitalizing the Health Professions for the Twenty-First Century.* San Francisco: Center for the Health Professions; 1995. This report is intended to be a guide to health care professionals, schools and governing policy bodies that direct their efforts in how to survive and thrive in a radically different health care world. It provides a broad assessment of the current state of reforms across the health professions, specific examples of those reforms, a set of recommendations, and an overall assessment of how far the overhaul of the health care system has come. Finally, the report makes recommendations generally for all health professionals and specifically for the fields of allied health practitioners, dentistry, medicine, pharmacy, public health, and nursing. Among its recommendations are decreasing the number of entrants to US medical schools by 20–25%; decreasing the number of pharmacy programs by 20–25% and nursing programs by 10–20%; tightening visa restrictions to assure that international medical graduates return to their home countries; and redirecting medical residencies so that 50% are in a primary care field.

Starfield B. *Primary Care: Balancing Health Needs, Services, and Technology.* Rev. ed. New York: Oxford University Press; 1998. This work examines the problems that arise in the implementation of effective primary health care. The book has four purposes: to help practitioners of primary care understand what they do and why; to provide a basis for the training of primary care practitioners; to stimulate research that will provide a more substantive basis for improvements in primary care; and to help policy makers understand the difficulties and challenges of primary care and its importance. The author addresses other important issues such as practitioner-patient communication, information systems and medical records, referral processes, personnel, managed care, financing, quality assessment and community orientation.

Stephens GG. *The Intellectual Basis of Family Practice.* Tucson: Winter Publishing; 1982. This collection of essays and presentations spans 15 years; it charts the development of the specialty of family practice and records the thinking of a man who has been at the forefront of this development. A theme running through the collection is a fundamental concern with the nature and role of the discipline of family practice in medicine and society.

World Health Organization. *Primary Health Care.* Report of the International Conference on Primary Health Care, Alma-Ata, Kazakh SSR, USSR, September 6–12, 1978. Geneva. A report on the historic Alma-Ata conference, jointly convened by WHO and UNICEF, that focused world attention on primary health care as the key to achieving an acceptable level of health throughout the world. Following an introductory chapter on the definition of primary health care, the report turns to topics of primary health care and development, operational aspects of primary health care, and national strategies and international support. Emphasis is placed on the importance of maximum community and individual self-reliance as the most reliable route to widespread, equitable, and sustained improvements in health.

# ARTICLES

Aiken LH, Lewis CE, Craig J, et al. The contribution of specialists to the delivery of primary care: A new perspective. *N Engl J Med.* 1979;300:1363–1370. This article reports on the results of two important studies. Based on these studies, the authors suggest that despite the current shortage of generalist physician services, continuing specialist participation in primary care will lead to sufficient generalist medical services by the mid-1980s. Whether specialist participation is the most appropriate or cost effective way to improve access to such care is unclear. Until this question is resolved, more governmental regulation of graduate medical education may be unwise. Offering all physicians more primary care experience during residency training might better deal with this aspect of American medical practice.

Alpert JJ. Providing primary pediatric care. *Postgrad Med J.* 1972;48:571–576. This article addresses three questions. First, does providing primary pediatric care make any difference to children and their families and can these differences be measured? Second, can primary pediatric care be described and can this help measure its quality? Third, are physicians, both general and pediatricians, being educated to deliver this care? Based on a survey of 1000 low income families in the Harvard Family Health Care Program (1972), the study found that primary pediatric care did not improve the short-term health of recipients, nor did it worsen it. Physician performance was measured in a limited way using a time-motion study on 50 experimental patients. There was significant variation between physicians in the style and content of their primary care practices (e.g. in the use of lab tests). With education concentrated in the hospital, physicians are not educated for primary care.

Alpert JJ. The future and primary care. *Pediatr Ann.* 1994;23:690–694. The author considers three pediatric megatrends that provide signposts for the 21st century: changing morbidity; the social, behavioral, and economic issues that children-at-risk will face; and spending limits. He examines why primary care is basic to the practice of medicine and discusses a definition of primary care first proposed by Alpert and Charney in 1973. He asks why we have failed to educate physicians as generalists and he argues that the hospital environment where education takes place was never designed for primary care. He suggests short-term strategies for correcting the primary care crisis, including increasing the non-physician role and educating more advanced nurse practitioners and physicians' assistants to deliver primary care; improving the work environment, reforming insurance, simplifying billing; increasing the income of the generalist; and changing medical education to make it more pertinent to practice. Long-term mechanisms include increasing reimbursement for primary care residencies and not funding subspecialties. He concludes with the idea that the future of primary care will be determined not just by what happens within the medical school setting, but also by what happens outside and that complex and large medical and social issues also need to be addressed.

Alpert JJ, Friedman RH, Green LA. Education of generalists: three tries a century is all we get! *J Gen Intern Med.* 1994;9(4 Suppl.1):S4–S6. The crisis in health care delivery presents a third opportunity to address the inadequate emphasis on generalism in the US medical system. The first opportunity occurred after World War II and led to experimental programs in comprehensive care. The second opportunity took place in the 1960s after a series of reports called for a national commitment to the education of "personal," "family," or "primary care" physicians. It led to the creation of family practice as a recognized specialty and federal support for departments of family medicine. A national focus on health reform offers a third opportunity. The authors conclude that the challenge is to create a system where specialists and generalists can coexist in a complementary balance and to restore generalism to its appropriate role in fulfilling the nation's primary care needs.

Altman DF. Revising the definition of the generalist physician. *Acad Med.* 1995;70: 1087–1090. Despite the growing recognition of the important role of generalist physician in the US, the author contends that there has been insufficient discussion of who generalists are and how their role is defined. Traditionally, generalists have been defined by their specialty, with physicians in general medicine, general internal medicine, and general pediatrics considered generalists. This approach, however, may not sufficiently recognize the specific competencies and therefore the specific training required of generalists. A new definition is based on the functional requirements of general practice and the central role that generalist physicians will play in comprehensive care.

Bindman AB. Primary and managed care: ingredients for health care reform. *West J Med,* 1994; 161:78–82. The author reviews the definition of primary care and the primary care physician, and shows how this delivery model can affect access to medical care, the cost of treatment, and the quality of services. To understand the delivery of primary care services and because the use of primary care is often greater in managed care environments than fee-for-service, the author compares the two insurance systems. Research suggests that primary care can help meet the goal of providing accessible, cost-effective, and high quality care, but that changes in medical education and marketplace incentives will be needed to encourage students and trained physicians to enter this field.

Block SD, Clark-Chiarelli N, Peters AS, Singer JD. Academia's chilly climate for primary care. *JAMA.* 1996;276:677–682. This study describes the attitudes toward and perceptions of primary care education and practice among academic health center constituents. Based on 2,293 telephone interviews with medical students and residents, faculty and administrators, the researchers found that respondents generally perceived primary care tasks as not requiring high levels of expertise; nearly half believed that generalists are not the best physicians to manage patients with serious illness, and that the quality of primary care research is inferior to that in other fields. The respondents also viewed the quality of their primary care training as inferior to that of specialty practice. The study concludes that despite changes in health care and education, students and residents encounter an atmosphere chilly towards primary care.

Brown JW, Robertson LS, Kosa J, Alpert JJ. A study of general practice in Massachusetts. *JAMA.* 1971;216:301–306. A study of 12,835 patient visits to 15 Massachusetts's general practitioners indicated that while illness was the reason for 75% of the visits, non-sickness accounted for 25% of the diagnoses. Fifty-two percent had multiple diagnoses and 20% raised problems about other family members. The study found that the youngest physicians had the highest percentage of younger patients. Study findings suggest that some tasks proposed for the new family physician are being accomplished although none of the participating physicians were trained for family medicine. Future family physicians will almost certainly require different training if they are to effectively respond to patient needs.

Budetti PP. Achieving a uniform federal primary care policy: opportunities presented by National Health Reform. *JAMA*. 1993;269:498–501. This article considers the obstacles to a coherent and consistent federal policy toward primary care and suggests possible ways to overcome them. The effects of the existing de facto policies are identified across four areas: education and training, physician payment, the service delivery system, and research. The author makes recommendations for developing a new federal primary care policy: (1) physician payment should incorporate incentives such as those used under the Medicare Resource Based Relative Value Schedule; (2) Graduate Medical Education payments should incorporate incentives that encourage an enhanced role for primary care residents; (3) changes in the health care delivery system, including the expansion of support for comprehensive primary care sites, should be more favorable to primary care; and (4) primary care research should be an integral aspect of outcomes and effectiveness research.

Eisenberg JM. Sculpture of a new academic discipline: four faces of academic general internal medicine. *Am J Med*. 1985;78:283–292. The author provides a commentary on the development of general internal medicine as an academic discipline. He describes four roles that its members have begun to play: primary care clinician-educator, secondary care clinician educator, clinical investigators, and generalists with an area of clinical expertise. The author observes that academic general internal medicine will need all the roles if it is to create a strong discipline. The challenge is diversification without disintegration.

Eisenberg JM. The internist as gatekeeper: preparing the general internist for a new role. *Ann Intern Med*. 1985;102:537–543. To reduce health care costs, some third party payers have enlisted primary care physicians as gatekeepers to medical care, where these physicians must approve all care provided to their patients. Payment for a medical service is conditional on the approval of the primary care physician, with the exception of a true emergency. This idea, sometimes called the case manager plan, extends the role of primary care physician from coordination to control of medical care. For the plan to stimulate cost effective medical care, it must overcome obstacles that threaten its ability to save money and provide high quality medical care. In addition, medical educators must ensure that the necessary attitudes, skills and knowledge are taught to students of internal medicine in order to perform this role.

Eisenberg JM. Cultivating a new field: development of a research program in general internal medicine. *J Gen Intern Med*. 1986;1(4 Suppl):S8–S18. This article presents the opinions of 15 leaders in general internal medicine about the factors that lead to the successful development of an individual's research career. He characterizes them under three headings: personal attributes, research design skills and the research environment. In addition to reporting the results of an informal survey, the author gives his personal views on what he considers to be two overrated factors— "protected time" and "local laboratory of clinical practice" and one underrated factor—learning to be a research manager. He then goes on to offer thoughts on how section chiefs and chairmen can develop active research programs in general internal medicine, and how to obtain funding for research projects.

Ferris TG, Saglam D, Stafford RS, et al. Changes in the daily practice of primary care for children. *Arch Pediatr Adolesc Med.* 1998;152:227–233.   The objective of this study was to identify aspects of primary care practice for children who are undergoing substantial change. An analysis was carried out of National Ambulatory Medical Care Surveys from 1979 to 1981, 1985, and 1989 to 1994. The study found that child visits to primary care physicians increased by 22% between 1979 and 1994. The mean age of children visiting primary care physicians decreased from 6.7 years in 1979 to 5.7 years in 1994. The ethnic diversity of child visits increased primarily as a result of increasing proportion of visits from Hispanic (6% in 1979; 12.6% in 1994) and Asian patients (1.6% in 1979; 4.1% in 1994). Medicaid and managed care increased dramatically as a form of payment. Changes in physician services included an increase in preventive services, changes in the most commonly prescribed medications, and an increased mean duration of patient visits (11.8 minutes 1979; 14.2 minutes 1994). The study concludes that a declining proportion of adolescent visits may present physicians with a challenge, that physician prescribing practices showed changes without evidence of benefits to child health and that increased ethnic diversity and provision of preventive services were associated with the increase in visit time.

Green LA. British general practice: a visiting American family medicine resident's view. *J Arkansas Med Soc.* 1977;73:457–461.   A visiting American family resident spends time in the United Kingdom to examine the encounter between the patient and the British general practitioner and the system that supports it. The style and content of the encounter is described in terms of national statistics as well as specific events of a day in a busy practice. He discusses training programs for the general practitioner. The author decides, after gaining some perspective on his visit, that he will make home visits in his practice and be available when patients need him. He perceives the major flaw in the National Health Service as the lack of incentive to be better; the inspired practitioner is inadequately rewarded. He also remains impressed that any person in the UK can receive all the medical care needed without fear of financial disaster.

Green LA. Science and the future of primary care. *J Fam Pract.* 1996;42:119–122.   In 1994, the Institute of Medicine (IOM) appointed a multidisciplinary committee to reexamine the future of primary care. The committee convened a workshop in 1995 at the National Academy of Sciences in Washington DC, to explore the scientific base of primary care. This paper discusses four themes that emerged from the workshop: (1) reasoning in primary care is complicated and differs in fundamental ways from referral/subspecialty clinical practice; (2) primary care can be improved through research to the benefit of many; (3) the United States lacks capacity to improve primary care just as it lurches toward greater reliance on primary care as the foundation of health services; and (4) primary care research is now an attractive investment. The author concludes with the notion that good primary care is interdependent with the rest of the health care system and other systems within communities. Organized responses to promoting health and preventing or treating disease and illnesses cannot be sufficient in the absence of excellent primary care.

Green LA. The view from 2020: how family practice failed. *J Fam Med.* 2001:33320–324. This article reports on the Keystone V Conference, convened in 2020, to discuss why family medicine had failed. The fantasy examines the world in 2020, and goes on to discuss the reasons why family medicine had proved insufficient, lost power, and failed the test of public opinion. The imaginary conference concludes by citing four possible answers: (1) family medicine had abdicated; (2) it had gone down with the old medical paradigm; (3) it had chosen the wrong tasks; and (4) it never became part of the culture.

Green LA, Fryer GE. The development and goals of the AAFP Center for Policy Studies in Family Practice and Primary Care. *J Fam Pract.* 1999;48:905–908. In this article, the authors describe the creation and role of the Center for Policy Studies in Family Practice and Primary Care established in 1999 by the American Academy of Family Physicians in Washington DC. Events leading to the decision to establish the Center are described, its guiding assumptions are listed, and its initial structure and function are explained. Three themes are identified that will guide the early work of the Center: sustaining the functional domain of family practice and primary care; investing in key infrastructures; and securing universal health coverage.

Green LA, Fryer GE, Yawn BP, Lanier D, Dovey SM. The ecology of medical care revisited. *N Engl J Med.* 2001;344:2021–2025. "The Ecology of Medical Care," by White et al, published in the *New England Journal of Medicine* in 1961 has provided a framework for thinking about the organization of health care, medical education and research. The report found that in a population of a 1,000 adults, in an average month, 750 reported an illness, 250 consulted a physician, 9 were hospitalized, 5 were referred to a physician and 1 was referred to a university medical center. The data has been updated in this new study, based on multiple sources, that focuses on the United States and also incorporates information on children. The new study finds some variation from the original but overall remarkable stability of the relationships proposed over 40 years ago.

Grumbach K, Fry J. Managing primary care in the U.S. and in the U.K. *N Engl J Med.* 1993;328:940–945. Many long established features of the British National Health Service (NHS), such as a strict system of referrals to specialists, a mixture of capitation and fee-for-service reimbursement, and responsibilities for defined populations in the community, are being introduced in managed care plans in the US. In this article, the authors compare primary care in the US and the UK, emphasizing similarities as well as differences in the overall health care systems and in the structure, processes, and outcomes of primary care in the two nations. The authors recommend joint cross-national thinking, planning and sharing of experiences to produce basic models of excellence in primary health care.

Grumbach K, Selby JV, Damberg C, et al. Resolving the gatekeeper conundrum: what patients value in primary care and referrals to specialists. *JAMA*. 1999:282: 261–266.   A cross sectional survey to determine the extent to which patients value the role of their primary care physicians was mailed in 1997 to 12,707 adult patients who were members of managed care plans, and received care from 10 large physician groups in California. The response rate was 71%. Ninety-four percent of patients valued the role of the primary care physician as a source of first contact care; depending on the medical problem, 75–91% preferred to seek care initially from their primary care physician; 23% reported that their primary care physician or medical group interfered with their ability to see specialists. Patients who had difficulty obtaining referrals were more likely to report low trust. The authors conclude that patients value the coordinating and first contact role of the primary care physician. However, managed care policies that emphasize the primary care physician as gatekeepers impeding access to specialists, undermine patients' trust and confidence in their primary care physician.

Haggerty RJ. Child health 2000: new pediatrics in the changing environment of children's needs in the 21st century. *Pediatrics*. 1995;96:804–812.   The author discusses how, in the next millennium, pediatric practice will require knowledge of new morbidities, such as AIDS and social and behavioral disorders, reemergent old disorders such as tuberculosis, and disorders rarely seen in the US but being brought by recent immigrants. Diversity in ethnic and cultural backgrounds and beliefs will continue to increase, and will need to be understood to treat children effectively. Changes in family structure will also require pediatricians to understand and accept diversity, e.g., gay and lesbian families. Increased isolation of individuals from society and their family of origin will require pediatricians to be more active in communities and schools and to participate with other disciplines and social support groups. The advancement of science and technology will continue to drive what the pediatrician does, and increase survival of children with fatal illnesses, requiring more emphasis on care of children with chronic illness. Pediatricians will need to partner with others in the fields of risk assessment and psychosocial disorders.

Igra V, Millstein SG. Current status and approaches to improving preventive services for adolescents. *JAMA*. 1993;269:1408–1412.   The authors analyze data from the National Ambulatory Medical Care Survey (NAMCS) to determine the current status of the provision of preventive services to adolescents and their findings suggest that it is suboptimal. Barriers (environmental and physician) to the provision of preventive services are examined, including: non-reimbursement from insurance companies; lack of time; lack of ancillary resources; absence of clearly defined non-controversial guidelines; lack of adequate physician training; the personal nature of many adolescent health problems (which physicians may deny as relevant to their practice); and physician forgetfulness.

Lamberts H, Hofmans-Okkes I. Episode of care: a core concept in family practice. *J Fam Pract.* 1996;42:161–167.   The Institute of Medicine's new definition of primary care requires that primary care clinicians address the majority of personal health care needs of their patients. The unit of assessment for this is called the "episode of care," defined as a health problem from its first encounter with a health care provider through the completion of the last encounter, distinct from an episode of disease or illness. In this article, episode-of-care data from Dutch family practice illustrates this approach using data from women 25–44 years old. The top twenty new reasons for encounter and new episodes of care, as well as the relationship between the reason for the encounter (headache) and the disease (sinusitis), support the potential of episode-oriented epidemiology.

Leader S, Perales PJ. Provision of primary-preventive health care services by obstetrician-gynecologists. *Obstet Gynecol.* 1995;85:391–395.   The objective of this study was to determine the extent to which obstetricians-gynecologists serve as primary care providers for women 15 years and older. Three national data bases were analyzed to see if differences existed in content of care during a general medical examination by three medical specialties. The study found that obstetrician-gynecologists provided more office-based general medical examinations to women 15 years and older than either general family practitioners or internists and that 48.3% of obstetrician-gynecologists considered themselves primary care providers as opposed to specialists.

Leopold N, Cooper J, Clancy C. Sustained partnership in primary care. *J Fam Pract.* 1996;42:129–137.   In 1994, the Institute of Medicine (IOM) convened the Committee on the Future of Primary Care. In the authors' opinion, one of the most striking additions to the 1978 definition of primary care made by this committee was the concept that primary care includes a sustained partnership with patients. The impact of a sustained partnership in a clinician-patient relationship remains largely unstudied. This paper reviews selected literature on this topic and proposes a theoretical basis for assessing the existence, antecedents, and outcomes of sustained partnerships.

Lipkin M, Levinson W, Barker R, et al. Primary care internal medicine: a challenging career choice for the 1990s. *Ann Intern Med.* 1990;112:371–378.   During the last decade, fewer medical students have selected training in internal medicine. This article attempts to inform medical students, their advisors, and other physicians about the field of primary care internal medicine. The authors define the discipline, compare it with traditional internal medicine and with family practice, and describe features of strong primary care internal medicine training programs. They discuss common misconceptions and concerns about training programs and give examples of the career paths chosen by graduates of primary care programs.

McWinney, IR. Core values in a changing world. *Br Med J.* 1998;316:1807–1809.   This article reflects on the core values underpinning the development of primary care.

The author notes that all key relationships in primary care—with patients, with colleagues in practices and in the wider health service, and with local communities—are underpinned by basic, core values passed down by tradition. Primary care practitioners must guard these values, recognizing that they may be affected by evolution in health care and its delivery. Primary care, must, however, ensure that this is a conscious and explicit evolution, rather than an erosion left too late to remedy.

Medalie JH, Zyzanski SJ, Langa D, Stange KC. The family in family practice: is it a reality? *J Fam Pract.* 1998;46:390–396. The purpose of this study was to describe from multiple perspectives the extent to which community family physicians focus on the family. Data was collected on 4,454 outpatient visits using direct observation, patient and physician questionnaires, and medical record review. The study found that, on average, 10% of the time intervals during patient visits was devoted to addressing family issues. Other family members were present during 32% of visits, and another family members' problems were discussed in 18% of visits. Seventy percent of patients reported that other family members see the same doctor. A family history was obtained during 51% of visits by new patients and 22% of visits by established patients. The presence or absence of a family history of breast or colon cancer was noted in 40% of the charts. A factor analysis showed two different physician styles: family history as a context for care of an individual patient, and the family as a unit of care. The authors conclude that family physicians show a high degree of emphasis on the family.

Mendenhall RC, Tarlov AR, Girard RA, Michel JK, Radecki S. A national study of internal medicine and its specialties: II. Primary care in internal medicine. *Ann Intern Med.* 1979;91:275–287. A nationwide study of practitioners in 24 medical and surgical specialties was conducted by the University of Southern California School of Medicine, Division of Research in Medical Education. This is the second report in a series of three. Internal medicine, general internal medicine and 10 subspecialties of internal medicine are compared using a care classification scheme designed for the study. The authors conclude that subspecialists in internal medicine are assuming ongoing and comprehensive responsibility for the management of very substantial numbers of their patients and have an appreciable commitment to entry-level care.

Mold JW, Green LA. Primary care research: revisiting its definition and rationale. *J Fam Pract.* 2000;49:206–208. Only 0.4% of NIH funding and only 4% of the funding from the Agency for Health Care Policy and Research goes to departments of family medicine. Many institutions and funding agencies have difficulty understanding what primary care research includes and what might be its potential value. This article attempts to define and describe the scope of primary care research. The authors explain the categories that primary care research has traditionally fallen under including theoretical and methodological research, health care research, clinical research, and health systems research. Three issues are mentioned that might benefit from primary health care research: night sweats; cognitive impairment in older people; and managing laboratory testing results.

Moore GT, Showstack J. Primary care medicine in crisis: toward reconstruction and renewal. *Ann Intern Med.* 2003;138:244–247. Primary care is in crisis. Despite its proud history and theoretical advantages, the field has failed to hold its own among medical specialties. While the rest of medicine promises technology and sophistication, the basic model of primary care has changed little over the past half-century. Why has the transition from general practice to today's primary care been so difficult? Many of the causes of this struggle may lie within primary care itself, ranging from failure to articulate to the public (and insurers and policymakers) what value it, and it alone, can offer to taking on an ever-broadening set of roles and responsibilities while all too often falling short of its promises. Perhaps most important, in the emerging health care system, the lack of a discrete definition of primary care has allowed managed care organizations and payers, among others, to define the role of primary care to suit their own interests. In response to a changing marketplace, political uncertainty, and shifting consumer expectations, primary care will need to reconstruct itself. The reconstruction will not be easy. Nevertheless, a process should begin that moves the field in the right direction. Building on its unique abilities, primary care can emerge as a redefined product that is attractive to patients, payers, and primary care practitioners alike.

Mullan F. The "Mona Lisa" of health policy: primary care at home and abroad. *Health Aff.* 1998;17:118–126. Briefly summarizing discussions on primary care at a four-nation conference, the author reviews the various definitions of the concept in the United States, beginning with Alpert and Charney's characterization as first-contact care, care over time, and coordination of care. He notes that in the United States, two philosophies—primary care as social justice and primary care as industrial efficiency—live side-by-side, often producing confusion and conflict. The author then reviews the practice of primary care in Germany, The Netherlands, Canada and the United States. He observes that the common theme that those responsible for paying are most interested in is the gatekeeping function of primary care.

Pellegrino ED. The identity crisis of an ideal. In: Ingelfinger FJ, Relman AS, Finland M, eds., *Controversy in Internal Medicine.* Vol. 2. Philadelphia: Saunders; 1974:41–50. Internal medicine, like general surgery and pediatrics, is today forced to confront a crisis of identity in which it may become lost as an entity or renewed as the synthesizing element in medical care. As it seeks to redefine itself in contemporary and future terms, it will find that some of the cherished attitudes and commitments are indeed, obsolete. It will gain new strength and identity, not by holding uncritically to its outworn elements or by extending itself into fields like family and community medicine that demand a wholly different orientation. Rather internal medicine must renew itself by cultivating those regions in which it is particularly adept and even unique. This renewal can grow easily and consciously by a redefinition of the ideals out of which internal medicine was originally generated.

Perkoff GT. General internal medicine, family practice or something better? *N Engl J Med.* 1978;299:654–657. In this article, the shortcomings of internal medicine in preparing its residents to attend to the primary care problems of patients are discussed. Despite attempts to make internal resident programs more oriented to primary care of the patient, the author contends that family medicine programs have made a commitment to the primary role of the generalist, in a way and to a degree that is far beyond what can be accomplished by internal medicine. He recommends that, instead of imitating family practice, departments of internal medicine should support departments of family practice and participate in the development of family-practice clinics. A cooperative endeavor would take cognizance of the deficiencies in general internal medicine and in family-practice training and work to correct both, to yield a new generalist of the future who would be better than either.

Robert Graham Center, Policy Studies in Family Practice and Primary Care. The importance of primary care physicians as the usual source of health care in the achievement of prevention goals. *Am Fam Physician.* 2000;62:1968.    This article confirms the importance of having a primary care physician as a usual source of care for achieving preventive goals. Data shows that having any usual source of care, either a facility or an individual provider, was uniformly associated with children less than six years old being immunized and adults receiving preventive services. In addition, adults with a general internist as their usual source of care received more preventive care in 1996 than those with a family physician. The reason for the difference could be related to time spent with the patient or the fact that more patients with family physicians lacked insurance and therefore did not seek out preventive care.

Rosenblatt RA, Hart LG, Gamliel S, et al. Identifying primary care disciplines by analyzing the diagnostic content of ambulatory care. *J Am Board Fam Pract.* 1995;8:34–45.    This study examines which medical specialties are primary care disciplines by analyzing the extent to which major physician disciplines provide comprehensive ambulatory care to large segments of the population, a characteristic central to the provision of primary care. Data was used from ambulatory visits to office-based physicians recorded in 1980–81 and 1989–90 versions of the National Ambulatory Medical Care Survey. The results showed that family medicine, general internal medicine, and general pediatrics provide the majority of non-referred ambulatory care for common conditions in the United States. Obstetrician-gynecologists tended to limit their care to obstetric and gynecologic problems; most care for adult women is provided by family physicians and general internists.

Sandy LG, Foster NE, Eisenberg JM. Challenges to generalism: views from the delivery system. *Acad Med.* 1995;70(1Suppl):S44–S46.    The declining interest in primary care among medical students is an ominous trend for the national health system. During a day-long meeting sponsored by The Robert Wood Johnson Foundation, representatives of group practices, HMOs, community health centers, and military medicine noted the universal shortage of primary care physicians, the fact that medical education does not prepare physicians for the realities of practice, the concern that "burnout" is a significant problem for physician satisfaction and retention, and the problem that the optimal design of primary care is not yet known. To reverse these trends, concerted action must take place within academic medicine, by policy makers and by the delivery system itself.

Schwenk TL, Woolley RF. The role of the community-oriented primary care physician. *Am J Prev Med*. 1986;2:49–58. This article attempts to clarify the role of community-oriented primary health care by applying systems theory to the concept of community-oriented primary care as first-contact medical care for the patient, in the context of the community. Relationships between the primary care physician and the following entities are defined: the patient; the physician's and patient's community, culture and the society; the physician's office; the medical care system; and the physician's and patient's families. The educational implication of the resultant role is discussed.

Sox HC Jr, Scott HD, Ginsburg JA. The role of the future general internist defined. *Ann Intern Med*. 1994;121:616–622. In this article, the American College of Physicians Task Force on Physician Supply examines the current and future roles of the ideal general internist. The following topics are discussed: characteristics shared by all internists, whether engaged in general or subspecialty practice; current trends and the growing crisis in the supply of primary care physicians; and the practices and patient characteristics of both general internists and family physicians. The Task Force proposed a new definition that reaffirms fundamental characteristics of today's general internists and adds characteristics that are shared by other generalist physicians. The new definition envisions the general internist as (1) a primary care physician: the patient's first contact and a provider of comprehensive, continuing care; (2) a physician who evaluates and manages all aspects of illness—biomedical and psychosocial—in the whole patient; (3) an expert in disease prevention, early detection of disease, and health promotion; (4) the patient's guide and advocate in a complex health care environment; (5) an expert in managing patients with advanced illness and diseases of several organ systems; (6) a consultant when patients have difficult, undifferentiated problems or when the general internist has special expertise to apply to their problems; (7) a resource manager who is familiar with the science of clinical epidemiology and decision-making and can bring a thoughtful lean practice style to evaluation and management; (8) a clinical information manager who can take full advantage of electronically stored data and can communicate using tools of modern technology; and (9) a generalist in outlook who also possesses special skills that respond to the needs of a particular care environment.

Spiegel JS, Rubenstein LV, Scott B, Brook RH. Who is the primary care physician? *N Engl J Med*. 1983;308:1208–1212. Several studies have concluded that specialists form a hidden system for primary care delivery. However, these studies assume that a specialist who provides the majority of care is the primary care physician. Using data from the Rand Health Insurance Experiment, the authors compared the effects of three definitions of a primary care physician on identification of the primary care provider: the physician who delivered the majority of care (34% were specialists), the physician designated by the patient to receive the results of a multiphasic-screening examination (12% were specialists), and the physician who treated common problems (9% were specialists). Use of the "majority of care" criterion overestimated by threefold the contribution of specialists. The authors conclude by saying that definitions of primary care should be more specific and include tasks frequently associated with primary care, as well as patients' perceptions of the physician providing their primary care.

St. Peter RF, Reed MC, Kemper P, Blumenthal D. Changes in the scope of care provided by primary care physicians. *N Engl J Med*. 1999;341:1980–1985. This study focuses on physicians' assessment of changes in the scope of care provided by primary care physicians and their assessment of the appropriateness of the care that primary care physicians are expected to provide. The analysis was based on telephone interviews from 7,015 primary care physicians and 5,092 specialists selected from the 1996–97 Community Tracking Study Physician Survey. Nearly one in four primary care physicians and 38% of specialists reported that the scope of care that primary care physicians were expected to provide was greater than it should be. The authors note that this raises questions about the effect of current changes in the health care system; as these changes create incentives for primary care physicians to play a more prominent role in caring for patients with complex conditions, it is important to monitor closely the quality of care they provide, as well as accessibility of service more appropriately provided by specialists.

Stafford RS, Saglam D, Causino N, et al. Trends in adult visits to primary care physicians in the U.S. *J Fam Med*. 1999;8:26–32. The investigators analyzed a nationally representative sample of 136,233 adult office visits to general internists, general practitioners and family physicians contained in the National Ambulatory Medical Care Survey conducted from 1978–1994. Data showed that patients visiting primary care physicians are older as a group and more ethnically and racially diverse, and have had a shift in their health coverage towards HMOs; but their clinical problems did not change. One of the most provocative findings was that visits to primary care physicians have diminished as a proportion of all adult visits from 52% in 1978 to 41% in 1994. The article concludes that the increasing role of primary care physicians, with its emphasis on productivity appears to be at odds with their increasing responsibility for prevention and the associated increase in the duration of primary care visits.

Stange KC, Zyzanski SJ, Callahan EJ, et al. Illuminating the "black box": a description of 4,454 patient visits to 138 family physicians. *J Fam Pract*. 1998;46:377–389. In this article, the content and context of community family practices, physicians, patients, and outpatient visits are described. Visits by 4,454 patients seeing 138 physicians in 84 practices were observed. The study demonstrated that outpatient visits to family physicians encompassed a wide variety of patients, problems, and levels of complexity. The average patient paid 4.3 visits to the practice within the past year. The mean visit duration was 10 minutes. Fifty-eight percent of visits were for acute illness, 24% for chronic illness, and 12% for well care. The most common uses of time were history-taking, planning treatment, physical examination, health education, feedback, family information, chatting, structuring the interaction, and patient questions. The study concludes that family practice and patient visits are complex, with competing demands and opportunities to address a wide range of problems of individuals and families over time and at various stages of health and illness.

Starfield B. Is primary care essential? *Lancet.* 1994;344:1129–1133.   The author considers whether primary care is the backbone of a rational health services system as is often perceived. After defining what she means by primary care—first contact, continuous, comprehensive, and coordinated care provided to populations undifferentiated by gender, disease, or organ system—the author suggests that primary care is more usefully seen as an approach to providing care rather than a set of specific services, with its practitioners or facilities judged on the degree to which they implement this approach. She reviews the proportion of practitioners needed for the adequate provision of primary care and assesses whether better health results when primary care forms the first level of care. Based on evidence available she concludes that a primary care orientation of the country's health service system is associated with lower costs, higher patient satisfaction, better health levels, and lower medication use.

Starfield B, Simpson L. Primary care as part of U.S. health services reform. *JAMA.* 1993;269:3136–3139.   The authors begin by discussing problems in the US health care service since the 1960s and emphasizing the importance of primary health care to the US system. They propose 12 avenues of approach (building on the content and form of the current health policy reform debate) to develop a primary care infrastructure in the US. Their approaches include: implementing mechanisms of reimbursement to facilitate primary care practitioners; establishing a more rational basis for referrals; restructuring licensing policies; providing financial incentives for training primary care providers; expanding and improving loan forgiveness for primary care physicians; restructuring fee schedules; replacing burdensome administrative work; providing bonuses for achieving preventative goals and team practice; rewarding high level of primary care practice by developing a national system of accountability; earmarking funding for primary care research; and involving residents in ongoing quality of care monitoring. The authors suggest that primary care should be one of the organizing focuses of health care reform, as it has been in other industrialized nations.

Stephens GG. The intellectual basis of family practice. *J Fam Pract.* 1975;2:423–428. Although progress is being made toward defining the family physician and specialty of family practice, there remains a need to describe more clearly a conceptual base for family medicine as an academic discipline. This paper explores common misconceptions and fallacies that have confused or prevented greater understanding of the intellectual basis of family practice. A thesis is presented and defended which holds that patient management is the quintessential skill of clinical practice and the unique field of knowledge of family physicians. The *sine qua non* of family practice is the knowledge and skill which allow the family physician to confront relatively large numbers of unselected patients with unselected conditions and to carry on therapeutic relationships with patients over time.

Stephens GG. Family practice and social and political change. *Fam Med.* 2001;33: 248–251. Reform in the US has been a longstanding process, intertwined with politics and social issues. Organizational medicine has resisted reform often, but despite this resistance, many changes took place in the US medical system in the 1960s. The establishment of the specialty of family practice coincided with these changes. Although family practice was established with many goals in mind, many of the goals did not match the public's perceived needs. One of family practice's current tasks is to examine its accountability to the public and decide what it can provide for the public good.

Stevens RA. The Americanization of family medicine: contradictions, challenges, and change, 1969–2000. *Fam Med.* 2001;33:232–243. Changing cultural and political environments have challenged the specialty of family medicine with pressures for reinvention with respect to identity, function and prestige. The most important impediment to a clear-cut role for family practice has been the lack of a formal administration structure for primary care practice on a nationwide basis. Family practice became one of several overlapping and competing primary care fields and its role is now less clear than the potential role envisioned for it in 1969. The author suggests that if family medicine is to be successful it must develop allies and work aggressively to establish its role in primary care.

Thomas P, Griffiths F, Kai J, O'Dwyer A. Networks for research in primary health care. *Br Med J.* 2001;322:588–590. In this article, the authors give an overview of primary care research networks. These networks were established as a way to enable diverse practitioners to engage in research. They start by defining and describing networks, using examples from the UK and elsewhere. They then go on to discuss the lessons learned from the UK experience and suggest how these lessons can be built on through better integration with emerging primary care structures.

Wagner EH. Chronic disease management: what will it take to improve care for chronic illness? *Eff Clin Pract.* 1998;1:2–4. Meeting the complex needs of patients with chronic illness or impairment is the single greatest challenge facing organized medical practice. If care is to be improved, evidence strongly suggests that the ambulatory care systems needs to be reshaped for this purpose. Patients and families suffering from chronic illness have unique needs. Efforts to improve care for patients with chronic illness fall into two groups: targeting and case management (the larger group) and comprehensive system change (the smaller group). On the basis of his work at Group Health Cooperative, and reviews of the literature, the author developed a model for improving care. The model assumes that the locus of care remains with the personal physician, supported by an integrated, and perhaps expanded, practice team.

Wagner EH. The role of patient care teams in chronic disease management: statistical data included. *Br Med J.* 2000;320:569–572. The author discusses the composition of a patient care team and how it might contribute to the care of a chronically ill patient. Successful teams will often include nurses and pharmacists with clinical and behavioral skills. Social workers and lay health workers can also play a part in team care. The article concludes that patient care teams have the potential to improve the care for patients with chronic illness, provided that the roles of team members are clearly defined and explicitly delegated, and the team members are trained for their roles.

Whitcomb ME, Desgroseilliers JP. Primary care medicine in Canada. *N Engl J Med.* 1992;326:1469–1472. In contrast to the United States, there is no shortage of primary care practitioners in Canada. Approximately half of Canadian physicians are general practitioners or family physicians whose practices are limited, for the most part, to primary care medicine. Furthermore, a large percentage of graduates (approximately half) in Canadian medical schools choose careers in primary care medicine. The authors contrast the Canadian approach to primary care medicine with that of the United States. They explain how primary care medicine in Canada evolved as a distinct form of practice with specialists practicing as consultants and payment policies that discouraged them from providing primary care services. The College of Physicians and Surgeons of Canada represents specialists and the College of Family Physicians represents family medicine. Canadian students have less financial debt after medical school than US medical students, and as a result do not look on the salary of a general practitioner as too low. In the US, the lack of prestige associated with primary care and the unfavorable economics of the practice create obstacles to US students choosing primary care as a career.

White KL. Primary medical care for families—organization and evaluation. *N Engl J Med.* 1967;277:847–852. The author proposes the development of health-services systems that would, like the airlines industry, be competitive at local and regional levels, regulated, franchised and subsidized when necessary. Each system would include a continuously available, accessible source of primary medical care, linked to a community hospital and to a medical center by common record, communication and referral systems. The author suggests that physicians work in pairs, or larger groups, that might include physician assistants, nurse practitioners or public health nurses. He concludes that the efforts of the health-services system should be evaluated not in terms of activities such as numbers of visits to doctors and admissions to hospital, or even of deaths postponed or diseases treated, but rather in terms of reduction in measures of disability, discomfort, and dissatisfaction.

Young LE. The broadly based internist as the backbone of medical practice. In: Ingelfinger FJ, Relman AS, Finland M, eds., *Controversy in Internal Medicine.* Vol. 2. Philadelphia: Saunders; 1974:51–63. This article discusses the role played by internists as personal physicians and describes it as grossly underestimated and poorly understood except by the patients who benefit from internist services. A study that considers functions and opinions of general internists in the Rochester region is analyzed to understand better the role of the internist in general medicine. Opinions are solicited from internists and patients. When internists were asked about recommendations for changes in post-doctoral education of personal physicians, 54 out of 83 respondents made a plea for more experience with ambulatory patient care. Other major issues considered in this article include: numbers of personal physicians needed; primary health care units; teamwork in primary health care; modernization of community and regional health care systems; and measurement of benefits and costs in health care.

CHAPTER THIRTEEN

# Improving the Health Care Workforce

*Perspectives from Twenty-Four Years' Experience*

Stephen L. Isaacs, J.D.; Lewis G. Sandy, M.D.; Steven A. Schroeder, M.D.
1997

The Robert Wood Johnson Foundation began operating as a national philanthropy in 1972. It was the year that Henry Kissinger and Le Duc Tho held secret peace negotiations in Paris, Richard Nixon was elected to a second term, and many people thought that national health insurance was right around the corner. Surveys conducted in the early 1970s indicated that access to basic ambulatory care was the nation's number one health care concern. Such concern attracted the immediate attention of the new foundation, and in its 1972 annual report David Rogers, the Foundation's first president, noted the relationship between access to services and the health care workforce:

> The uneven availability of continuing medical care of acceptable quality is one
> of the most serious problems we face today. The problem is twofold. First, there
> are too few health resources in rural and urban poverty areas. Thus, we have
> too many people—particularly our poor, our elderly, and our isolated—lacking
> ready access to appropriate services. Second, the specialty balance of physicians
> and their associated personnel is significantly out of line with needs. There is a

This chapter originally appeared as Isaacs SL, Sandy LG, Schroeder SA. Improving the health
care workforce: perspectives from twenty-four years' experience. *To Improve Health and Health
Care 1997: The Robert Wood Johnson Foundation Anthology* (Chap. 2). San Francisco: Jossey-
Bass, 1997. Copyright © 1997, The Robert Wood Johnson Foundation. Reprinted with permission.

sharp shortage of those who deliver primary care and increasing evidence to suggest a relative oversupply of physicians in certain medical and surgical specialties.[1]

To increase Americans' access to a physician or some other health care professional, and to prepare for national health insurance, the Foundation made a commitment to expanding and improving the health care workforce—a commitment that continues to this day. The Foundation has funded programs to increase the number of health professionals who can provide primary care to communities in need: generalist physicians, nurse practitioners, physician assistants, and family dentists. In addition, it launched fellowship programs to develop a cadre of health care professionals with interdisciplinary knowledge and breadth of vision who could be leaders in shaping health care policy. Since 1972, the Foundation has allocated $520 million—more than one out of every five dollars it has awarded—to workforce programs. National programs carried out at a number of sites have received $419 million; these are listed and described in the Appendix at the end of this chapter. Another $101 million has been given in ad hoc, or single site, grants.

The Foundation does not, of course, act in isolation. Other foundations also fund programs to make the health care workforce more responsive to national needs. For example, the W. K. Kellogg Foundation was an early supporter of family practice; the Commonwealth Fund supported innovative projects like the WAMI program, designed to bring primary care to underserved communities in Washington, Alaska, Montana, and Idaho; the Kaiser Family Foundation supported faculty fellowships in general internal medicine; and the Pew Charitable Trusts offer health policy fellowships and operate a Health Professions Commission that examines workforce issues.

Governments have also become more active in reshaping the workforce. Many states now promote primary care initiatives within their own borders. The federal government, through Titles VII and VIII of the Public Health Service Act, supports the education of health professionals. Through the National Health Service Corps, it places physicians in underserved areas in return for scholarships or forgiveness of student loans. The federal government currently spends more than $400 million a year in forty-four workforce initiatives that encourage health professionals to study primary care and to practice in underserved areas.[2] Even greater federal funding goes toward specialization and high technology. This includes $6 billion a year that Medicare spends annually for graduate medical education and $8.5 billion that the National Institutes of Health spend annually for medical research and training.[3]

Then there are market forces—perhaps the most crucial factor in determining what and where health professionals practice. The rise of managed care, for example, is persuading an increasing number of medical students to consider careers as generalists. However, since there are few financial incentives to serve chronically ill, poor, or geographically isolated individuals, managed care may do little to increase access for underserved populations.

Although the resources of any one foundation may be relatively modest in terms of the total available for health care issues, philanthropy can play a unique and catalytic role. Rogers said of this role, "A foundation can offer people, institutions, and communities the opportunity to test a new approach and then give others the chance to prod it, examine it, and see if it fits their particular set of circumstances, and whether it can have yet broader application. Fear of the new is sometimes allayed by taking an idea out of the abstract and seeing it in operation."[4]

# 1970s WORKFORCE PROGRAMS

## Primary Care Physicians

Since its earliest days, the Foundation has given high priority to promoting primary care and making it a more attractive career for physicians. In the 1970s, it launched programs (Figure 13.1) intended to attract top internists and pediatricians to primary care, so as to enhance the credibility and the standing of primary care in the medical community. This approach—training a small number of key individuals, particularly academics, to serve as agents of change in a high-priority area—was to serve as a model for the Foundation. The *Primary Care Residency Program,* begun in 1973, gave training in primary care to general pediatric residents and internal medicine residents at nine hospitals and outpatient clinics. Six years later, the Foundation began the *General Pediatric Academic Development Program,* which awarded two-year fellowships to prepare pediatric faculty members to conduct research on the more common childhood illnesses such as ear infections that were not, at the time, covered in medical school curricula. The third program, the *Family Practice Fellowship Program,* attempted to establish a firmer academic base for family medicine by training a small core of highly respected faculty members. Begun in 1978, it complemented the federal government's short-term fellowships in family practice by offering two-year postresidency fellowships in family medicine.

These three programs helped develop the field of primary care, giving it more respectability in academic medicine. The Primary Care Residency Program served as a model for the federal government, which began funding primary care training for internists and pediatricians in 1977. The General Pediatric Academic Development Program led to the inclusion of general pediatrics as a normal part of pediatricians' training. An evaluation of the Family Practice

Fellowship Program found that four years after it ended 65 percent of the graduates held medical school appointments and more than 90 percent, including those not affiliated with a medical school, spent some of their time teaching.

## Nurse Practitioners, Physician Assistants, and Health Associates

When the Foundation began its philanthropic efforts, it recognized that if health care were to be made accessible to underserved populations, health professionals other than physicians would have to be trained to deliver primary care. As a result, it began supporting the training of nurse practitioners and physician assistants in the early 1970s, a time when both fields were in their infancy.

**Figure 13.1**. Foundation National Workforce Programs Begun in the 1970s.

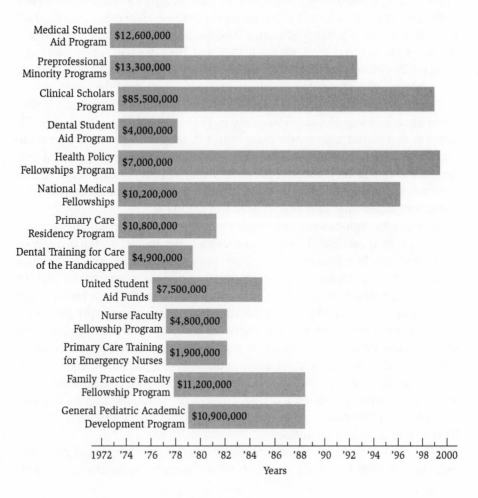

Initially, grants were made to a number of demonstration programs. The Utah Valley Hospital in Provo, for example, received funds to establish a network of rural clinics that would be staffed by nurse practitioners backed up by physicians who flew in every week. At the same time, the Foundation supported several pilot programs to train physician assistants.

Acceptance of nurse practitioners did not come easily. (Physician assistants were less threatening to people, since their profession grew out of efforts within the medical profession, and they worked directly under the supervision of doctors.) Many people in the medical community saw nurse practitioners as unqualified upstarts eager to encroach on the territory of physicians. To placate these concerns and give credibility to advanced-degree primary care nursing, the Foundation adopted two approaches to bring nurse-practitioner training into the mainstream of graduate nursing education. In the mid-1970s, it awarded ad hoc grants to six nursing schools to establish primary care training for nurse practitioners at the master's degree level. Next, it initiated a *Nurse Faculty Fellowship Program* to develop a core of nursing educators who would be able to train nurse practitioners at the master's level. Between 1977 and 1982, ninety-nine fellows—the pioneers in a movement that led to the acceptance of nurse-practitioner training as an integral part of graduate nursing education—completed the program.

Before the Foundation established its successful nursing programs, it provided funds to Johns Hopkins University in 1973 to establish a school of health services that would train a new class of health professional—similar in some ways to physician assistants—called health associates. These newly minted professionals were to be the model for the delivery of primary care services at a time when the debut of national health insurance seemed imminent. However, the school closed after only four classes had graduated.

This was the Foundation's most visible workforce failure: an admittedly high-risk idea that, if successful, might have had a major impact on the delivery of health services. In retrospect, it may have been unrealistic to expect a medical school whose reputation depended on training specialists to throw its support behind an approach to health care that would rely on people who were not physicians. Moreover, the timing for such a program was simply not right. National health insurance was not enacted in the 1970s, and the huge infusions of federal money to train physician assistants and other health professionals as part of health care reform never materialized. Within the university, the new school had little political leverage. Given these factors, it is not surprising that when the university suffered a budget crisis in the seventies and the Foundation's funding also ended, Johns Hopkins decided not to commit any more of its scarce resources to the school.

With this exception, the Foundation's early nurse practitioner and physician assistant programs have been among its more successful undertakings. Its funding helped establish these two fields as viable career options at a time when the idea of such programs was under attack. The Foundation decided to withdraw its support for these programs in the late 1970s, after Congress began earmarking money to train nurse practitioners, physician assistants, and generalist physicians. The Foundation reasoned that once the models it had helped develop were adopted by the federal government, it should move on to new endeavors. Although nurse practitioners and physician assistants still faced formidable legal, political, and financial obstacles, for twelve years beginning in 1982 the Foundation did not develop any new national programs directed toward these health professionals.

## Dentistry

Another field that attracted the early attention of the Foundation was dentistry. The *Program for Training Dentists in the Care of Handicapped Patients,* 1974–1979, led to the inclusion of dentistry for handicapped patients in the standard dental school curriculum. The *Dental Research Scholars Program* aimed at developing a cadre of dental faculty members knowledgeable in health care services and administration. It awarded two-year postdoctoral fellowships for research in dental health services. The Foundation did not fund any new national workforce programs for dentists after 1982, although it did provide partial support for an Institute of Medicine study on the future of dental education and continued to provide ad hoc grants to the dental profession.

## Fellowships

The Foundation also has sought to improve the American health care climate by developing health professionals—primarily physicians—who understand health services, the social sciences, and health policy making, and who could become leaders in their home institutions, professional societies, and state and federal government. To train these leaders, the Foundation established two fellowship programs.

Established by the Commonwealth Fund and the Carnegie Corporation in 1969, the *Clinical Scholars Program* was taken over and expanded by The Robert Wood Johnson Foundation shortly after the Foundation became a national philanthropy. This program, which continues to flourish, gives young physicians who are committed to clinical careers the opportunity to acquire skills and knowledge in areas such as epidemiology, economics, law, biostatistics, management, ethics, and anthropology. Currently, thirty-four scholars (eight of whom are funded by the Department of Veterans Affairs) are chosen annually to spend two years studying and conducting research at one of seven leading academic medical centers. Outside evaluators have praised the program as "a national treasure"[5] and "exceptionally influential."[6] Many of its more than seven hundred graduates have become leaders in academic institutions, managed health care programs, and government agencies.

The second program, begun in 1973 and still in operation, is the *Health Policy Fellowships Program.* Every year, it gives six outstanding midcareer health professionals an in-depth look at the federal health policy process. The fellowships begin with a three-month orientation in Washington, D.C., followed by a nine-month placement in the office of a senator, representative, or senior member of an executive department.

# 1980s WORKFORCE PROGRAMS

In the 1980s, the federal government turned away from the role it had played since the 1930s in addressing the nation's social problems. Rising health care costs became a national concern; the maldistribution of the health care workforce worsened, particularly as more young physicians chose careers in medical specialties. During this period, the Foundation solidified its commitment to training minority health professionals, developed national programs to strengthen the nursing profession, and established a new fellowship program for health care finance (Figure 13.2).

## Minority Physicians

The Foundation has allocated more than $100 million to date to minority health professionals. Although this commitment began with its very first program—medical school scholarships for women, students from rural areas, and minorities—it was in the mid-1980s that the Foundation launched its first national initiatives to bring more minorities into the health professions. What the Foundation hopes to achieve is increased access: if everyone is to have access to medical care, there must be more minority health professionals, for studies show that they choose careers in primary care, serve other minorities, and provide care to poor patients to a greater degree than nonminority physicians. African Americans, Mexican Americans, Native Americans, and mainland Puerto Ricans make up 22 percent of the United States population, but only a small proportion of the health care workforce.

In addition to its early scholarship programs for needy minority medical students, the Foundation addressed the fact that many minority applicants had not been adequately prepared to enter medical school. Many of these students had not taken the right premed courses and had not been adequately prepared for the Medical College Admission Test (MCAT); as a result, they could not compete successfully for admission with other college students. To overcome these disadvantages, the Foundation supported a wide variety of enrichment programs for minority college students in the 1970s and early 1980s.

**Figure 13.2.** Foundation National Workforce Programs Begun in the 1980s.

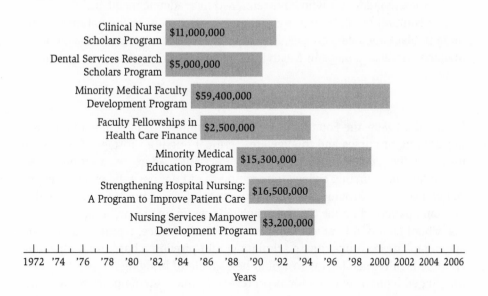

In 1985, a report issued by the Educational Testing Service found that summer programs increased the chances that minority students would be accepted into medical school. The Foundation combined its various enrichment programs into one national program, the *Minority Medical Education Program,* which continues today. Guided by a mentor, students learn about medical care and research, take courses in math and science, and are counseled in practical matters such as how to complete a medical school application and improve their interview skills. Currently, eight academic medical centers participate, each providing a six-week summer program for approximately 125 minority college students. An in-house evaluation found that the summer enrichment program doubles a student's chances of being admitted to a medical school.[7]

Even highly qualified and well-prepared minority students have been hesitant to apply to medical schools that did not have minority faculty members who could ease the difficulties that minority students sometimes encounter. So the *Minority Medical Faculty Development Program* was developed to increase the number of full-time minority faculty members in nonminority medical schools. Begun in 1984, this program helps promising junior faculty members who are committed to academic careers move up the academic ladder by offering them four-year postdoctoral research fellowships. Research can be in the biomedical, clinical, or health services area. Initially, eight fellows a year were appointed; this number was increased to twelve in 1991. A recent evaluation concluded that the program played a pivotal role in developing the potential for advancement of its program graduates who have remained in academic medicine.[8]

The Foundation also supported faculty development at the nation's traditionally black medical colleges. The bulk of Foundation support has gone to Meharry Medical College in Nashville, Tennessee, primarily to strengthen its faculty.

## Nursing

During the 1980s, the Foundation launched a number of programs to improve the training of nurses and to alleviate a critical nursing shortage. The first of these was the *Clinical Nurse Scholars Program,* which addressed a serious problem of hospital nursing: college-trained nurses did not have the practical experience needed to provide adequate patient care. The Foundation designed a program, patterned on the Clinical Scholars Program, to prepare a cadre of nursing school faculty for careers combining clinical practice, research, and management. These clinical nurse scholars would provide a base of notable and credible faculty members who would be capable of bridging the gap between nursing education, with its focus on research, and nursing practice, with its focus on patient care and management.

As the program was originally designed, nine midcareer fellows were to be chosen every year to conduct clinical or health sciences research. The first nurse scholars were selected in 1982. As it developed, however, the program shifted direction and became a basic research fellowship program for postdoctoral students. This led the Foundation to reconsider the program, and to end it three years earlier than planned. The last group of fellows completed its studies in 1991.

The 1980s witnessed a severe shortage of nurses; a commission established by the Secretary of Health and Human Services characterized this shortage as "real, widespread, and of significant magnitude."[9] In response, the Foundation funded three new national programs. The first, *Strengthening Hospital Nursing: A Program to Improve Patient Care,* was a six-year, $26.8 million effort begun in 1989. Funded jointly with the Pew Charitable Trusts, the program attempted to make hospital nursing a more attractive career choice by restructuring medical and support services around the nursing staff. More than a thousand hospitals and consortiums submitted applications, eighty of which received planning grants, and twenty of which were awarded five-year implementation grants.

The two other programs—the *Nursing Services Manpower Development Program,* begun in 1989, and *Ladders in Nursing Careers,* begun in 1993—aimed at increasing the number of nurses by attracting and supporting disadvantaged students and health care workers who wanted to pursue nursing careers. The seven Nursing Services Manpower Program grantees adopted approaches ranging from counseling minority seventh graders to setting up a cooperative recruitment program among nursing schools to attract minority students. Under the Ladders in Nursing Careers Program, grants were awarded to nine hospital associations to help employees, especially nurses' aides, overcome financial, educational, and other barriers to becoming nurses.

For a variety of reasons, the Foundation has not succeeded in developing a coherent and consistent approach to its nursing programs. Some of the reasons have to do with the characteristics of nursing: the gulf between the academic focus of nursing education and the clinical focus of its practice; three distinct entry levels (diploma, associate degree, and baccalaureate degree) leading to what many employers consider the same job; the lack of agreement about nurses' roles and the skills nurses need to fill their roles; and the recurring scarcity and surplus of nurses.[10]

Other reasons have their roots in the Foundation's approach. Perhaps reflecting the bias of an organization whose three presidents have been internists from academic medical institutions, the Foundation single-mindedly pursued its goal of training primary care physicians. In contrast, its nursing programs addressed short-term labor crises rather than long-term needs; supported activities with diffuse, conflicting, or unclear objectives; and lacked follow-through. The Clinical Nurse Scholars Program was probably terminated prematurely; although it had veered from its original objectives, it might have been redesigned to overcome its problems.[11] The Strengthening Hospital Nursing program had unclear and perhaps unrealistic objectives. Not only did it focus exclusively on process but its twin goals—one having to do with reorganizing hospital care around nursing, the other having to do with improving patient care—were not necessarily compatible. (In addition, it had the misfortune to begin just as many hospitals were laying off nurses in a wave of downsizing.) Similarly, the objectives of the Nursing Services Manpower Training and Ladders in Nursing Careers programs were overly broad: on the one hand they were supposed to increase the supply of nurses, and on the other they were supposed to attract minorities to nursing careers.

## Health Care Finance

As health care evolved in the 1980s from the fee-for-service care offered by nonprofit institutions to managed care provided by for-profit entities, and as cost became a public policy issue, it became increasingly clear that health care finance was the key to understanding the system—and perhaps to reforming it. It became equally clear that the number of people who could claim expertise in this complex field was limited. In 1985, the Foundation began its *Program for Faculty Fellowships in Health Care Finance*. It offered thirty-month fellowships to six faculty members a year. An evaluation found that even though the program changed the lives of many of its fellows, its target audience was unclear; for example, it was not clear whether the purpose was to increase the knowledge of professors of health care finance, introduce health policy faculty to financing issues, or train professors of finance in health policy issues. Concern was also raised about the narrowness of an approach that trained faculty in health care financing apart from overall health policy. The program ended in 1994.

# 1990s WORKFORCE PROGRAMS

The early 1990s were characterized by concern about escalating health care costs, President Clinton's failed attempt to reform the system, and the growth of for-profit managed care. Within the Foundation, a new board chairman took office in 1989, a new president in 1990. These appointments led to a refocusing of the Foundation's workforce programs: renewed emphasis on educating primary care physicians, reinvigorated efforts to train other health care professionals, and concentration on entire systems of health care rather than individual components. At the same time, the Foundation reasserted its commitment to minorities and opened its fellowship programs to a wider group of recipients (Figure 13.3).

## Generalist Physicians

In the early 1990s, as part of a $100 million strategy to improve access to basic health care, the Foundation launched a second cluster of programs to bring primary care into the mainstream of academic medicine and to attract more medical students to general medicine. The goal was no less than to change the thrust and the focus of medical education. Unlike the programs of the 1970s, which added more generalists to the pool of physicians without reducing the number of specialists, these programs sought more fundamental change: shifting the balance between generalists and specialists.

Under the *Generalist Physician Initiative,* the Foundation gave grants to medical schools that made a commitment to training generalist physicians and to increasing the proportion of generalists to specialists they graduated. Working in collaboration with state agencies, HMOs, and other partners, the grantees devised strategies aimed at four critical points in medical education: admissions, undergraduate medical curriculum, residency, and entry into practice. Beginning in 1991, the Foundation awarded planning grants to eighteen medical schools and consortiums, followed by six-year awards to fourteen of them to carry out the programs they had designed. The initiative stimulated a number of innovative partnerships and served as a model for New York and Pennsylvania to develop their own grant programs to increase the supply of primary care physicians.

**Figure 13.3.** Foundation National Workforce Programs Begun in the 1990s.

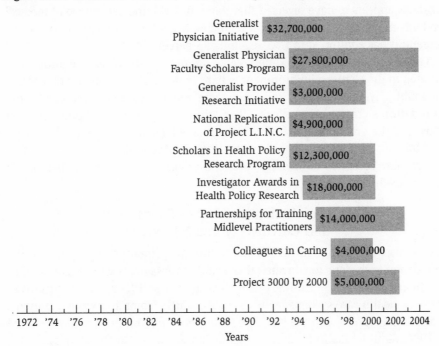

A parallel program, the *Generalist Physician Faculty Scholars Program,* started in 1993, aimed at increasing the prestige and credibility of generalist faculty members at medical schools. Recognizing that published research is the key to respect and seniority in academia, the program awarded four-year research grants to up to fifteen junior faculty members annually.

In lieu of evaluating each of its programs to encourage generalist medicine, and to place its efforts in a larger context, the Foundation funded the *Generalist Provider Research Initiative,* a five-year program also begun in 1993. Awards were made to carry out research on issues such as how to increase the number of physicians entering the three generalist fields, reduce the number of specialists, and attract more physicians to underserved areas.

Until the managed care revolution changed the way that professionals viewed health care, American medical students looked askance at careers in general medicine. The percentage of medical students selecting one of the three generalist fields—general internal medicine, general pediatrics, and family practice—as their first choice dropped from 36 percent in 1982 to less than 17 percent in

1991 and 1992. But the need for primary care physicians by managed care organizations appears to have reversed that trend. In 1993, the percentage of medical students making one of the general medicine fields their first choice rose to 19 percent; it has continued to rise, reaching 35 percent in 1996.

The extent to which The Robert Wood Johnson Foundation programs contributed to the changed environment is hard to determine. While market forces no doubt played a dominant role, they were augmented and reinforced by the Foundation's efforts. At the least, through its programs and a phenomenon known as the brochure effect, the Foundation's long commitment helped validate the idea of training generalists, made medical school faculty and administrators more receptive to primary care, and prepared medical schools to teach general medicine.

## Physician Assistants, Nurse Practitioners, and Certified Nurse Midwives

Beyond its work with medical schools in training primary care physicians, the Foundation took steps to educate other health professionals who might practice in underserved areas. Unlike the programs of the 1970s, these initiatives involved health care systems: state agencies, HMOs, community organizations, professional schools, and the like. The *Partnerships for Training Program,* started in 1996, required institutions in a region—universities, HMOs, state agencies, employers—to collaborate in the use of nontraditional techniques such as distance learning to train nurse practitioners, certified nurse midwives, and physician assistants in their home communities. Since these health professionals are being educated in the underserved communities where they live, they are expected to practice in those communities when their training is completed.

## Minority Health Professionals

The 1990s also saw an expansion of the training of minority health care professionals. In part because of the Foundation's Minority Medical Education Program, academically qualified minority students had a good chance of being admitted to medical school. But the number of minority students is small relative to their proportion in the population. To reach a far wider pool at an earlier point in their lives, the Association of American Medical Colleges (AAMC) began *Project 3000 by 2000* in 1991. This program tries to attract and prepare high school students for medical careers. The goal of the AAMC is to more than double—from thirteen hundred to three thousand—the number of underrepresented minority students entering medical school by the year 2000.

In 1994, with Foundation support, the project expanded to include other health professionals. Working in partnerships with colleges, school systems, and communities, ten academic centers offer enrichment courses, collaborate in creating magnet health sciences programs in high schools, provide mentors, and strengthen the science skills of elementary and secondary teachers. As mentioned earlier, the Foundation also is attempting to increase the number of minority nurses through two other programs: the Nursing Services Manpower and the Ladders in Nursing Careers programs.

### Expanding Fellowship Opportunities in Health Policy

Responding to changes in the health care system, in the 1990s the Foundation expanded the eligibility requirements for people who might become fellows. At mid-decade, amid concerns that bright junior members of social science faculties were not drawn to health policy research and that senior investigators were not receiving sufficient support, the Foundation initiated two new fellowship programs. Under the *Scholars in Health Policy Research Program*, which started in 1993, twelve two-year postdoctoral fellowships are awarded annually to promising young economists, political scientists, and sociologists. The *Investigator Awards in Health Policy Research*, which began in 1994, broadens the pool of health policy researchers even further: applicants may come from any discipline. The program provides salary support for ten outstanding young researchers or eminent senior scholars for up to three years.

# PERSPECTIVES FROM TWENTY-FOUR YEARS OF EXPERIENCE

From its very earliest days, the Foundation had a vision of a health care system that would be available to all Americans. As a result, it funded a multitude of programs to improve the health care workforce in the belief that this would result in more available care. Some, such as the Clinical Scholars Program, succeeded spectacularly. Others, such as the bold attempt to establish a new class of health associates at Johns Hopkins, failed utterly.

Where the Foundation worked with academic medicine, it has been successful. Through its programs with academic medical centers, it has been a major force in developing the field of general internal medicine, in introducing primary care into the medical school curriculum and residency training, and in making medical education more relevant. Perhaps more important than the specific programs it funded, the Foundation served as what one commentator called "a moral compass."[12] It pursued its vision of primary care as the key to health services, even when the idea seemed hopelessly unfashionable.

The Foundation showed similar determination in fostering a core of physicians to assume positions of leadership in the health care field. The Clinical Scholars Program, now nearly a quarter of a century old, is considered to be its flagship program, boasting a large constituency within the Foundation, among the program directors at the schools that train the fellows, and in academic medicine generally. The Foundation has also stayed the course in preparing minority students for medical school and training minority medical faculty.

When it came to nonphysician health professionals, however, the Foundation showed little of the same clear vision and steely devotion that characterized its programs for improving the physician workforce. After taking the lead in developing nurse practitioners and physician assistants as viable professions, it pulled back support in the early 1980s. Its nursing programs have lacked coherence and long-term perspective. The flow of money speaks loudly here: national programs to train physicians consumed 70 percent of the Foundation's workforce budget, leaving 30 percent for training all other health professionals (Figure 13.4).

Perhaps reflecting its comfort with academic medical institutions, the Foundation was slow to recognize that the shift in health care from the medical community to corporations and business concerns presented an opportunity to offer training to individuals from disciplines such as economics, management, and law that are not normally associated with health care.

As the twenty-first century approaches, the question is how the nation's workforce programs will respond to a health care system that was barely envisioned in the relatively recent past. Twenty-some years ago, "health maintenance organization" was a concept known to only a smattering of academicians, policy wonks, and health professionals. Now most people with medical needs enter the world of managed care, where large conglomerates buy and sell health services, generalist physicians serve as gatekeepers, and the bottom line is paramount. Government can no longer be counted on to ensure that services are provided for the neediest citizens, and federal subsidies for graduate medical education are threatened. With the graying of the population, more chronic care is provided in homes and outpatient facilities. At the same time, the amount of acute care in hospitals is declining as these services are delivered on an outpatient basis. Advances in communications technology are changing the way information is transmitted and received.

This is the context in which workforce programs intended for the early twenty-first century operate. The *content* of the programs depends on how these factors are addressed. While it is premature to draw definitive conclusions from recently initiated programs, the Foundation's cumulative experience over nearly a quarter of a century suggests four principles that can serve as guidelines for the development of future workforce programs.

## Invest in Individuals

Investments in people provide great returns to the health care field. To date, the Foundation has already devoted nearly half of its workforce funds to fellowships and faculty development awards (Table 13.1).

**Figure 13.4.** National Workforce Programs for Physicians and Other Health Professionals, by Dollar Amount and Percentage.

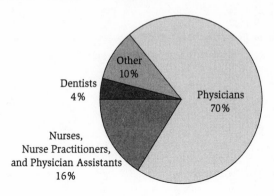

Although these are expensive (each clinical scholar and health policy fellow costs the Foundation more than $100,000 a year),[13] often invisible to trustees and staff, and difficult to evaluate (how much credit, for example, does a fellowship contribute to an individual's success later in life?), they are a productive investment. They give talented individuals the freedom to take risks and enter careers that the market is not yet willing to support.

What's more, there is a professional advantage in being awarded an esteemed fellowship. Such a plum often leads to enhanced career opportunities and to greater influence on the institutions where fellows work, the professional societies to which they belong, and health policy in general. It may be that the Foundation has had more effect on academic medicine and the public policy process indirectly through its fellows and scholars than directly through its institutional support.

## Broaden Fellowships to Other Disciplines

As professionals other than physicians play a greater role in health care, fellowship programs should be broadened to include people from a wide range of disciplines. The Foundation's fellowship programs during the 1970s and 1980s reflected the dominance of physicians in the health care system. During these years, the Foundation invested heavily in training physicians, particularly internists. It made a smaller but still substantial investment in nursing and dental fellows.[14] Of the programs initiated in those decades, only the health policy fellowships (which, in practice, have been awarded mainly to physicians) and the faculty fellowships in health care finance were open to a broader range of disciplines.

*(continued on page 246)*

**Table 13.1. Foundation Fellowship—Faculty Scholar Programs.**

| Program | Dates | Fellows | Training or Research Focus | Fellows per Year | Length of Awards | Number of Graduates Through 1996 | Funding ($ million) |
|---|---|---|---|---|---|---|---|
| Clinical Nurse Scholars | 1982–1991 | Nurses | Nursing research, clinical practice and management | 9 | 2 years | 62 | 11.0 |
| Clinical Scholars | 1973–1998 | Physicians | Nonbiological health sciences | 34<br>26 RWJF<br>8 Dept. of<br>Veterans Affairs | 2 years | 707 | 85.5 |
| Dental Services Research Scholars | 1982–1990 | Dentists | Health services | 5 | 2 years | 30 | 5.0 |
| Faculty Fellowships in Health Care Finance | 1985–1994 | Health administration faculty | Health care financing | 6 | $1\frac{1}{2}$ years | 60 | 2.5 |
| Family Practice Fellowship | 1977–1988 | Doctors training to be family practitioners | Family practice | 12 | 2 years | 101 | 11.2 |

Table 13.1. Foundation Fellowship and Faculty Scholar Programs. (continued)

| | | | | | | | |
|---|---|---|---|---|---|---|---|
| General Pediatric Development | 1979–1988 | Pediatricians | Developmental pediatrics | 12 | 2 years | 111 | 10.9 |
| Generalist Physician Faculty Scholars | 1993–2004 | Physicians | Primary care | 15 | 4 years | 0 | 27.8 |
| Health Policy Fellows | 1973–1998 | Mainly physicians—some nurses and others | Staff work in Congress or executive branch | 6 | 1 year | 133 | 7.0 |
| Investigator Awards in Health Policy Research | 1994–1999 | All disciplines except medicine | Broad health policy | 10 | Up to 3 years | 1 | 18.0 |
| Minority Medical Faculty Development | 1984–2000 | Minority physicians | Biomedical, clinical health services | 12 | 4 years | 67 | 59.4 |
| Nurse Faculty Fellowships | 1977–1982 | Nurses | Develop nurse-practitioner faculty | 20 | 1 year | 99 | 4.8 |
| Scholars in Health Policy Research | 1993–1999 | Economists, political scientists, sociologists | Multidisciplinary health policy | 12 | 2 years | 12 | 12.3 |

In the 1990s, the role of business executives, economists, lawyers, and other nonphysicians in shaping health policy has expanded, while the dominance of physicians has diminished. Whatever one might think of this trend, it does offer an opportunity to broaden the network of people who receive fellowships, and indeed, recent Foundation programs have opened up fellowships to individuals from nonmedical, nonnursing disciplines. In light of this change, and in recognition of the changes in the health care sector, it is time to explore an increased focus on training professionals who can play important roles but do not come from disciplines traditionally associated with health care.

## Attend to Total Systems

With the rapid and dramatic changes in health services, workforce programs should involve total systems of health care rather than focusing on specific components such as medical centers. In the 1970s, the power to affect health care lay substantially with academic medicine. This led The Robert Wood Johnson Foundation to concentrate its resources in medical centers. Since then, health care has changed dramatically. New organizations—HMOs, health centers, hospital and health care networks, and state agencies—have joined academic medical centers in shaping the careers of health professionals.

Any institution that strives to influence the supply and distribution of health professionals must design programs to work with these organizations. Currently, three programs support consortiums of health providers and training institutions: the Generalist Physician Initiative, Practice Sights, and Partnerships for Training. Systemwide and cross-cutting approaches that move beyond academic medicine in the training and placement of health professionals are the logical way to respond to and influence an increasingly complex health care system.

## Improve Distribution of Health Professionals

To increase access to health care requires emphasizing more equitable distribution, as well as an increased supply, of health professionals. Even with increased numbers of generalist and minority physicians, nurse practitioners, and physician assistants, the scarcity of health professionals in underserved areas remains critical, and in the current economic and political climate this is likely to worsen. So far, nobody has found the key, if one exists, to overcoming the barriers that discourage health professionals from serving inner city and rural communities. Although it may be, as some commentators have argued, that nothing short of an expanded National Health Service Corps will resolve the problem,[15] the Foundation has made some limited attempts to encourage physicians to practice in underserved areas.

In the 1970s and 1980s, the Foundation addressed the distribution of health professionals as a peripheral part of programs designed to restructure health care delivery, for example, by establishing networks of rural physicians and group practices allied with community hospitals. In the mid-1990s, the Foundation began to address some of the structural and social factors that discourage health care professionals from practicing in rural areas and inner cities: the poor reimbursement, the isolation, and the lack of social amenities and professional opportunities for a spouse that keep health care professionals, no matter how well trained, from serving in rural areas. *Practice Sights,* a five-year program begun in 1993, focuses directly on reducing such barriers. It requires participating health care systems—such as state agencies, academic institutions, and HMOs—to work together. Under this program, health care systems have set up loan forgiveness programs, provided technical assistance in practice management, worked to increase reimbursement rates, and offered other incentives to attract health professionals to inner city and rural practices. A second program, *Reach Out,* is discussed in Chapter One [of *To Improve Health and Health Care 1997: The Robert Wood Johnson Foundation Anthology*]; in the present context we note how it builds on the medical profession's tradition of community service.

Investments in training the health care workforce are necessary, but not sufficient, to increase access by underserved populations to basic health care. As the creation of such programs as Practice Sights and Reach Out suggests, it is important to address the inequitable distribution of health professionals directly.

# CONCLUSION

The lessons of the past twenty-four years are both simple and complex. They are simple in demonstrating that an unwavering commitment to improving the health care workforce is required to effect change, or to prepare for it when change comes about for other reasons. The lessons are complex insofar as any single foundation's resources can have only a limited impact in a health care system that is rapidly changing and has many more key players than it did even five years ago.

The challenge for the future is to develop workforce programs that further a vision of universal access within the context of an evolving American health care system where business rather than social values predominate, where incentives to avoid serving sick and vulnerable populations are inherent, and where power has shifted out of the hands of medicine. How institutions, including The Robert Wood Johnson Foundation, meet this challenge will determine the course of health care in the United States.

## Notes

1. D. Rogers, Robert Wood Johnson Foundation, *Annual Report 1972,* pp. 11–12.

2. N. Kassebaum, "Federal Health Professions Training and Distribution Initiatives: Foundations for a Targeted Approach," *Academic Medicine* 70 (1995), 296–297.

3. National Institutes of Health, *Data Book 1994,* tab. 20; U.S. Senate Committee on Labor and Human Resources, *Health Professions Education Consolidation and Reauthorization Act of 1995: Report* (1995); R. Rosenblatt and others, "The Effect of Federal Grants on Medical Schools' Production of Primary Care Physicians," *American Journal of Public Health* 83 (1993), 322–328; A. Epstein, "U.S. Teaching Hospitals in the Evolving Health Care System," *JAMA* 273 (1995), 1203–1207.

4. D. Rogers, *Annual Report,* p. 28.

5. R. Fein and J. Rowe, *A Review of the RWJF Clinical Scholars Program,* unpublished (1992), p. 10.

6. J. Evans and C. Royer, *The Robert Wood Johnson Foundation: A Twenty-Year Assessment,* unpublished (1992), p. 10.

7. J. Cantor and others, *Evaluation of the Minority Medical Education Program,* unpublished (1994).

8. K. Bridges and L. Smith, *An Evaluation of the Minority Medical Faculty Development Program of the Robert Wood Johnson Foundation,* unpublished (1995).

9. U. S. Department of Health and Human Services, *Secretary's Commission on Nursing: Final Report* (1988), p. 175.

10. See T. Keenan and others, *Nurses and Doctors: Their Education and Practice* (Cambridge, Mass.: Oelgeschlager, Gunn & Hain, 1992); L. Aiken and M. Gwyther, "Medicare Funding of Nurse Education," *Journal of the American Medical Association* 273 (1995), 1528–1532; C. Fagin, "The Visible Problems of an 'Invisible' Profession: The Crisis and Challenge for Nursing," in *The Nation's Health* (3rd. ed.), P. Lee and C. Estes, eds. (Boston: Jones & Bartlett, 1990), 190–192; U.S. Department of Health and Human Services, *Secretary's Commission on Nursing, Final Report* (1988).

11. The project's final report—written in 1990, when fifty-three scholars had completed training—found that "all of the scholars have remained active in nursing in a leadership role. With three exceptions, all of the scholars are actively involved in academic careers in a major school of nursing." R. de Tornyay, *Final Report on the RWJF Clinical Nurse Scholars Program,* unpublished (1990).

12. R. Bulger, *The Robert Wood Johnson Foundation and Human Resources for Health: Some Observations on the First Twenty Years and Some Proposals for the Next Ten,* unpublished (1992).

13. S. A. Schroeder, "The Institute of Medicine's Review of the Health Policy Fellowship Programs," in *For the Public Good: Highlights from the Institute of Medicine, 1970–1995* (Washington, D.C.: National Academy Press, 1995), 161–167.

14. Nearly one thousand physicians and two hundred nurses, nurse practitioners, dentists, and physician assistants were trained or received fellowships under the Foundation's programs.

15. R. Reynolds, "Make Health Reform Work. Draft Doctors," *New York Times* (June 1, 1993), p. A17.

# APPENDIX: NATIONAL WORKFORCE PROGRAMS, BY DATE

**Medical School Student Aid Program**
- Financial aid for women, minority, and rural medical students
- 1972-1978
- $12,600,000 awarded

**Pre-professional Minority Programs**
- Enrichment programs for potential medical school candidates
- 1972-1992
- $13,300,000 awarded

**Clinical Scholars Program**
- Two-year postresidency fellowships in nonbiomedical health sciences for physicians committed to clinical medicine
- 1973-1998
- $85,500,000 authorized
- Currently, thirty-four Clinical Scholars a year are appointed (eight are funded by the Department of Veterans Affairs); 707 scholars completed the program through 1996
- Training is offered at the following medical centers: Chicago, Johns Hopkins, Michigan, University of California-Los Angeles, North Carolina, Washington, and Yale. It was offered in the past at University of California-San Francisco and Stanford (a joint program that ran between 1974 and mid-1996), Case Western Reserve (1970-76), Columbia (1975-78), Duke (1969-75; this site was funded under the original program of the Carnegie Corporation and Commonwealth Fund and was not continued when The Robert Wood Johnson Foundation took over the program), George Washington (1975-79), McGill (1970-81), and Pennsylvania (1974-mid-1996)

**Dental School Student Aid Program**
- Financial aid for women, minority, and rural dental students
- 1973-1978
- $4,000,000 awarded

**Health Policy Fellowships Program**
- One-year fellowships (three-month orientation organized by the

Note: Programs with an end date of 1997 and beyond may be extended.

Institute of Medicine followed by a nine-month assignment in Congress or executive branch) in Washington, D.C.

- 1973-1998
- $7,000,000 authorized
- Six fellowships a year are awarded; 60 fellows completed the program

### National Medical Fellowships
- Financial aid for minority medical students
- 1973-1996
- $10,200,000 authorized

### Primary Care Residency Program
- Primary care training for internal medicine and pediatric residents
- 1973-1981
- $10,800,000 awarded to the following medical centers or hospitals: Boston City Hospital, Florida, Harvard, Missouri, Pennsylvania, Rochester, UCLA, UCSF, Washington

### Dental Training for Care of the Handicapped
- Development of training programs to improve dental treatment of handicapped patients
- 1974-1979
- $4,900,000 awarded to eleven dental schools: Alabama, UCLA, Columbia, Kentucky, Maryland, Michigan, Minnesota, Nebraska, New York, Tennessee, and Washington

### United Student Aid Funds
- Financial assistance
- 1977-1985
- $7,500,000 awarded

### Nurse Faculty Fellowship Program
- One-year fellowships to develop core nurse-practitioner faculty
- 1977-1982
- $4,800,000 awarded to four nursing schools: Colorado, Indiana, Maryland, and Rochester
- Twenty fellowships a year were awarded; ninety-nine fellows completed the program

### Primary Care Training for Emergency Nurses
- Certificate training in primary care for nursing staff of rural hospitals

- 1977-1982
- $1,900,000 awarded to six hospital training sites

**Family Practice Faculty Fellowships Program**
- Two-year postresident fellowships in family practice for physicians planning academic careers
- 1978-1988
- $11,200,000 awarded. Five medical centers offered fellowship training initially: Case Western Reserve, Iowa, Missouri-Columbia, Utah, and Washington-Seattle. It was later reduced to three (Washington-Seattle, Missouri-Columbia, and Case Western Reserve)
- Twelve fellowships a year were awarded; 101 fellows completed the program

**General Pediatric Academic Development Program**
- Two-year fellowships to train future pediatric faculty in general pediatrics
- 1979-1988
- $10,900,000 awarded to six academic medical centers: Duke, Johns Hopkins, Pennsylvania, Rochester, Stanford, and Yale
- Twelve fellowships a year were awarded; 11 pediatricians completed the program.

**Clinical Nurse Scholars Program**
- Two-year scholarships to develop a core nursing faculty skilled in research, clinical practice, and management
- 1982-1991
- $11,000,000 awarded for training at three sites: Pennsylvania, Rochester, and UCSF
- Nine scholarships a year were awarded; sixty-two scholars completed the program

**Dental Services Research Scholars Program**
- Two-year fellowships to train dental faculty in nonclinical health sciences and health services
- 1982-1990
- $5,000,000 awarded for training at two sites (Harvard and UCLA)
- Five scholarships a year were awarded; thirty scholars completed the program

**Minority Medical Faculty Development Program**
- Four-year postdoctoral research fellowships for minority physicians committed to careers in academic medicine
- 1984-2000
- $59,400,000 authorized
- Currently, twelve fellowships a year are awarded; sixty-seven fellows completed the program through 1996

**Faculty Fellowships in Health Care Finance**
- Thirty-month fellowships—three-month (later changed to four) orientation at The Johns Hopkins University, followed by a nine-month (later changed to eight) assignment to a health care financing organization and up to eighteen months' research
- 1985-1994
- $2,500,000 awarded
- Six fellowships a year were awarded; sixty fellows completed the program

**Minority Medical Education Program**
- Six-week summer program for minority college students considering medical school
- 1988-1999
- $15,300,000 authorized. As of 1996, eight sites offer training: Alabama, Baylor, Case Western Reserve, Chicago Consortium led by Rush University, United Negro College Fund (Fisk University/Vanderbilt), Virginia, Western Consortium led by the University of Washington School of Medicine, and Yale. The Illinois Institute of Technology was a site between 1988 and 1995.
- 125 students a year are selected per site; 5,500 students have completed the program through 1996

**Strengthening Hospital Nursing: A Program to Improve Patient Care**
- Grants to hospitals to improve patient care by restructuring services around the nursing staff
- 1989-1995
- A $26.8 million joint program with the Pew Charitable Trusts. RWJF awarded $16,500,000 for twenty planning grants, fifteen phase one implementation grants, and fourteen phase two implementation grants

**Nursing Services Manpower Development Program**
- Four-year grants, on average, to institutions to attract more minorities and others (older women, single mothers) to nursing careers and to overcome the barriers to their entering the profession

- 1989-1994
- $3,200,000 awarded to institutions in seven states: California, Illinois, Iowa, Indiana, New York, Pennsylvania, and Texas

**Generalist Physician Initiative**
- Grants to academic medical centers, in collaboration with HMOs, state governments, private insurers, hospitals, and community health centers, to increase the number of general internists, general pediatricians, and family practitioners
- 1991-2000
- $32,700,000 authorized planning grants were awarded to eighteen medical centers or consortiums in 1992; of these, fourteen received implementation grants: Boston, Case Western Reserve, Dartmouth, East Carolina, Hahnemann, Massachusetts, Georgia, Nevada, New Mexico, New York Medical College, Pennsylvania State, Texas-Galveston, SUNY/Buffalo, Virginia

**Generalist Physician Faculty Scholars Program**
- 1993-2004
- $27,800,000 authorized
- Fifteen scholars a year are selected

**Generalist Provider Research Initiative**
- Research on generalist/specialist mix and distribution and to evaluate the Foundation's generalist programs in a larger context
- 1993-1998
- $3,000,000 authorized

**Ladders in Nursing Careers (National Replication)**
- National replication of program developed in 1988 by the Greater New York Hospital Foundation. Grants to hospital associations to assist minority and other disadvantaged (e.g., single parents) housekeeping staff, nurses' aides, and nurses to advance their careers.
- 1993-1997
- $4,900,000 authorized. Through the end of 1995, awards were made to hospital associations in nine states: Georgia, Iowa, Maryland, Minnesota, North Dakota, Ohio, Rhode Island, South Carolina, and Texas

**Scholars in Health Policy Research**
- Two-year postdoctoral fellowships to economists, political scientists, and sociologists to conduct health care research

- 1993-1999
- $12,300,000 authorized
- Twelve scholars a year are selected

### Investigator Awards in Health Policy Research
- Three years' salary support for outstanding young researchers or eminent senior scholars to pursue health care research
- 1994-1999
- $18,000,000 authorized
- Ten investigators are selected each year

### Partnerships for Training: Regional Education Systems for Nurse Practitioners, Certified Nurse-Midwives, and Physician Assistants
- Support of innovative and collaborative education models for training nurse practitioners, certified nurse-midwives, and physician assistants in their own communities
- 1995-2001
- $14,000,000 authorized
- Planning grants were made to organizations in twelve states: Arkansas, California, Colorado, Idaho, Illinois, Michigan, Minnesota, New Mexico, New York, North Carolina, Pennsylvania, and Wisconsin

### Colleagues in Caring Regional Collaboratives for Nursing Workforce Development
- Grants to regional consortiums of nursing schools, hospitals, and nursing service providers and associations to assess and meet the nursing needs in the region
- 1996-1999
- $4,000,000 authorized

### Project 3000 by 2000: Health Professions Partnership Initiative
- Grants to academic medical centers, working in partnership with local schools, colleges, and community organizations, to attract minority high school students to health professions and to nurture their interest
- 1996-2001
- $5,000,000 authorized for grants to the following medical centers: Connecticut, Georgia, Louisville, Massachusetts, Nebraska, North Carolina, Oregon, Pennsylvania/Hahnemann, South Carolina, and Wisconsin-Madison. Up to five additional sites will be selected in the future.

# Grant Report Summaries from
# The Robert Wood Johnson Foundation

## SUPPORT FOR A CITY-STATE PARTNERSHIP TO
## DEVELOP PRIMARY CARE FACILITIES IN NEW YORK CITY
(last updated 2001)

### Grantees

Primary Care Development Corporation (New York, New York)
New York City-State Partnership for Primary Care Facility Development

### Summary

These grants from The Robert Wood Johnson Foundation (RWJF) were part of a multifoundation New York City-State effort to improve access to basic health services to New York City residents through a program focusing on planning, development, and construction of new primary care facilities. The initiative provided start-up support for a new, independent organization, the Primary Care Development Corporation (PCDC), set up by New York City (NYC). A total of $35.1 million from a variety of public and private sources supported the PCDC's operations, project development, and capital development; with $17 million of this funding, received as a capital grant from the city, the PCDC set up and administered the Primary Care Development Fund, a revolving loan fund. The bulk of the loan fund proceeds were used for planning and development costs for sponsors of new facilities, including costs for facility design and obtaining regulatory approvals, and special reserve funds to provide additional security for facility capital financing. PCDC staff also provided technical assistance to the primary care facilities sponsors for identifying sites, completing required land use and environmental reviews, program and facility design, and obtaining health care regulatory approvals. By the end of the second RWJF grant, twenty-one facilities were in operation and seven more were under construction, representing a total investment of approximately $100 million. All twenty-eight facilities were located in underserved communities throughout the city's five boroughs. At full capacity, the facilities were projected to provide 730,000 patient visits annually and generate nearly a thousand jobs, many in the city's most economically distressed areas. In collaboration with four of the city's largest banks—Chase, Citibank, Republic, and JP Morgan—the PCDC also created a $20 million primary care loan pool to finance small projects (defined as those under $3 million). Called the Primary Care Capital Fund (PCCF), it was intended to assist small projects for which the PCDC's tax-exempt bond program was inappropriate. In spring 1999, the PCCF received an award for innovation from Social Compact, a Washington-based national community development organization. In fall 1999, the PCDC's governing board decided to expand the organization's mandate by increasing the number of loans to modernize existing primary care facilities and expanding its programs to improve facilities' operational efficiency, effectiveness, and quality.

# STUDY OF BARRIERS TO PRIMARY CARE IN CALIFORNIA

(last updated April 2001)

## Grantee

University of California, San Francisco

## Summary

These grants from The Robert Wood Johnson Foundation enabled researchers at the University of California, San Francisco, to study access to primary care in selected urban California communities. The research was designed to assess whether hospitalization rates for certain chronic conditions typically managed by timely outpatient care are valid and useful measures of community access to care. Using hospital discharge and census data, the researchers calculated hospitalization rates for five "ambulatory care–sensitive" (ACS) conditions—asthma, hypertension, congestive heart failure, chronic obstructive pulmonary disease, and diabetes—among 250 ZIP code clusters in California. The project also included surveys of patients, residents, and community physicians to determine whether variations in hospitalization rates for ACS conditions could be explained by variations in the health-seeking behavior of individuals, the disease prevalence in a community, or the patterns of physician practice. Among the investigators' key findings: (1) communities where people perceive their access to care as the lowest have the highest rates of hospitalization for ACS conditions; (2) hospitalizations for ACS conditions were higher in communities with greater proportions of uninsured and Medicaid patients and higher in areas where greater proportions of residents said they had no regular place to obtain health care; (3) variations in physician practice styles or in patients' propensity to seek care for medical symptoms could not explain variations in hospitalization rates for ACS conditions. The strong positive association between hospitalization rates for ACS conditions and perceived access to care suggests that these rates can serve as a valid measure of access to care, the investigators say. Findings from the project were reported in several major medical journals, including the *Journal of the American Medical Association* and the *New England Journal of Medicine,* and in presentations at several national meetings. The principal investigator and his colleagues are currently conducting a longitudinal analysis of how managed care penetration in the community affects hospitalization rates for ACS conditions.

# STUDY OF BARRIERS TO PRIMARY CARE
# LEADING TO UNNECESSARY HOSPITALIZATION

(last updated July 2001)

## Grantee

United Hospital Fund of New York (New York, New York)

## Summary

These grants from The Robert Wood Johnson Foundation provided support to the United Hospital Fund of New York to develop, validate, and implement a research technique called small-area analysis, used to identify communities with high rates of unnecessary hospitalization and limited access to primary care. During the first phase of the project, investigators refined the small-area analysis technique and used it to study differences in hospitalization rates for "ambulatory care–sensitive" (ACS) conditions, such as bacterial pneumonia and otitis media (a severe ear infection), which can be reduced with timely and effective outpatient care. Key findings included the following: (1) hospitalization for these ACS conditions was two to ten times greater in low-income than in high-income neighborhoods in New York City, and (2) poor African American areas in New York City had consistently higher hospital admission rates than other low-income areas. During the second phase of the project, investigators further analyzed data on preventable hospitalization in New York City and applied the small-area analysis technique to urban areas throughout the country. Key findings included the following: (1) more than half of all low-income patients in New York City reported access problems that delayed or prevented them from obtaining care, and (2) low-income areas in urban communities of Massachusetts, New York, New Jersey, Florida, Oregon, California, and Washington State had substantially higher admission rates for ACS conditions than high-income areas did. These replications validated the use of small-area analysis as a technique to identify and measure differences in hospitalization rates for ACS conditions. Articles based on the results of this study have appeared in the *Journal of the American Medical Association, Health Affairs,* and *HRP Reports.* A book, *Anatomy of a Safety Net,* is forthcoming. The investigators continue to assist other researchers and local planning officials in employing small-area analysis to identify barriers to primary care and to conduct analyses to more accurately pinpoint areas with high hospital utilization for ACS conditions.

# STUDY OF PRIMARY CARE FOR NURSING HOME RESIDENTS IN THREE HEALTH MAINTENANCE ORGANIZATIONS

## Grantee

School of Medicine, University of California, Los Angeles

## Summary

With this grant from The Robert Wood Johnson Foundation, the project team at the UCLA School of Medicine studied the long-term care being provided to nursing home residents using different models of HMO primary care. Case studies were conducted of three HMO programs covering 402 nursing home residents. Two basic models of providing care were found: the "dedicated team" model, which relies on a cadre of four physicians whose responsibilities are limited to nursing home, hospice, and home care and who are paired with full-time nurse practitioners or physicians assistants, and the "augmentation" model, which uses physicians who perform more conventional roles and provide primary care to nursing home residents in addition to their usual responsibilities and whose capabilities are augmented by nurse practitioners who also provide nursing home care. Findings include that (1) total primary care visits per month were higher among HMO residents than fee-for-service residents, (2) the use of the "dedicated team" approach provided more care than the other plans, and (3) in the plans using the "dedicated team" model, nursing home residents were transferred less often to the emergency department and a smaller number of residents were hospitalized compared to fee-for-service Medicare residents in the same nursing homes. The plan that used the "augmentation" model had similar health care utilization compared to fee-for-service in the same homes.

# ASSESSMENT OF THE NEEDS OF COMMUNITY-BASED PRIMARY CARE CENTERS MOVING INTO MANAGED CARE

(last updated January 1999)

## Grantee

Institute for Public Policy and Management, University of Washington (Seattle)

## Summary

The ability of community-based primary care centers to make the transition to managed care is important to their survival. Medicaid is a key source of revenue for these facilities, many of which are at risk of losing their Medicaid clients, who are increasingly moving into managed care. The first grant from The Robert Wood Johnson Foundation provided funding for an assessment of the needs of community-based primary care centers to participate successfully in managed care. The report was to include suggestions for how the Foundation could assist primary care centers in this process. A supplemental grant was necessary to complete the work because of unexpected delays. The principal investigator interviewed 111 individuals knowledgeable in community health centers or managed care, reviewed related literature, and surveyed activities in this area by other charitable foundations. He found that state Medicaid policies are critical in determining whether community-based primary care centers move successfully into managed care. The final report identified seven critical determinants of community health center success in managed care and recommended twelve projects for funding to address health center needs, including two national demonstration programs. None of the twelve has been funded. The Foundation is continuing to study the broader "safety net" system and wants to better understand its role in health care access before taking action on any one component. The report provided a snapshot of the nation's community-based primary care system. The principal investigator distributed approximately twenty copies of the report and made a presentation on the project at the National Association of Community Health Centers' annual convention.

SECTION THREE

# SUPPLY AND DISTRIBUTION

# Editors' Introduction to Section Three

In the 1960s, physicians, economists, and politicians began to express concern about the decreasing percentage of generalist physicians and the increasing percentage of physicians in specialty practices. They argued that this would result in uneven access to medical care and high costs. Since then, the composition of the health care workforce has attracted the attention of government, academics, and the medical and nursing communities. The debate raises questions about whether there was a current or impending shortage of generalist physicians (or physicians as a whole), what a proper percentage of generalist physicians would be, whether it is an appropriate area for government action, whether the market alone should determine physicians' career choices, and whether primary care should be provided by U.S.-trained or foreign-trained doctors.

The American Medical Association, the Association of American Medical Colleges, and other organizations concerned with the medical workforce and patient care have given great attention to the supply of physicians. Among the most influential voices has been the Council on Graduate Medical Education, which issued a series of reports on the health care workforce. To begin Section Three, we are reprinting in Chapter Fourteen the findings from its influential 1992 report, *Improving Access to Health Care Through Physician Workforce Reform.* The Institute of Medicine has been another prominent voice. The introduction to and summary of its 1978 study, *A Manpower Policy for Primary*

*Health Care,* are reprinted in Chapter Fifteen. A great many excellent articles were written in the 1990s—some of them based on research using sophisticated forecasting techniques. The 1993 article by David Kindig, James Cultice, and Fitzhugh Mullan titled "The Elusive Generalist Physician: Can We Reach a 50 Percent Goal?" (Chapter Sixteen) is illustrative. Using a computer model that forecasts physician supply, the authors suggested that even if it were possible to agree that a goal of 50 percent generalist physicians is desirable, reaching it would present a great challenge.

Although the rise of managed care in the mid-1990s tempered, at least for a while, the worry that there would be insufficient numbers of primary care physicians, the issue has not gone away. In 2002, Richard Cooper and colleagues published an article concluding that a physician shortage—and particularly a shortage of specialists—was impending. This article is reprinted in Chapter Seventeen and is followed in Chapter Eighteen by Kevin Grumbach's response.

A frequently asked question is what factors influence physicians to choose careers in primary care. Much has been written on the topic, and we are reprinting in Chapter Nineteen an article by Michael Rosenthal and his colleagues, published in 1994, that summarizes the state of knowledge about factors such as potential income, hours worked, and debt repayment on physicians' decisions to practice primary care.

Although a great deal of the literature has been devoted to the supply of primary care physicians, a considerable literature exists as well about their distribution: How do you attract physicians to traditionally underserved rural areas and, to a lesser extent, inner cities? The 2000 article by Roger Rosenblatt and Gary Hart, reprinted in Chapter Twenty, provides a fine summary of the factors that lead physicians to practice in rural areas.

The reprints are followed by abstracts from the literature on the supply and the distribution of primary care physicians.

The Robert Wood Johnson Foundation has attempted to increase the supply of primary care physicians and to improve their distribution through a number of national programs. One of them, Practice Sights: State Primary Care Development Strategies, was the subject of a chapter by Irene Wielawski in volume 6 of *To Improve Health and Health Care: The Robert Wood Johnson Foundation Anthology,* which we reprint as Chapter Twenty-One. It is followed by summaries of reports done by the Foundation's Grant Results Reporting Unit on relevant Foundation grants.

CHAPTER FOURTEEN

# Improving Access to Health Care Through Physician Workforce Reform

## Directions for the Twenty-First Century

Council on Graduate Medical Education
1992

## FINDING NO. 1:

The Nation has too few generalists and too many specialists.

- The growing shortage of practicing generalists (i.e., family physicians, general internists, and general pediatricians) will be greatly aggravated by the growing percentage of medical school graduates who plan to subspecialize. The expansion of managed care and provision of universal access to care will only further increase the demand for generalist physicians.

- A rational health care system must be based upon an infrastructure consisting of a majority of generalist physicians trained to provide quality primary care and an appropriate mix of other specialists to meet health care needs. Today, other specialists and subspecialists provide a significant amount of primary care. However, physicians who are trained, practice, and receive continuing education in the generalist disciplines provide more comprehensive and cost-effective care than nonprimary care specialists and subspecialists.

## FINDING NO. 2:

Problems of access to medical care persist in rural and inner-city areas despite large increases in the number of physicians nationally.

This chapter originally appeared as Council on Graduate Medical Education. *Third Report: Improving Access to Health Care Through Physician Workforce Reform: Directions for the 21st Century.* Rockville, Md: U.S. Department of Health and Human Services; 1992.

- Access to primary care services is especially difficult in rural and inner-city areas. Many factors contribute to the problems of access, including economic and social circumstances of rural and inner-city areas as well as the shortage of minority and generalist physicians. Minority physicians and physicians in the three primary care specialties (family practice, general internal medicine, and general pediatrics) are more likely to serve inner-city populations.

- Family physicians and general surgeons are more likely than other specialties to serve rural populations. The decline in numbers of general surgeons entering rural practice is little recognized and has significant implications for access to trauma, obstetrical, and orthopedic services in rural settings and to the fiscal viability or rural hospitals.

- Consequently, more minority and generalist physicians must be educated, and educational programs should specifically address skills needed in these settings. This must be accompanied by sufficient incentives to enter and remain in inner-city and rural practice and by the development of adequate health care systems in which they can practice.

- Access to one important component of primary medical care, obstetrical services, has been in the national spotlight. Problems are greatest in rural and inner-city areas. Causes include economic and sociocultural factors and the availability of obstetricians, family physicians, and nurse midwives. While the total number of obstetricians continues to increase, the proportion providing obstetrical services decreases dramatically with the number of years in practice. Less that 10 percent of obstetricians practice in rural settings. Consequently, family physicians historically provide the majority of rural obstetrical care. In recent years, however, the proportion of family physicians providing obstetrical services has also declined markedly. While rising malpractice claims clearly have contributed to the decreasing provisions of obstetrical care, other factors, such as unpredictable hours, also seem to have contributed to these decisions.

# FINDING NO. 3:

The racial/ethnic composition of the Nation's physicians does not reflect the general population and contributes to access problems for underrepresented minorities.

- Although African Americans, Hispanic Americans, and Native Americans compose 22 percent of the total population and will constitute almost one-fourth of all Americans by the year 2000, they represent only 10 percent of practicing physicians and 3 percent of medical faculty.

- Increasing the percentage of underrepresented minorities in the medical profession is vital as a means of improving access to care and health status of these vulnerable and underserved populations. Minority physicians tend to practice more in minority/underserved areas, reduce language and cultural barriers to care, and provide much needed community leadership.

- Strategies to increase minority enrollment must emphasize increasing and strengthening the applicant pool, the acceptance rate from within this pool, and the student retention rate. These strategies must take into account disproportionately high rates of poverty, poor health status, poor schools, and a continued lack of access to educational and career opportunities. They must include both traditional short-term efforts and long-term strategies targeting younger students early in the education pipeline.

# FINDING NO 4:

Shortages exist in the specialties of general surgery, adult and child psychiatry, and preventive medicine and among generalist physicians with additional geriatrics training.

- The future growth in general surgical services is likely to exceed the growth in the supply of general surgeons. Aging of the U.S. population will increase demand for surgical services, and the number of physicians in general surgery is inadequate to meet a growing need for trauma care services and for surgical care in rural areas. The training curricula for general surgery need to be broad-based to ensure that graduates have sufficient knowledge and skills to manage the wide array of surgical problems that may be seen in rural and inner-city areas.

# FINDING NO. 5:

Within the framework of the present health care system, the current physician-to-population ratio in the Nation is adequate. Further increases in this ratio will do little to enhance the health of the public or to address the Nation's problems of access to health care. Continued increases in this ratio will, in fact, hinder efforts to contain costs.

- Efforts to solve problems of access to health care by increasing the total physician supply have been largely unsuccessful. A growing physician oversupply is projected, which will hinder efforts to contain costs.

Consequently, the number of physicians educated should be reduced. Strategies to improve access to care should, instead, focus on altering the specialty mix, racial/ethnic composition, and geographic distribution of physicians.

# FINDING NO. 6:

The Nation's medical education system can be more responsive to public needs for more generalists, underrepresented minority physicians, and physicians for medically underserved rural and inner-city areas.

- The Nation's system of undergraduate and graduate medical education, taking place in 141 osteopathic and allopathic medical schools and in more than 1,500 institutions and agencies, has responded effectively to many of the Nation's health care needs. During the past 25 years, our Nation's medical education system has responded to public demands to increase the numbers of physicians, advance biomedical research, and develop new medical technology. These responses have resulted in a doubling of the physician supply and the establishment of a biomedical research and medical technology infrastructure that is unsurpassed.

- Today, the medical education system must respond to the Nation's health care and physician workforce needs in the 21st century. These include the need for more primary care research and increased access to primary care, particularly in underserved rural and urban communities. Changes in the institutional mission, goals, admissions policies, curriculum, faculty composition and reward system, and the site for medical education and teaching are necessary to respond to these needs.

# FINDING NO. 7:

The absence of a national physician workforce plan combined with financial and other disincentives are barriers to improved access to care.

- There is no national physician workforce plan for the United States to meet the current and projected future health care needs of the American people. In addition, there is no coordinated financing strategy and integrated medical education system to implement such a plan. Instead, such critical policy issues as the aggregate physician supply and specialty mix are the result of a series of individual decisions make by the 126 allopathic and 15 osteopathic medical schools and nearly 1,500 institutions and agencies that currently sponsor or affiliate with GME training programs. The medical education financing and health care reimbursement systems create significant disincentives to students who wish to become generalists, physicians who wish practice in underserved areas, and to the provision of basic primary and preventive services to all Americans.

CHAPTER FIFTEEN

# A Manpower Policy for Primary Health Care

*Introduction and Summary*

Institute of Medicine
1978

The complexity of the health services industry in the United States has, in recent years, heightened public and professional interest in primary health care. Access to the entire range of health services has its focus on the primary care practitioner, who also is expected to coordinate the services and to assure continuity of care.

The importance of an adequate supply of primary care practitioners in the U.S. began to receive increased public attention during the 1960s. By 1976 the Congress declared, in the statutory preamble to the Health Professions Educational Assistance Act, that the availability of health care in general depends largely on the availability of primary care practitioners.

Because appropriate manpower resources are essential to an effective primary care strategy, the Institute of Medicine undertook the study reported here to propose recommendations that would coordinate many important aspects of primary care manpower policy and to help assure that the development of that policy is based on appropriate information. An interest in contributing to the development of a national health manpower policy was initially expressed by Institute of Medicine members considering the Institute's own program in the spring of 1972. A work group on health manpower proposed a study to examine the place of primary care in the U.S. health care system, and particularly the roles of different categories of primary care professionals. This report presents the conclusions of that study, begun in 1975.

---

# POLICY ISSUES IN PRIMARY CARE

Primary health care is defined in this report as accessible, comprehensive, coordinated, and continual care provided by accountable providers of health services. It is generally recognized as the first level of personal health services (as distinguished from public, environmental and occupational health services), where initial professional attention is paid to current or potential health problems. Frequently, primary care is associated with care of the "whole person" rather than care for an illness.

The term *primary care* has gained wide usage in the present decade, although the concept is not new. In the United States, national attention began to be focused on primary care in the mid-1960s. At that time a series of commission reports by health leaders in the private sector proposed the development of training programs to prepare physicians to deliver comprehensive and continual care.[1] These reports reflected a conviction that more socially oriented care, responding to a wide range of patients' problems, was needed to complement the growing medical use of highly specialized services and technological procedures.

An increase in programs to train physicians for primary care has been accompanied by increased interest in having coordinated care delivered by an interdisciplinary team of physicians, nurses, and other therapists who can provide diverse services to the patient.[2] To supplement physician services and make primary care available to medically underserved populations, programs have been established with federal support to train nurse practitioners and physician assistants.[3]

A growing body of literature[4] indicates that a small number of issues have been paramount in discussions of primary care policy:

1. What is the scope of primary care? How should primary care be *defined*? What categories of health professionals are primary care practitioners?

2. What would be an adequate *supply* of primary care practitioners? What are the dimensions of any current or projected national shortage of primary care practitioners?

3. How can an appropriate *distribution* of manpower be attained in order to meet nationwide primary care needs? What public financial incentives and education policies are appropriate to help assure the availability of primary care in rural areas and inner cities? What financial incentives and education policies should be used to help assure the commitment of sufficient professional manpower to primary care vis-à-vis "secondary" or "tertiary" care?

4. How and where should primary care practitioners be *educated* and trained? What attention should be paid to primary care in the education of physicians and other health professionals? What efforts are needed, if any, to devote sufficient educational resources to primary care? How should primary care practitioners and training programs be *credentialed*?

As a whole, these issues require the development of a comprehensive health manpower policy for primary care. Manpower considerations have been prominent in the evolution of primary care policy, partly because of the importance of education and other health manpower considerations to the reduction of primary care shortages. Also, manpower considerations are basic to primary care policy because primary care is highly labor-intensive, relying more on personal communication and perhaps less on sophisticated equipment than do "secondary" or "tertiary" levels of care.

Unfortunately, primary care manpower issues must still be considered without the benefit of knowing where health care stops and social services begin. Preventive and promotional health education, counseling of patients, and continuity of care are all features of primary care with important social as well as medical implications. Therefore, manpower policies developed in this and earlier reports on primary care may have to be reconsidered when the bounds of health care are more clearly defined and the effects of primary care services on health outcomes are better understood. In this report, health manpower policy concerns are linked with a range of services that includes diagnostic and therapeutic procedures and health education.

# SCOPE AND METHODOLOGY OF THE STUDY

The conduct of this study has been based on the belief that a reasoned choice among objectives is necessary for the development of primary care manpower policy. Alternative goals and strategy options have been considered by the study steering committee and are presented in this report along with the committee's recommendations.

The study mandate was to develop an "integrated" primary care manpower policy. In the committee's view, an integrated policy embraces all major categories of primary care practitioners and serves to coordinate all important policy actions affecting their use. This report therefore addresses not only such traditional manpower concerns as public funding of education, credentialing of practitioners, and qualitative and quantitative aspects of training programs, but also the scope of primary care services, their reimbursement, and health services research. These latter issues so deeply affect the use and supply of primary care manpower that they must be included, in the committee's judgment, in any comprehensive and integrated, primary care manpower policy.

# FUNCTIONS AND ROLES

The output of the study was originally intended to be a determination of both the functions of primary care and the roles of different types of professionals in primary care. Functions and roles were thought to be the appropriate bases of an integrated primary care manpower policy. Consequently, the committee's first product, a definition of primary care, is an attempt to delineate primary care *functions* as fully as can now be done for purposes of public policy. That definition has been published as an interim report.[5]

The committee, however, came to believe that an explication of the *roles* of different professional groups was not now a practical, policy-oriented undertaking. In primary care, such roles overlap greatly and vary among practice settings and geographic locations. Roles often are not commensurate with training and experience. Occupational roles only now are being developed for the relatively new professional categories of family physicians, nurse practitioners, and physician assistants. Moreover, the activities of different professions may be merged in a team approach to health care.[6]

# ACTIVITY OF THE COMMITTEE

The committee began its two-year inquiry with a general goal of recommending policy toward an appropriate supply of trained practitioners providing high quality primary care to all populations in the country. In order to refine that goal, the committee developed a definition of primary care and a checklist with which to determine whether a provider is delivering primary care as defined.[7]

Because of the importance of the topic and wide interest in the study, the committee early in its deliberations formally solicited ideas and opinions from nearly one hundred concerned organizations and individuals. Statements by 18 organizations and individuals were presented at a one-day open meeting of the committee at the National Academy of Sciences in Washington, D.C., in January 1976.[8]

The committee met regularly to formulate a definition of primary care and to develop recommendations about the credentialing of primary care practitioners and their legal liability, the use and acceptance of nurse practitioners and physician assistants, and the financing of primary care services. Recommendations also were developed on the supply and distribution of primary care practitioners, the day-to-day content of primary care practice, and the contribution to primary care made by professional groups other than physicians in primary care disciplines, nurse practitioners, and physician assistants.

Policy options and research needs were considered in each of these areas. The committee made its conclusions on the basis of the best available data and research findings; in some areas, however, it was compelled to exercise judgment in the absence of numerical data. Information used by the committee in arriving at recommendations included published and unpublished material, papers prepared by the staff at the committee's request, presentations at the 1976 open meeting, and knowledge based on the committee's own expertise. No original research was undertaken by the committee.

# SUMMARY OF RECOMMENDATIONS

Chapters 2 through 5 of this report present background discussion, policy options, and recommendations in each major area that the committee considers important to the development of primary care manpower policy. The concluding section (Chapter 6) proposes a schedule for implementing the recommendations. Each recommendation is meant to be feasible, broad enough to guide activity for several years, and important for meeting the nation's primary care needs.

In Chapters 2 through 5, the essential data and evidence about the major topics are presented. These are followed by a description and evaluation of each of the policy options considered by the committee. Committee judgments, opinions, and beliefs are noted, as are the intended effects of each recommendation.

## Chapter 2: Primary Health Care Defined

Opinions of various interested groups and existing definitions were reviewed to reach a consensus on the definition of primary care. The committee agreed that primary care should be accessible, comprehensive, coordinated, continual care delivered by an accountable provider of health services. The chapter also includes a checklist for determining whether a given health care provider is delivering primary care as defined.

## Chapter 3: Practice Arrangements for Primary Health Care

The health problems and diagnoses most frequently recognized by physicians in primary care disciplines indicate the range of primary care services. Twenty-four diagnoses accounted in 1975 for about half of all office visits to general practitioners, family physicians, internists, pediatricians, and obstetricians and gynecologists in the United States. Visits to these physicians account for two-thirds of all office-based physician visits. Primary care is also delivered by nurse practitioners and physician assistants, approximately three-fourths of whom are employed in primary care settings.

Prototypes of primary care practice arrangements include single specialty units (including family physicians), multispecialty units, family practice teams, and multispecialty teams. Teams include physicians and new health practitioners. Currently, three-fourths of practicing U.S. physicians work in solo or two-physician practices. The committee recommends that (Recommendation #1) *because no practice arrangement has been found consistently superior to any other, primary care as defined in this report should continue to be delivered by various combinations of health care providers in a variety of practice arrangements.* Diversity in delivery methods is advocated so that a flexible primary care system can benefit from a pluralistic approach to the needs of different types of communities.

## Chapter 4: The Supply and Distribution of Primary Health Care Practitioners

Primary care manpower supplies and needs now constitute a major health policy consideration. The manpower issues include the overall supply of physicians and new health practitioners, physician specialty and geographic distribution, and monitoring and research priorities.

The committee notes that the supply of physicians in the United States will increase more than 60 percent by 1990 if total medical and osteopathic school enrollments continue at their current level. Physician productivity, population needs, and financial considerations make the adequacy of physician supply difficult to measure and evaluate, but the committee finds no reason to continue to increase the number of medical students across the country. However, it believes that an increasing number of future physicians should be in primary care. Pending progress in determining the adequacy of physician supply, it is urged that (Recommendation #2) *for the present, the number of entrants to medical school should remain at the current annual level.*

The supply of new health practitioners—nurse practitioners and physician assistants—is expected to exceed 40,000 in 1990, although only 9,500 new health practitioners had graduated from DHEW formal training programs by 1976. The committee is impressed by the quality of care delivered by new health practitioners. Their productivity, potential use to medically underserved populations, ability to deliver health education and counseling, and cost-containment potential justify financial support of their training. Because of the projected rise in physician supply, however, an increase in the training rate of nurse practitioners and physician assistants now appears undesirable. In the committee's judgment (Recommendation #3), *for the present, the number of nurse practitioners and physician assistants trained should remain at the current annual level.*

Reimbursement strategies were considered as a method for making primary care practice more attractive to physicians. The proportion of physicians in primary care disciplines has fallen from 94 percent in 1931 to 42 percent in 1963 and 38 percent in 1975. The committee rejects the option of increasing the number of physicians in primary care disciplines by increasing total physician supply. The committee instead proposes the following changes in reimbursement policies:

(Recommendation #4) *Third-party payors (federal, state, and private) should reimburse all physicians at the same payment level for the same primary care service.* This change would assure that physicians in primary care disciplines receive the same fees as other physicians for equivalent services. Higher fees would be justified only for specialty services provided on physician referral. Fee levels would be statewide under Recommendation #8.

(Recommendation #5) *Third-party payors (federal, state, and private) should reduce the differentials in payment levels between primary care procedures and non–primary care procedures.* The committee is not satisfied that current reimbursement practices provide adequate compensation for primary care services compared with surgery and other non–primary care services.

(Recommendation #6) *Third-party payors (federal, state, and private) should institute payments to practice units for those necessary services delivered by primary care providers and currently not reimbursed, such as commonly accepted health education and preventive services.* The delivery of comprehensive care stressing health maintenance is inhibited by a failure to reimburse for the full range of primary care services. Tests for efficacy and demonstration or special projects are suggested in initiating reimbursement of primary care providers for work in the prevention of illness and health education.

The geographic distribution of primary care physicians is another subject addressed in Chapter 4. In the committee's judgment (Recommendation #7), *training programs for family physicians, nurse practitioners, and physician assistants should continue to receive direct federal, state, and private support, because these practitioners are the most feasible providers of primary care to underserved populations.* Also, some changes in reimbursement policies are advocated to encourage primary care practitioners to serve in shortage areas, although the committee recognizes a dearth of available evidence linking reimbursement levels to physician location. The suggested changes are the following:

(Recommendation #8) *Third-party payors (federal, state, and private) should discontinue all geographic differentials in payment levels for physician services within a state.* This recommendation would eliminate any payment practice affording greater reimbursement to physicians in adequately served areas than to physicians in rural, underserved areas.

(Recommendation #9) *Third-party payors (federal, state, and private) should reimburse the practice unit for the same primary care services at the same payment level regardless of whether the services are provided by physicians, nurse practitioners, or physician assistants.* Lower reimbursement for new health practitioners suggests a two-tiered system of care, overlooks the high quality of services provided by nurse practitioners and physician assistants, and could hinder their employment. Practice units eligible for reimbursement could be owned by physicians, other health professionals, and private or public organizations.

The committee also examines the importance of monitoring and researching the success of an integrated primary care manpower policy. The committee believes (Recommendation #10) that *there should be an active, continuous program for monitoring a number of factors, including the numbers and specialty and geographic distribution of physicians, nurse practitioners, and physician assistants, and also for monitoring the perceptions of the patient population regarding the adequacy and availability of primary care services.* To expand and improve the knowledge base used in making decisions in primary care manpower policy, the committee finds (Recommendation #11) that *an increased emphasis should be given to health services research in primary care manpower.* Such research could be especially helpful in determining primary care manpower needs. It could also reveal why physicians choose to seek training and continue to practice in primary care or other specialties.

## Chapter 5: Education for Primary Health Care Practice

Primary care education policy should assure both an adequate supply of primary care practitioners and levels of competency suitable for the task to be performed. At this time, major educational issues include percentage goals for primary care residencies, public support of primary care residency programs, the nature of primary care medical education and team training, and credentialing.

Although the committee did not find an adequate data base for establishing a percentage goal for residency programs in primary care disciplines, it is inclined to believe that most physicians should be primary care practitioners, because primary care includes the management of the great majority of problems presented by patients. Therefore (Recommendation #12), *the committee recommends a substantial increase in the national goal for the percent of first-year residents in primary care fields.* Most committee members believe that perhaps the goal should be in the range of 60 to 70 percent while the current shortage exists.

To develop graduate medical education in primary care disciplines, training facilities must be designed and faculties compensated. In the committee's view, government financial incentives are preferable to public action requiring that medical schools contribute prescribed portions of their resources to primary care training programs. The committee recommends (Recommendation #13) that *federal and state governments should continue to promote primary care partly by using financial incentives for the creation and support of primary care residency programs.*

The nature of medical education in general inhibits the development of primary care. A broad, simultaneous set of actions is recommended to assure an atmosphere better suited to primary care development. These actions include the following:

(Recommendation #14) *It is desirable that all medical schools direct or have a major affiliation with at least one primary care residency program in which residents have responsibility under faculty supervision for the provision of accountable, accessible, comprehensive, continual, and coordinated care.* A majority of the committee asserts that qualified medical school graduates should be able to receive graduate training in primary care in programs affiliated with their schools.

(Recommendation #15) *In selecting among applicants for admission, medical schools should give weight to likely indicators of primary care career selection.* Although the data and evidence are incomplete, such indicators now being investigated include an affinity for personal service, interpersonal skills, ability to function as part of a team, and performance in behavioral and social sciences. Continued special attention should be given to admission of minority students.

(Recommendation #16) *Undergraduate medical education should provide students with a knowledge of epidemiology and aspects of behavioral and social sciences relevant to patient care.* Medical students should be presented with an array of course material helpful to understanding and communicating with patients. This may require new courses or the integration of new material into existing courses and clinical training.

(Recommendation #17) *Medical schools should provide all students with some clinical experience in a primary care setting.* This experience might be obtained in academic medical centers, in nearby clinics or offices under faculty supervision, or under preceptorships. Primary care is a vital feature of medical education because primary care, as defined by the committee, is the level of care at which the great majority of health problems is managed. Experience in primary care clinical settings can provide medical students with role models useful for leading the students into primary care careers.

(Recommendation #18) *Medical schools and primary care training programs should teach a team approach to the delivery of primary care.* The committee believes that primary care is best taught in a setting that offers patients combined professional skills and access to such services as mental health care, eye care, social support, allied health services, and efficient communication among different types of professionals.

In proposing credentialing policies, the committee is interested in assuring opportunity for innovation as well as promoting quality of care. (Recommendation #19) *Amendments to state licensing laws should authorize, through regulations, nurse practitioners and physician assistants to provide medical services, including making medical diagnoses and prescribing drugs when appropriate. Nurse practitioners and physician assistants in general should be required to perform the range of services they provide as skillfully as physicians, but they should not provide medical services without physician supervision.* There are various opinions about the degree of physician supervision required.

Also on credentialing, the committee would promote development by the nursing profession of more uniform standards for nurse practitioner programs. The committee believes (Recommendation #20) that *the nursing profession should continue to have accreditation responsibility for nurse practitioner education programs and should establish requirements for nurse practitioner education and training, in collaboration with physicians and other health professionals.*

## Chapter 6: Conclusions: The Schedule of Implementation

The final chapter of the report emphasizes the importance of coordinating all aspects of primary care manpower policy. Chapter 6 also presents a schedule of implementation, suggesting prerequisites, time frames, and responsible groups for each recommendation of the report.

## Notes

1. Citizens' Commission on Graduate Medical Education, Report, *The Graduate Education of Physicians,* by John S. Millis, Chairman (Chicago: American Medical Association, 1966); Ad Hoc Committee on Education for Family Practice of the Council on Medical Education of the American Medical Association, Report, *Meeting the Challenge of Family Practice,* by William R. Willard, Chairman (Chicago: American Medical Association, 1966); Committee on Medical Schools and the Association of American Medical Colleges in Relation to Training for Family Practice, Report, "Planning for Comprehensive and Continuing Care of Patients Through Education," by Edmund S. Pellegrino, Chairman, *Journal of Medical Education* 43 (1968): 751–759.

2. Lowell T. Coggeshall, Report, *Planning for Medical Progress Through Education* (Evanston, Ill.: Association of American Medical Colleges, 1965).

3. See *Manpower Policy,* chap. 4. In this report, the term *nurse practitioner* refers to a graduate of an approved continuing or graduate education program to train registered nurses to become nurse practitioners. *Physician assistants,* including MEDEX, are either graduates of approved physician assistant programs or other persons certified as physician assistants. Nurse practitioners and physician assistants are referred to collectively as "new health practitioners."

4. Particularly significant works on primary care include Joel J. Alpert and Evan Charney, *The Education of Physicians for Primary Care,* DHEW Publication No. (HRA) 74-3113 (1973); Spyros Andreopoulos, ed., *Primary Care: Where Medicine Fails* (New York: John Wiley and Sons, 1974); Association of American Medical Colleges, "Proceedings of the Institute of Primary Care" (Washington, D.C.: 1974); and Philip R. Lee, Lauren Le Roy, Janice Stalcup, and John Beck, *Primary Care in a Specialized World* (Cambridge, Mass.: Ballinger, 1976).

5. Institute of Medicine, *Primary Care in Medicine: A Definition* (Washington, D.C.: National Academy Press, 1977).

6. See staff papers, "Education of Primary Care Practitioners," "Data on the Supply and Distribution of Primary Care Physicians," "A Compilation of Data on the Content of Primary Care Practice," "Data on the Roles of the Physician Assistant and Nurse Practitioner," and "Licensure of Primary Care Practitioners."

7. See *Manpower Policy,* chap. 2.

8. Each organization or individual invited to the open meeting was asked to submit a paper suggesting references, areas of inquiry, and important policy considerations. Submitted papers were reviewed by the committee, which selected 18 of the papers for presentation at the meeting. In addition, all 73 of those who attended were afforded the opportunity to address the committee with brief statements or questions.

# CHAPTER SIXTEEN

# The Elusive Generalist Physician

## Can We Reach a 50 Percent Goal?

David A. Kindig, M.D., Ph.D.; James M. Cultice; Fitzhugh Mullan, M.D.
1993

Determining and achieving an appropriate balance of generalist and specialist physicians in the United States has been a policy interest recently. (The term *generalist* includes all active allopathic physicians in the fields of general and family medicine, general internal medicine, and general pediatrics. We acknowledge that these generalist disciplines are technically specialties and are recognized as such in certification and practice.) In the late 1960s and early 1970s, the expansion in physician demand stimulated by the passage of Medicare and Medicaid and concern over physician shortages in rural and inner-city areas resulted in a number of federal initiatives, including construction and capitation grants to medical schools, direct support for training in family medicine, general internal medicine, and pediatrics, and sponsorship of nurse practitioner and physician assistant training programs. Service-linked programs, such as community health centers, area health education centers, and the National Health Service Corps, were also enacted.[1] Taken as a whole, these programs provided unprecedented federal incentives for increasing the number of medical school graduates with an emphasis on generalist disciplines. It was intended that these innovations would result in increased access to generalist physicians in all areas of society, with special emphasis on traditionally underserved populations.

Many of these initiatives and programs slowed in the late 1970s and 1980s due to decreased federal appropriations and to the findings of the Graduate Medical Education National Advisory Committee (GMENAC), which predicted an aggregate physician surplus by 1990 and a physician "balance" in family practice, general medicine, general pediatrics, and osteopathy.[2] These findings resulted in the widespread belief that the overall increase in the number of physicians would solve the continued problems of specialty imbalance and geographic maldistribution. This belief was reinforced by emphasis on a competitive market approach to health care that came to public prominence with the election of Ronald Reagan in 1980.

The methods and conclusions of the GMENAC report were criticized when they first appeared,[3,4] and several analysts warned that excessive numbers of specialists would lead to potential problems.[5] Kindig and Cross-Dunham[5] projected in 1985 that by the year 2020 there would be a 55% (81,000) increase in generalists and a 111% (260,000) increase in specialists and suggested that it might be difficult to absorb that number of specialists in a cost-effective manner. Tarlov,[6] who had chaired the GMENAC, calculated in 1986 that by the year 2000 there might be three times as many physicians in the fee-for-service sector as in the managed care sector and that the multiplier was even higher for most subspecialties.

Schroeder[7] observed in 1987 that "it is indisputable that we are training too many internal medicine subspecialists and also likely too many general internists, although uncertainties about changes in physician effort and the future role of internists in health maintenance organizations makes this point more debatable." He had earlier noted from comparative studies done in Europe that when physicians are in excess supply, "underutilized physicians trained in medical and surgical subspecialties have insufficient opportunities to keep their technical skills," thereby increasing the risks of adverse consequences of care. Often, to take up slack time, they were forced to do primary care for which they were not "temperamentally or educationally prepared."[8] A number of specialty-specific studies in dermatology, neurology, and surgery raised concerns about excessive specialist production.[9-11] Schwartz and colleagues[12] had contrary projections for internal medicine; they asserted that every city with a population greater than 50,000 needed a board-certified specialist in each field and that small towns needed more specialists. Their projections concluded that there would be 7,000 too few medical specialists by the year 2000 in cities of these sizes.

None of these studies, however, provides definitive methods or figures for determining the appropriate or adequate number, percentage, or number per capita of generalists needed in the national pool or in subnational areas or populations. The GMENAC report, certainly the most exhaustive physician workforce study to date, projected a nearly balanced supply of generalists by 1990. Recently, however, policy observers have indicated increasing concern about the continuing imbalance of generalists and specialists as well as the low absolute number of generalists entering practice.

Among the many reasons for the increased attention to this imbalance is the erosion of generalist preferences among practitioners and students. The growth in total physician supply from 1970 to the present has been accompanied by a drop in the number of generalists from 40% to less than one third in 1991.[13] Moreover, medical student preferences for generalist careers fell during the 1980s[14] to a current level of about 20%. (The Association of American Medical Colleges [AAMC] 1992 graduation questionnaire[15] indicates that only 14.6% of graduating seniors specifically indicate generalist career preference; however, an additional 6.6% indicate "certification plans" for a general specialty. We have therefore arbitrarily taken "about 20%" as an estimate of current generalist preference.)

Also contributing to the concern about the generalist to specialist mix is the widely documented shortage of generalist physicians in rural and inner-city areas.[16,17] The Department of Health and Human Services Health Resources and Services Administration estimates that at least 4,550 physicians are needed to bring the areas they have designated as having the most critical health workforce shortages up to the minimal quartile of generalist physician supply.[18] Added to this demand has been the growth in managed care plans, which are hiring generalists in record numbers and are emerging as advocates for increased generalist production nationally and regionally.

In addition, the relative number of specialists is frequently cited as contributing to increasing overall health expenditures; the fact that Canada has lower costs and a national share of 50% generalists has added to this perception. One recent study by Grumbach and Lee[19] indicated that $55 billion could be saved if the supply of generalists was increased. Results from the Medical Outcomes Study[20] indicated that after controlling for patient mix, specialists use more resources than general internists, and general internists use more than family physicians. Recently, the AAMC has endorsed increases in generalist training,[21,22] and the American Medical Association (AMA) has also expressed concern about the lack of generalist practitioners.[23,24]

All of these studies and forces have resulted in a revived interest in the supply of generalist physicians, unprecedented since 1967. The Council on Graduate Medical Education has recommended moving to a system with 50% physicians practicing in generalist disciplines[25]; major foundations have announced initiatives to produce more generalists; there is increased interest in providing financial incentives through graduate education and other payment sources; and editorial comment on the subject is increasing monthly.[26,27] The 50% goal has generated attention because it is easy to grasp, it reflects the percentages within the Canadian physician workforce, and it would represent a substantial turnabout from the specialty selection pattern of recent U.S. graduates.

However, making major changes in the physician practice pool is a task of considerable magnitude given the size of that pool and the length of physicians' working lives. The aggregate physician supply is still increasing from the enrollment increases of the 1970s and 1980s and will not peak until around 2020. The protracted periods required to alter the composition of the aggregate pool of physicians have not been carefully analyzed. We therefore conducted a study to calculate the time it would take to achieve a goal of 50% practicing generalist physicians under a series of hypothetical conditions. In addition, we have analyzed future projections of generalists and specialists per 100,000 population since achieving a goal of 50% generalists in 2020 and beyond produces quite a different number of generalists and specialists per 100,000 population than the current figures because of the increased aggregate physician supply. We believe that the results of this modeling exercise will be useful for policymakers considering educational, practice, or regulatory incentives to modify the composition of the nation's medical workforce in future years.

# MATERIALS AND METHODS

This study's projections are based on results from the Bureau of Health Professions' physician supply forecasting model.[28] The model, in use by the bureau since 1982, forecasts the nation's supply of allopathic physicians both in the aggregate and by specialty and professional activity. We are currently conducting similar projections for osteopathic physicians; these data are not included herein since the sources are not totally comparable. We expect that their inclusion would add about 2% to the national percentage of generalists.

In the first stage of the forecasts, we used the aggregate model to project the number of active physicians to the year 2040. The aggregate projections model augments the active supply of physicians in the base year (1986) with annual new entrants and subtracts annual losses due to deaths and retirements. Graduates from U.S. medical schools were projected using estimates of first-year enrollments and 4-year retention rates in medical school. We used immigration information on international medical graduates (IMGs) and Canadian medical graduates to project foreign-trained additions to the supply.

The model builds on the AMA Physician Masterfile data for its 1986 base-year population of physicians; data elements include age, gender, year of graduation from medical school, country of medical education (United States, Canada, or foreign trained), medical specialty, and major professional activity. Enrollment projections were obtained from extrapolations of the AAMC applicant and matriculant trend data. Projected estimates of foreign-trained new entrants, including foreign nationals and U.S. citizens who trained abroad, are based on recent trends in total numbers of new IMGs added to the AMA Physician Masterfile each year. This group is assumed to number about 4,800 annually; the number of new U.S. physicians graduating from Canadian medical schools is expected to be around 200 each year. Age- and gender-specific mortality and retirement rates are based on the "average" separation experiences of physicians between 1979 and 1983. Population projections were obtained from the U.S. Bureau of the Census.[29]

The aggregate projections distinguish physicians by age, gender, and country of medical education. In the next stage of the forecasts, we distributed the aggregate numbers by medical specialty and professional activity using the Bureau of Health Professions' physician specialty forecasting model. The distribution of the aggregate totals into specialty categories depends on the physician's number of years since graduation. The specialty forecasting model first projects specialty distributions for the 10th year since graduation (YSG-10) of new entrant cohorts (graduating classes). The projections focused on YSG-10 because it is the year by which most graduates are expected to reach their eventual practice specialty. We estimated current and future YSG-10 distributions based on data from the AMA Masterfile, Physician Characteristics and Distribution information from the AMA, the annual medical education issues of the *Journal of the American Medical Association*, the AAMC graduation questionnaire results, the National Residency Matching Program results, and other sources. These data were combined to give a general indication of trends in specialty choice and then were applied to formulate predictions of the YSG-10 distributions in the model. The YSG-10 distributions are specific for U.S. medical graduates, U.S. citizen IMGs, and foreign national IMGs.

Next, we developed training-path proportions for each specialty and applied them to trace the pathways in each of the earlier years since graduation that would lead to the ultimate practice specialty distributions in YSG-10. In the Physician Masterfile, specialty designations are drawn from self-report surveys of the AMA and a physician is assigned to that primary specialty in which the most hours per week are indicated.

Training-path proportions were estimated from minimum training requirements set forth in the Directory of Graduate Medical Education together with unpublished data collected by the AAMC on the residency experiences of 1983 medical school graduates. Since not all residents follow a direct path in training for a specialty, the AAMC data were used to model appropriate lags in achieving a practice specialty. The training-path proportions of U.S. medical graduates through YSG-9 were applied to IMG new entrants without further adjustment. Although the YSG-10 training-path proportions are based on a single cohort (1983 graduates), they are assumed to be constant over time, i.e., the same distribution was applied to each succeeding cohort as it enters postgraduate year 1.

In the third step, we simulated the specialty transitions that occur annually among cohorts beyond YSG-10. Specialty transitions are relatively rare in these later years but they do occur. Since the transitions are based on self-designated specialty choice, they may reflect late transitions occurring without formal retraining. A method was developed that used AMA Masterfile data for 1983 and 1986 to infer changes in the YSG-11 through YSG-41 specialty distributions; these were then applied to redistribute cohorts of newly entering U.S. medical graduates in their later years since graduation in each projection year. The 3-year gap between observation years prohibited direct estimation of 1-year transition rates; instead, 3-year transition rates were calculated and 1-year rates were inferred from them. Data limitations prevented making career change adjustments for IMG new entrants. The specialty transitions beyond YSG-10 appear most pronounced for those in internal medicine subspecialties who are projected to increase their shares from 5.5% to 6.0% from YSG-11 to YSG-21, for those in diagnostic radiology whose numbers would increase from 4.9% to 5.2%, and for those in general internal medicine who are projected to decrease their share from 12.3% to 10.9% during the same period.

In the final step, we added the forecasted numbers of new entrants after 1986 by specialty and demographic detail to corresponding numbers in the 1986 base of active physicians. In a separate procedure, the base was "aged" to account for shifts in specialty and activity expected to occur in the projection period. The following data summarize major assumptions underlying the Bureau of Health Professions' Supply Model forecasts:

1. First-year enrollments in U.S. medical schools are expected to reach 17,000 (including those repeating the first year) by 1995 and to remain at this number, leading to 16,160 graduates each year after 1998.

2. Residents were counted as 50% of a practicing physician.

3. About 4,800 new IMGs will enter the physician supply each year in the projection period; the fraction of IMGs among total physicians will fall from about 22% today to 17% by 2020 and will remain at this share for the balance of the projection period. Around 200 new Canadian medical graduates will be added to the physician supply each year, holding the total supply of Canadian-trained physicians in the United States to 7,500. The IMGs will continue to enter generalist practice at somewhat higher rates than U.S. medical graduates.

4. Physicians' death and retirement patterns have not significantly changed since the 1979 to 1983 period and are held constant over the projection period.

5. The percentage of female physicians is projected to rise from about 18% currently to 24% by 2000; their share would increase to 33% by 2020 and would reach 37% by 2040. They will choose generalist careers at the same rate as they do now; about 36% of women and 25% of men will practice as generalists.

6. Patterns of specialty switching after the YSG-10 year will not change from the pathways observed in the 1983 graduating class.

To forecast future changes in the physician pool, five alternative scenarios were modeled to suggest what the mix of specialists and generalists in the total supply might be if graduates were to enter generalist practice at different rates. The first three alternative scenarios were chosen to represent (1) 30% generalists, an assumption that 30% of 1993 and subsequent graduates are in generalist practice in YSG-10; (2) 20% generalists, an assumption that only 20% of 1993 and subsequent graduates are in generalist practice by YSG-10; and (3) 50% generalists, an assumption that the proportion of graduates practicing as generalists in YSG-10 increases to 50% by 1997.

Additionally, we explored two extreme conditions to illustrate the outer bounds of changes in specialty balance. The first is a 100% generalists situation that assumes that all graduates after 1993 will enter generalist practice, and the second is a 0% generalists model that places all graduates after 1993 into specialties.

These results must be viewed with respect to certain limitations imposed by the forecasts' underlying assumptions. First, as previously noted, had osteopaths been included, the forecasted share of physicians in primary care would have risen in all scenarios except the one in which all physicians are trained as generalists. We estimate that inclusion of osteopaths would add about 2% to the share of generalists by 2020. Second, we assume that all current and future graduates experience interspecialty switching identical to that observed for the 1983 graduating class. To the degree that interspecialty movement has shifted or that future graduates follow different paths through graduate medical education, the forecasted mix of specialists and generalists may be distorted. Finally, we assume that each physician is completely a generalist or a specialist. There is evidence that some generalists do specialty work, and vice versa.[30] The model assumes that these events cancel each other, but we have no empirical evidence on this point.

# RESULTS

The results of the five projections are displayed in Figure 16.1; the line with open triangles indicates a 50% generalist goal. Under conditions like those in the mid-1980s, with approximately 30% of physicians practicing as generalists by YSG-10, the number of generalists will grow from 173,940 in 1990 to 232,000 in 2040—a slight percentage decrease, from 32.8% to 30.2%. Where only 20% of physicians enter generalist practice, the proportion of all generalists would fall to 21% by 2040. The projections in the 50% model show that if 50% of

**Figure 16.1.** Projections of Generalist Physician Supply, 1990–2040.

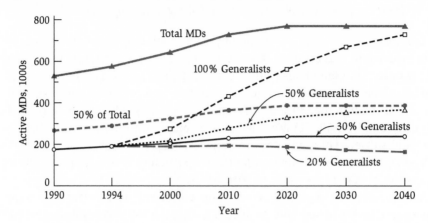

graduates were entering generalist practice, just less than 50% of the physician pool would be generalist practitioners in 2040. The fourth and fifth models present the extreme modeling possibilities. If 100% of graduates enter generalist practice after 1993, their proportion would exceed 90% in 2040; alternatively, if no graduates entered generalist practice after 1993, the share of all generalists would decline to nearly zero by 2040.

Because aggregate physician supply is projected to grow until about 2020, it is important to consider the relationship between generalists and specialists not only as a percentage of the total pool but as generalist and specialist ratios of physicians per 100,000 to indicate their relative availability to the population. Table 16.1 displays these data for the 30%, 20%, and 50% scenarios.

Under the 30% projection, the generalist ratio per 100,000 population increases from 69.5 to about 77, while the specialist ratio increases from 142 to about 178. Under the 20% scenario, the generalists per 100,000 would fall to about 53, whereas the specialists would grow from 142 to more than 200. Finally, the 50% scenario predicts an increase in generalists to about 124 per 100,000, while specialists increase to a peak of 160 per 100,000 in 2010 and then decline to about 132 per 100,000 by 2040.

# COMMENT

We had expected that the results of this modeling exercise would confirm the substantial time required to alter the overall specialty composition of the U.S. physician pool, but the number of years shown in our projections is considerably longer than anticipated. The finding that the unrealistic and extreme pro-

Table 16.1. Generalist and Specialist Availability per 100,000 Population,
1990–2040: Alternative Scenarios.

| | | | Year | | | |
|---|---|---|---|---|---|---|
| Projection | 1990 | 2000 | 2010 | 2020 | 2030 | 2040 |
| 30% Generalists | | | | | | |
| Generalists | 69.5 | 75.0 | 79.7 | 79.8 | 77.5 | 76.8 |
| Specialists | 142.0 | 163.9 | 177.8 | 180.9 | 178.9 | 177.8 |
| 20% Generalists | | | | | | |
| Generalists | 69.5 | 69.9 | 67.8 | 62.4 | 56.0 | 53.2 |
| Specialists | 142.0 | 168.7 | 189.3 | 197.9 | 200.0 | 201.1 |
| 50% Generalists[a] | | | | | | |
| Generalists | 69.5 | 79.7 | 97.9 | 109.5 | 116.8 | 123.5 |
| Specialists | 142.0 | 159.7 | 160.3 | 151.9 | 140.3 | 131.8 |

[a]Denotes percentage of graduates after 1993 who are assumed to be practicing as generalists 10 years
after graduation.

jection of 100% post-1993 graduates choosing generalist careers would result
only in a 50% generalist supply by 2004 is sobering. Achieving even a 50% rate
of graduates entering generalist practice by 1997 would be a considerable challenge requiring major educational, financial, and regulatory initiatives; yet it
would still leave us shy of a 50% generalist practice target by 2040. If generalist entry rates drop to the 20% level, as seems to be suggested by current medical student interest, the overall generalist practice percentage would fall to less
than 25% by 2020 and would hit 20% by 2040 as older physicians are replaced
by post-1990 graduates.

Underlying these ratios is the difficult but important question of what the
appropriate supply of total physicians and generalists should be. There is no
consensus in answer to this question. The GMENAC requirements projections,
which were regarded as "needs-based" and professionally ideal, called for an
aggregate target of 191 per 100,000 population, with approximately 36%
(69/100,000) in the generalist specialties.[2]

On the demand side, most studies of health maintenance organization physician use are dated or do not allow for confident extrapolation to the national
supply owing to limitations of plan type, part-time physicians, out-of-plan use,
panel age composition, and exclusion of teaching and research physicians. Staff
and group model plans use about 130 total full-time physicians per 100,000
enrollees, of which 73% (95/100,000) are generalists. Of full- and part-time

physicians combined, 49% are generalists.[31] There are no adequate data for IPA-type plans, which have the largest enrollment and growth rates.

Despite their limitations, these figures raise questions about the appropriateness of future aggregate physician supply and the level of specialists that, if current inputs remain constant, will reach levels considerably higher than the GMENAC standards or the reported health maintenance organization experience. Fifty percent (191/100,000) of the 1990 GMENAC total requirements would call for 95.5 generalists and 95.5 specialists per 100,000. The 30% scenario never reaches higher than this generalist target but consistently projects more specialists than did the GMENAC report. The 50% scenario approaches generalist targets by 2010 but then continues to increase, while specialist ratios remain above the GMENAC targets for the entire projection period.

These projections raise concerns similar to those expressed by Tarlov[6] and Schroeder[7] about the physician workforce of the near future. Growth in the number of specialists seems inevitable and particularly problematic. The magnitude of the problem will in part be determined by the extent to which cost-effective managed care plans capture the U.S. health care market and whether physicians are used at rates comparable to those of staff and group model health maintenance organizations described herein.

At the least, public and private policymakers should seriously consider setting an ideal target of generalists and specialists per 100,000 population. If increases in generalists are indicated, policy options can be suggested to achieve this goal. If generalist supply seems appropriate but specialists are in excess, alternative policies will be required.

Additional analysis needs to be done at state, rural, and urban levels since the distribution and needs for generalist and specialists vary geographically. Currently, a considerable range of generalist and specialist supply exists across the states; national policy changes could have different effects across the country.[32] Different numbers of generalists and specialists are distributed to and perhaps needed in rural and inner-city areas. Similarly, we need to analyze the extent to which nurse practitioners and physician assistants can substitute for and enhance both generalists and specialists and to determine their potential cost-effective impact on the aggregate physician pool. A study also needs to be undertaken of the effect of reducing domestically trained physicians and IMG entrants on aggregate physician supply and specialty balance.

The five projections presented herein describe possible outcomes of generalist practitioner supply without specifying what blend or choice of educational, financial, or regulatory policies might be used to produce such outcomes. If a 50% generalist supply is desired, it is unlikely that changes in the educational system alone will be adequate. Physician payment reform, such as the Medicare Resource-Based Relative Value Scale, may have some impact, particularly if applied to all payers, but it is too early to tell to what extent the current incentives will effect future specialty choice. If the 20% projection represents generalist specialty choice at present, significant intervention will be required simply to maintain current numbers of generalists.

Given the long periods required to change the composition of the existing physician pool, other possibilities for increasing generalist practitioners should be considered, such as increasing the number of nonphysicians or increasing the generalist capability of specialists. Schroeder[33] has identified the latter as one potential scenario for correcting the imbalance. He indicates that certain specialties like gynecology could hold residency programs and certifying boards accountable for generalist competencies such as "interviewing, patient compliance, and principles of screening and for the diagnosis and management of common syndromes." He also indicates that existing specialists could be retrained as generalists through continuing education courses, but the disadvantages of this approach are that it does not automatically decrease the costs associated with specialist care and it is not "at all clear that most specialists really wish to be held accountable for general clinical care." These alternatives will have to be more seriously developed and critiqued if changes from initial specialty choice are desired more rapidly than our model suggests. A starting point for such thinking should be to determine those physicians, primarily internal medicine specialists with mixed practices, who might most easily increase their generalist capability with appropriate incentives.

Because of the long time required for most policy changes to affect the size or composition of the physician workforce, quantitative goals and policy directions need to be set now if we are to have an appropriate national physician workforce in the first decades of the 21st century.

# Notes

1. Politzer R, Harris D, Gatson M, Mullan F. Primary care physician supply and the medically underserved. *JAMA*. 1991;266:104–109.

2. Graduate Medical Education National Advisory Committee. *The Report of the Graduate Medical Education National Advisory Committee (GMENAC)*. Washington, DC: U.S. Department of Health and Human Services; 1980;1–7.

3. Bowman MA, Walsh WB Jr. Perspectives on the GMENAC report. *Health Aff.* 1982;1:55–60.

4. Reinhardt U. The GMENAC forecast: an alternative view. *Am J Public Health.* 1981;1:1149.

5. Kindig DA, Cross-Dunham N. Physician specialist growth into the twenty-first century. *J Med Educ.* 1985;60:558–559.

6. Tarlov AR. HMO enrollment growth and physicians: the third compartment. *Health Aff.* 1986;5:23–35.

7. Schroeder SA. The health manpower challenge to internal medicine. *Ann Intern Med.* 1987;106:768–770.

8. Schroeder SA. Western European responses to physician oversupply: lesson for the United States. *JAMA*. 1984;52:373.

9. Stern RS. Dermatologists in the year 2000. *Arch Dermatol*. 1986;122:675–678.

10. Menken M, Sheps CG. Consequences of an oversupply of specialists: the case of neurology. *JAMA*. 1985;253:1926–1928.

11. Moore FD. Surgical manpower, past and present reality, estimates for 2000. *Surg Clin North Am*. 1982;62:579–602.

12. Schwartz WB, Williams AP, Newhouse JP, Witsberger C. Are we training too many subspecialists? *JAMA*. 1988;259:233–239.

13. American Medical Association. *Physician Characteristics and Distribution in the U.S.* Chicago: American Medical Association; 1993.

14. Colwill JM. Where have all the primary care applicants gone? *N Engl J Med*. 1992;326:387–393.

15. Kassebaum DG, Szenas MA. Specialty preferences of graduating medical students: 1992 update. *Acad Med*. 1992;67:800–806.

16. Kindig DA, Movassaghi H. The adequacy of physician supply in small rural counties. *Health Aff*. 1989;81:61–76.

17. Kindig DA, Movassaghi H, Cross-Dunham N, Zwick DI, Taylor CM. Trends in physician availability in ten urban areas from 1963 to 1980. *Inquiry*. 1987;24:136–146.

18. Bureau of Primary Health Care. *Selected Statistics on Health Professional Shortage Area as of September 30, 1992*. Washington, DC: U.S. Department of Health and Human Services; 1992.

19. Grumbach K, Lee PR. How many physicians can we afford? *JAMA*. 1991;265:2369–2372.

20. Greenfield S, Nelson EC, Zubkoff M, et al. Variations in resource utilization among medical specialties and systems of cure: results for the Medical Outcomes Study. *JAMA*. 1992;267:1624–1630.

21. Petersdorf RG. Primary care's time has come. *Acad Med*. 1992;67:377.

22. AAMC policy on the generalist physician. *Acad Med*. 1993;68:1–6.

23. Todd JS. Health care reform and the medical education imperative. *JAMA*. 1992;268:1133–1134.

24. Martini C. Graduate medical education in the changing environment of medicine. *JAMA*. 1992;268:1097–1105.

25. Council on Graduate Medical Education. *Third Report: Improving Access to Health Care Through Physician Workforce Reform: Directions for the Twenty-First Century*. Washington, DC: U.S. Department of Health and Human Services; 1992.

26. Rosenblatt RA. Specialists or generalists: on whom should we base the American health care system? *JAMA*. 1992;267:1165–1666.

27. Ginzberg E. Caring for the uninsured and underinsured: physician supply policies and health reform. *JAMA*. 1992;268:3115–3118.

28. Vector Research Inc, revision of BHPR Physician Forecasting Models, unpublished report prepared under contract HRSA 240-88-0048 by C. Roehrig and A. Turner for the Bureau of Health Professions, Rockville, Md, December 1989.

29. Spencer G. *Projections of the Population of the United States by Age, Sex, and Race, 1988–2080.* Current Population Reports, Series P-25, No. 1018. Washington, DC: U.S. Government Printing Office; 1989.

30. Aiken L, Lewis CH, Craig J, et al. The contribution of specialists to the delivery of primary care. *N Engl J Med.* 1979;300:1363–1385.

31. Hodges D, Camerlo K, Gold M. *HMO Industry Profile: Physician Staffing and Utilization Patterns, Group Health Association 1991 Industry Survey.* Washington, DC: Group Health Association of America; 1991.

32. Riportella-Muller R, Kindig DA. Predictors of state variation in primary care physicians. Paper presented at the AHCPR Primary Care Research Conference, January 12, 1993, Atlanta.

33. Schroeder SA. Training and appropriate mix of physicians to meet the nation's needs. *Acad Med.* 1993;68:118–122.

CHAPTER SEVENTEEN

# Economic and Demographic Trends Signal an Impending Physician Shortage

Richard A. Cooper, M.D.; Thomas E. Getzen, Ph.D.;
Heather J. McKee, M.D.; Prakash Laud, Ph.D.
2002

For people interested in the physician workforce, 2000 was an important year, since it was the year in which it was generally accepted—indeed feared—that there would be a vast surplus of physicians, particularly of specialists. The increased expenditure associated with this was to have been detrimental to the overall economy. Instead, we are beginning to see shortages of physicians, principally of specialists, and an economic decline that would be much deeper than it is, if not for sustained levels of health care spending.[1]

Why was the current need for physicians so underestimated? How can future requirements be more reliably discerned? And what do shortages and surpluses of physicians mean for the health care system and for the profession of medicine itself? This chapter attempts to find answers to these questions in the context of the long-term trends that underlie physician supply and utilization. It leads ultimately to the question of whether it is time for the nation to begin to increase its medical training capacity to meet the demands for physicians that are evolving.

## PAST PREDICTIONS OF SURPLUSES

Concerns about potential physician surpluses were prominent during the debate over medical school expansion in the 1960s. In 1981 the report of the Graduate Medical Education National Advisory Committee (GMENAC) gave these concerns a quantitative basis, which was reinforced by a series of studies conducted in the 1990s on behalf of the Council on Graduate Medical Education (COGME).[2] The message from these various studies was consistent: Surplus numbers of specialists equal to 15–30 percent of all physicians would develop by the year 2000, to be accompanied by shortages in the number of primary care physicians.

While differing in detail, these studies shared a common framework, which was based on quantifying the "tasks" (that is, physician visits and procedures) and associated "times" (expressed as full-time-equivalent, or FTE, physicians) that constituted "good" patient care, an approach that was first developed in the 1920s by the Committee on the Costs of Medical Care (CCMC).[3] This methodology was based on the assumption that more detail would lead to greater accuracy. Therefore, these studies required that physician services be disaggregated into microunits according to such factors as disease prevalence, demographic subgroups, or insurance products, a requirement that exceeded the available data and confounded the results. However, their greatest deficit was not methodological, but conceptual. It was their adoption of a social planning perspective that centered on what ought to occur, rather than an analytic approach that sought to define what most likely would occur. Nonetheless, despite challenges from some, the surpluses predicted by these studies gained wide acceptance, and they formed the theoretical basis for subsequent actions, including the termination of federal support for undergraduate medical education and a progressive decrease in support for graduate medical education.[4]

# THE TREND MODEL

We have developed an alternative approach to physician workforce planning, based not on microanalyses of tasks and times but on macroanalyses of the long-term trends that underlie the supply and use of physician services.[5] Four such trends were considered. First is economic expansion, the dominant factor that drives the use of health care.[6] Second is population growth, which directly affects the need for physicians. Third is the work effort of physicians, which has been declining.[7] And fourth are the services provided by non-physician clinicians (NPCs), which have been increasing.[8] These four trends have been combined into a model termed the "Trend Model," which we have used to assess the adequacy of physician supply over the next twenty years.

The Trend Model differs from earlier models in several ways. First, it is a macroanalysis with relatively few data requirements, based on the notion that simpler and more aggregate models are more effective and readily reproducible. Second, it relies on long-term trends, which tend to dominate short-term fluctuations. Third, by assuming that historical trends in physician supply reflect the historical demand for physician services, it creates a conceptual link between supply and demand. This allows projections of future demand to be based on past trends and compared with separate projections of supply. Finally, while it makes assumptions about what is likely to occur, it does not base its projections on what ought to occur.

In striking contrast to earlier predictions, the Trend Model indicates that if the pace of medical education remains unchanged, the United States will soon be facing shortages of physicians and that these shortages will become progressively more severe over time. This echoes the conclusions reached by William Schwartz and colleagues, who, using a conceptually similar approach, predicted more than a decade ago that surpluses of the magnitude predicted by GMENAC and COGME for the year 2000 would not materialize.[9]

# ECONOMIC TRENDS

## Longitudinal Trends

The major trend affecting the demand for physician services is the economy. In developed countries throughout the world, health care spending has been closely tied to levels of economic development, as reflected by a country's real (inflation-adjusted) gross domestic product (GDP) or national income.[10] Since labor is the principal health care expense component, it is not surprising that growth of GDP has also correlated with growth of the health care labor force.[11] However, most of this growth in the workforce has involved ancillary personnel, so physicians have become a proportionately smaller component.[12] The composite result of these interrelated trends is depicted in Figure 17.1, which displays the close, long-term relationship that has existed in the United States between growth of GDP and growth of physician supply over a period of more than seventy years. The data diverged in the direction of physician undersupply in the 1960s, when most policymakers agreed that shortages were occurring, but it returned to the trend line in the 1980s following an increase in the number of physicians being trained.

Similar correlations among GDP, health spending, and physician supply were observed in other Western democracies over the shorter time span from 1960 to 1998, as well as in most states over the period 1980–1998.[13] The power of these regressions was greater when the known temporal lags between changes in GDP and changes in health care spending were also considered.[14] Moreover, they remained strong even after GDP was adjusted for the linear effects of time.[15] Taken together, these observations are consistent with the notion that a causal relationship exists between economic expansion and growth of physician supply.

**Figure 17.1.** Physician Supply and Gross Domestic Product, 1929–2000 and Projections to 2020.

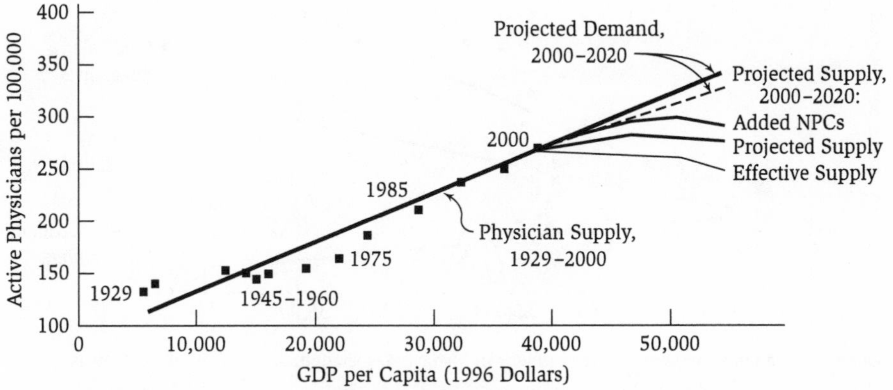

*Sources:* Physician supply: R. I. Lee and L. W. Jones, *The Fundamentals of Good Medical Care* (Chicago: University of Chicago Press, 1933); W. H. Steward and M. Pennell, "Health Manpower, 1930–75," *Public Health Reports* 75, no. 3 (1960): 274–280; American Osteopathic Association; and Bureau of Health Professions. Population: Bureau of the Census. Gross domestic product: Bureau of Economic Analysis. Supply projections based on authors' model.[4]

*Notes:* "Physician supply, 1929–2000" includes active physicians only ($r^2$ = 0.94). "Projected supply" includes all active physicians. "Effective supply" represents the number of active physicians reduced by the decrements in work effort associated with increasing numbers of female and older physicians in the workforce. "Added NPCs" represents the sum of "effective supply" plus the incremental contributions of nonphysician providers (NPCs). Per capita GDP is expressed in chained 1996 dollars. "Physician demand" is projected based on average GDP growth rates of 1.5 percent (dotted line) and 2 percent (solid line).

## Cross-Sectional Analyses

Evidence supporting the role of economic factors in determining physician supply also emerged from cross-sectional analyses of the fifty states (Figure 17.2). Physician supply correlated with state per capita income, as had been noted earlier.[16] The slopes (that is, betas) of these regressions were virtually identical at various time points over a period spanning almost thirty years. However, they were not the same for all specialties of medicine. The medical specialties (including both general and subspecialty internal medicine and pediatrics) were most responsive to income effects, while the surgical specialties were less affected, and family/general practice displayed a slightly negative relationship with per capita income. These observations not only confirm the link between economic growth and the demand for physician services but also suggest that geographic differences in physician supply are likely to persist as long as regional differences in income exist.

**Figure 17.2.** Physician Supply in States, by Major Specialty Group and State Per Capita Income.

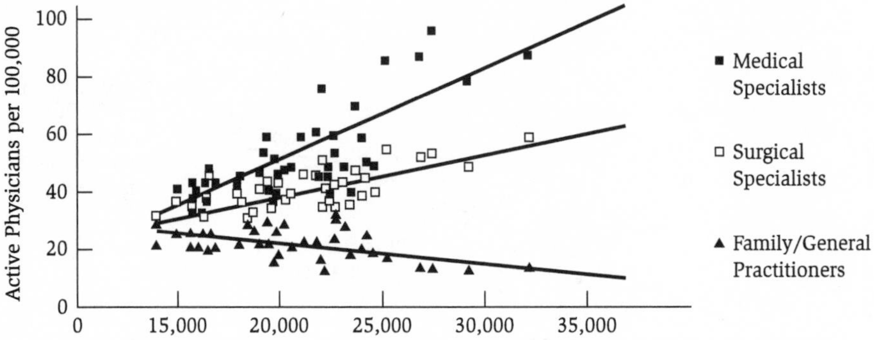

*Sources:* Bureau of Economic Analysis; American Medical Association; and Bureau of the Census.

## The Economic Chain

Throughout this series of analyses, physician supply correlated with economic growth. On average, the magnitude of this relationship was equivalent to a difference in physician supply of approximately 0.75 percent for each 1 percent difference in GDP or personal income. However, there are several important points to consider in interpreting this relationship. First, it is not a simple mathematical relationship that always holds true. It is a macrotrend that only applies to physicians in the aggregate over broad periods. While microturbulence, such as changes in payment schemes, governmental regulation, or the structure of health plans, may induce deviations from the trend lasting as long as five to ten years, such factors do not influence the slope of the trend, which is affected by macroeconomic dynamics.

Second, it is not a simple relationship. It results from a complex set of interrelationships that begins with increases in GDP, which (with a lag of several years) induces further demand for health services, thereby causing health care spending to rise. This leads to growth of the health care labor force, of which physicians are an important component. The fact that strong correlations exist across this entire spectrum, from GDP to physician supply, speaks to the systematic nature of the intervening steps.

Finally, the relationship between GDP and the demand for physician services does not exist in isolation. It is the consequence of countervailing societal forces that both promote and constrain utilization. For example, the perceived triumphs of technology contribute to a culture that is willing to devote more resources to health care. Similarly, although population aging does not itself cause health care spending to rise above its established trends, the elderly constitute a political force that can influence the allocation of societal resources.[17] In each instance, efforts to push health care use higher are balanced by public and private "reforms" that work to constrain spending and limit access. The striking observation is that the net of these counterbalancing factors yields such stable results, infrequently allowing physician supply to deviate by more than 10 percent from its long-term relationship with GDP.

# POPULATION TRENDS

Population growth is a second major factor that affects the demand for physicians. Unfortunately, most previous workforce analyses used unmodified population forecasts from the Census Bureau, which have proved to be low, and, therefore, the resulting projections of physicians per capita were excessively high. Indeed, this error accounts for approximately 25 percent of the physician surpluses that were previously predicted.[18] To place this into perspective, the total output of ten to twelve medical schools would be required to service the population that was omitted from consideration by these earlier studies.

Using a modification of Census Bureau estimates, we have forecasted that the U.S. population will grow from 285 million in 2000 to 325 million in 2010 and that it will reach 345 million in 2020. These values are similar to those that both we and the Centers for Medicare and Medicaid Services (CMS, formerly HCFA) have used previously.[19] Although 6–8 percent higher than current Census Bureau forecasts, they are within 2 percent of the projections that can be derived using data from the year 2000 census.[20]

# PHYSICIAN SUPPLY AND SUFFICIENCY TRENDS

## Current Supply

The starting point in all workforce supply projections is an estimate of the current physician labor force. Unlike most earlier analyses, the Trend Model avoids the errors that are inherent in deciding what constitutes "one FTE physician" by basing its measures on a "head count" of all active physicians, including residents, irrespective of their level of activity. Applying this definition to data from the period of seventy years that was analyzed, physician supply increased fivefold, from 144,000 in 1929 to 772,000 in 2000.[21] This represents more than a doubling of physicians per capita, from 119 physicians per 100,000 of population in 1929 to 270 in 2000 (Figure 17.1).

## Sufficiency

To use current "head counts" of physicians for projecting future supply, one must first assess both the adequacy of physician supply and the degree to which physicians are utilized. Recent surveys of physicians and the public, combined with information on physician recruitment, yield a picture of marginal sufficiency, with a strong demand for specialists, lengthening of waiting times in many specialties, and sporadic reports of physician shortages.[22]

## Future Supply

The method used by the Trend Model to project physician supply into the future follows the general form used by others.[23] For operational purposes, it holds inputs steady by assuming that the number of first-time, first-year residents will remain fixed at 23,000 (126 percent of U.S. medical graduates) and that 20 percent of international medical graduates (IMGs) will return to their countries of origin, as has been true over the past decade. The model also assumes that current patterns of retirement will continue.[24] Based on these assumptions, and using the population projections discussed above, we project that the "head count" of active physicians will increase from 772,000 (270 per 100,000 of population) in 2000 to a peak level of 887,300 (283 per 100,000 of population) in 2010 (Figure 17.1). Thereafter, the total number will continue to grow, reaching 964,700 in 2020, but the population will grow even faster, and the number of physicians per capita will actually decrease slightly, to 280 per 100,000 of population. Thus, for most of the next twenty years per capita physician supply will be essentially flat.

# PHYSICIAN WORK EFFORT

Because physician work effort is changing, these projections must be modified to reflect the existing trends. All are in the direction of reduced effort. This includes the aging of the physician workforce (with its associated decrease in hours worked), the increasing number of female physicians, the lesser work effort of physicians who are employees, the tendency of younger physicians to place a greater emphasis on personal time, the increasing frequency of early retirement, and the decreasing hours that residents are permitted to work.[25] Although all are important, only the first two were factored into the model, by assuming reductions of 10 percent and 20 percent, respectively, in the efforts of physicians ages 55–65 and over age 65, and a 20 percent reduction in the effort of female physicians. This resulted in a decrease in the "effective supply" of physicians by 5 percent in 2010 and 7 percent in 2020 (Figure 17.1). Because these adjustments do not include consideration of other factors that also reduce work effort, they probably overstate the amount of physician effort that will actually be available in the future.

# SUBSTITUTION TRENDS

The final trend that we considered is the substitution of NPCs in the provision of "physician services." Until recently NPCs' ability to substitute for physicians was limited by their licensed prerogatives and by their total numbers, but both of these limitations are diminishing.[26] Most NPCs now provide not only adjunctive services but also services that broadly overlap those provided by physicians, and their potential for substitution is substantial.[27] And their numbers are growing. By 2015 there are likely to be as many as 275,000 nurse practitioners, physician assistants, and nurse-midwives; 150,000 chiropractors and acupuncturists; and 100,000 other NPCs engaged in specific specialties, such as psychology, anesthesia, and optometry. Their combined output will be equivalent to the services of approximately 65 physicians per 100,000 of population. More than one-third of this output is in place already. Therefore, the incremental growth of NPCs over the next fifteen years was taken to be equivalent to 40 physicians per 100,000 of population (Figure 17.1), which is equal to approximately 15 percent of the physician work force. Paradoxically, most of this growth will be concentrated in primary care, which has shown relatively stable needs, whereas the greatest growth of demand for physician services is in the nonprimary care specialties, to which NPCs can be expected to contribute proportionately less.

# APPLYING THE TREND MODEL

## Projections

Projections based on the Trend Model build from these separate trends. On the demand side, health care spending has tended to outpace GDP by a ratio of approximately 1.5 to 1.0. If this differential continues, as has been projected, and if real per capita economic growth continues at 1.5–2.0 percent annually, as also has been projected, the fraction of GDP devoted to health care will increase from approximately 14 percent in 2000 to 18 percent in 2020.[28] Based on an increase in physician supply of approximately 0.75 percent for each 1 percent increase in GDP, as discussed above, the Trend Model projects a growth in the demand for physician services of approximately 1.1–1.5 percent annually (Figure 17.1), a rate of increase that is similar to the job opportunities for physicians that have been projected by the Bureau of Labor Statistics.[29]

Comparing this growth in the demand for physician services with the number of active physicians that has been projected reveals a shortfall of substantial magnitude (Figure 17.1). This shortfall widens further when work effort is considered and demand is compared, instead, with the "effective supply" of physicians, but the incremental contributions of NPCs more than compensate for changes due to physician work effort, leaving a projected deficit in 2010 of only 50,000 physicians, less than 6 percent of the projected demand. Some of this is within the margin of error of the trends that were analyzed, and much of it could be accommodated by the elasticity of the health care labor force. However, by 2020 the deficit is projected to exceed 200,000 physicians, an amount that represents more than 20 percent of the projected demand. In percentage terms, this is greater than the shortages that existed during the 1960s.

## Assumptions

To properly assess these estimates of shortages, they must be interpreted in the context of the errors and uncertainties that are inherent in the Trend Model. The assumption that the number of physicians being trained would remain constant was simply operational, since the purpose of this exercise is to determine whether that number should change. Other assumptions were in the direction of overestimating physician supply. Thus, it was assumed that the current rates of attrition would continue, although anecdotal evidence suggests that attrition is increasing. Similarly, in projecting "effective physician supply," the model assumed decrements in work effort attributable to aging and sex, but it did not consider other, less well defined factors that also have a negative impact on physician work effort. The major error in the population projections was also in the direction of overestimating per capita physician supply (by underestimating population growth), because it was assumed that the rate of immigration would not change, whereas increases seem likely. Subsequent applications of the Trend Model will have to incorporate alternative projections and assumptions as these various issues are clarified.

More ambiguity is associated with estimates of substitution, particularly since any protracted shortages of physicians are likely to cause an expansion in the autonomy and scope of practice of NPCs in those states in which these prerogatives are still limited, thereby increasing NPCs' ability to provide "physician services." However, unless new disciplines emerge or existing disciplines vastly expand their scope of activities, substitution is ultimately limited by the range of tasks that NPCs now can reasonably assume. Thus, under most scenarios the supply of physicians plus NPCs is likely to remain relatively unchanged over the next twenty years (Figure 17.1).

The greatest uncertainty rests with the demand for physician services and with the economic growth that underlies it. While there were no indications in our analyses that the trends defining this relationship were changing, it seems inevitable that, at some point, the relative rates of economic growth and the growth of health care services will have to narrow. However, even if that occurs, or if overall economic growth slows, the inevitable divergence between an essentially flat physician supply and the rising demand that any significant economic expansion will induce predicts progressively increasing physician shortages.

# THE NATION'S FUTURE PHYSICIAN SUPPLY

These projections are made against a background of concern that health care spending is excessive and that physicians may exacerbate the problem, either by actually inducing demand or by facilitating utilization in a system in which they exert control over most expenditures, a conclusion that is not supported by contemporary data.[30] Among those who hold this perspective, constraining the growth of physician supply is seen as a means of limiting spending. Canada followed such a policy throughout the 1990s. Physician supply in the United States has remained lower relative to GDP than in most Organization for Economic Cooperation and Development (OECD) countries, and managed care has been used to further limit access. However, as revealed both by the backlash against managed care in the United States and by the recent recognition in both Canada and California that physician shortages are looming, such constraints inevitably conflict with long-term economic trends and with the perceptions of need that flow from them.[31]

Thus, physicians are at the nexus of a health care system that is shaped in large measure by exogenous trends. Their role is broad. It bridges an expanding universe of medical science and a long tradition of compassion and healing. But are the trends consistent with the continuation of this duality? Faced with the "taut supply" that Eli Ginzberg has advocated, it seems more likely that physicians will be drawn to those complex areas of specialty medicine that demand their attention most and that they will find it increasingly difficult to "lavishly dispense time, sympathy and understanding," as Francis Peabody urged they should.[32] Patients desire the most advanced treatments, but they also seek a caring physician. Ironically, attempts to impede patients' access to the former have had the unintended consequence of squeezing out the latter.

The sociologist Andrew Abbott has observed that "a profession whose jurisdiction is excessive must increase its productivity or expand its numbers." Conversely, "when a powerful profession ignores a potential clientele, paraprofessionals appear to provide the needed services."[33] These statements characterize the dilemma that physicians now face. Their ability to increase their productivity is limited by their declining work effort. Their ability to grow their numbers is hostage to the belief that surpluses exist. And organized medicine has embarked on a vigorous campaign to thwart expansion of the NPC disciplines.[34] Yet it was shortages in the past that motivated state legislatures to remove the barriers to licensure for NPCs and to enlarge their range of privileges, and it is perceived professional opportunities that stimulated the creation of new disciplines and the expansion of existing ones.

The last debate about physician shortages continued well into the 1960s. Ultimately, the Health Professions Education Assistance Act of 1963 led to a doubling of medical school slots, but it was another fifteen years before appreciably more physicians were available to the public. It is doubtful that this process could occur any more rapidly today. While the recruitment of additional IMGs could shorten the response time, the wisdom of even our current dependency on IMGs has been questioned.[35] If, instead, the infrastructure of medical education were expanded to alleviate just one-third of the projected shortages, more than twenty-five additional medical schools would be required over the next decade, a formidable undertaking. But to do nothing invites public discontent and forces the profession of medicine to redefine itself in an ever more narrow scientific and technological sphere while other disciplines evolve to fill important gaps. Although the path is uncertain, the choices are clear. We believe that a dialogue regarding these choices is imperative.

## Notes

1. On physician shortages, see J. H. Sunshine, "Employment Among Recent Residency Program Graduates," *Journal of the American Medical Association* 281, no. 7 (1999): 611; D. C. Angus et al., "Current and Projected Workforce Requirements for Care of the Critically Ill and Patients with Pulmonary Disease," *Journal of the American Medical Association* 284, no. 21 (2000): 2762–2770; California Medical Association, *And Then There Were None: The Coming Physician Supply Problem* (San Francisco: California Medical Association, 2001); and A. Schubert et al., "Evidence of a Current and Lasting National Anesthesia Personnel Shortfall: Scope and Implications," *Mayo Clinic Proceedings* 76, no. 10 (2001): 995–1010.

2. Graduate Medical Education National Advisory Committee, *Report of the Graduate Medical Education National Advisory Committee to the Secretary, Department of Health and Human Services* (Washington, D.C.: U.S. Department of Health and Human Services, 1981); J. P. Weiner, "Forecasting the Effects of Health Reform on U.S. Physician Workforce Requirement: Evidence from HMO Staffing Patterns," *Journal of the American Medical Association* 272, no. 3 (1994): 222–230; S. Gamliel et al., "Managed Care on the March: Will Physicians Meet the Challenge?" *Health Affairs* (Summer 1995): 131–142; R. M. Politzer et al., "Matching Physician Supply and Requirements: Testing Policy Recommendations," *Inquiry* (Summer 1996): 181–194; and L. Greenberg and J. M. Cultice, "Forecasting the Need for Physicians in the United States: The Health Resources and Services Administration's Physician Requirements Model," *Health Services Research* 31, no. 6 (1997):

723–737. See also the *Third, Fourth,* and *Sixth Report of the Council on Graduate Medical Education* (Washington, D.C.: U.S. Department of Health and Human Services, 1992, 1994, 1995).

3. R. I. Lee and L. W. Jones, *The Fundamentals of Good Medical Care* (Chicago: University of Chicago Press, 1933).

4. Challenges to the reports from GMENAC, COGME, and related studies include U. E. Reinhardt, "The GMENAC Forecast: An Alternative View," *American Journal of Public Health* 71, no. 10 (1981): 1149–1157; J. E. Harris, "How Many Doctors Are Enough?" *Health Affairs* (Winter 1986): 74–83; W. B. Schwartz, F. A. Sloan, and D. N. Mendelson, "Why There Will Be Little or No Physician Surplus Between Now and the Year 2000," *New England Journal of Medicine* 318, no. 14 (1988): 892–897; E. P. Schloss, "Beyond GMENAC—Another Physician Shortage from 2010 to 2030?" *New England Journal of Medicine* 318, no. 14 (1988): 920–922; R. A. Cooper, "Seeking a Balanced Physician Workforce for the Twenty-First Century," *Journal of the American Medical Association* 272, no. 9 (1994): 680–687; and R. A. Cooper, "Perspectives on the Physician Workforce to the Year 2020," *Journal of the American Medical Association* 274, no. 19 (1995): 1534–1543. Organizations endorsing these studies and their proposals included Josiah Macy Jr. Foundation, *Report of the Josiah Macy Jr. Foundation for July 1, 1991, through June 30, 1992* (New York: Josiah Macy Jr. Foundation, 1992); Physician Payment Review Commission, "Graduate Medical Education Reform," in *Annual Report to Congress, 1994* (Washington, D.C.: Physician Payment Review Commission, 1994), 237–263; Institute of Medicine, *The Nation's Physician Workforce: Options for Balancing Supply and Requirements* (Washington, D.C.: National Academy Press, 1996); and Association of American Medical Colleges, *AMA, AOA, AAMC, AACOM, AAHC, NMA Consensus Statement on Physician Workforce,* AAMC Advisory no. 97-9 (Washington, D.C.: Association of American Medical Colleges, 1997).

5. R. A. Cooper, "Conceptual Framework," in *Evaluation of Specialty Workforce Methodologies* (Washington, D.C.: Council on Graduate Medical Education, U.S. Department of Health and Human Services, 2000), D1–D2; and R.A. Cooper, "Forecasting the Physician Workforce," in *Papers and Proceedings of the Eleventh Federal Forecasters Conference* (Washington, D.C.: U.S. Department of Education, 2000), 87–96.

6. J. R. Seale, "A General Theory of National Expenditure on Medical Care," *Lancet* 2 (October 1959): 555–559; J. P. Newhouse, "Medical Care Expenditure: A Cross-National Survey," *Journal of Human Resources* 12, no. 1 (1977): 115–125; T. E. Getzen, "Forecasting Health Expenditures: Short, Medium, and Long (Long) Term," *Journal of Health Care Financing* 263, no. 3 (2000): 56–72; and T. E. Getzen, "Health Care Is an Individual Necessity and a National Luxury: Applying Multilevel Decision Models to the Analysis of Health Care Expenditures," *Journal of Health Economics* 19, no. 2 (2000): 259–270.

7. W. B. Schwartz and D. N. Mendelson, "No Evidence of an Emerging Physician Surplus: An Analysis of Changes in Physicians' Work Load and Income" *Journal of the American Medical Association* 263, no. 4 (1990): 557–560; P. R. Kletke,

W. D. Marder, and A. B. Silberger, "The Growing Proportion of Female Physicians: Implications for the U.S. Physician Supply," *American Journal of Public Health* 80, no. 3 (1990): 300–403; and P. R. Kletke, "The Projected Supply of Physicians, 1998–2020," in *Physician Characteristics and Distribution in the U.S., 2000–2001 Edition*, ed. T. Pasko, B. Seidman, and S. Birkhead (Chicago: American Medical Association, 2000), 361–375.

8. R. A. Cooper, P. Laud, and C. L. Dietrich, "Current and Projected Workforce of Nonphysician Clinicians," *Journal of the American Medical Association* 280, no. 9 (1998): 788–794; and R. A. Cooper, T. Henderson, and C. L. Dietrich, "Roles of Nonphysician Clinicians as Autonomous Providers of Patient Care," *Journal of the American Medical Association* 280, no. 9 (1998): 795–802.

9. Schwartz et al., "Why There Will Be Little or No Physician Surplus"; and Schwartz and Mendelson, "No Evidence of an Emerging Physician Surplus."

10. Getzen, "Forecasting Health Expenditures"; Newhouse, "Medical Care Expenditure"; and M. Pfaff, "Differences in Health Care Spending Across Countries: Statistical Evidence," *Journal of Health Politics, Policy and Law* 15, no. 1 (1990): 1–67.

11. Organization for Economic Cooperation and Development, *OECD Health Data 2000: A Comparative Analysis of Twenty-Nine Countries* (Paris: Organization for Economic Cooperation and Development, Health Policy Unit, 2000).

12. M. Kendix and T. E. Getzen, "U.S. Health Services Employment: A Time Series Analysis," *Health Economics* 3, no. 3 (1994): 169–181.

13. International data were obtained from *OECD Health Data 2000*. State data were from the AMA and the Bureau of Economic Analysis, U.S. Department of Commerce.

14. T. E. Getzen, "Macroeconomic Forecasting of National Health Expenditures," *Advances in Health Economics and Health Services Research* 11 (1990): 27–48; and T. E. Getzen and J. P. Poullier, "International Health Spending Forecasts: Concepts and Evaluation," *Social Science and Medicine* 34, no. 9 (1992): 1057–1068.

15. The trend variable was adjusted for time by calculating the partial coefficient of multiple determination, which in various analyses ranged from 0.27 to 0.38 ($p <$ .0001); see C. R. Rao, *Linear Statistical Inference and Its Applications* (New York: John Wiley and Sons, 1965), 225.

16. U. E. Reinhardt, *Physician Productivity and the Demand for Health Manpower* (Cambridge, Mass.: Ballinger, 1975); W. B. Schwartz et al., "The Changing Geographic Distribution of Board-Certified Physicians," *New England Journal of Medicine* 303, no. 18 (1980): 1032–1038; and R. L. Ernst and D. E. Yett, *Physician Location and Specialty Choice* (Ann Arbor, Mich.: Health Administration Press, 1985). Correlation coefficients relating per capita income and total active physician supply ranged from .50 to .55 at six time points between 1970 and 1998.

17. T. E. Getzen, "Population Aging and the Growth of Health Expenditures," *Journal of Gerontology: Social Sciences* 47, no. 3 (1992): S98–S104; and T. R. Marmor, "How Not to Think About Medicare Reform," *Journal of Health Politics, Policy, and Law* 26, no. 1 (2001): 107–117.

18. For a critique of the use of Census Bureau projections in workforce analyses, see Cooper, "Perspectives on the Physician Workforce."

19. Ibid.; Cooper, "Seeking a Balanced Physician Workforce"; and Centers for Medicare and Medicaid Services, "National Health Expenditures Projections: 1998–2008," < www.hcfa.gov/stats/NHE-Proj/proj1998/default.htm > (15 June 2001).

20. U.S. Department of Commerce, U.S. Census Bureau, "National Population Projections," < www.census.gov/population/www/projections/natproj.html > (10 June 2001). Projections were derived using population estimates from the 2000 census and the bureau's prior forecasting algorithm.

21. Kletke, "The Projected Supply of Physicians"; and Bureau of Health Professions, "Total and Active Physicians and Physician-to-Population Ratios, Selected Years, 1950–1997," < http://bhpr.hrsa.gov/healthworkforce/factbook.htm > (10 June 2001). For physician supply data before 1950, see Lee and Jones, *Fundamentals of Good Medical Care;* and W. H. Stewart and M. Pennell, "Health Manpower, 1930–75," *Public Health Reports* 75, no. 3 (1960): 274–280.

22. Physician surveys and estimates of sufficiency include Commonwealth Fund, *Multinational Comparisons of Health Systems Data, 2000* (New York: Commonwealth Fund, 2000); Sunshine, "Employment Among Recent Residency Program Graduates"; Angus et al., "Current and Projected Workforce Requirements"; California Medical Association, *And Then There Were None;* and Schubert et al., "Evidence." Surveys of the public include R. J. Blendon and J. M. Benson, "Americans' Views on Health Policy: A Fifty-Year Historical Perspective," *Health Affairs* (March-April 2001): 33–46; and H. Smith, *Critical Condition: Health Care in the 2000 Election* (Princeton, N.J.: Princeton Survey Research Associates, 2000). Recruitment experiences are from Merritt, Hawkins, and Associates, "Summary Report, 2000: Review of Physician Recruitment Incentives," < www.merritthawkins.com/compensation/comp_index.htm > (5 January 2001).

23. Kletke, "Projected Supply of Physicians"; Cooper, "Seeking a Balanced Physician Workforce"; and Bureau of Health Professions, *Forecasting the Future Supply of Physicians: Logic and Operation of the BHPr Physician Supply Model* (Rockville, Md.: U.S. Department of Health and Human Services, 1992).

24. Merritt, Hawkins, and Associates, "Summary Report, 2000: Review of Physicians 50 Years Old and Older," < www.merritthawkins.com/compensation/comp_index.htm > (15 January 2001); and C. Hogan, J. H. Sunshine, and B. Schepp, "Hiring of Diagnostic Radiologists in 1998," *American Journal of Roentgenology* 176, no. 2 (2001): 307–312.

25. For a discussion of these factors, see Kletke et al., "Growing Proportion of Female Physicians"; Kletke, "Projected Supply of Physicians"; and Merritt, Hawkins, "Summary Report . . . Physicians 50 Years Old and Older."

26. Cooper et al., "Roles of Nonphysician Clinicians"; Cooper et al., "Current and Projected Workforce"; and E. S. Sekscenski et al., "State Practice Environments and the Supply of Physician Assistants, Nurse Practitioners, and Certified Nurse-Midwives," *New England Journal of Medicine* 331, no. 19 (1994): 1266–1271.

27. M. O. Mundinger et al., "Primary Care Outcomes in Patients Treated by Nurse Practitioners or Physicians: A Randomized Trial," *Journal of the American Medical Association* 283, no. 1 (2000): 59–68; S. L. Krein, "The Employment and Use of Nurse Practitioners and Physician Assistants by Rural Hospitals," *Journal of Rural Health* 13, no. 1 (1997): 45–58; R. S. Hooker and L. F. McCaig, "Use of Physician Assistants and Nurse Practitioners in Primary Care, 1995–1999," *Health Affairs* (July-August 2001): 231–238; and T. H. Dial et al., "Clinical Staffing in Staff- and Group-Model HMOs," *Health Affairs* (Summer 1995): 168–180.

28. Centers for Medicare and Medicaid Services, "National Health Expenditures Projections"; Congressional Budget Office, "The Economic Outlook," in *The Budget and Economic Outlook: Fiscal Years 2001–2010,* < www.cbo/showdoc.cfm?index = 1824&sequence = 0&from = 7 > (15 January 2001); and S. Heffler et al., "Health Spending Growth Up in 1999; Faster Growth Expected in the Future," *Health Affairs* (March-Apr 2001): 193–203.

29. D. Braddock, "Occupational Outlook, 1998–2008: Occupational Employment Projections to 2008," *Monthly Labor Review* (November 1999): 51–77.

30. E. Ginzberg, "Physician Supply Policies and Health Reform," *Journal of the American Medical Association* 268, no. 21 (1992): 3115–3118; K. Grumbach and P. R. Lee, "How Many Physicians Can We Afford?" *Journal of the American Medical Association* 265, no. 18 (1991): 2369–2372; and S. A. Schroeder and L. G. Sandy, "Specialty Distribution of U.S. Physicians: The Invisible Drivers of Health Care Spending," *New England Journal of Medicine* 328, no. 13 (1993): 961–963. For a critique of supplied-induced demand, see S. Folland, A. C. Goodman, and M. Stano, *The Economics of Health and Health Care* (Upper Saddle River, N.J.: Prentice Hall, 2001), 204–216.

31. P. Sullivan, "Concerns About Size of M.D. Workforce, Medicine's Future Dominate CMA Annual Meeting," *Canadian Medical Association Journal* 161, no. 5 (1999): 561–562; and California Medical Association, *And Then There Were None.*

32. E. Ginzberg, "A Hard Look at Cost Containment," *New England Journal of Medicine* 316, no. 18 (1987): 1151–1154; and F. W. Peabody, "The Care of the Patient," *Journal of the American Medical Association* (19 March 1927): 877–882.

33. A. D. Abbott, *The System of Professions: An Essay on the Division of Expert Labor* (Chicago: University of Chicago Press, 1988).

34. J. Greene, "Physicians Win Big in States over Scope-of-Practice Issues," *American Medical News* (2 July 2001): 1–2.

35. F. Mullan, "The Case for More U.S. Medical Students," *New England Journal of Medicine* 343, no. 3 (2000): 213–217.

CHAPTER EIGHTEEN

# The Ramifications of Specialty-Dominated Medicine

Kevin Grumbach, M.D.
2002

Reading [Chapter Seventeen] by Richard Cooper and colleagues is like watching a television commercial for a sport-utility vehicle (SUV). "Buy more physicians" is the marketing pitch—and not just any physician, but the four-by-four (as in four years of medical school plus four or more years of residency training), gas-guzzling specialist model that creates an irresistible buying frenzy among American consumers eager to spend their discretionary income.

When I watch advertisements showing a mud-splattered SUV careening along a dirt road and coming to rest atop an impossibly remote mountain peak, I confess that I feel no automotive lust. I think about ruined natural habitats, global warming, depletion of natural resources, the nation's economic addiction to petroleum, and the poor guy in the Honda Civic about to collide with the SUV. I rue the distortedly low sticker price of buying and operating an SUV that fails to account for the true social costs associated with SUVs. And I ponder the "utility" of an SUV that so often seems to carry only a single passenger on urban commutes.

Nonetheless, SUVs are an undeniably popular item in the United States, with sales continuing to soar. Lots of people desire them (some of my best friends even own them). As Sen. Trent Lott (R-Miss.) recently asserted, "The American people have a right to drive a great big road hog SUV if they want to, and I'm gonna get me one."[1]

In the view of Cooper and colleagues, Americans also appear to have the right to an ever bigger and more expensive health system featuring a steadily increasing supply of physicians per capita, especially of specialists. The authors interpret their study as "consistent with the notion that a causal relationship exists between economic expansion and the growth of physician supply." Based on the historical association between trends in physician supply and economic activity in the United States, they calculate that each 1 percent increase in gross domestic product (GDP) per capita produces a 0.75 percent increase in physicians per capita. Of note, virtually all of the growth in U.S. physician supply per capita in the past half-century has been in the supply of specialists.[2] The high elasticity between GDP per capita and specialist supply suggests that specialty care (like SUVs) functions as a luxury good.

In the interpretation of the authors, this relationship is not merely a description of past trends but a rule for projecting future demand for physicians. Presented this way, the relationship between economic growth and increasing specialist supply takes on the properties of natural law. Social planners can attempt to tamper with this natural law and impose constraints on growth of specialist supply. But like the protagonists of a Greek tragedy, social planners reveal their hubris in challenging the national destiny for more physicians and must inevitably discover, to their dismay, that their efforts to thwart the will of the market deity can come to no good. We might as well ask Americans to stop buying so many SUVs.

There are several reasons to take issue with this fatalistic view. Consumer demand for physicians is not the exogenous force implied by Cooper and colleagues. Physicians are able to induce demand for their services, creating a self-replicating cycle of more physicians begetting more demand begetting more physicians.[3] Nor is the preponderance of health care purchased in an individual consumer market. Public funds pay for about 40 percent of health care, and funds pooled through private insurance purchase another 40 percent. The 20 percent of patients who generate 80 percent of health expenditures every year are for the most part spending someone else's money on health care. (That's the whole point of health insurance.) Collective financing of health care calls for collective decisions about how much to spend. Endowing individual consumer demand for health care with a preeminent role in determining the proper equilibrium level of health care spending and physician supply is as flawed a concept as promoting a universal automotive coverage plan that would give every household a third-party payment to purchase an SUV. The market and social objectives for health care are very different from those for automobiles.

The "Americans have a right to buy more specialists" view also raises the question of whether people are actually buying anything of benefit. Cooper and colleagues portray their analysis as one free of value judgments about what "ought" to be. The consumer is sovereign; social planners are presumptuous to question this sovereign being about how it wishes to spend its (or in the case of health care, someone else's) hard-earned cash. But as a taxpayer contributing to Medicare and Medicaid, and as a subscriber in my employer's group health insurance plan, I do want to know whether the extra tariff on my income that Cooper and colleagues would levy to pay for more specialists will in fact purchase better health for me and for the nation.

The evidence on this score is not reassuring. Many studies indicate that a greater supply of specialists is not associated with better population health. Leiyu Shi has conducted a series of studies comparing physician supply and health indicators across U.S. states and substate regions, controlling for a variety of population characteristics.[4] The studies have shown that a greater supply of primary care physicians is associated with lower mortality rates as well as lower disease-specific death rates in some categories. A greater supply of specialists has either no association with these health indicators or in some instances an association with worse health outcomes.

A second example is neonatology, a specialty that has proliferated in recent decades. And yet recent research by David Goodman has found that regions in the country with above-average numbers of neonatologists per capita do not have better outcomes for high-risk newborns than do regions with a lower supply.[5]

A third example, appendicitis, is a common condition that has attracted greater specialist involvement in recent years. Many patients with clinical findings suggestive of possible appendicitis who formerly went straight to the operating room now make a detour to the radiology suite for a diagnostic sonogram or computed tomography (CT) scan of the abdomen. However, a statewide study of appendectomies in Washington State over the past decade found no reduction in rates of removal of normal appendices.[6] Elliot Fisher and Gilbert Welch have cogently discussed the general case for "how might more be worse" in health care.[7]

One final problem of unmitigated growth of physician supply and health spending is that it will accentuate inequities in health care. Who is going to pay for that rising "projected demand" in Cooper's Figure 17.1 that looks as if it will never bend toward an asymptotic slope? Not most employers, who are moving to defined contribution plans to limit their health care outlays. Not government, in an era of investing in antiterrorism measures and tax rebates. Not the uninsured, clinging as best as they can to what's left of the health care safety net. And probably not the public at large, facing an economic downturn bordering on a recession. Unmitigated growth in health care spending means a widening gap between the medical haves and have-nots, producing more uninsured Americans as employers, individuals, and government find insurance less affordable, while the affluent and well-insured consume an ever greater share of the nation's health care resources.

The future that Cooper and colleagues project is the SUV-ification of U.S. health care. It is a future of more specialists, more high-tech care, higher costs, and greater disparities, of a system built out of proportion of the true needs of the public for efficient and effective health care. It threatens the proper ecology of medical care.[8] It may even be harmful. Many nations have people driving automobiles of modest size and excellent fuel efficiency. Many nations have health care systems that provide health care for all residents in a less specialty-oriented manner and with better health outcomes than is true of the United States. It would be a mistake to believe that the future predicted by Cooper and colleagues is either preordained or desirable.

# Notes

1. "Energy Policy Briefing, Roll Call Q&A, Lott Lights Up the Democrats," *Roll Call*, 12 March 2001.

2. Council on Graduate Medical Education, *Eighth Report: Patient Care Physician Supply and Requirements: Testing COGME Recommendations* (Rockville, Md.: Council on Graduate Medical Education, 1996).

3. T. H. Rice and R. J. Labelle, "Do Physicians Induce Demand for Medical Services?" *Journal of Health Politics, Policy, and Law* 14, no. 3 (1989): 587–600; and R. J. Labelle, G. Stoddart, and T. H. Rice, "A Reexamination of the Meaning and Importance of Supplier-Induced Demand," *Journal of Health Economics* 13, no. 3 (1994): 347–368.

4. L. Shi et al., "Income Inequality, Primary Care, and Health Indicators," *Journal of Family Practice* 48, no. 4 (1999): 275–284; L. Shi and B. Starfield, "Primary Care, Income Inequality, and Self-Rated Health in the United States: A Mixed-Level Analysis," *International Journal of Health Services* 30, no. 3 (2000): 541–555; and L. Shi and B. Starfield, "The Effect of Primary Care Physician Supply and Income Inequality on Mortality Among Blacks and Whites in U.S. Metropolitan Areas," *American Journal of Public Health* 91, no. 8 (2001): 1246–1250.

5. D. C. Goodman et al., "Regional Variation in Neonatal Intensive Care: The Association Between Capacity, Need, and Mortality," 2000 AAP Abstract, *Journal of Perinatology* 20, no. 7 (2000): 463.

6. D. R. Flum et al., "Has Misdiagnosis of Appendicitis Decreased over Time? A Population-Based Analysis," *Journal of the American Medical Association* 286, no. 14 (2001): 1748–1753.

7. E. S. Fisher and H. G. Welch, "Avoiding the Unintended Consequences of Growth in Medical Care: How Might More Be Worse?" *Journal of the American Medical Association* 281, no. 5 (1999): 446–453.

8. L. A. Green et al., "The Ecology of Medical Care Revisited," *New England Journal of Medicine* 344, no. 26 (2001): 2021–2025.

# Influence of Income, Hours Worked, and Loan Repayment on Medical Students' Decision to Pursue a Primary Care Career

Michael P. Rosenthal, M.D.; James J. Diamond, Ph.D.;
Howard K. Rabinowitz, M.D.; Laurence C. Bauer, MSW, M.Ed.;
Robert L. Jones, D.Ed., MCP; Gary W. Kearl, M.D.;
Robert B. Kelly, M.D., M.S.; Kent J. Sheets, Ph.D.; Arnold Jaffe, Ph.D.;
A. Patrick Jonas, M.D.; Mack T. Ruffin IV, M.D., M.P.H.

1994

Within the current climate of health system reform, experts agree that a national shortage of generalist physicians exists and that 50% of the physician workforce should include primary care specialists (family physicians, general internists, and general pediatricians).[1–4] Currently, only one third of physicians practicing in the United States are generalists, and less than one fifth of recent medical school graduates are planning generalist careers.[1,5] Successful health system reform must include targeted strategies to produce more generalists.[1–6]

Although the need to increase the number of generalist physicians is clear, the means of accomplishing this goal are not. Choosing a specialty is a complex process, dependent on a variety of intrinsic and extrinsic factors that operate from premedical education through residency.[4,7–10] Medical students' specialty preferences on entrance into medical school and their educational experiences clearly are contributors to their eventual specialty choices.[5,11,12] In addition, economic and lifestyle considerations are becoming increasingly important factors in students' choices of specialties and have a significant effect on specialty distribution.[5,9,11,13] In particular, higher student indebtedness seems to discourage pursuit of a generalist career, but the effect of indebtedness on specialty choice has been more difficult to demonstrate.[2,5,6,11,14–16]

Would the ratio of generalists to specialists increase if economic and lifestyle incentives for generalist physicians were improved? Based on a pilot project,[17] colleagues at six institutions with an interest in primary care conducted a

This chapter originally appeared as Rosenthal MP, Diamond JJ, Rabinowitz HK, et al. Influence of income, hours worked, and loan repayment on medical students' decision to pursue a primary care career. *JAMA*. 1994;271(12):914-917. Copyright © 1994, American Medical Association. Reprinted with permission.

collaborative study to assess the specialty plans of their current fourth-year medical students and, for those not choosing primary care, to investigate students' reports of the potential effect that alteration of key economic or lifestyle factors could have in attracting such students to the primary care specialties.

# METHODS

This study surveyed the 1993 graduating classes of six U.S. medical schools (Jefferson Medical College, Thomas Jefferson University, Philadelphia; Ohio State University College of Medicine, Columbus; The Pennsylvania State University College of Medicine, Hershey; State University of New York at Stony Brook School of Medicine; University of Kentucky College of Medicine, Lexington; and University of Michigan Medical School, Ann Arbor). A survey was mailed to all 901 fourth-year students at the six schools in the fall of their senior year, the time when most students were solidifying their career plans and preparing their applications for residency positions. A standardized cover letter was included, along with a stamped, self-addressed envelope. There were two mailings and one telephone follow-up. The confidentiality of responses was assured.

Students were asked which specialty they eventually planned to practice by indicating the one they would "choose today," even if they were undecided and forced to make a decision. They were also asked to indicate their expected average yearly income in their chosen specialty, how many hours they expected to work in an average week, and their estimated debt for education when they graduated from medical school.

Primary care specialties were defined as family practice, general internal medicine, and general pediatrics, in accordance with prior national reports.[1,3,4] All other specialties, including "internal medicine, subspecialty" and "pediatrics, subspecialty," were defined as non–primary care (NPC). The NPC students were asked which (if any) of three specific factors would cause them to change to a primary care specialty and to designate the one most important factor that would cause them to change. The three specific factors investigated in this study were annual income, number of work hours per week, and debt alleviation via medical school loan repayment.

Descriptive statistics were used to summarize the overall findings. Strata were formed using selected variables such as debt for additional descriptive analyses. All data were analyzed using SAS software for personal computers.[18]

# RESULTS

Of the 901 surveys mailed, 688 were received for an overall response rate of 76% (range among schools, 70% to 84%). Only three students did not answer the question regarding their planned specialty, and these three surveys were removed from the analysis. Responders were similar to nonresponders in terms of demographic variables. Primary care specialties were chosen by 27% of the students ($n$ = 188): 15% chose family practice, 6% chose general internal medicine, and 6% chose general pediatrics.

Little difference existed between the primary care and NPC students' estimates of their mean debt for education ($49,000 vs. $49,000) and anticipated weekly work hours (62 hours vs. 64 hours). However, the primary care students' mean expected income was $60,000 less than the mean expected income of the NPC students ($92,000 vs. $152,000). The primary care students showed a 50:50 male-to-female gender distribution, and the NPC students' male-to-female ratio was 69:31.

The survey also centered on the potential incentives (specific factors) that might attract those students pursuing NPC specialties to primary care. The NPC students were asked to indicate at which salary (if any) they "would change to a primary care specialty." They were given a choice of potential salaries ranging from $120,000 to $220,000 in $20,000 increments. Seventeen percent of the NPC students indicated they would change for one of the salaries, with a mean salary incentive of $180,000. The NPC students were also asked to indicate whether they would change to a primary care specialty if their "number of work hours per week (not including residency) would be . . .," and they were given a choice of 30 hours to 80 hours (in 10-hour increments). Nineteen percent of the NPC students indicated they would change for one of the choices, with a mean incentive of 50 work hours per week. In addition, 10% of the NPC students indicated that they "would change to a primary care specialty if all my medical school loans would be repaid."

Given the three factors surveyed, the NPC students were then asked to "check the ONE most important factor that would cause you to change to a primary care specialty." A total of one quarter ($n$ = 125) of the NPC students indicated one of the three options of income (10%), hours worked (11%), or loan repayment (4%). Overall, no gender difference existed in percentage of NPC students who would change to primary care. However, men found the income option more attractive (13% men vs. 6% women) and women found the hours worked option slightly more attractive (13% women vs. 11% men). The other 75% (both men and women) indicated that they "would not change to a primary care specialty for any of these reasons" ($n$ = 337) or left the item blank ($n$ = 35).

The willingness of NPC students to change to primary care and the most important reason to change varied according to the students' planned specialties (Table 19.1). Almost one third of students choosing internal medicine and pediatric subspecialties or "other, not surgical" specialties said they would change to primary care, whereas only 7% of students planning careers in the surgical specialties would change. Students planning to pursue internal medicine or pediatric subspecialties showed a preference for change based on income; while of those planning to pursue "other, not surgical" specialties, more

Table 19.1. Percentage of Non–Primary Care Students Who Would Change to Primary Care, by Incentive for Change and Planned Specialty

| Specialty | Income | Work Hours | Loan Repayment | Total |
|---|---|---|---|---|
| Internal medicine ($n$ = 84) and pediatric subspecialties[a] | 18 | 8 | 6 | 32 |
| Other, not surgery ($n$ = 299)[b] | 10 | 15 | 5 | 30 |
| Surgery and surgical subspecialties ($n$ = 110)[c] | 6 | 1 | 0 | 7 |

[a]Does not include four students with specialties that could not be classified.

[b]"Other, not surgery" indicates allergy and immunology, anesthesiology, dermatology, emergency medicine, obstetrics and gynecology, neurology, ophthalmology, otolaryngology, pathology, physical medicine and rehabilitation, preventive medicine, psychiatry, radiation oncology, or radiology.

[c]"Surgery" indicates general surgery, maxillofacial surgery, neurosurgery, orthopedics, plastic surgery, thoracic surgery, or urology.

students preferred switching to primary care for the number of work hours per week. For the few students planning surgical careers who would change to primary care, the income factor was predominant. The loan repayment option was the least preferred reason for change in all groups. However, for students whose debt was $50,000 or greater, the loan repayment option was much more important than for students with lesser debt. In fact, as debt levels increased, the percentage of NPC students who would change for loan repayment increased while the income and hours worked factors decreased in relative importance (Figure 19.1).

In all, a total of 45% (313/688) of the students said that they would pursue primary care careers. This 45% included the 188 students who reported plans to enter primary care, as well as the 125 NPC students who indicated that they would change to a primary care specialty with appropriate adjustments in income, hours worked, or loan repayment.

# COMMENT

The results of this multi-institutional study are consistent with other studies,[9,11,19,20] which indicate that many students who have recently chosen NPC specialties have, at least in part, made those choices based on economic or lifestyle considerations. Furthermore, this study suggests that changing eventual economic or lifestyle factors could directly affect the ability to attract students to the primary care specialties. In fact, if students' reports were borne out

**Figure 19.1.** Percentage of Non–Primary Care Students Who Would Change to Primary Care, by Incentive for Change at Differing Levels of Debt.

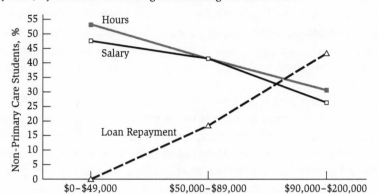

*Note:* Does not include non–primary care students unwilling to change specialty who had estimated debt levels of $0 to $49,000 ($n$ = 181), $50,000 to $89,000 ($n$ = 129), and $90,000 to $200,000 ($n$ = 57) or five non–primary care students who did not estimate their levels of debt.

in practice after such changes were made, the United States could approach the goal of graduating 50% generalist physicians.

The senior students surveyed appeared to have a good understanding of the financial aspects of specialty choice, since the primary care and NPC students' estimates of their earning potential were consistent with the current earnings of such physicians,[21,22] and the mean salary ($180,000) that might be expected to induce the NPC students to change to primary care is similar to the typical income that could be achieved in most NPC specialties.[21,22] Interestingly, more than 50% of the NPC students who said they would change from internal medicine or pediatrics subspecialties identified income as the most important factor, implying that their subspecialist vs. generalist choice was significantly related to their income expectations. Conversely, 50% of the NPC students who said they would change from the "other, not surgery" specialties identified hours worked as their most important factor; this group closely corresponds to the "controllable lifestyle" specialties noted in other studies.[23–25]

This study also suggests that amount of debt plays a role in specialty selection. Of all the NPC students with debt less than $50,000 ($n$ = 234), none said they would change to primary care if their loans would be repaid, but 7% of those with debt of $50,000 or more ($n$ = 258) said they would change for loan repayment. In addition, Figure 19.1 indicates that for NPC students who would change to primary care, the loan repayment incentive becomes much more important with increasingly higher debt loads. Recent data show that the mean debt of medical students is now approximately $50,000 and is increasing yearly, as is the number of students with debts of $50,000 or more.[14,26,27] Difficulties in prior efforts to identify debt as a significant factor in specialty choice may have been related to lower levels of debt, to grouping debts by specialty, and to studying the combined, mean debt of all students (including students with no or low debt). In the future, the escalating costs of medical education and medical student indebtedness will likely become even more significant factors in specialty choice.

From a policy perspective, the costs and benefits of changing different "adjustable" factors in order to address the physician-specialty mix need to be considered, since both the income enhancement and loan repayment incentives could be expensive. Indeed, increasing the annual income of all primary care physicians to $180,000, the mean level to entice NPC students to change to primary care, would be extraordinarily costly, especially since that income would need to be maintained over a 30- to 40-year career. However, the cost to society of a loan repayment program, even to finance high levels of debt, would actually be much less, since the cost would only be paid once during a physician's career.

Could there be a combination of income and loan repayment incentives?[2] Linking incentives to preferential admissions programs (which have proven success in recruiting students to primary care[5,12]) and/or public service[6] could also be considered. A national preferential loan assistance program (low-percentage loans) has recently been redesigned to support students choosing primary care careers.[28] We believe this program is an important first step, but our data suggest that a greater economic and widespread societal commitment is necessary to attract more students to primary care specialties.

This study, which identified key factors that could attract more students to primary care, has some limitations. First, we evaluated the self-reported career plans and hypothetical career changes of senior students, not their actual specialty choices. Second, the factors studied were evaluated as independent variables, although interactions among these factors undoubtedly exist. However, if combinations of these adjustments were implemented, even more students would likely be attracted to primary care specialties. Finally, there may be some question about the generalizability of our results. Although the six collaborating institutions represent several regions of the United States, they are notable for having established family practice departments and role models who teach in the preclinical and clinical years of medical school and have a combined 10-year average of students entering family practice (13%) that is somewhat above the national average (11%).[29] Although students at all medical schools would likely consider a primary care career if appropriate economic and lifestyle changes were made, a supportive primary care environment where students have generalist role models and can assess their lifestyles would likely increase these effects.[28,30–32]

In conclusion, the need to attract more students to primary care specialties is a national health care priority. It is encouraging to find that many students interested in other NPC specialties might change to primary care if important economic or lifestyle factors were addressed: nearly 50% of the students in this study indicated they would have chosen primary care specialties if offered the proper incentive. Further delineation of these factors and how to change them most effectively are important considerations for the U.S. health care system.

## Notes

1. Council on Graduate Medical Education. *Third Report: Improving Access to Health Care Through Physician Workforce Reform: Directions for the Twenty-First Century.* Rockville, Md.: U.S. Department of Health and Human Services; 1992.

2. Starfield B, Simpson S. Primary care as part of U.S. health services reform. *JAMA.* 1993;269:3136–3139.

3. Task Force on the Generalist Physician. *Executive Summary.* Washington, DC: Association of American Medical Colleges; 1992.

4. Primary Care Task Force. Report of the Medical Schools Section Primary Care Task Force. *JAMA.* 1992;268:1092–1094.

5. Colwill J. Where have all the primary care applicants gone? *N Engl J Med.* 1992;326:387–393.

6. Petersdorf RG. Financing medical education: a universal "Berry plan" for medical students. *N Engl J Med.* 1993;328:651–654.

7. Babbott D, Baldwin DC Jr, Killian CD, Weaver SO. Trends in evolution of specialty choice: comparison of U.S. medical school graduates in 1983 and 1987. *JAMA.* 1989;261:2367–2373.

8. Mowbray RM. Research in choice of medical specialty: a review of the literature, 1977–1987. *Aust N Z J Med.* 1989;19:389–399.

9. Rogers LQ, Fincher R-ME, Lewis LA. Factors influencing medical students to choose primary care or non–primary care specialties. *Acad Med.* 1990;65(September suppl):S47–S48.

10. Rabinowitz HK. The change in specialty preference by medical students over time: an analysis of students who prefer family medicine. *Fam Med.* 1990;36:62–63.

11. Rosenthal MP, Turner TN, Diamond JJ, Rabinowitz HK. Income expectations of first-year students at Jefferson Medical College as a predictor of family practice specialty choice. *Acad Med.* 1992;67:328–331.

12. Rabinowitz HK. Recruitment, retention, and follow-up of graduates of a program to increase the number of family physicians in rural and underserved areas. *N Engl J Med.* 1993;328:934–939.

13. Fincher R-ME, Lewis LA, Rogers LQ. Classification model that predicts medical students' choices of primary care or non–primary care specialties. *Acad Med.* 1992;67:324–327.

14. Kassebaum DG, Szenas PL. Relationship between indebtedness and the specialty choices of graduating medical students. *Acad Med.* 1992;67:700–707.

15. Bernstein DS. Medical student indebtedness and choice of specialty. *JAMA.* 1992;267:1921–1922.

16. McLaughlin MA, Daugherty SR, Rose WH, Goodman LJ. The impact of medical school debt on postgraduate career and lifestyle. *Acad Med.* 1991;66(September suppl):S43–S45.

17. Rosenthal MP, Yoon MY, Diamond JJ, Rabinowitz HK. The potential influence of income, hours worked, and loan repayment on medical student specialty selection. Paper presented at the 25th Annual Spring Conference of the Society of Teachers of Family Medicine; April 27, 1992; St Louis, Mo. Abstract.

18. *SAS/STAT Users' Guide.* Version 6.03. Cary, NC: SAS Institute Inc; 1988.

19. Lieu TA, Schroeder SA, Altman DF. Specialty choice at one medical school: recent trends and analysis of predictive factors. *Acad Med.* 1989;64:622–629.

20. Tardiff R, Cella D, Seiferth C, Perry S. Selection and change of specialties by medical school graduates. *J Med Educ.* 1986;61:790–796.

21. Clark L. Which non-surgeons are doing best in earnings? *Med Econ.* 1989;66:94–110.

22. Owens A. What's the recession done to your buying power? *Med Econ.* 1992;69:194–206.

23. Schwartz RW, Jarecky RK, Stodel WE, et al. Controllable lifestyle: a new factor in career choice by medical students. *Acad Med.* 1989;64:606–609.

24. Schwartz RW, Haley JV, Williams C, et al. The controllable lifestyle factor and students' attitudes about specialty selection. *Acad Med.* 1990;65:207–210.

25. Jarecky RK, Schwartz RW, Haley JV, Donnelly MB. Stability of medical specialty selection. *Acad Med.* 1991;66:756–761.

26. Park R. Graduating medical students debt and specialty choices. *Acad Med.* 1990;65:485–486.

27. Jolin LD, Jolly P, Krakower JY, Beran R. U.S. medical school finances. *JAMA.* 1992;268:1149–1155.

28. Rivo ML. Internal medicine and the journey to medical generalism. *Ann Intern Med.* 1993;119:146–152.

29. American Academy of Family Physicians. *Facts About Family Practice.* Kansas City, Mo: American Academy of Family Physicians; 1993.

30. Rabinowitz HK. Sixteen years' experience with a required third-year family medicine clerkship at Jefferson Medical College. *Acad Med.* 1992;67:150–156.

31. Rabinowitz HK. The relationship between career choice and a required third-year family practice clerkship. *Fam Med.* 1988;20:118–121.

32. Politzer RM, Harris DL, Gaston MH, Mullan F. Primary care physician supply and the medically underserved. *JAMA.* 1991;266:104–109.

# CHAPTER TWENTY

# Physicians and Rural America

Roger A. Rosenblatt, M.D., M.P.H.; L. Gary Hart, Ph.D.
2000

Many rural Americans have limited access to health care. This problem stems from two characteristics of the health care system: the many Americans without health care insurance and the tendency of health care professionals to locate and practice in relatively affluent urban and suburban areas.

The relative shortage of physicians in rural areas of the United States is one of the few constants in any description of the U.S. medical care system. About 20% of the U.S. population—more than 50 million people—live in rural areas, but only 9% of the nation's physicians practice in rural communities.[1]

Crude comparisons of the physician-to-population ratio in rural versus urban areas can be extremely misleading and provide almost no information about whether shortages or surpluses exist in either location.[2] In 1995—the latest year for which data are available—gaps existed between the supply of active physicians in counties of different size (Figure 20.1). As can be seen in this figure, major differences persist between the aggregate supply in urban and rural areas, with the larger counties having many more physicians per 100,000 population.

But this information obscures the fact that the physician supply has grown in rural areas in the past 20 years, although the growth has not been uniform. The supply of rural physicians has increased modestly in the past few decades, with most of the increase in the larger rural communities adjacent to metropolitan areas (Figure 20.2). Rural supply lags far behind the current urban supply of physicians, but the urban supply of physicians is, in the opinion of many, excessive.

---

This chapter originally appeared as Rosenblatt RA, Hart LG. Physicians and rural America. *West J Med.* 2000;173:348–351. Reprinted with permission from the BMJ Publishing Group. This chapter was adapted, with permission, from Ricketts III TC: *Rural Health in the United States.* New York: Oxford University Press; 1999.

**Figure 20.1.** Active Physicians per 100,000 Population, 1995, by Location.

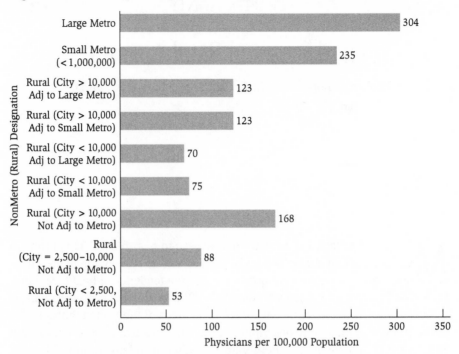

*Source:* Data provided by American Medical Association, 1997.

Physician supply in rural areas is closely tied to the specialty mix of American physicians. Specialty has a powerful effect on physician location choice for each of the major specialty groups (Figure 20.3). Family physicians distribute themselves in proportion to the population in both rural and urban locations and are the largest single source of physicians in rural areas. All other specialties are much more likely to settle in urban areas.

Given the expansion of the rural physician supply, it is important to distinguish between rural areas that have definite shortages of critical health professionals and those that have fewer health professionals relative to oversupplied urban areas. Historically, the government has designated areas as seriously underserved based on the physician-to-population ratio within a specific health service area. Populations with too few physicians have been categorized as health professional shortage areas, thus becoming eligible for a broad array of governmental assistance.

**Figure 20.2.** Active Physicians per 100,000 Population, 1940–1995, by Year and Location.

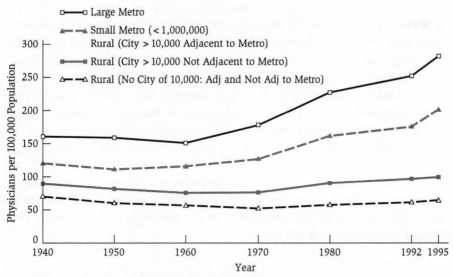

*Source:* Data provided by American Medical Association, 1997.

**Figure 20.3.** Patient Care Physicians per 100,000 Population, 1995, by Location and Specialty.

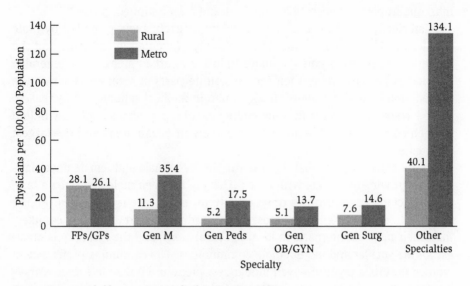

*Source:* Data provided by American Medical Association, 1997.

# EFFECT OF SPECIALTY CHOICE AND DISTRIBUTION

Nothing affects the location decision of physicians more than specialty. The more highly specialized the physician, the less likely he or she will settle in a rural area. As a consequence, the growth of specialization is a major contributor to the geographic maldistribution of physicians. Many of the shortages in communities with fewer than 10,000 residents could have been reduced or eliminated if even a small fraction of subspecialists produced over the past 15 years had chosen to become primary care physicians in rural or underserved areas.[3]

The recently revived interest in family medicine and the other generalist disciplines is a major factor in addressing rural geographic maldistribution. The decreasing proportion of generalist physicians leveled off in the 1980s (Figure 20.4).[4] Despite recently increased interest in primary care, the percentage in generalist disciplines has not yet shown a substantial increase. An improvement in the balance of generalists and specialists is a necessary precondition for eliminating rural physician shortages.

# EFFECT OF GENDER ON CHOICE OF PRACTICE LOCATION

Starting a decade ago, the proportion of women attending medical school increased rapidly. The number of female physicians in the United States more than quadrupled between 1970 and 1991 and has continued to rise.[5]

Historically, rural medical care was almost exclusively provided by male physicians. This was a product of the paucity of women in medicine and the tendency of the few female graduates to locate in urban areas. Male generalist physicians far outnumber their female counterparts in rural areas across the United States. As the proportion of women in medical schools has increased, there have been concerns that the supply of rural physicians might dwindle if women continue to settle almost exclusively in urban areas and the largest rural cities.

Recent work suggests that the disparity between male and female physicians may be growing less acute with time.[6] The gap between male and female family physicians has narrowed dramatically for more recent graduates (Figure 20.5). Still, even women in the most recent graduate cohort are much less likely than their male counterparts to locate in rural areas, and the disparity is greatest for the smaller and more remote communities. The continuing preference of women for urban practice—even though less pronounced than in earlier years—may still pose a problem for the future recruitment of rural physicians.

**Figure 20.4.** Percentage of Primary Care and Non–Primary Care Physicians for Selected Years, 1931–1996.

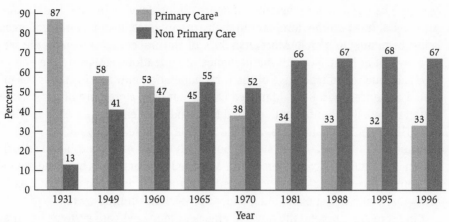

*Source:* Data provided by American Medical Association, 1997.

[a]Family physicians, general internists, and general pediatrics. The AMA reclassified MDs in 1968, causing a 3.5% change in the primary care/non–primary care mix.

**Figure 20.5.** Ratio of Male to Female Family or General Physicians, 1997, by Graduation Cohort.

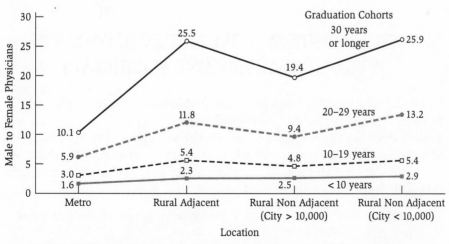

*Source:* Ellsbury KE, Doescher MP, Hart LG. U.S. medical schools and the rural family physician gender gap. *Fam Med.* 2000;32:331–337.

# INFLUENCE OF MANAGED CARE

Managed care is a major emerging influence on the delivery of rural health care. Although it has become dominant in many urban areas, its effect in rural areas is just beginning to be felt. More than 80% of all rural counties were in the service area of at least 1 health maintenance organization (HMO) by the end of 1995, although the percentage of the rural population enrolled in HMOs is estimated to be less than 8%.[7] Managed care is not only a creature of the private sector; nationally, about a tenth of rural Medicaid recipients are enrolled in Medicaid HMOs and prepaid plans, and the number is increasing rapidly.

Managed care is a 2-edged sword, both with regard to geographic maldistribution and rural medical underservice. Managed care networks have the potential to provide organizational vehicles for hiring and deploying physicians in areas that could not support independent physicians on their own.

But there are 2 potentially adverse effects of managed care systems on rural health: the loss of local control of health care systems and the reluctance of private managed care systems to provide care to the uninsured. Most managed care systems are sponsored by large metropolitan organizations, and these entities may have little understanding of or empathy for isolated rural areas. The presence of physicians hired through vertically integrated systems may mean that the community has health professionals, but they may be of little use to the working poor who have neither Medicaid nor conventional health insurance. The managed care industry is in rapid flux, and the extent to which managed care will ultimately dominate rural areas as it has dominated some urban ones is difficult to predict.

# POSSIBLE SOLUTIONS TO THE PROBLEM OF INEQUITIES IN RURAL HEALTH EDUCATIONAL INITIATIVES

One of the most powerful ways to remedy problems of rural geographic maldistribution is to change the medical education system so that it selects, trains, and deploys more health care workers who choose to practice in rural areas. Much of the federal support incorporated within the Title VII programs—the major federal vehicle for generalist training—is based on the premise that this is an achievable goal. Talley has discussed the 4 basic "truths" about rural health[4]:

- Students with rural origins are more likely to train in primary care and return to rural areas,

- Residents trained in rural areas are more likely to choose to practice in rural areas,

- Family medicine is the key discipline of rural health care, and
- Residents practice close to where they train.

To the extent that these relationships are accurate—and evidence supports associations between these characteristics and the decision to practice in rural areas—modifications of the training milieu to incorporate these factors make sense.

The advantage of this approach is that it takes optimum advantage of free-market solutions to the problem of geographic physician maldistribution. Rather than requiring the establishment of federal or state delivery systems that may be controversial, complex, and expensive, graduating residents gravitate to underserved areas to fill their personal desires.

Although this type of intervention does not lend itself to controlled experiments, ample evidence exists that such an approach works. Publicly owned medical schools in rural states, particularly those that see their mission as training future family physicians, have high proportions of their graduating classes ultimately practicing in rural areas. By contrast, research-intensive private schools in metropolitan areas with no commitment to family medicine have virtually no rural graduates.[5]

# CHANGES IN REIMBURSEMENT STRATEGIES OF MEDICARE AND MEDICAID

A powerful mechanism to improve the flow of health professionals to rural areas is the use of targeted incentives. Central to this approach is the belief that physicians and others act as rational economic beings. If some form of economic inducement enhances the reimbursement for rural services, then physicians are more likely to locate in these areas. This approach has been used with some success in Britain, Canada, and Australia, where a variety of bonuses increase reimbursement for selected rural practitioners.

# CHANGES IN EXISTING DIRECT FEDERAL AND STATE PROGRAMS

When educational interventions and economic incentives fail to remedy geographic maldistribution, the major recourse is the creation of programs that provide direct services to underserved areas. There are numerous examples of such programs, the largest of which are the community health centers and the

National Health Service Corps (NHSC). There is no question that these 2 federal programs remain the preeminent safety net programs for rural America. Studies by the Rural Health Research Centers in Chapel Hill, NC, and Seattle demonstrate that about 1 in 4 of every new primary care physician entering a health professional shortage area in the late 1980s was placed there under NHSC auspices[8] and that 1 in 5 physicians practicing independently in many of the smallest rural communities was initially brought to those areas through their service in the NHSC.[9]

Given the realities of the current system, future efforts should concentrate on improving the fit between need and services, enhanced coordination—and reduced duplication—of services provided, better identification of students to ultimately serve in the NHSC and state programs, and improved effectiveness and efficiency of governmentally sponsored health care services, including those of rural health clinics.[10] The wide variety of programs available—and the natural variability in the way they are organized and administered—leads to enormous complexity in the provision of services. It is certainly worth the effort to simplify programs and their administration and to ensure that governmental resources follow human need, not the administrative prowess of officials who excel at the bureaucratic skills that can obtain these services for their communities.

# NEW TECHNOLOGIES: POSSIBLE EFFECT OF TELEMEDICINE

Telemedicine is an emerging technology with enormous potential for mitigating the effects of the geographic maldistribution of health professionals. Although telemedicine has a legitimate, important, and growing role in rural medicine,[11] the path to the future is uncertain. As pointed out in the 2nd Invitational Consensus Conference on Telemedicine and the National Information Infrastructure, multiple and significant obstacles exist that make the current efforts uncoordinated, expensive, inaccessible, and at times even illegal.[12]

The current state of telemedicine could be characterized as creative but relatively unstructured, with a wide variety of public and private sector experiments proceeding simultaneously. Some applications, such as reading electrocardiograms at a distance, have become commonplace. Others, such as dermatology consultations, are being performed in many different places but without standard protocols for transmission, interaction, evaluation, or charging. And others, such as doing an appendectomy at a distance, remain in the realm of science fiction, if just barely. From the standpoint of geographic maldistribution, there are 3 key issues in improving the delivery of telemedicine to rural areas:

- Resolution of the professional licensure regulations, allowing physicians in metropolitan areas to make their expertise available to remote rural areas, even across state lines

- Clear protocols for a unified technologic infrastructure to reduce costs and to allow rural providers to have the option of communicating with multiple providers of these distant services without being captives of any single information provider

- Reasonable reimbursement by third-party payers for providing medical services at a distance

# CONCLUSIONS

Geographic maldistribution of health providers is one of the most deep-seated characteristics of the American health care system. Even though the 1990s have been marked by rapid expansion in the absolute and relative number of practicing physicians, substantial rural shortages have persisted. Rural areas will continue to have structural barriers that will require special programs to assist in the training, deployment, and support of health professionals.

## Notes

1. Bureau of Health Professions. *Rural Health Professions Facts: Supply and Distribution of Health Professions in Rural America.* Rockville, MD: Health Resources and Services Administration; 1992.

2. Center for the Evaluative Clinical Sciences, Dartmouth Medical School. *The Dartmouth Atlas of Health Care.* Chicago: American Hospital Publishing; 1996.

3. Konrad TR. "Shortages of Physicians and Other Health Professionals in Rural Areas: Background Paper Produced for COGME" (unpublished). Chapel Hill: Cecil G. Sheps Center for Health Services Research, University of North Carolina; 1997.

4. Talley RC. Graduate medical education and rural health care. *Acad Med.* 1990;65:522–525.

5. Rosenblatt RA, Whitcomb ME, Cullen TJ, Lishner DM, Hart LG. Which medical schools produce rural physicians? *JAMA.* 1992;268:1559–1565.

6. Doescher MP, Ellsbury KE, Hart LG. The distribution of rural female generalist physicians in the United States. *J Rural Health.* 2000;16:111–118.

7. Casey MM. Rural managed care. In: Ricketts TC III, ed. *Rural Health in the United States.* New York: Oxford University Press; 1999:113–118.

8. Konrad TR. *The Rural HPSA Physician Retention Study: Final Report for Grant No. RO HS 06544-0 from Agency for Health Care Policy and Research.* Chapel Hill:

Cecil G. Sheps Center for Health Services Research, University of North Carolina; 1994.

9. Cullen TJ, Hart LG. Whitcomb ME, Lishner DM, Rosenblatt RA. The National Health Service Corps: rural physician service and retention. *J Am Board Fam Pract.* 1997;10:272–279.

10. General Accounting Office. *Rural Health Clinics: Rising Program Expenditures Not Focused on Improving Care in Isolated Areas.* Washington, DC: General Accounting Office; 1996.

11. Balas EA, Jaffrey F, Kuperman GJ, et al. Electronic communication with patients: evaluation of distance medicine technology. *JAMA.* 1997;278:152–158.

12. Bashshur RL, Puskin D, Silva J. Telemedicine and the national information infrastructure. *Telemed J.* 1995;1:321–375.

# Abstracts from the Literature

## Supply and Distribution

## BOOKS AND REPORTS

American Medical Association Center for Health Policy Research, Kletke P, Marder WD, Silberger A. *The Demographics of Physician Supply: Trends and Projections.* Chicago: American Medical Association; 1987. This monograph sets out to achieve two goals. The first is to analyze trends in a number of areas that have influenced and will continue to influence the supply and career choices of future physicians. The second and more important goal, is to introduce the AMA Demographic Model of the Physician Population. This model makes it possible to project the size and composition of the physician population under a number of different policy scenarios.

Center for the Health Professions. *Considering the Future of Health Care Workforce Regulation.* San Francisco: Center for the Health Professions; 1997. Responses from the field to Pew Health Professions Commission's December 1995 report: *Reforming Health Care Workforce Regulation.*

Council on Graduate Medical Education. *Fourth Report: Recommendations to Improve Access to Health Care Through Physician Workforce Reform.* Rockville, Md: U.S. Department of Health and Human Services; 1994. This report addresses the mismatch between physician supply and health care requirements. COGME believes that the following physician workforce goals should be attained by 2000: first year residency positions limited to 10% more than the number of 1993 US medical school graduates; at least 50% of `residency graduates should enter practice as generalist physicians (family physician, general internist and general pediatrician); the number of underrepresented minority students should be doubled; and primary care shortage areas should be eliminated. If these goals were attained, there would be 25% fewer physicians produced annually, of whom at least half would be practicing generalists. This output is projected to produce a balanced generalist physician workforce in the year 2020 and a much smaller specialty surplus. The Council recommends that all third party payers explicitly pay for GME. A centerpiece of the COGME proposal is that funds and slots would be allocated through medical school coordinated consortia, functioning as "accountable education partnerships." Each consortium would collectively determine the specialty mix of residency positions based on local, state and regional health care needs under broad national guidelines which specify the number of residency positions and mandate that 50% of graduates be generalists.

Council on Graduate Medical Education. *Eighth Report: Patient Care, Physician Supply, and Requirements: Testing COGME Recommendations.* Rockville, Md: U.S. Department of Health and Human Services; 1996.

Council on Graduate Medical Education.*Tenth Report: Physician Distribution and Health Care Challenges in Rural and Inner-City Areas.* Rockville, Md: U.S. Department of Health and Human Services; 1998.

Council on Graduate Medical Education. *Eleventh Report: International Medical Graduates, the Physician Workforce, and GME Payment Reform.* Rockville, Md: U.S. Department of Health and Human Services; 1998.

Council on Graduate Medical Education. *Fourteenth Report: COGME Physician Workforce Policies: Recent Development and Remaining Challenges in Meeting National Goals.* Rockville, Md: U.S. Department of Health and Human Services; 1999.

General Accounting Office. *Progress and Problems in Improving the Availability of Primary Care Providers in Underserved Areas: Report to the Congress by the Comptroller General of the United States.* Washington, DC: General Accounting Office; 1978. In addition to examining trends in the geographic distribution of physicians that have recently established practice, this report considered the following topics: (1) factors newly established physicians considered important in selecting practice locations; (2) progress made by federal programs to improve the availability of physician services in underserved areas; and (3) projects which rely on physician extenders (Physician Assistants and Nurse Practitioners) for increasing the availability of health care services in underserved areas.

Graduate Medical Education National Advisory Committee. *Policy Analysis for Physician Manpower Planning.* Proceedings of a symposium held in conjunction with the Joint National Meeting of the Institute of Management Sciences and Operations

Research Society, San Francisco. Washington, DC: U.S. Department of Health, Education and Welfare; 1977.

Graduate Medical Education National Advisory Committee. *Supply and Distribution of Physicians and Physician Extenders.* Background paper. Washington, DC: U.S. Department of Health, Education and Welfare; 1977.

Graduate Medical Education National Advisory Committee, Jacoby I. *Physician Requirements Forecasting: Need-Based Versus Demand-Based Methodologies.* Washington, DC: U.S. Department of Health, Education and Welfare; 1978.

Graduate Medical Education National Advisory Committee, Pollitt A. *Social and Psychological Characteristics in Medical Specialty and Geographic Decisions.* Washington, DC: U.S. Department of Health, Education and Welfare; 1978.

Health Resources Administration. *Model for Estimating Physician Supply in 1990.* Washington, DC: Health Resources Administration, Office of Graduate Medical Education; 1981. This report describes a model for projecting supply of active physicians in the US and then applies the model to forecast the number of doctors, by specialty, in 1990.

Health Resources Administration. *The Current and Future Supply of Physicians and Physician Specialists.* Washington, DC: U.S. Department of Health and Human Services; 1980. The characteristics of current physician practice in the US are varied and often difficult to interpret, and the characteristics of future practice are subject to even more question. The Physician Supply Model described in this report represents the latest in the Division of Health Professions Analysis efforts to develop analytical information on physician resources to aid officials in policy decisions.

Institute of Medicine. *A Manpower Policy for Primary Health Care.* Washington, DC: National Academy Press; 1978.

Institute of Medicine. *Access to Health Care in America.* Millman M, ed. Washington, DC: National Academy Press; 1993.

Institute of Medicine. *The Nation's Physician Workforce: Options for Balancing Supply and Requirements.* Lohr KN, Vanselow NA, Detmer DE, eds. Washington, DC: National Academy Press; 1996.

Pew Health Professions Commission. *Shifting the Supply of Our Health Care Workforce: A Guide to Redirecting Federal Subsidy of Medical Education.* San Francisco: Center for the Health Professions; 1995.

Pew Health Professions Commission. *Reforming Health Care Workforce Regulation: Policy Considerations for the Twenty-First Century.* San Francisco: Center for the Health Professions; 1995.

# ARTICLES

Association of American Medical Colleges Generalist Physician Task Force. AAMC policy on the generalist physician. *Acad Med.* 1993;68:1–6.   In 1992, the Association of American Medical Colleges created the Generalist Physician Task Force to develop a policy statement for the AAMC and to recommend ways to help reverse the trend away from generalism. The task force strongly endorsed using private-sector initiatives exerted through consensus and voluntary cooperation, although recognizing the indispensable role of government in defining the magnitude of the need for generalist physicians, and in eliminating barriers to meet those needs. As a policy, the AAMC advocates an overall national goal that a majority of graduating medical students be committed to generalist careers (family medicine, general internal medicine, or general pediatrics) and that appropriate efforts be made by all schools so that this goal can be reached within the shortest possible time. To further this goal, the task force recommended strategies for the AAMC, schools of medicine, graduate medical education, and the practice environment.

Cohen JJ, Whitcomb ME. Are the recommendations of the AAMC's task force on the generalist physician still valid? *Acad Med.* 1997;72:13–16.   In 1992, the AAMC Taskforce called for at least half the graduates of US allopathic medical schools to enter practice as generalists and for medical schools to design their educational programs to promote affinity for generalism among their students. Since that time, research findings have suggested that the current size of the country's generalist physician workforce in relation to projected need may be adequate. In light of these observations, the authors ask if the Taskforce's major recommendations remains valid. In this article, they state their reasons for thinking that they do.

Colwill JM. Where have all the primary care applicants gone? *N Engl J Med.* 1992;326:387–393.   This article considers the shrinking pool of applicants for primary care training programs, discusses factors associated with these trends, and explores the role of medical schools in meeting future needs for primary care physicians. Using data from the Association of American Medical Colleges and the Medical Admission Test questionnaire, the author suggests that fewer than 20 percent of graduates are currently planning careers in primary care. He goes on to discuss factors associated with changing specialty preferences (such as income, payment of debt and quality of life) and the effect of the academic medical center on specialty preferences. The author concludes by saying that solutions to enhancing the selection of careers in primary care (including the dominance of sub-specialties) must lie in medical education, in patterns of remuneration, and in the practice environment. Government and other third parties also have a role to play through reimbursement reform, the reduction of bureaucracy, and support of primary care education.

Colwill JM, Perkoff GT, Blake RL Jr, Paden C, Beachler M. Modifying the culture of medical education: the first three years of the RWJ Generalist Physician Initiative.

*Acad Med.* 1997;72:745–753. The Generalist Physician Initiative created by the Robert Wood Johnson Foundation helped schools modify the culture in which medical education occurs so that they may increase their production of generalists. Fourteen grants for six years were made to 16 US medical schools in 1994. This article reports on the program at its half way mark. It describes the conceptual bases for the program, identifies common approaches to intervention chosen by the schools and explores issues facing the schools as they implement change.

Cooper RA. Seeking a balanced physician workforce for the 21st century. *JAMA.* 1994;272:680–687. This article presents a broad overview of the conditions and context of the physician workforce environment into the next century. The author questions the rationale for the "50% percent solution" which proposes that the proportion of medical graduates entering the primary care disciplines be increased from 20–25% to 50%, in order to achieve a better balance between primary care physicians and specialists. Noting that the primary care workforce has remained stable at 75 to 85 primary care physicians per 100,000 people, he proposes a less dramatic shift to a 33%-67% mix of primary care and specialists. Recognizing the impact of current proposals on specialty training programs, he identifies distribution deficiencies that are a system problem rather than a workforce problem, and acknowledges the future contribution of primary care by mid-level practitioners. He concludes by noting that achieving a balanced workforce will require a balancing of governmental intervention with initiatives undertaken by the profession, a balancing of regulation with the dynamic forces of the market, and a balancing of near term objectives with long-term goals.

Cooper RA. Perspectives on the physician workforce to the year 2020. *JAMA.* 1995;274:1534–1543. Physician supply and demand to 2020 is assessed from three perspectives: physician utilization in group- and staff-model health maintenance organizations, physician distribution, and the future supply of non-physician clinicians. The national norm for physician demand in 1993 was estimated to be 205 per 100,000 population. Although demand is projected to increase by 2020, supply will initially increase more rapidly, resulting in a surplus of 31,000 physicians (5% of patient care physicians) in the year 2000 and 62,000 physicians (8%) in the year 2010, after which the gap will narrow. Relative to the national norm, surpluses already exist in some states and shortages exist in others. In addition, the number of non-physician clinicians is projected to double by 2010, equaling 60% of the number of patient care physicians. The author concludes that in terms of physicians alone, there is no evidence of an impending surplus. The major determinant of overall surplus may be the extent to which patients seek services from non-physician clinicians.

Darley, W. Physicians for the future. *J Med Educ.* 1965;40:1086–1095. In 1959, the Surgeon General's Consultant Group on Medical Education carried out a study to determine the nation's future need for physicians, and to assess the expansion of educational programs and facilities necessary to satisfy this need. The Group recommended that in order to maintain the existing physician population ratio, an additional 3,600 medical graduates would be necessary, 4,000 taking into account the attrition rate between the time a class starts and graduation. The author reports that at mid-point in the 12-year span covered in the study, only 20% of the goal had been reached: only 750 new student places had been created. He suggests a thorough reappraisal of ways to increase the resources for the production of physician manpower in the US, including the following methods: federal aid for the construction and operation of undergraduate medical facilities; increasing the enrollment of existing schools; developing new schools; making medical schools integral parts of universities; and reducing the rate of attrition by allowing students in two-year programs to transfer to four-year schools, and fill existing vacancies in the third and fourth years. The author also discusses the influx of foreign-trained physicians, how they should be developed and used to their full potential; at the same time he cautions using them as a substitute for personnel developed and trained in the US.

Dwinnell B, Adams L. Why we are on the cusp of a generalist crisis. *Acad Med.* 2001;76:707–708.   The National Residency Matching Program ("the Match") in 2000 and 2001 showed that in 2001, 51% of graduates chose primary care fields, the same percentage as 2000. However, fewer graduates are choosing primary care careers. Compared with 2000 Match results, primary care medicine positions filled by US graduates in 2001 declined 16.7% and family medicine positions 17.3%. The authors note that these statistics are particularly disappointing in light of effort expended in the 1990s to foster generalist medicine. They attribute the trend to a number of factors: the economic boom in the 1990s offered unprecedented opportunities in high technology fields; continuing disparity of pay between generalists and specialists; student debt issues; and primary care physicians losing control of deciding what is right for their patients. Underlying the reasons given above for the decline in interest in primary care careers is a more fundamental one: Medicine is increasingly becoming a business, eroding the noble qualities that most physicians recognize as inherent and essential to the profession they chose. The authors note that there is an increased interest in subspecialty training and that it is imperative that medical schools and residency programs re-examine what they can do to make generalist careers more desirable. Otherwise, there will be a shortage of primary care physicians that will likely rival, if not surpass, what was encountered in the early 1990s.

Fryer GE, Green LA, Dovey SM, Phillips RI Jr. The United States relies on family physicians unlike any other specialty. *Am Fam Physician.* 2001;63:1669.   Designation of a county as a Primary Care Health Personnel Shortage Area (PCHPSA) depends on the ratio of physicians to people. This article finds that without family physicians an additional 1,332 of the United States' 3,082 rural counties would qualify under the designation. In contrast, if all internists, pediatricians and obstetricians-gynecologists in aggregate were withdrawn from the statistics an additional 176 counties would meet the criteria for designation. This demonstrates how much the United States relies on family physicians in rural areas.

Geyman JP. Training primary care physicians for the 21st century: alternative scenarios for competitive vs. generic approach. *JAMA*. 1986;255:2631–2635. The author reviews the ongoing problem of the shortage of primary care physicians in the US and examines the outcomes of recent initiatives that have attempted to address this issue. He summarizes future needs for primary care physicians and suggests three alternative scenarios for dealing with the problem: (1) a continuation of the open, unregulated system of primary care; (2) a competitive approach by the three primary care specialties whereby each specialty expands its market share at the expense of others; or (3) a generic approach whereby a system evolves for training generic primary care physicians capable of providing personal and comprehensive health care, regardless of age and setting. Advantages and disadvantages of each scenario are given and recommendations are made if options 2 or 3 are to be pursued.

Goodman DC, Fisher ES, Bubolz TA, et al. Benchmarking the U.S. physician workforce. *JAMA*. 1996;276:1811–1817. The objective of this study was to propose population-based benchmarking as an alternative to needs- or demand-based planning for estimating a reasonable sized, clinically active physician workforce for the United States and its regional healthcare markets. The physician workforce was compared with four benchmarks: the staffing within a large health maintenance organization (HMO); a hospital referral region dominated by managed care; a hospital referral region dominated by fee-for-service; and the proposed "balanced" physician supply (50%) generalists. The study found that the proportion of the US population residing in hospital referral regions with a higher per capital generalist workforce than the benchmark was 96% for the HMO benchmark, 60% for fee-for service; and 27% for managed care. The specialist workforce exceeded all three benchmarks for 74% of the population. The per capita workforce of generalists was not related to the proportion of generalists among regions. The authors conclude that population-based benchmarking offers practical advantages to needs- or demand-based planning.

Kindig DA. Policy priorities for rural physician supply. *Acad Med.* 1990;65:S15–S17. A number of efforts can be made in rural education initiatives in recruitment, socialization, curricular reform, and community technical assistance. Further work is needed in identifying strategies that are most appropriate and cost effective in different states and regions that may have different needs. Careful consideration should be given as to why such ideas have not moved forward in the past twenty years; the article suggests that without substantial reform of payment systems favoring rural and primary care, educational reform will have marginal effectiveness and remain at the demonstration stage.

Kindig DA. Counting generalist physicians. *JAMA*. 1994;271:1505–1507. The Council on General Medical Education has called for a 50:50 generalist to specialist mix. In order to consider the impact of various proposals to achieve a balance in the workforce, the author argues for an agreement on the definitional and analytic framework for counting physicians and generalists, so that valid comparisons across proposals can be made. The author discusses use of data, unit of analysis, and analytic issues. The author suggests the following standard working definition of generalist production: the number of active physicians, minus residents and fellows, in the self-designated primary specialties of general/family practice, internal medicine minus subspecialties, and pediatrics minus subspecialties entering practice in the first post residency/fellowship year.

Kindig DA, Libby DL. How will graduate medical education reform affect specialties and geographic areas? *JAMA.* 1994;272:37–42.  The objective of this study was to project specialty and geographic impacts of workforce reform proposals on the practice output of graduate medical education (GME). A demographic life-table model was designed to predict GME output (allopathic and osteopathic programs) using 1987 cohort data from the Association of American Medical Colleges Annual GME Census. The 1992 cohort was used as a baseline to compare the simulated impact of alternate specialty and regional policies. The study found that if GME input is reduced to 110% of US medical graduates with 55% entering practice as generalists, then the total number of first year positions will decline from 24,433 to 18,783, and the total number of residents in GME would decline from 103,858 to 80,699. Even with a 110% reduction on GME input, the overall physician to population ratio will continue to grow, albeit at a slower rate. The number of generalists leaving GME annually would increase by 742 (9%) and the number of specialists would decline by 6517 (44%). At the regional level, allocating GME positions by prorating to the current distribution, results in less change than would prorating positions to regional populations.

Kindig DA, Libby DL. Domestic production vs. international migration: options for the U.S. physician workforce. *JAMA.* 1996;276:978–982.  The objective of this study was to determine alternate combinations for reductions in US medical school graduates (USMGs), international medical graduate (IMG) immigration, and graduate medical education (GME) residencies, based on future physician-to-population ratio targets. A demographic projection model of the physician supply was constructed and calibrated to fit observed AMA Physician Masterfile data and current supply forecasts. The main outcome measures were the annual number of new physicians added to supply from domestic or international sources needed to reach future physician-to-population ratio targets. Results showed that because of the low rate of attrition from the physician supply, it takes up to 50 years for workforce policy to stabilize the physician-to-population ratio at a target level. All target numbers considered required immediate reductions in GME positions. These reductions must be followed be gradual annual increases to account for population growth. The size of USMG and IMG reductions are interrelated and depend on how many IMGs remain to practice in the US. Based on their projections, the authors conclude that reductions in future physician supply can come from either the UMSG or IMG component of physician production or both. This model allows the estimation of multiple combinations of both GME components.

Kindig DA, Ricketts TC. Determining adequacy of physicians and nurses for rural populations: background and strategy. *J Rural Health* 1991;7(4 Suppl):313–326. When considering the issue of the supply of health professionals in rural areas, planners have been more likely to accept as a given the organizational structures and practice forms that already exist in those areas and concentrate on training and placement programs as the best way to increase the number of health professionals. The authors suggest that both the structural formulations of the system and the training-related typologies do not directly link the needs of the communities to the number and mix of health care professionals, the two anchor points in the whole issue of professional maldistribution for rural America. The article outlines an approach that links the two in the construction of system guidelines to provide adequate care for rural people as well as introduces regional considerations into the process of developing a health professional supply-needs calculation for rural America.

Lannon CM, Oliver TK Jr, Guerin RO, Day SC, Tunnessen WW Jr. Internal medicine–pediatrics combined residency graduates: what are they doing now? Results of a survey. *Arch Pediatr Adolesc Med.* 1999;153:823–828. 1,005 graduates of internal medicine-pediatric residency programs, whose names came from the computer databases of the American Board of Pediatrics and the American Board of Internal Medicine, were surveyed to determine the career outcomes of graduates of these programs. 87.3% of these graduates were certified by the American Board of Internal Medicine; 91.3% by the American Board of Pediatrics, and 81.6% by both Boards. The principle activity of 70% of the graduates was direct patient care. Most graduates cared for patients of all ages. More than half noted that their principal clinical site is a community office practice. 85% managed patients who require hospitalization. 50% had a medical appointment. The study provides strong evidence that most meds/peds graduates are practicing generalists who care for adults and children.

Lundberg GD, Lamm RD. Solving our primary care crisis by retraining specialists to gain specific primary care competencies. *JAMA.* 1993;270:380–381. The authors address the issue of the decline in numbers of physicians graduating from US medical schools who are declaring generalist fields, which has gone down from 36% in the graduating class of 1982 to only 14% in 1992. They suggest four options for fixing the system: (1) increase the number of medical school graduates who enter generalist fields, (2) curtail the number of resident physicians in specialties and subspecialties and increase the number in primary care fields, (3) allow primary care to be provided by physicians currently in the field and let the remainder of care be given by non physicians such as nurse practitioners, physician's assistants, homeopaths, and chiropractors, (4) create a system of incentives and disincentives that encourages a huge shift of practicing specialists and subspecialists into primary care. The authors propose that primary care leaders review the Pew Health Professions Commission's suggestions and establish primary care competencies and that curriculum planners develop curricula for specialist and subspecialist phsycians. They support the idea that the national health service be made mandatory to encourage work at the community level.

Lurie JD, Goodman DC, Wennberg JE. Benchmarking the future generalist workforce. *Eff Clin Pract.* 2002;5:58–66.   The objective of this study was to predict the future supply of generalist physicians relative to future requirements. A model was developed that projects the supply of generalists into the future on the basis of the annual number of physicians entering and leaving the workforce based on the physician master-files of the American Medical Association and the American Osteopathic Association, the 1999 to 2000 AMA Annual Survey of Graduate Medical Education, and data provided by the Bureau of Health Professions. The study found that the supply of generalists is projected to grow from its current level of 69 per 100,000 population to nearly 88 per 100,000 population by the year 2025. Adjusting for the changing age-sex structure of the physician workforce decreases the "effective" supply to 85 generalists per 100,000 population. According to these calculations, by the year 2025, the effective supply of generalists will exceed the Council on Graduate Medical Education's upper estimate of generalist requirements (80 generalists per 100,000), resulting in an excess of about 18,000 full-time equivalent generalists

Moore, GT. The case of the disappearing generalist: does it need to be solved? *Milbank Q.* 1992;70:361–374.   In this article, the author explores the importance of the decline in the number and status of generalist physicians from three different perspectives: the generalist, the specialist, and the market. He concludes, after considering the arguments, that each perspective is inconclusive and unlikely to provide a solid foundation for policy choice. He suggests that one solution to halting the decline of the generalist physician may be to use the power of the market to create and promote a better product. Generalist physicians must perform impeccably and should also identify new supplementary functions that build upon their traditional role. For example, generalists might provide highly technical home care services to meet the special needs of the elderly and homebound.

Moscovice IS, Rosenblatt RA. Rural health care delivery amid federal retrenchment: lessons from The Robert Wood Johnson Foundation's Rural Practice Project. *Am J Public Health.* 1982;72:1380–1385.   This paper examines the experience of the Robert Wood Johnson Foundation's Rural Practice Project (RPP), a major non-governmental effort in the last decade concentrating on the direct delivery of rural health services. After four years of operation, all nine RPP sites had completed their period of grant support; the practices survived in all cases with almost all retaining community sponsorship, salaried physicians and a commitment to comprehensive care. Practices in sparsely populated areas grew more slowly than those set in rural areas with a higher population density and more ancillary resources. The authors concluded that the use of time-limited subsidies is an effective way to start new rural practices in undeserved areas, and that those practices have a good chance of surviving their start-up phase.

Petersdorf RG. The doctors dilemma. *N Engl J Med.* 1978;299:628–663.   Studies show that there is a surplus of specialists and not enough primary care physicians, as well as a shortage of doctors in the inner cities and rural areas. The specialty of family medicine, which grew rapidly during the 1970s, has probably plateaued. Thus, a major onus for redressing physician manpower imbalance rests on the specialty of internal medicine. The author considers the issue from the perspectives of the medical student, the house officer, the subspecialty program director, the departmental chairman, the teaching hospital, the American Board of Internal Medicine, the accrediting agencies and the private sector, and the government. He concludes with a number of recommendations including, at the academic level, maintaining the ratio of generalist to subspecialist trainees constant at a ratio of 2:1, while cutting the number of specialty trainees in half; and at the government level, instituting a service requirement to assure an adequate number of physicians in underserved areas.

Politzer RM, Hardwick KS, Cultice JM, Bazell C. Eliminating primary care Health Professional Shortage Areas: the impact of Title VII on generalist physician education. *J Rural Health.* 1999;15:11–20.   This study estimates the impact that Title VII support for generalist training has on reducing and eliminating health professional shortage areas (HPSAs) under multiple scenarios, that either vary the Title VII funding level or the percentage of Title VII-funded program graduates who practice in medically underserved areas (MUAs). For each scenario, the number of Title VII-funded graduates who initially practice in MUAs, and the time it would take to eliminate HPSAs are estimated. Using 1996 rates, the analysis predicts that 1,214 generalist physicians will enter practice in HPSAs annually, leading to the elimination of HPSAs in 25 years. Doubling the funding for these programs would increase the number of generalist physicians entering MUAs and eliminate the HPSAs in as little as 6 years. The study concludes that eliminating HPSAs requires broader Title VII influence and continuous improvement in rates of production of graduates who practice in MUAs. Without this improvement of the Title VII program, the number of Americans with reduced access to essential health care will continue to grow.

Rabinowitz HK, Diamond JJ, Veloski JJ, Gayle JA. The impact of multiple predictors on generalist physicians' care of underserved populations. *Am J Public Health.* 2000;90:1225–1228.   This study examined the relative and incremental importance of multiple predictors of generalist physicians' care of underserved populations. Survey results from a 1993 national random sample of 2,955 allopathic and osteopathic generalist physicians who graduated medical school in 1983 and 1984 were analyzed. The results showed four independent predictors of providing care to underserved populations: (1) being a member of an underserved ethnic/minority group; (2) having participated in the National Health Service Corps; (3) having a strong interest in practicing in an underserved area prior to attending medical school; and (4) growing up in an underserved area. Eighty-six percent of physicians with all 4 predictors were providing substantial care to underserved populations, compared with 65% with 3 predictors, 49% with 2 predictors, 34% with 1 predictor, and 22% with no predictors.

Rivo ML, Henderson TM, Jackson DM. State legislative strategies to improve the supply and distribution of generalist physicians, 1985–1992. *Am J Public Health.* 1995;85:405–407. State laws enacted between 1985 and 1992 were reviewed to examine state involvement in influencing the supply and distribution of generalist physicians. 47 states enacted 248 relevant laws during this period. In 1991 and 1992, 36 states enacted 98 laws, as compared with 1985 and 1986, when 8 states enacted 12 laws. Legislation addressed planning and oversight; financial incentives to institutions, students and residents; and strategies to enhance the practice environment. A new strategy is to link funding to measurable outcomes, such as the career choices of a state medical school's graduates. Few states devoted resources to evaluate their efforts.

Rivo ML, Kindig DA. A report card on a physician work force in the United States. *N Engl J Med.* 1996;334:892–896. The authors present a report card on the physician workforce in the United States. The report card looks at the supply of physicians, the mix of generalist and specialists, the geographic distribution and physicians' skills. The article suggests that the United States now has a moderate need for more generalists and a substantial surplus of specialists. It recommends that goals be set for the representation of minority groups in order to address the health needs of minorities and that less graduate medical training be done in hospitals and more in community, primary care and managed care settings.

Rivo ML, Satcher D. Improving access to health care through physician workforce reform: directions for the 21st century. *JAMA.* 1993;270:1074–1078. This article summarizes the findings, goals and recommendations contained in the Third Report of the Council on Graduate Medical Education (COGME) to Congress and the Health and Humn Services Secretary, October 1992. The COGME limited its review to general and family practice, general internal medicine, general pediatrics, general surgery, adult and child psychiatry, obstetrics-gynecology, preventive medicine, and geriatrics, partly based on considerations of primary care orientation, specialty size and supply-requirement imbalances. The report lists seven deficiencies in the physician workforce, medical education system and public policy that hinder strategies to provide affordable health care to all US citizens. The Council recommends the establishment of a national physician workforce plan and financing strategy to address the nation's future physician needs. In addition, specific recommendations are made for medical educators.

Rosenblatt RA. The potential of the academic medical center to shape policy-oriented rural health research. *Acad Med.* 1991;66:662–667. Rural communities continue to have problems in gaining access to basic health care services, a problem exacerbated by persistent shortages of physicians, financially threatened rural hospitals and weak local economies. The author suggests that academic health centers can help to address these issues, not only by increasing the flow of graduates to rural areas, but also by supporting health services research designed to shape public policy that affects rural United States. Such research includes experiments designed to influence locational decisions of medical students and residents, studies of the quality and cost-effectiveness of care in rural hospitals, and the testing of new ways to provide emergency medical care in rural areas.

Rosenblatt, RA, Whitcomb ME, Cullen TJ, Lishner DM, Hart LG. Which medical schools produce rural physicians? *JAMA*. 1992;268:1559–1565.   The objective of this study was to examine the hypothesis that medical schools vary systematically and predictably in the proportion of their graduates who enter rural practice. The December 1991 version of the American Medical Association Physician Masterfile was used to examine the rural and urban practice locations of physicians who graduated from American medical schools between 1976 and 1985. The study found that 12.6% of the practicing graduates were located in rural counties; family physicians were more likely than members of other specialties to select rural practice, particularly in the smallest and most isolated counties. Women were more likely than men to enter rural practice. Medical schools varied greatly in the percentage of graduates who entered rural practice, ranging from 41.2% to 2.3% of the classes studied. Four variables were strongly associated with a tendency of a medical school to produce rural graduates: location in a rural state; public ownership; production of family physicians; and smaller amounts of funding from the National Institute of Health. The authors conclude that increasing policy coordination among medical schools and state and federal government entities would most effectively address residual problems of rural physician shortages.

Rosenblatt RA, Whitcomb ME, Cullen TJ, et al. The effect of federal grants on medical schools' production of primary care physicians. *Am J Public Health*. 1993;83:322–328.   This study explores recent trends in the proportion of US medical school graduates entering primary care, in relationship to Title VII of the Health Professions Educational Assistance Act of 1976 funding. The American Medical Association Physician Masterfile was used to determine the specialty of all students graduating from American medical schools between 1960 and 85. Results showed that the proportion of graduates entering primary care rose from 19.7% in 1967 to 31.1% in 1976 and remained stable for the subsequent decade. The increase occurred before implementation of Title VII. Rural, state-owned medical schools tended to produce a greater proportion of primary care physicians than urban private schools without family medicine departments. The authors conclude that the values of American medical schools and the reward structure of medical practice favor specialists over primary care physicians. Although Title VII has helped to encourage and sustain the development of educational programs related to primary care, an increase in the proportion of primary care physicians requires fundamental changes.

Schroeder SA. Western European responses to physician oversupply. *JAMA*. 1984;252:373–384.   The supply and specialty distribution of physicians in Belgium, West Germany, the Netherlands, and the United Kingdom were compared with those in the United States. The numbers of physicians per 10,000 population in 1980 was 24 (Belgium), 22.9 (West Germany), 19.1 (United States), 19 (The Netherlands), and 16.2 (United Kingdom). Projections for 1990 were 34 (Belgium),

32.6 (West Germany), 24.3 (United States), and 17.1 (United Kingdom). The United States and the United Kingdom produce about half as many physicians per population but have a much higher proportion (26%) of foreign physicians. The US has a much higher rate of specialists to generalists. Official recognition of oversupply exists in Belgium, which is restricting specialty training, and the Netherlands, which is reducing both medical school intake and specialty training, but not yet in West Germany. The European experience suggests that the United States' most pressing health manpower problem is oversupply of specialists.

Schroeder SA. The making of a medical generalist. *Health Aff.* 1985;4(2):22–46.   The author makes the case for increasing the number of generalist physicians in relationship to the number of specialty physicians. He states that there are four basic reasons why decreasing the relative supply of specialists makes sense: to increase the quality of care; to decrease the costs of care; to increase patient satisfaction; and to increase physician satisfaction. He reviews the factors involved in producing generalist physicians, including uncertainty over the definition of a generalist, the multiplicity of providers who function as generalists, various factors that might stimulate production of generalists, and areas where philanthropic foundations and federal and state governments might exert influence.

Schroeder SA, Mitchell T. Employment choices in conditions of physician oversupply. *J Gen Intern Med.* 1988;3:25–31.   The authors surveyed 297 internists who had completed their residency or fellowship training at six San Francisco institutions from 1979 through 1984, to assess how the recently expanded supply of physicians has affected the intensity of their practice and their decisions about location. The vast majority of internists (93%) settled in metropolitan areas, with 56% staying in the Bay Area, despite that region's high concentration of physicians. Although subspecialists earned more income than generalists, this was because they worked longer hours. Those who graduated later were significantly less likely to be in private practice in 1985, mainly because they selected salaried institutional work more often than earlier graduates. Women worked 85% of men's work week and subspecialized significantly less often. The results suggest that internists will continue to settle in "over doctored" areas.

Schwartz WB, Newhouse JP, Bennett BW, Williams AP. The changing geographic distribution of board certified physicians. *N Engl J Med.* 1980;303:1032–1038.   The authors studied the distribution of board-certified specialists among cities and towns of different sizes. Between 1960 and 1977, diplomates of the eight specialty boards appeared for the first time in many small non-metropolitan towns. The percentage increase in numbers of specialists in small towns exceeded that in cities, but the absolute increase was greatest in metropolitan areas. The authors conclude that the increased supply of specialists activated market forces that caused the change in distribution. In addition, a preference for small-town living may have been a contributing factor.

Shelov SP, Alpert JJ, Rayman I, et al. Federally supported primary care training programs and pediatric careers. *Am J Dis Child.* 1987;141:65–66.   The purpose of this article is to report the results of a survey of the federally supported pediatric programs to determine whether or not pediatrics has achieved results similar to family practice and internal medicine in producing primary care practitioners. Federally funded residency programs were mailed a questionnaire. Forty-two of the 53 programs responded. Career information was available on 599 graduates. 449 graduates (75%) were reported to be in practice while the remaining 150 (25%) had pursued training, largely in fellowship positions. Of the graduates in practice, 434 (97%) were reported to be practicing pediatrics, and only 15 (3%) were in subspecialty pediatrics. The majority practiced in large or medium-sized cities. 42% were reported to be practicing general pediatrics in economically deprived areas. The results of the descriptive survey indicated that pediatricians participating in federally funded programs were pursuing primary care careers.

Sox HC Jr. Supply, demand, and the workforce of internal medicine. *Am J Med.* 2001;110:745–749.   The purpose of this article is to understand the determinants of the internal medicine workforce (general internists, family physicians, internal medicine, sub-specialists, nurse practitioners and physician assistants) well enough to predict its future direction. The author suggests that for each group to be successful, there must be a reasonable balance between the supply of practitioners and demand for their services. He observes that the most important workforce trend is the growth of the non-physician clinician. Graduates of physician assistant training programs numbered 1,360 in 1992; 3,400 will graduate in 2001. Newly graduated nurse practitioners numbered 1,500 in 1992; 7,250 will graduate in 2001. By comparison medical school graduates numbered 15,548 in 1992 and 15,824 in 2000. General internists also feel pressure from subspecialists who claim to provide better care for patients with medical problems that fall within their domain of expertise. The author concludes that internal medicine subspecialties are likely to remain an attractive career choice because the supply of subspecialists is relatively stable and appears to be in balance with demand. Although general internists have some cause for concern relating to a potential decline in demand for their services, several trends provide important opportunities for them including the role of the hospitalist, caring for patients with progressive serious illness, and caring for older patients.

Weiner JP. Forecasting the effects of health reform on U.S. physician workforce requirement: evidence from HMO staffing patterns. *JAMA.* 1994;272:222–230. This article provides an estimate of the effects of health reform on the US physician workforce requirement. Its basic methodology is to extrapolate current patterns of staffing within managed care plans to the reshaped health care system of the year 2000. In this analysis, it is assumed that 40% to 65% of Americans will be receiving care from the integrated managed care networks in the near future, and that all citizens will be covered by some type of health insurance. On the basis of these assumptions, this article forecasts that in the year 2000, (1) there will be an overall surplus of about 165,000 patient care physicians; (2) the requirement and supply of primary care physicians will be in relative balance; and (3) the supply of specialists will outstrip the requirement by more than 60%. In conclusion, it appears that national health reform will have a significant impact on the US physician workforce requirement and that the evidence presented in this article suggests that the issue is not so much a primary care provider shortage as a specialty surplus.

Williams AP, Schwartz WB, Newhouse JP, Bennett BW. How many miles to the doctor? *N Engl J Med.* 1983;309:958–963.   The objective of this study was to determine the distance that residents of outlying areas (or of towns less than 25,000 population, outside metropolitan areas) have to travel to receive various types of medical care. For both 1970 and 1979 the study found that approximately 80% of residents lived within ten miles driving distance of a physician and 98% lived within 25 miles. Most of the remaining 2% lived in places so sparsely populated that physicians would not find these areas economically attractive as practice locations. During the 1970s, the distance of members of the studied population from medical and surgical specialists was substantially reduced. The greatest improvement occurred for the specialties that had the largest increase in numbers. The authors conclude that as the physician pool expands further during the 1980s, geographic access to specialty care should show a further improvement. However, this improvement may not suffice to fulfill the medical needs of the economically deprived or the geographically isolated.

# CHAPTER TWENTY-ONE

# Practice Sights

## State Primary Care Development Strategies

Irene M. Wielawski
2003

David Adams is a recent recruit to the health care system of Fairbury, Nebraska, population four thousand. An M.D., he works with four other family practitioners at the Fairbury Clinic, which is the source of primary care for most of Jefferson County—a large, rectangular chunk of farmland on the Nebraska-Kansas border. People travel an hour or more in all kinds of weather to get to the clinic, but they rarely complain of inconvenience. You don't have to go back many generations in rural America to hear firsthand what it was like when there was no doctor.

The inconveniences, moreover, are not borne entirely by patients. Adams and his colleagues must deliver twenty-first-century medicine in a setting that lacks the backup specialists and high-tech equipment they took for granted in training. The nearest specialists are in Beatrice, about fifty minutes from Fairbury. Lincoln, the state capital, where Adams trained, is more than a two-hour drive, and Omaha is three.

"We have to be able to do just about everything—the sore throat, the heart attack, the car wreck," says Adams, who happens to relish the challenge. Rural practitioners also speak of personal rewards that come through knowing their patients as fellow members of a community rather than as strangers passing through a busy urban practice.

Yet Adams and his sort are a scarce commodity. Only 2.6 percent of medical school graduates choose practice in a small town or rural area, according to the Association of American Medical Colleges. Over the years, this has resulted in

---

This chapter originally appeared as Wielawski, IM. Practice sights: state primary care development strategies. *To Improve Health and Health Care: The Robert Wood Johnson Foundation Anthology, Vol. VI* (Chap. 3), San Francisco: Jossey-Bass, 2002. Copyright © 2002, The Robert Wood Johnson Foundation. Reprinted with permission.

a lopsided scenario in which fifty-one million rural Americans—roughly 20 percent of the nation's population—are being cared for by less than 10 percent of the nation's practicing physicians. Poor inner-city neighborhoods are similarly underserved because of a scarcity of health care providers.

This is not a new problem. The provider imbalance has worried academicians, government leaders, and health policy experts for more than thirty years. Periodically, efforts are launched to correct it, but there has been little measurable long-term improvement. Between 1980 and 1990, the number of federally designated Health Professional Shortage Areas, or HPSA, remained constant, at 1,956. The number of HPSAs steadily rose through the 1990s, despite an overall increase in the U.S. physician supply. By 2002, they totaled 3,168, of which 2,209 (70 percent) were in "nonmetropolitan" areas, as designated by the U.S. Health Resources and Services Administration. To eliminate these rural shortages would require successful recruitment and retention of 3,327 additional primary care physicians.[1]

There are several reasons for the continuing shortage. Income potential for a physician is lower in an underserved area, and many physicians today emerge from training with significant debt. Long hours, professional isolation, and lifestyle preferences are also cited as factors. Beyond these, however, rural health experts point to the absence of a national plan to improve the geographic distribution of health care providers. Efforts to date have been largely piecemeal, with little coordination among government and private sector initiatives.

Perhaps the best known of these initiatives is the National Health Service Corps, made up of physicians who agree to be posted to underserved areas of the United States in exchange for repayment of medical education loans. The Corps has been an excellent source of physicians for localities that would have had a hard time recruiting on their own. Unfortunately, Corps physicians tend to leave when their contracts are up, sending these communities scurrying once again for what is still the most essential component of any health care system: a doctor.

Historically, states have not, until recently, paid much attention to their medically underserved areas, often considering them a federal responsibility, similar to the provision of health insurance (Medicaid and Medicare), welfare, or housing support for the very poor. Some states have experimented with home-grown solutions, such as loan repayment and locum tenens (substitute doctor) programs, to ease the economic and workload burden on providers. The majority, however, simply clamored for more National Health Service Corps doctors, more federally funded clinics for poor and uninsured patients, more federal response in general.

Finger-pointing at the feds may be convenient for governors, but it didn't sit well with state public health professionals. Just as poverty and a lack of insurance have measurable consequences for the health of individuals, so does a medically underserved area have consequences for population health. Population health is the means by which public health professionals measure their own performance. As the provider shortages persisted, it became apparent that medically underserved areas were dragging down population health statistics. People in these communities are sicker than residents of communities with sufficient doctors and health centers.[2] They also tend to have a lower immunization rate, higher infant mortality, and other measurable deficits. Smart program design, compelling health promotion campaigns, determined outreach workers—all fail without health care providers to deliver the goods.

It was against this backdrop that The Robert Wood Johnson Foundation decided to offer a challenge to states to come up with more comprehensive approaches to recruitment and retention of rural and inner-city health care providers. The $16.5 million program was called Practice Sights: State Primary Care Development Strategies. Its overriding goal was to improve access to primary health care by increasing the number of providers in underserved areas. Physicians were only one type of provider envisioned by those designing Practice Sights. The program also sought to introduce physicians' assistants, nurse practitioners, and nurse midwives into underserved communities, and to improve the regulatory climate in states that restricted these mid-level practitioners from fully using their skills.

Success in landing recruits is only half the task; the other half is, How do you get them to stay? The Foundation had more ambitious goals than to merely duplicate underserved communities' experience with the National Health Service Corps. To this end, Practice Sights challenged states to come up with ways to make medical practice in these communities economically viable and to ameliorate the conditions that lead health care providers to leave, among them professional isolation and excessive workload.

Practice Sights was authorized by the Foundation in the fall of 1991 and ran through 1998. A National Program Office, or NPO, was established at the North Carolina Foundation for Alternative Health, under the direction of James D. Bernstein. Practice Sights clearly struck a chord with state health officials eager to emancipate themselves from dependence on disparate federal programs: forty-four of the fifty states responded to the NPO's request for proposals. Of these, fifteen were successful in winning Practice Sights planning grants of up to $100,000.

The planning grant was to be used to lay the groundwork for effective recruiting and retention of physicians and midlevel practitioners. Planning activities included assembling interagency working groups; building liaison between state entities and underserved communities; developing statewide information systems to track vacancies and advertise for candidates; and removing licensing or other barriers to effective use of physician assistants, nurse practitioners, and other non-M.D. primary care providers.

Practice Sights moved into its second phase, implementation, in the summer of 1994. The Foundation authorized a new round of grants averaging $800,000 that states could use over three years to carry out ideas honed in the planning phase. Of the fifteen states that received planning grants, ten were successful in winning implementation grants: Idaho, Kentucky, Minnesota, Nebraska, New Hampshire, New Mexico, New York, Pennsylvania, South Dakota, and Virginia. These states mostly focused on underserved rural areas, even though Practice Sights originally aimed at addressing human resource shortages in both rural and inner-city settings. As a result, the collective Practice Sights effort emphasized rural issues.

# PROGRAM OVERVIEW

Practice Sights swam against the economic and cultural tide of American medicine and long-established trends among medical school graduates to head for metropolitan practices, where pay and prestige are greatest. The program set three goals for grantees:

- To increase the number of primary care providers in underserved areas
- To improve reimbursement levels and working conditions in underserved areas so they have a better chance of attracting and keeping providers
- To increase the state's capacity to support primary care systems

For a single site to achieve even one of these goals in the relatively short run of the program would have been impressive. To make headway during the particular years of Practice Sights is nothing short of amazing, for there has probably been no period of greater upheaval in the history of the American health care system.

Practice Sights' debut coincided with widespread public and political concern about the plight of the medically uninsured and the unreliability of the private insurance system. Passage of some type of national health reform was considered imminent. The universal health coverage included in most proposals before Congress was especially important in the context of Practice Sights, since medically underserved areas have a relatively high proportion of uninsured or inadequately insured patients. If federal reform gave these patients a means to pay for medical treatment, health systems and providers in underserved areas would benefit as well. This could only enhance the prospects for successful recruiting and retention. No one designing Practice Sights in the early 1990s or applying for one of its grants could have anticipated the failure of President Bill Clinton's Health Security Plan in 1994, and the domino effect on all other reform proposals. The timing was particularly onerous; congressional leaders declared health reform dead only a month after Practice Sights' most adventuresome states entered the high-risk implementation phase.

There followed a dizzying period of health care system reorganization and consolidation, in anticipation of a managed care juggernaut. Rural health systems were caught up in the general frenzy. New Hampshire, for one, saw its rural hospitals scrambling to buy out physician practices, or to affiliate with neighboring hospitals. These local health systems believed their best defense against the shrewd deal making of gigantic multistate managed care companies was to array patients and other assets into a unified front. The feared alternative was to be picked off one by one and lowballed on reimbursement rates. These turned out to be costly strategies, fueled by fear. By the late 1990s, it was clear that managed care companies had little interest in rural markets. But Practice Sights was already well along by then.

"There were pluses and minuses to that period," says Jonathan Stewart, director of the Community Health Institute in Concord, New Hampshire, a collaborator on that state's Practice Sights project. Pluses included an unusual receptivity to new ideas among normally tradition-bound rural physicians and hospitals. On the other hand, with day-to-day survival a foremost concern, it was difficult to get people focused on long-term systemic improvements.

Another wild card in Practice Sights was the character of rural medicine in each of the participating states. It is a running joke among rural providers that the only people who can comfortably generalize about their working conditions are researchers studying them from the climate-controlled comfort of an urban think tank. That said, rural providers themselves tend to generalize from their own experience, which may not be the norm for others. The Practice Sights states exemplified this variation in functional definitions of rural and medically needy. New Hampshire, for example, has a hospital every thirty miles or so in its underserved North Country. Providers and patients in larger states such as South Dakota and Nebraska would consider this pure luxury (that is, until they tried driving New Hampshire's twisty North Country roads in January). As for the needs of Virginia's rural communities, well, it depends upon which part of the state you're talking about. Says Deborah D. Oswalt, executive director of the Virginia Health Care Foundation and a Practice Sights collaborator:

> Our southwest tail—that's Appalachia—has such difficult terrain that it can take you an hour to go ten miles, especially if you get behind a coal truck. We've got Southside Virginia, which is a very different place with very different people. It is still very agricultural. More than a third of the population over age twenty-five in Southside has not completed high school. There is still housing in some places with dirt floors and no indoor plumbing. Then we have the Northern Neck, which is in eastern Virginia near Chesapeake Bay. We have a lot of watermen there who make their living by fishing and crabbing and oystering, and

their health issues and travel issues are very different from those of the mountain and Southside people. You simply cannot generalize about rural health needs, not even in a single state.

Practice Sights had a final twist. In addition to traditional grant funding, the Foundation offered participating states a highly atypical business deal. Essentially, the Foundation took on the role of a bank, sending seed money to grantees so that they in turn could create a loan fund to give rural providers access to low-interest capital. The Foundation loans—called Program-Related Investments, or PRIs—ranged from $700,000 to $1.5 million.[3] Payback with interest was required within ten years. Only four of the ten Practice Sights grantees took the PRI option, and it proved to be a rocky experiment for all concerned, with mixed results.

# A SHOWCASE OF LESSONS FROM THREE STATES

The lessons of Practice Sights found their best showcases in three states: New Hampshire, Nebraska, and Virginia. These states exemplify the rural diversity that characterized the program, and their experiences underscore the importance of local fine-tuning if a national workforce strategy ever materializes. These states also emerged as unusually illustrative of how the Practice Sights program played out. New Hampshire used Practice Sights to build a strong statewide provider recruitment system, but it did not develop a loan program and had limited success in other areas of the project, such as improved working conditions. Nebraska's greatest accomplishments came in organizing balkanized rural providers into mutually supportive hospital and physician networks, thereby reducing professional isolation and improving economic stability. But its PRI loan program was a colossal failure. Virginia made little progress in moving recruiting to the state level; the rural physician workforce continues to be replenished through direct recruiting by local practices. However, the Virginia project took a $700,000 seed loan from the Foundation and leveraged it into a successful revolving fund that to date has issued nearly $6 million in low-interest financing for health-related investments in underserved communities.

## Recruiting

Why would your average debt-laden medical school graduate choose to work in a setting with limited income potential, long hours, and gravely compromised social options? This was the challenge to Practice Sights leaders. In New Hampshire, the sales job belongs to Stephanie Pagliuca.

Pagliuca is program manager of the New Hampshire Recruitment Center. Located in Concord, the state capital, the Recruitment Center is a not-for-profit enterprise created through Practice Sights. Its track record is impressive. By the end of 2001, the state had filled just about every vacancy in its medically under-served areas, including the North Country, a sparsely populated region that bor-ders Canada. Overall, since the inception of Practice Sights, a total of 131 physicians and nurse practitioners have been successfully recruited in New Hampshire. Twenty-six percent of those recruited went to HPSAs, a federal des-ignation for regions where the ratio of patients to physicians is greater than 3,500:1. Twenty-nine percent went to Medically Underserved Areas, so-called because population and health demographics—including age, poverty, and a high rate of low-birth-weight babies—show a need for more doctors. The remaining 45 percent went to practices elsewhere in the state.

The Recruitment Center was part of a broad Practice Sights-fueled effort to address a patchwork health care infrastructure in New Hampshire, especially in its North Country. Population and the lion's share of health care professionals and facilities were concentrated in the southern half of the state. Public health workers were scattered and poorly coordinated. The state used the umbrella of Practice Sights to join forces with local community health care organizations. Besides the Recruitment Center, New Hampshire's Practice Sights leaders created the Community Health Institute, which provided consulting services to medically needy communities, administered a state loan repayment fund to enhance recruiting of health care providers with sizeable school debt, and developed pre-ceptor programs with local colleges and universities, through which medical and nursing students were placed in underserved areas. The Institute, in collabora-tion with the state health department, gained new federal support for New Hampshire by qualifying communities for community health center grants.

The standout legacy of Practice Sights in New Hampshire, however, is the Recruitment Center. Initially supported by Practice Sights grant money and state contributions, the Recruitment Center today is largely self-sustaining. It oper-ates on a fee-for-service basis, charging hospitals, clinics, and physician prac-tices about half what they would pay for commercial recruiting assistance.

Ironically, one of New Hampshire's strongest assets is the relative weakness of what Practice Sights architects thought would be the program's anchor: state health departments. New Hampshire's history is one of decentralized govern-ment; its state agencies are bare-bones, and the electorate consistently votes against anything that would expand the power of state government over local community rule.

"The basic social and decision-making unit in New Hampshire is the town—the community," says James W. Squires, a surgeon and former state senator. He currently heads the Endowment for Health, a foundation working to improve health care access in New Hampshire. "It is not the county; it is not a hospital catchment area; it is not a demographic unit; and it is certainly not state gov-ernment. Every town has its own police force; every one has its own ambulance, fire department, and education system."

A single town is not the ideal unit for advancing statewide improvements in health systems or workforce, but state officials in New Hampshire are used to modest stature and are adept at getting around the handicap.

"We know right off that we will never have the expertise in state government to guide each community to fulfill its health care needs," says John Bonds, a state health services planner and a Practice Sights project director. "So we are very good at creating community and statewide coalitions to help formulate and carry out programs. Everything is done under contract to existing community-based agencies: visiting nurses, home health care agencies, and the rest."

As a result, Practice Sights in New Hampshire spent almost no time bottled up in health department bureaucracy; instead it immediately began to work with mostly private sector coalitions with established credibility in the health care community. (By contrast, Nebraska's project lacked staff for more than two years because of a statewide hiring freeze that barred health officials from filling the grant-funded position.) Bonds, Pagliuca, and other Practice Sights leaders were able to turn to these community-based coalitions for ideas and practical assistance in implementing the goals of Practice Sights.

For example, at the outset of the 1990s, New Hampshire had only one federally funded community health center, even though numerous localities met the criteria to qualify for federal assistance. What they lacked was the leadership necessary to mount a successful application. This was the genesis of the New Hampshire Practice Sights' consulting arm, the Community Health Institute. State and private sector health leaders saw an opportunity to mobilize communities under the aegis of Practice Sights, since new health centers with funded staff positions for underserved communities would be consistent with the program's goals. The applications were carefully timed to prevent one New Hampshire community from knocking another out of contention. The collaborative approach resulted in nine new health centers—a significant accomplishment for a small state in a competitive federal program.

In building the recruitment center's capacity, Pagliuca and her colleagues took a similarly collaborative approach. She recalls:

> We started out simply responding to requests for candidates to fill vacancies. We did some educating of practices to think about using nurse practitioners, because the University of New Hampshire had an emerging training program. Then we started to link up with other organizations in New Hampshire that were getting similar calls: the medical society, the hospital association. Then we got the nurse practitioner and physician assistant societies joining. Then we linked up to our state loan repayment program, and strengthened our relationship with the National Health Service Corps. That gave us a more comprehensive package to offer candidates.
>
> We also helped create marketing materials for the practices, advertisements for publications read by physicians such as the *New England Journal of Medicine,* the *Family Physician Recruiter* newsletter, *OBG Management,* and so on.

Gavin Muir was one of the recruiting successes. Muir graduated from Temple University's medical school in 1995 and trained in family practice in a Pueblo, Colorado, residency program strongly oriented to rural practice. He began talking to Pagliuca about job possibilities in August 1997, which was eleven months before he completed training.

"I had some very specific requirements and after that I was flexible," Muir says. "Number one, I wanted to work some place where I could practice obstetrics because I put so much blood, sweat, and tears into the advanced obstetrics program in Pueblo. Number two, I wanted some place that would help me with my loans. I had $160,000 in medical school debt. Number three, my wife and I wanted to be reasonably close to our families—she's from Buffalo. Number four, I wanted a decent quality of life."

All of these criteria were met by the Manchester Community Health Center, where Muir is currently medical director. The health center is one of New Hampshire's new ones, located in a rare pocket of urban need. A manufacturing city of about one hundred thousand residents, Manchester is home to a large immigrant community, with a recent influx of Bosnian and Sudanese refugees. Muir is delighted with his job for professional, practical, and personal reasons.

"I work a four-day week," he says, which enables him to spend time with his wife and four-year-old daughter. "I'm in the fourth year of federal loan repayment because I work in a federally designated underserved area. This means $120,000 in loans paid off so far by the feds. I love what I am doing; I enjoy living where I am. All my friends who did National Health Service Corps got out as soon as they could because their spouses were ready to kill them. But this is a place where people would love to live. An hour from the beach, an hour from the mountains, a couple of hours from Boston."

Pagliuca acknowledges recruiting advantages for New Hampshire in the state's natural beauty and its relative proximity to a major city like Boston. The Recruiting Center's Web site emphasizes these attributes on each informational screen, with luscious photographs of lakes, mountains, and majestic forests. Of course, the appeal is not universal.

Pagliuca recalls a deluge of job seekers from 1996 to 1997, all foreign-born and looking to bypass immigration requirements that they return to their own country after training. A loophole was the J-1 visa program, which exempted foreign physicians working in medically underserved areas of the United States. Pagliuca's experience with one of these physicians illustrates another recruiting responsibility: screening out an unqualified applicant or, simply, a poor fit. As she recalls:

Many of them I could barely understand over the phone, their English was so poor. How could they practice in our rural areas? We were recruiting for retention, and the lack of cultural outlets for these physicians really didn't make it realistic. There were no appropriate places of worship, no ethnic food stores, that sort of thing.

I had one physician from a Middle Eastern country who was interested in a position in our North Country. But he was a vegetarian. There is a real problem getting fresh produce up there in winter. That's a genuine concern, although a lot of times the physicians don't really think about these things. It is our job to bring up these lifestyle and cultural issues with every candidate. Think about this: "You are going to a rural town. What does that mean in terms of social outlets? Does your spouse want to work? Are there opportunities there?"

Initially, I felt a little uncomfortable asking these questions about spouses, or dealing with issues of same-sex couples or racial and cultural issues. How many of these questions are discriminatory? We worry about this, but then we realize that the physicians are just as interested in going to a community that will be a good fit for them. We do an awful lot of handholding on both sides.

In the case of the Middle Eastern physician, a site visit helped clarify realities for all concerned. What Pagliuca could not convey during the office interview was amply demonstrated during the visit, which included a stop at the local grocery store. The physician was dismayed by the skimpy produce section, which his family would depend upon to uphold cultural and religious dietary practices. In subsequent interviews with local physicians and hospital officials, he brought this up as a concern. Eager for help with the patient load, the physicians assured him that he and his family would soon love meat. They even offered to supply his wife with recipes and take him on moose hunting trips.

"He came back to Concord and withdrew his application," Pagliuca recalls. "He told me, 'I am not going to change my beliefs and practices just for a job.' It was a satisfactory conclusion. It wasn't going to be a good fit for anyone."

In Nebraska and Virginia, recruiting continues to be a function of local practices, although Practice Sights did help to establish statewide databanks cataloguing the characteristics of locales, provider needs, and other considerations. Unlike New Hampshire, which is a relatively small state, Nebraska and Virginia must contend with significant distance and diversity in their health systems. The experience of Practice Sights leaders there suggests that a regional approach to recruiting might work better in a larger state, or even that several states with common geography and demographics might collaborate in recruiting. In Nebraska, for example, practices like the one David Adams joined in Fairbury are the easiest to recruit for because the community has a full-service local hospital, urban centers are relatively close, and the Fairbury practice has enough doctors for collegiality and a reasonable work schedule. It is more difficult to sell physicians on a remote community such as Benkelman, six hours' drive from Lincoln, or Calloway, where the district hospital's medical staff consists of a single doctor—a 24/7 job if there ever was one. "I wouldn't say Benkelman is exactly the end of the world," says Dennis Berens of Nebraska's Office of Rural Health. "But you can see it from there."

Even to recruit someone who is as ideal on paper as David Adams was takes creativity. The body of research on rural physicians suggests that those who work out best grow up in a small town; marry someone from a small town; and have a self-confident, take-charge personality. David Adams is all of these. But he brought requirements to the table that typify expectations of the newest medical school graduates—a reality for rural recruiting no less than for a large group practice. His negotiations with the Fairbury Clinic underscore the personal and highly individualized dynamic that Stephanie Pagliuca has found essential to success in New Hampshire.

Adams didn't want to work the twelve-hour days that his seniors in the Fairbury practice considered routine, and he was equally tough-minded about night and weekend duty. He wanted an income sufficient to meet lifestyle and financial goals. Indeed, most states are finding they cannot recruit rural physicians without a guaranteed first-year income of $100,000 to $125,000. And though it's true that Adams has a spouse to help in his transition to small-town America, that's not her complete job description, as it might have been a generation ago. Mrs. David Adams also happens to be a physician. Any practice hoping to recruit David Adams, M.D., had to come up with an equally appealing position for Kari Adams, M.D. The physician partners in the Fairbury Clinic decided it was worth it to go up to five doctors from four to accommodate both Adamses.

Virginia's rural areas are experimenting with private recruiting on a larger scale. In its southwestern Appalachia region, the not-for-profit Carilion Medical Group handles recruiting for forty-four affiliated private practices. The group has 175 physician members and is a subsidiary of the Carilion Health System, the largest hospital network in western Virginia. The health system provides income subsidies for new physician recruits and for members of the medical group working in extreme poverty areas. For its part, the medical group runs educational workshops and has linked the practices to computerized information systems to keep its members up to date on the latest developments in medical science.

This last element is critical, says James G. Nuckolls, a rural physician in Galax, who is the group's medical director. He emphasizes what so often is left out of the numbers discussion dominating conventional thinking on rural recruitment: rural populations need good doctors, not just warm bodies.

"We do our best to recruit the people that seem to be good, but then we watch them real close during the first year," Nuckolls says. "We want to make sure they are real doctors, not just playing at being a doctor to fulfill lifestyle needs. It's like that saying: 'He ain't no cowboy till you seen him ride.' We support them every way we can, but we've got to see that they are hard workers and team players."

Landing quality recruits, however, is only the first step. Keeping them sharp is as much a part of the retention formula as income and lifestyle support, according to Nuckolls. "The thing that happens to rural doctors is that they get isolated and can no longer measure the true quality of their work," he says. "They start to measure themselves by the compliments they receive from patients. Pretty soon, the doctor's head gets so swelled that he's a walking deity. The fact is, medical quality is best judged by one's peers. You've got to be in contact with peers, challenged on the science and so forth, to keep yourself sharp and interested."

## Improving Economic Conditions

The dream of Nebraska's rural health planners is to have a dozen networks scattered about the state, mimicking the Carilion system in southwest Virginia. But with Practice Sights they were starting from scratch, and with two strikes against them. First, the historic evolution of the state's rural health system had left individual hospitals and physicians unusually isolated from one another, compared with smaller and more populous states. Second, many of them were struggling financially at the launch of Practice Sights and had little capital to invest in systems change.

Nebraska is very rural. Its two urban centers, Lincoln and Omaha, are on the eastern edge, about an hour apart. These cities are also the center of tertiary care medicine and medical education. As you head west toward the Panhandle region, bordering Wyoming, towns become smaller and farther apart. Large sections of the state don't even qualify as rural, falling instead into the public health definition of frontier. No statewide entity—no health department, hospital association, or medical society—can generalize about the characteristics and needs of Nebraska's rural health systems. They pretty much operate as a collection of local fiefdoms, some good, some less so, all fiercely independent in character. This defining ethos goes back to pioneer times, when an isolated community had to develop self-sufficiency or perish. It continues today for remarkably similar reasons. Of 534 incorporated communities in Nebraska, 90 percent have fewer than twenty-five hundred people. But with an area of 77,355 square miles, Nebraska is more than eight times the size of New Hampshire. The one-on-one handholding that Stephanie Pagliuca can do from Concord is not possible from Lincoln. Just to sit down with physicians in the Panhandle means an eight-hour drive.

"You do not come in as a state person in Nebraska and say, 'This is how it is going to be,'" says David Palm of the state Department of Health and Human Services, who led the Practice Sights project in Nebraska and has folded his lanky 6'6'' frame into state cars for many such trips. "You have to soft-pedal everything, and be very respectful of how the communities have traditionally done things, and think carefully about what we at the state level can do to help them accomplish their goals."

Dennis Berens, who heads Nebraska's Office of Rural Health and was the mild-mannered Palm's colleague on Practice Sights, adds, "People here don't like outsiders coming in and telling them what to do—not from Lincoln, not from Washington, and not from some big foundation in Princeton. If we tried to do that, it would be 'Just put the money in a bag and leave it at the outskirts of town. . . .'"

Nebraska's health officials used the Practice Sights grant to organize the state's diverse and far-flung regions into five provider networks. With varying degrees of success, the networks worked collaboratively to recruit additional health care providers and to provide educational forums for members—both goals of Practice Sights. The networks also joined forces with the University of Nebraska and various state agencies to expand scholarship, loan repayment, and locum tenens programs for health care providers willing to work in an underserved area. Practice Sights leaders were also successful in spurring legislative action to eliminate certain practice restrictions on physicians' assistants so they could help alleviate the provider shortage.

As in New Hampshire, Nebraska's Practice Sights leaders got unexpected momentum from rural providers' panic over managed care, which spurred interest in collaborative action. In southeast Nebraska, physicians had already formed the Southeast Rural Physicians Alliance to negotiate managed care contracts and explore other business-oriented group activities such as bulk purchasing of supplies and better rates for malpractice insurance. Similarly, the hospitals in that region had formed the Blue River Valley Hospital Network. Seeing an opportunity for fully integrating the health care delivery system, Palm suggested that the organizations take the next step of collaborating with one another. This led to formation of the Rural Comprehensive Care Network, a physician and hospital alliance made up of local health systems in seventeen counties in Nebraska's southeastern corner.

The southeast network—which today remains the strongest of those organized under Practice Sights—undertakes a variety of projects for its members, including negotiating lower-cost bulk purchase of supplies and better rates on malpractice insurance. It has also started some medical quality-improvement projects. But there is no mistaking the driving force behind these activities: the economic survival of local hospitals and physicians. Even the medical quality-improvement projects are oriented to the bottom line; one purpose is to prove to local residents that they needn't drive all the way to Lincoln for first-rate primary medical care.

Palm, Berens, and other Practice Sights leaders sought to sell the program's goals—improved recruiting, better use of midlevel practitioners, and so on—in the context of these overtly financial concerns. Indeed, Practice Sights stripped down was very much about economic survival. At some point in the program's five-year course, every grantee realized the need to meld principle—improving health care access for rural populations—with the practical: ensuring the financial viability of rural physicians and hospitals. In Nebraska, however, cold reality was a companion from Day One. Consider:

- Pushed to explore the possibility of expanding the capacity of his solo practice with a nurse practitioner, an older rural physician was shocked to discover that the going rate for a salary—about $60,000 a year— exceeded his own income. He gave up, unable to imagine how to fund the position, given the general poverty of his community.

- In the Panhandle, where state health officials hoped to stimulate formation of a rural health coalition similar to the one in southeast Nebraska, nine of the region's thirteen hospital administrators turned over in two years, a leadership instability related to the very conditions Practice Sights sought to alleviate for physicians.

- Reimbursement rates set by Medicare, the dominant payer in rural Nebraska, were among the worst in the country because of historically low fees charged by physicians and hospitals.

"We had older physicians who were still charging five, eight, and ten dollars a visit," Palm says. "That was going to be a real problem if managed care came in and tried to negotiate on the basis of that rate. We realized we needed to lay some building blocks for improving recruiting and many other aspects of rural health in Nebraska. You can't look just at recruitment and retention as a single issue. The solutions really have to be multifaceted, and you can't attribute them to one program or one set of goals."

Just about everything Nebraska experimented with under Practice Sights came down to money—mostly the lack of it. In its effort to lay building blocks, the health department, as Practice Sights' lead agency, brought in a variety of partners, including the Nebraska Economic Development Corporation, the medical school at the University of Nebraska, the Office of Rural Health, and even private community entities such as the Saint Elizabeth's Foundation. The latter was asked to develop a locum tenens program, through which medical residents and emergency room or retired physicians in Lincoln and Omaha would cover for rural physicians who needed a break. Surveys of doctors and potential recruits showed enthusiasm for such a program, but Nebraska's rural health systems could pay only twenty to thirty dollars an hour, which was about fifteen dollars under market. Moonlighters could earn more—and conveniently— by filling openings in the cities or suburbs. "Fifty miles was about the limit of what they wanted to travel," says Donna K. Hammack, of the Saint Elizabeth's Foundation. "Our rural areas were a lot farther than that."

The failure of the experiment convinced Practice Sights leaders of the necessity of locally based human resource solutions. But human resources could not be bolstered without significant improvement in rural health's bottom line—exactly the focus of the program's constituents. Practice Sights leaders redirected their efforts from the specific goals articulated by the grant program to Palm's building blocks. Specifically, they set out to help rural hospitals take advantage of federal programs—designation as a Critical Access Hospital or Rural Health Clinic—that would vastly improve the revenue stream for providers. Both programs afford an opportunity for qualified providers to secure higher reimbursement under Medicare and Medicaid.

The strategy had remarkable success, similar to New Hampshire's with gaining federally funded health centers. The number of physician practices earning Rural Health Clinic status went from five to seventy-seven in Nebraska; the number of Critical Access Hospitals went from zero to fifty-five, largely as a result of the momentum gained from Practice Sights.

Other building blocks include the startup of three additional hospital/physician networks modeled on southeast Nebraska's Rural Comprehensive Care Network. Practice Sights leaders also gave support to University of Nebraska efforts aimed at creating a supply of health professionals. As it is, the majority of physicians practicing in Nebraska are graduates of the University of Nebraska or its medical school. But to build a supply of rural physicians, the university's medical center now sponsors an eighth grade science fair to identify talented students in rural areas. These youngsters become eligible for scholarships to state colleges and, if successful there, are guaranteed admission to a health profession graduate program at the University, including medicine, pharmacy, dentistry, physical therapy, and occupational therapy. The medical school has a special Rural Health Opportunities Program, which rotates students through rural practices to give them hands-on experience. An added benefit is courtesy faculty status for the students' physician mentors, giving these relatively isolated practitioners a connection to the university.

## The Loan Program

Virginia was one of only four Practice Sights grantees that dared to tango with The Robert Wood Johnson Foundation's Program-Related Investment idea. The Virginia project was ultimately successful, but only after protracted and dizzying negotiations that left other Practice Sights grantees badly winded. Nebraska had the worst experience and ended up returning the Foundation's money.

The PRI was a relatively new undertaking for the Foundation when program officers made it part of Practice Sights, though conceptually it had been a recognized vehicle for charitable funding since the Tax Reform Act of 1969. Instead of a grant, the Foundation proposed to lend seed money to Practice Sights grantees for a revolving loan fund that would give health care providers access to capital at a favorable interest rate. Unlike a grant, whose use is restricted to project personnel and operating costs, a loan fund could legitimately finance bricks-and-mortar-type investment consistent with program goals. In Practice Sights, one could imagine many such uses, from upgrading a rural physician's office equipment to rehabilitating a Main Street storefront for use as a primary care clinic. The Foundation expected grantees to round up local partners to match the seed loan, five to one. It also required payback of the Foundation's loan plus 3 percent interest within ten years.

The loan arrangement was the problem. It saddled Practice Sights grantees with an unusual and intimidating management task. Most of their experience was with grants, which, once you land them, can be freely spent for defined purposes. About the only way you can get into trouble is if you take a Hawaiian vacation or otherwise abuse a funder's trust. The essence of successful grant management is prudence and integrity. Practice Sights leaders were confident that they could manage the grants part of the program.

The PRI requirements, however, challenged their financial acumen, of which they were less confident. Among several noteworthy consequences was unusual timidity in this area of Practice Sights. The grantees stuck the loan money in bank certificates of deposit, the most conservative form of investment. Their primary concern was safeguarding the Foundation's money and earning the required interest before even a penny went out into the field. In this, the PRI experiment contrasted sharply with The Robert Wood Johnson Foundation's long-avowed mission of stimulating innovation and risk taking in the field, which unquestionably occurred in Practice Sights grant-funded areas.

Peter Goodwin, the Foundation's vice president for finance, acknowledges conceptual miscalculations with the PRI. "It was a new business for us, and at the time we weren't very good at it," he says. Among other things, Foundation staff members did not think through the operational difficulties conferred by the loan repayment conditions. The staff members thought the loan would be educational for grantees, stimulating greater financial sophistication than a grant could about how to use money to greatest effect. But neither the Foundation nor the grantees joining in this experiment realized the complexity of the world they were entering. Fluctuating interest rates during Practice Sights' tenure were only one problem. There was also the surprising naïveté of the loan program's intended beneficiaries: rural health care providers. The PRI experience was instructive for the Foundation and grantees alike, but its structural complexity interfered with program goals.

In Nebraska's case, it utterly defeated them. "We probably spent eight or nine months negotiating the terms with Robert Wood Johnson, the legal and finance people," recalls George Frye, executive vice president of the Nebraska Economic Development Corporation, or NEDCO, which handled the rollout of the loan fund. By the time agreement was reached, in December 1996, interest rates had dropped too low for NEDCO to offer a competitive rate and still make the money necessary to pay back the Foundation. Moreover, Nebraska found that it needed to sell the idea of borrowing to rural providers and then walk them through the loan process. They needed much more help than NEDCO's usual business customers did.

"We basically were trying to do this in a place as big as Nebraska with the existing NEDCO staff, which is pretty small," Frye said. "It's me, and I'm part-time, one full-time loan packager, and one portfolio manager. There was no money for marketing or extra staff. If we could have just had one person dedicated to going around and acquainting people with this program, I think we could have done better."

In the end, Nebraska's Community Primary Care Loan Program made only two loans. The first one ended in default; the second one financed a bailout of the first one. At that point, Practice Sights leaders concluded that the experiment was too high-risk, especially with only a ten-year loan cycle. They retrenched to priority number one: paying back the Foundation. In December 2000, their investments succeeded in restoring the full loan amount plus 3 percent. Nebraska promptly cut a check to the Foundation and withdrew from the experiment.

Virginia encountered many of the same structural problems but overcame them. The loan program established under Practice Sights, called the Healthy Communities Loan Fund, continues to grow in volume and scope. It is run under the auspices of a private philanthropy, the Virginia Health Care Foundation, which was a collaborator with the Virginia Department of Health in Practice Sights. The fund surpassed the $4 million mark in late 2001 and recently extended eligibility for a loan to mental health professionals and pharmacists. Ironically, at $700,000, Virginia's seed loan was the smallest in the program. Nebraska, by contrast, got $1.5 million.

Why was Virginia's experience so different from Nebraska's? Deborah D. Oswalt, of the Virginia Health Care Foundation, has a quick answer: "We had real bankers with commercial lending experience helping us every step of the way." Getting "real bankers" on board was an idea forged by Oswalt's concern over the PRI's complexity, which also raised eyebrows on her governing board.

"The fact that it was a loan and that we had to repay it and pay interest and so on definitely influenced how we handled the $700,000," Oswalt says. "It is not as if we were some banking gurus. We're a nonprofit foundation. What did we know about any of that sophisticated high-finance stuff? My board wanted to be sure I wasn't sitting there making loan decisions. This helped us develop a real working partnership with the banking community."

Oswalt and her staff came up with an ingenious method of identifying the best bank for their purposes. They superimposed a map of Virginia's underserved areas on the branch networks of Virginia-based banks and found that

First Virginia Banks had 310 branches in Virginia, many of them in the areas Practice Sights deemed eligible for lending. Says Oswalt:

> I can't overemphasize the importance of the relationship with the bank to our success. We learned so much from them and got help in ways we never expected. When we ran into declining interest rates, we actually questioned whether we should continue. It was getting impossible to offer the favorable loan terms we wanted: prime rate, no points, no prepayment penalties to make this a really good deal for our rural providers. But the bank was able to come through with special package deals like free checking and all those other extras banks offer good customers. So, yes, maybe the doctors could go elsewhere and get a better rate, but they wouldn't get the individual attention and help they get from us.

The bank also prints and mails the health care foundation's informational brochures, subsidizes other marketing costs, and works closely with Lilia Mayer, the Healthy Communities Loan Fund's indispensable point person. As in Nebraska, Virginia found that it needed a dedicated staff person to promote the project and respond to inquiries. The expertise that they assumed highly educated people such as doctors would bring to the transaction simply wasn't there.

"We learned to our surprise that some physicians are poor businessmen," Oswalt says. "Their bookkeeping was very rudimentary. They just wanted to treat patients, and they really did not know how to assess their assets or how much of a loan they could handle or how to develop a business plan. So Lilia began to incorporate the literature of the Small Business Administration in our mailings to help them out. It was never envisioned that we would be a technical assistance program in addition to a loan program, but that is how it turned out."

First Virginia Banks has reaped rewards as well. Tentative at first, the bank has steadily ramped up its support, recognizing the loan program's benefit to core business. First Virginia competes with larger banks by cultivating grassroots customers as opposed to major national corporations, according to John P. Salop, a senior vice president and liaison to the Healthy Communities Loan Fund. The bank recently received the American Bankers Association's ACTION Award in recognition of its Practice Sights contributions. Still, Salop admits to some early qualms.

"This was new, it was different, so, sure, there were people at the bank with reservations," he says. "The biggest fear was that you would be spinning your wheels, that it would never get going because the underpinnings were weak. You don't want to waste your time. We said we would be willing to accept less"—in the way of interest and collateral, for instance—"but they still had to be profitable loans if this was going to be a long-term thing. Everything has to make economic sense."

With the experience of Practice Sights as a guide, The Robert Wood Johnson Foundation took another look at the economic sense of requiring loan repayment plus interest. Specifically, in the case of Virginia's Healthy Communities Loan Fund, the Foundation decided in early 2002 to forgive the 3 percent interest requirement entirely. Bank interest rates had dropped so precipitously during 2001 that the loan fund barely earned enough to cover program operating costs, never mind the Foundation's fee. Recognizing this difficulty, the Foundation essentially converted the terms of the PRI agreement to those of an interest-free loan.

Current Foundation programs are experimenting with PRIs whose seed money comes in the form of grants, not loans. The term of the grant may also be indefinitely extended, eliminating the inflexibility of a short loan cycle.

# CONCLUSIONS

Practice Sights aimed at improving health care by easing conditions that discourage health care providers from working in underserved rural or inner city settings. The program also sought to build capacity at the state level to address workforce issues, thus reducing states' dependence upon federal initiatives.

Collectively, grantees succeeded in recruiting 867 health care providers; the total includes physicians, nurse midwives, nurse practitioners, and physician assistants. New Hampshire had a net increase in physicians. Nebraska, by contrast, finished the project with exactly the same number of rural physicians as when Practice Sights started. But the state's success in shoring up the financial underpinnings of rural health systems via Critical Access Hospital and Rural Health Clinic designations resulted in hiring a significant number of midlevel providers, where before there had been none.

To the numerical scorecard, Practice Sights added valuable insights into the alchemy of successful recruiting and retention of health care providers. Notably, it illustrated the links between the rural health care workforce and larger economic, political, and workforce trends in the United States. If a local hospital is too cash-strapped to hire a mid-level health professional to help with night and weekend emergency room coverage, there isn't much hope for improving the physician's call schedule. Similarly, a revolving door of providers and administrators bodes ill for any health system's ability to meet community needs. As Nebraska's David Palm observed, no single program or initiative can tackle all of the factors that discourage providers from working in certain areas. But Practice Sights shed new light on the dimensions of the problem and challenged conventional thinking in some areas.

The connection between health care and the larger environment plays out daily in recruiting. Success depends upon nimbly tailoring a pitch to current market demands. However, recruiters seasoned by Practice Sights learned to take the stated expectations of today's medical school graduates with more of a grain of salt than health systems researchers or senior physicians seem to. This last group is uniformly exasperated by recent candidates' determined negotiation of limits to night and weekend duty, privately grumbling about a declining work ethic in their profession. Some researchers echo this sentiment. Practice Sights recruiters, by contrast, attributed the focus on perks and work schedules to be a combination of naïveté and of competing opportunities in the larger job market. Anyone starting a career brings to it the hopes of Gavin Muir: good location, comfortable hours, challenging work, nice life. Those who succeed professionally usually do so because, at some level, they love the work and commit what it takes to do it well. His four-day workweek notwithstanding, Muir ended up being interviewed for this chapter at 11:00 P.M., after medical emergencies had forced him to cancel several earlier appointments. He still loves his job.

As for the larger job market, its influence was palpable during Practice Sights. Recruiters saw in many candidates a reflection of the expectations of their generational peers during a period of record-breaking prosperity in the United States. During the mid-1990s, many of the so-called best and brightest of college-educated young people flocked to quick wealth on Wall Street or in a dot com startup. The number of economics and business majors at the undergraduate level soared, while medical schools saw a precipitous drop in applicants, from a high of 46,965 in 1996 to 34,859 in 2001, according to the Association of American Medical Colleges. In this context, the emphasis on perks as opposed to the "working where I can make a difference" ethos of a previous era is less surprising—and also less predictive of future trends. It's worth noting that since Practice Sights, the dot com bubble has burst, Wall Street is laying off, and recent college graduates are beating the bushes for jobs. This is the sobering reality of today's medical school students: a context that could make job security in a medically underserved area sound very nice indeed.

That said, Practice Sights leaders identified workforce changes that are more likely to be long-term. The single-breadwinner family is becoming a rarity. Time and again, grantees found that success in recruiting and retaining providers required attention to a spouse's career or avocational interests. Married physicians are not necessarily a doctor-and-doctor package, as with David and Kari Adams. In Littleton, New Hampshire, Jessica Thibodeau, a nurse practitioner recruited from Boston, had to be sold on the area's opportunities for her husband, Scott Brumenschenkel, a self-employed furniture maker and designer of custom cabinetry. Her job would provide the family's steady income, but for the relocation to work in the long run he needed a market for his high-end skills. Although the immediate area is poor, Thibodeau reports that Brumenschenkel was able to find customers among those with seasonal vacation homes in New

Hampshire, and by way of local galleries. The couple's final concern was whether Littleton would be a good match for their school-aged daughter. The quality of the local school system was a significant draw, illustrating yet again the importance of the larger community infrastructure to health care improvements.

Another insight from Practice Sights is the need for more up-to-date and integrated national databases to guide recruiting strategies for underserved areas. The enthusiastic response of state health departments to Practice Sights stemmed in part from frustration with the disjointed status quo in health care workforce initiatives. The research field reflects this history. Much of the published data fall into isolated niches of inquiry and significantly lag behind the conditions driving decision making on the front line of recruitment and retention. The most comprehensive data sets—compiled by the federal Office of Rural Health and the Council on Graduate Medical Education—date to 1997. Any wisdom that researchers can offer a front-line recruiter is accordingly handicapped by lack of timeliness. During Practice Sights, the NPO developed computer software to assist states or small agencies in accomplishing recruiting tasks. The National Health Service Corps subsequently provided funding to make the software available to all fifty states. Similar coordination in updating and integrating disparate data sets would be helpful to those on the front line.

A final observation from the platform of Practice Sights is that there's no such thing as recruiting for permanence. Television dramas depict the silver-haired rural practitioner, beloved by his community, delivering the babies of babies he helped into the world at the start of his career. This romantic scenario is not borne out statistically. The average stay for a rural practitioner is six years. Some leave because of the specific hardships that Practice Sights sought to alleviate: long hours, isolation, and inadequate income. But others leave for the reasons that lead other professionals to jump from company to company or to move about the country: a better opportunity, family needs, or perhaps just to try something different. This mobility—part of a general workforce trend that took hold in the later years of the twentieth century—can work both ways. Rural areas occasionally benefit from providers' disenchantment with urban practice. During the 1990s, for example, California physicians left the state by the thousands rather than accept changes in practice conditions and reimbursement imposed by managed care plans. How to capitalize on the many intersecting trends and crosscurrents illustrated by Practice Sights remains a challenge for those seeking to improve access to health care in underserved communities.

## Notes

1. Health Research and Services Administration. *Health Professional Shortage Areas by Metropolitan/Non-Metropolitan Classification as of March 31, 2002.* Washington, D.C.: U.S. Department of Health and Human Services, 2002), tab. 2.

2. H. K. Rabinowitz, J. J. Diamond, F. W. Markham, N. P. Paynter. "Critical Factors for Designing Programs to Increase the Supply and Retention of Rural Primary Care Physicians." *Journal of the American Medical Association,* 2001, *286,* 1041–1048.

3. Marco Navarro and Peter Goodwin discuss the Foundation's PRIs in "Program-Related Investments," in *To Improve Health and Health Care: The Robert Wood Johnson Foundation Anthology, Vol. V* (San Francisco: Jossey-Bass, 2002).

# Grant Report Summaries from The Robert Wood Johnson Foundation

## ESTABLISHMENT OF
## A MODEL VOLUNTEER PRIMARY CARE CLINIC
(last updated May 1997)

### Grantee

The Volunteers in Medicine Clinic (Hilton Head Island, South Carolina)

### Summary

Two grants, one for planning and one for implementation, supported the establishment of a model volunteer clinic on Hilton Head Island, providing care to medically underserved residents and low-income people employed on the island. The new 7,000-square-foot clinic opened in June 1994 and is staffed by more than 280 professional and lay volunteers, many of them retired physicians, nurses, and dentists. The clinic provided 10,370 visits in 1996 at no cost to patients.

Representatives of the Volunteers in Medicine (VIM) clinic have met or communicated with over a thousand people from around the country who have expressed interest in starting volunteer medical clinics. The promotional efforts of project director Jack B. McConnell, M.D., have brought visibility to the project and made it a model for others. Communities without Hilton Head's supply of retirees have adapted the prototype, using a mix of retirees and employed health care workers. This project has received extensive coverage locally and nationally and has called attention to the value of retired physicians as a resource.

# STUDIES OF THE MIX OF GENERALISTS AND SPECIALISTS IN THE PHYSICIAN WORKFORCE

(last updated May 1998)

## Grantee

University of Wisconsin-Madison Medical School (Madison, Wisconsin)

Policy Studies on Generalist-Specialist Physician Mix

## Summary

During the early 1990s, as policymakers began to express concern about the size of the physician workforce and its mix of generalist and specialist physicians, a number of national institutions and commissions recommended various strategies to reduce the growth of physician supply and alter the mix of generalists and specialists. With these two grants, researchers conducted policy studies using different mathematical models designed to test the effects of these proposals. Among the key findings reported in the more than twenty articles and papers produced are (1) achieving a 50–50 mix of generalist and specialist physicians could take fifty years or longer; (2) nurse practitioners and physician assistants are already used extensively as substitutes for medical residents in teaching and other hospitals; (3) HMOs use fewer physicians per 100,000 enrollees compared with the ratio of physicians to the total U.S. population; (4) large sustained cuts in the number of first-year residents being trained are needed in order to achieve targeted ratios both for the overall physician supply and for the ratio of generalists to specialists; (5) cutting residency slots currently occupied by international medical graduates alone would not sufficiently curb the growth in U.S. physician supply; and (6) improving minority representation in the physician workforce would require huge increases in the numbers of blacks, Hispanics, and Native Americans as first-year medical residents. These findings, among others, have been published in peer-reviewed journals such as the *Journal of the American Medical Association, Health Affairs, Academic Medicine,* the *American Journal of Medicine,* and the *Journal of Community Health.* The investigators are currently researching changes in physician supply in twenty-five U.S. cities under a subsequent Robert Wood Johnson Foundation grant.

# STUDY OF THE DECLINING SUPPLY OF RURAL PHYSICIANS

(last updated January 1999)

## Grantee

People-to-People Health Foundation, Inc. (Millwood, Virginia)

## Summary

This grant from The Robert Wood Johnson Foundation supported the design and execution of a 1993–1994 national survey of rural physicians. The purpose of the survey was to examine the availability and practice characteristics of physicians who were working in severely medically underserved areas and to identify related implications for access to basic health care. The survey also attempted to identify the level of rural physicians' participation in managed care plans and their attitudes and opinions about health care reform. Survey results reflected the complex nature of physicians' decisions to remain in rural medicine as well as to stay in their current practice. Approximately 40 percent of the 1,601 rural physicians surveyed planned to leave their *current* practice at some point in the future, 22 percent of them within five years. Of the rural physicians sampled, 44 percent planned to remain in rural medicine indefinitely while another 38 percent planned to leave rural medicine altogether. The practice patterns of a general probability sample of rural physicians and those of a subsample of physicians who practiced in "crisis areas" (areas with extremely low physician-to-population ratios) were similar. The survey also found that rural physicians made use of nonphysician providers, such as nurse practitioners and physician assistants, and expected to increase their use of these health care professionals. The grantee made two presentations on rural physician practice patterns and one on the design of the survey. A number of papers were in preparation at the end of the grant.

# PRACTICE SIGHTS:
# STATE PRIMARY CARE DEVELOPMENT STRATEGIES

(last updated March 2000)

## Grantee

National Program Office, North Carolina Foundation for Alternative Health (Raleigh)

## Summary

Uneven distribution of primary care physicians, as well as inadequate use of mid-level providers—physician assistants, nurse practitioners, and nurse midwives—creates barriers to access for many rural and inner-city residents. The Robert Wood Johnson Foundation (RWJF) launched Practice Sights: State Primary Care Development Strategies in 1991 to strength state efforts to recruit and retain primary care providers, including physicians and mid-level providers, and develop and sustain practice sites in underserved areas, authorizing up to $16.5 million for the purpose. Fifteen states (Arizona, Arkansas, Idaho, Kentucky, Maine, Minnesota, Nebraska, New Hampshire, New Mexico, New York, Pennsylvania, South Dakota, Texas, Virginia, and Wisconsin) received planning grants; ten of these states (Idaho, Kentucky, Minnesota, Nebraska, New Hampshire, New Mexico, New York, Pennsylvania, South Dakota, and Virginia) continued with three-year implementation grants. Four of these states (Idaho, Minnesota, Nebraska, and Virginia) also received program-related investments (PRIs) allowing them to create loan funds totaling $19.7 million for capital projects that will increase the availability of health care in underserved areas.

States pursued a variety of strategies that helped improve access in underserved areas in the following ways:

- Creation of recruitment centers helped publicize openings and matched providers with practice sites.

- Provision of technical assistance helped practice sites in underserved areas improve their financial viability.

- Adoption of financial incentives such as loan repayment programs encouraged providers to practice in underserved areas.

- Establishment of locum tenens programs, which provided temporary backup for practitioners in underserved areas, giving them the opportunity to attend conferences or take vacations.

- Expansion of the scope of practice for mid-level practitioners—physician assistants, nurse practitioners, and nurse midwives—increased the services these providers could offer.

In addition, the National Program Office (NPO) created recruitment-tracking software and provided technical assistance through regular workshops and site visits. During the program, recruitment centers in the ten implementation states placed 867 providers in underserved areas; not all of these placements can be attributed to Practice Sights, however.

In 1998, RWJF provided a grant to the NPO to upgrade the Practice Sights software, disseminate it to more states, and integrate it with an Internet recruitment tool called the National Rural Recruitment and Retention Network (3R Net).

# ALTERNATIVE MODELS TO ENSURE PRIMARY CARE ACCESS IN NURSING HOMES

## Grantee

Health Research, Inc. (Albany, New York)

## Summary

This three-year demonstration project examined differences in cost and quality among four alternative staffing models allowed under Medicaid for delivering primary care services in nursing homes. It found that the experimental closed staffing model showed both cost savings and improved quality of care when compared to the open staffing model control group. Nursing home residents in the closed staffing model facilities experienced fewer total hospital admissions, shorter lengths of stay when hospitalized, and fewer visits to the emergency room. The total cost savings to Medicaid and Medicare in these facilities was $1.7 million, or approximately $508 per patient per year. The investigators determined that the process of care was significantly better in the experimental group during the demonstration period. In addition, a survey of residents showed that significantly more patients in the experimental group felt that they were examined more carefully, were able to express feelings, had better access to care, and felt that the doctor cared and was friendly during the demonstration period. The researchers concluded that having primary care providers on staff ensures that nursing homes can provide care to residents as soon as it is needed.

# STUDY OF URBAN PHYSICIAN SUPPLY TRENDS

(last updated February 2001)

## Grantee

University of Wisconsin-Madison Medical School

## Summary

This grant from The Robert Wood Johnson Foundation (RWJF) funded a study of changes in the availability of physicians in U.S. urban areas from 1980 to 1997. Using data from eight sources, the investigators sought to update and extend previous research on the physician workforce and improve the knowledge base for physician workforce policy. One particular focus was the period between 1990 and 1997, when many states enacted policies that aimed to improve the availability of physicians, particularly those in primary care practice, in underserved areas. Key findings included that (1) the number of office-based primary care physicians grew in all areas from 1980 to 1997 and availability continued to be higher in nonpoverty areas than in poverty areas; (2) the number of specialists and hospital-based physicians grew much faster in poverty areas than in nonpoverty areas during this period; (3) physician availability in any given U.S. census tract is most strongly associated with the concentration of hospitals; (4) no single policy aimed at altering the medical workforce had a dramatic impact on physician availability; and (5) in 1997, the availability of office-based primary care physicians in both high- and low-poverty areas was below levels considered adequate by a panel of eleven medical workforce experts polled by the principal investigator. Study findings were presented informally at the 1999 national meeting of the Council on Graduate Medical Education (COGME), an advisory panel authorized by Congress to make recommendations on physician workforce policy. The investigators are currently preparing manuscripts for publication that will focus on physician availability in urban areas.

# GENERALIST PROVIDER RESEARCH INITIATIVE

## Grantee

University of Wisconsin-Madison Medical School

## Summary

Due to the emphasis given to specialty training in U.S. medical education since World War II, specialty medicine had by the 1980s acquired a dominant position in the U.S. health care system at the expense of general medicine. Many in the health policy community thought the resulting shortage in generalist providers relative to specialist providers contributed to restriction of access to primary care and to an increase in the cost of care. The Generalist Provider Research Initiative (GPRI) was one of four programs launched by The Robert Wood Johnson Foundation (RWJF) in the early 1990s to address that issue. The other three programs were the Generalist Physician Faculty Scholars Program, the Generalist Physician Initiative, and Practice Sights: State Primary Care Initiative. Collectively, the programs focused on the development, analysis, and implementation of strategies aimed at increasing the number of generalist physicians relative to specialists.

Authorized by RWJF's board of trustees in April 1993 for up to $3 million, GPRI supported a series of research projects that addressed determinants of the generalist-specialist ratio and opportunities for and constraints to change. RWJF staff thought the findings of the projects would in turn provide policymakers, educators, and health care providers with information needed for these parties to take action to strengthen the role of generalists in the delivery of primary care and alter the imbalance in generalist versus specialist services.

Managed internally by RWJF staff with technical assistance early on from the University of Wisconsin-Madison School of Medicine, GPRI funded a total of twelve studies. Some of the projects were developed as solicited proposals; others were selected by means of competitive calls for proposals. In all cases, RWJF staff exercised a great deal of influence on the topics to be addressed and the character of the research to be carried out. The intent was both to focus expert attention on areas of health care manpower policy in which little research had been done and to direct researchers to areas in which new knowledge was likely to contribute to the policy debate.

The research agenda consisted of the following nine topic areas:

1. The consequences of generalist versus specialist care on the costs of care and medical outcomes

2. The market dynamics of the use of various forms of labor resources in the health care sector

3. Possible public and private actions to be taken to limit the number of specialists

4. Determinants of patient preferences for generalist versus specialist care

5. Determinants of residency choice

6. Factors that influence the job satisfaction of generalist physicians

7. Factors that affect the choice of generalists to practice in underserved areas

8. The relative impact of changes in medical school admission processes, medical training environments, and practice entry incentives on the supply and distribution of generalist physicians

9. The impact of changes in the organization of health care on the demand and need for generalists

RWJF staff also wanted the findings from the studies to be widely disseminated among policymakers, scholars, and educators. Project directors accomplished that dissemination goal largely through numerous publications they generated—many of them in refereed journals such as the *Journal of the American Medical Association,* the *Journal of General Internal Medicine,* and the *American Journal of Public Health.* Some of the findings received widespread coverage in medical newsletters and in mass media such as the *New York Times,* the *Boston Globe,* and National Public Radio.

# STUDY OF BARRIERS TO PRIMARY CARE IN CALIFORNIA

(last updated April 2001)

## Grantees

University of California, San Francisco

Thomas Jefferson University, Jefferson Medical College (Philadelphia)

## Summary

These grants from The Robert Wood Johnson Foundation (RWJF) enabled researchers at the University of California, San Francisco, to study access to primary care in selected urban California communities. The research was designed to assess whether hospitalization rates for certain chronic conditions typically managed by timely outpatient care are valid and useful measures of community access to care. Using hospital discharge and census data, the researchers calculated hospitalization rates for five "ambulatory care sensitive" (ACS) conditions—asthma, hypertension, congestive heart failure, chronic obstructive pulmonary disease, and diabetes—among 250 ZIP code clusters in California. The project also included surveys of patients, residents, and community physicians to determine whether variations in hospitalization rates for ACS conditions could be explained by variations in the health-seeking behavior of individuals, the disease prevalence within a community, or the patterns of physician practice. Among the investigators' key findings: (1) communities where people perceive their access to care as the lowest have the highest rates of hospitalization for ACS conditions; (2) hospitalizations for ACS conditions were higher in communities with greater proportions of uninsured and Medicaid patients and higher in areas where greater proportions of residents said they had no regular place to obtain health care; and (3) variations in physician practice styles or in patients' propensity to seek care for medical symptoms could not explain variations in hospitalization rates for ACS conditions. The strong positive association between hospitalization rates for ACS conditions and perceived access to care suggests that these rates can serve as a valid measure of access to care, the investigators say. Findings from the project were reported in several major medical journals, including the *Journal of the American Medical Association* and the *New England Journal of Medicine,* and in presentations at several national meetings. The principal investigator and his colleagues are currently conducting a longitudinal analysis of how managed care penetration in the community affects hospitalization rates for ACS conditions.

SECTION FOUR

# EDUCATION AND TRAINING

# Editors' Introduction to Section Four

Whereas Section Three dealt with questions of how to attract physicians to practice primary care and to serve in rural and inner-city areas, Section Four looks at a complementary question: how to educate and train them. As far back as the 1960s, the failure of medical schools to promote generalist medicine—particularly the placement of medical residents in tertiary care hospitals, where they saw patients with complex conditions not encountered in normal practice—was attracting attention within the medical profession, and it has continued to do so through the work of groups such as the Pew Health Professions Commission, the Council on Graduate Medical Education, the Graduate Medical Education National Advisory Committee, the American Medical Association, and the Association of American Medical Colleges. Several national programs funded by The Robert Wood Johnson Foundation, such as the Generalist Physician Initiative and the Generalist Physician Faculty Scholars Program, attempted to encourage academic medical centers to incorporate generalism within the mainstream of medical education.

To place the issues in context, we have chosen to reprint relevant parts of two influential reports written in the 1960s and 1970s. The first, reprinted in Chapter Twenty-Two, is the 1966 Report of the Citizens' Commission on Graduate Medical Education of the American Medical Association (known as "The Millis Commission Report," after its chairman, John Millis). Along with The Willard Committee Report, a portion of which is reprinted in Chapter Five, it had a significant impact on medical education. The second report, *The Education of*

379

*Physicians for Primary Care,* written by Joel Alpert and Evan Charney, was published by the U.S. Department of Health, Education and Welfare in 1973. We reprint in Chapter Twenty-Three the portion of the report in which the authors lay out a concrete plan for educating generalist physicians.

Many scholars and practitioners have focused on the inappropriateness of training medical residents for primary care in tertiary hospitals where they see patients with rare and complex disorders. Among the most influential exponents of this position has been Steven Schroeder. In Chapter Twenty-Four, we reprint "Residency Training in Internal Medicine: Time for a Change?" in which Schroeder and his colleagues Jonathan Showstack and Barbara Gerbert, in a conclusion reflecting that of the pioneering study of Kerr White, Franklin Williams, and Bernard Greenberg (reprinted in Chapter Three), call for at least some internal medical residencies to be shifted out of hospitals and into outpatient settings.

Two more recent articles follow. They take a look back on the education and training of generalist physicians. The first, written by Evan Charney in 1995, "The Education of Pediatricians for Primary Care: The Score After Two Score Years," is reprinted in Chapter Twenty-Five. The second, written by Thomas Inui and his colleagues in 1998, summarizes the report of a subgroup of the Advisory Panel on the Mission and Organization of Medical Schools sponsored by the Association of American Medical Colleges. Reprinted in Chapter Twenty-Six, it reviews the growth of primary care education in medical schools and offers a plan to sustain it.

Abstracts of reports and articles on education and training of primary care physicians come next.

Following the abstracts, we look at investments The Robert Wood Johnson Foundation has made to improve the education of primary care physicians. These have largely involved Foundation support of academic medical centers. Chapter Twenty-Seven, "Influencing Academic Health Centers: The Robert Wood Johnson Foundation Experience" by Lewis Sandy and Richard Reynolds, is reprinted from *To Improve Health and Health Care, 1998–1999: The Robert Wood Johnson Foundation Anthology.* It is followed by summaries of grant reports on relevant programs by the Foundation's Grant Results Reporting Unit.

# CHAPTER TWENTY-TWO

# The Graduate Education of Physicians (The Millis Commission Report)

## Chapter 5—Comprehensive Health Care

Citizens' Commission on Graduate Medical Education
1966

The general practitioner of revered memory knew his patients, did whatever he could to cure or ease their varied ailments, and provided continuing care through the course of minor ailments and major emergencies. His deficiencies—and they were many—were partly offset by intimate knowledge of his patients, the support he gave them, and the trust and confidence his services engendered.

Now he is vanishing. Time has changed both him and his patients. Patients now have access to a richer variety of medical services, and many of them have insurance to help pay for hospital and specialist services. In medicine, the major advances, the major triumphs of biomedical research, have not dealt with man as a whole but with his individual bodily systems or organs. As the science and art of medicine devoted to understanding and treating individual organs and systems have outrun the science and art of understanding and treating the whole man, specialty practice has become more necessary and more attractive.

There are no satisfactory statistics on the number of physicians in general practice. Some physicians who started as general practitioners now limit their practice, wholly or partially, to a specialty, and some with specialty training engage in general practice. There is no doubt, however, that the number and the percentage in general practice are declining. In 1931, 84 percent of all physicians in private practice reported themselves to be general practitioners. In 1960, the corresponding percentage was 45; and in 1965, 37. The percentage is sure

This chapter originally appeared as Citizens' Commission on Graduate Medical Education. *The Millis Commission Report/Comprehensive Health Care*, 1966; used by the permission of the American Medical Association.

to decline further, for of all general practitioners in private practice in 1965, 18 percent were over 65 years of age, a proportion of oldsters much higher than in any other area of practice, and in recent classes of medical school graduates, only some 15 percent have planned to enter general practice.

The general practitioner leaves behind him a vacuum that organized medicine has not decided how to fill.

One result of this vacuum has been that the patient becomes his own diagnostician, and decides which kind of specialist he should approach. Or he seeks the advice of a pharmacist or a friend, or follows his own ideas of what constitutes proper treatment. Other patients—in increasing numbers—take their problems to the hospital emergency room. It is always open; all are received; and good medical care and facilities are there available, at least for emergencies. This solution, however, offers little continuity, and the relationship is less than satisfactory either to the patient or the hospital staff.

In the meantime, discussions of "general practice," or "family medicine," or "personal physicians" go on. Some physicians recommend a two- or three-year graduate program as a means of improving and perpetuating the general practitioner. Specialists, in contrast, often think of the general practitioner as being chiefly useful as a "referral service or a clearinghouse for important medical problems the G.P. can't handle." A few medical schools and teaching hospitals have offered programs in family medicine, but most of these programs have been halfway measures that proved to be less than halfway successful.

There are, of course, some excellent general practitioners, and there are some specialists who administer continuing and comprehensive care of high quality. But there are not enough such men, and there is not enough of the service they offer—as most patients, physicians, and legislators agree. The patients give their evidence by waiting in line at hospital emergency rooms. The House of Delegates of the American Medical Association has attempted to reverse the trend away from family medicine. And the medical legislation adopted by the 89th Congress differs from earlier federal legislation, which was designed to stimulate and improve medical research, by placing great emphasis upon improving medical care.

Many leaders of medical thought have proclaimed the desirability of training physicians able and willing to offer comprehensive medical care of a quality far higher than that provided by the typical general practitioner of the past. The physician they conceive of is knowledgeable—as are other physicians—about organs, systems, and techniques, but he focuses not upon individual organs and systems but upon the whole man, who lives in a complex social setting, and he knows that diagnosis or treatment of a part often overlooks major causative factors and therapeutic opportunities.

One of his qualifications must be a thorough knowledge of and access to the whole range of medical services of the community. Thus he is able to call upon the special skills of others when they can help his patient. If the full range of medical competence is to be made effectively and efficiently available, it is mandatory that means be found to increase the supply of physicians willing and properly trained to serve in this comprehensive role.

What is wanted is comprehensive and continuing health care, including not only the diagnosis and treatment of illness but also its prevention and the supportive and rehabilitative care that helps a person to maintain, or to return to, as high a level of physical and mental health and well being as he can attain. Few hospitals and few existing specialists consider comprehensive and continuing medical care to be their responsibility and within their range of competence; and not many of the present general practitioners are qualified to fill this role. A different kind of physician is called for.

There is an annoying semantic problem in talking about this kind of physician. What should he be called? The title *general practitioner* has lost its once honored status. Dr. Russell Lee suggests that we "Build a monument to him and . . . start now with a new concept of the personal physician."

But *personal physician* also presents difficulties. The relation of physician to patient should never be impersonal. Surgeons and psychiatrists and obstetricians and dermatologists are all personal physicians to their patients, whether the relationship is temporary or sustained.

*First-contact physician* has been suggested, but here again there are difficulties. There is always a first contact, and the choice depends upon the patient. It may be an internist, an obstetrician, a pediatrician, or a surgeon. The title merely indicates a temporal relationship and sometimes a temporal accident, not a definitive kind of medical service.

*Family physician* is an often-suggested title, and there are some advantages in having the same physician serve all members of a family. But the family relationship is by no means necessary, and although the term sounds appropriate for informal and individual use ("Dr. Jones is our family physician"), it does not describe the qualifications that should be involved.

*Comprehensive care* probably best indicates the nature of the medical and health service involved. But *comprehensive-care physician* is an awkward title.

We suggest that he be called a *primary physician*. He should usually be primary in the first-contact sense. He will serve as the primary medical resource and counselor to an individual or a family. When a patient needs hospitalization, the services of other medical specialists, or other medical or paramedical assistance, the primary physician will see that the necessary arrangements are made, giving such responsibility to others as is appropriate, and retaining his own continuing and comprehensive responsibility.

Perhaps a better name will emerge as the function—which is the truly important element—becomes more generally recognized and more widely available.

In the meantime, and for the purposes of this report, we will use the title *primary physician.*

Medical literature is full of articles lamenting the failure to develop a substantial corps of well-trained primary physicians. Why, then, are there so few of them?

We find three major reasons:

1. General practice, once the mainstay of medicine, has gradually lost prestige as the specialties have risen in honor and accomplishments. In deciding upon his own career, the young physician may never see excellent examples of comprehensive, continuing care or highly qualified and prestigious primary physicians. He is certain, however, to see a variety of specialists and to observe that they usually enjoy higher prestige, greater hospital privileges, and more favorable working conditions than do general practitioners.

2. Educational opportunities that would serve to interest students in family practice and provide interns and residents with appropriate training are few in number and often poorer in quality than the programs leading to the specialties.

3. The conditions of practice for a general practitioner or a physician interested in family practice are thought to be less attractive than the conditions and privileges enjoyed by a specialist.

All three of these difficulties can be overcome, but heroic work will be required. It is time for a revolution, not a few patchwork adaptations.

# THE POSITION OF COMPREHENSIVE MEDICINE IN THE MEDICAL HIERARCHY

The first necessity is for organized medicine to recognize—not merely in a formal sense, but sincerely—that comprehensive health care is a high calling, different from specialization in thoracic surgery or hematology or something else, but not inferior—not inferior in training, in rewards, or in position within the house of medicine.

The lip service routinely paid to the importance of comprehensive, continuing health care does little to offset the powerful inducements to specialization. Family or personal physicians are said to be important. The House of Delegates has repeatedly emphasized the need for more of them. But in defining their functions and their relations with other physicians, the family or personal physician not infrequently is described in such condescending terms as these: "He provides medical care within the limits of his competence," "He refers to other physicians those patients who have problems beyond his competence," or "His practice gives emphasis to the frequent and commonplace ailments."

The attitude conveyed by such statements is more likely to repel than to attract able and ambitious students to careers in comprehensive family practice.

There is a kind of arrogance in specialized medicine that runs deeper than such attitudes do in other fields. The president of a company often defers to his comptroller on fiscal matters and to his legal counsel on legal matters. He utilizes their specialized knowledge without anyone talking about "referring problems beyond his competence." On the contrary, he is regarded as the epitome of over-all competence. Or, as another analogy, if the quarterback holds the ball for a place-kick specialist or calls upon the fullback to make a needed final yard, he is commended for utilizing effectively the talents of different members of the team. No one makes derogatory remarks about problems "beyond his competence." The practice of law, like the practice of medicine, now requires specialization. But in a modern law office it is a generalist rather than a narrow specialist who takes the leading role and earns at least equal prestige.

The analogies are relevant because the patient wants, and should have, someone of high competence and good judgment to take charge of the total situation, someone who can serve as coordinator of all of the medical resources that can help to solve his problem. He wants a company president who will make proper use of the skills and knowledge of more specialized members of the firm. He wants a quarterback who will diagnose the constantly changing situation, coordinate the whole team, and call on each member for the particular contributions that he is best able to make to the team effort.

In contrast, the words used in medical discussions often seem to assign to the family practitioner the inferior status of a routing clerk rather than that of an important member of the team.

In these attitudes, medicine has adopted and perhaps exaggerated the values of the scientific specialist. In the academic world, it is customary to put a greater premium on depth of knowledge in a specialized area than on more comprehensive wisdom covering a wider field. Within their own guilds, the most highly respected mathematicians, physicists, or economists are those who have penetrated most deeply into specialized and restricted domains. Perhaps these attitudes are proper among scientists or in the university, where the men most honored are the ones who are extending the frontiers of knowledge. But medicine, although intimately based upon science, is not science. It is an application of science.

What happens to the patient is the measure of success in medical practice. He brings the physician a problem, often a complex one. The factors that contribute to it may be physiological, anatomical, psychological, social, economic, genetic, or describable in still other terms. Sometimes he needs many kinds of help. At other times the proper remedy is as specific as the contents of a single bottle from the pharmacy. In either case, the problem of diagnosing the situation, weighing the several factors, and determining the appropriate course of action is a complex one that calls for breadth of view. One ulcer patient may properly be sent to surgery, a second to a psychiatrist, and a third treated by medicine. All three patients should be able to feel confident that they get first attention from a physician who is aware that there may be several alternatives, not from a physician who knows only one.

Harvey Brooks, dean of engineering and applied physics at Harvard, has described the similar dilemmas of engineering and medicine as they have come to be more and more firmly based on science:

> In both medicine and engineering the importance of the underlying sciences has become so great that medical and engineering faculties are increasingly populated with basic scientists who do research or teaching in sciences which are relevant to but by no means identical with the practice of medicine or engineering. The old form of teaching primarily by practicing physicians or engineers was found wanting because practical knowledge was too rapidly being made obsolete by new scientific developments which could not be fully absorbed or appreciated by the mature practitioner. Yet in the process something of the spirit and attitude of the skilled practitioner was lost, particularly his willingness to deal with problems whole rather than in terms of the individual contributing disciplines.

The Flexner report gave medical education a timely and healthy push in the biological and biochemical direction. Growing scientific knowledge furthered the trend. And the availability of large funds for biomedical research accelerated it. Medicine has been greatly strengthened by these developments. They should be supported and continued. The problem is not that these aspects of medicine have grown too rapidly. The problem now is to add a new dimension to the practice of medicine that will help to utilize this growth and to bring the practice of medicine up to its high potential. The needed new dimension is continuing and comprehensive care of high quality. Medical education must produce competent and broadly trained physicians to give that care.

We have already made a start. The House of Delegates, the Academy of General Practice, the College of Physicians, and many individual leaders of medical thought—albeit with differences in the particular remedies and approaches they recommend—have all agreed upon the urgency of greater and more widespread provision of comprehensive medical services. Of course there are difficulties, but the change is necessary for the welfare of patients and for the future standing and respect, including self-respect, of the profession. It is time for decisive action to increase greatly the number of physicians who will devote their professional careers to the highly competent provision of comprehensive and continuing medical services. If organized medicine does not take the leadership in meeting this problem, others will.

# EDUCATION FOR COMPREHENSIVE MEDICAL CARE

Medical schools and teaching hospitals are generally organized along discipli-nary and specialty lines. There are departments of anatomy and physiology and other disciplines; there are pediatric and surgical and other services; but there are few services or clinics of comprehensive medicine. If students are to see comprehensive medicine practiced at its best, major changes in curricula and a major addition to teaching facilities must be made, starting in the medical school. It is in the medical school that the student first begins to make realistic comparisons between different kinds of medical careers, and it is there that he finds the first models upon which he patterns his own career aspirations. At pre-sent, medical schools provide excellent models of the scientist-research scholar and the hospital-based specialist, but rarely if ever do they provide models of comprehensive health care or of physicians who are successful and highly regarded for providing that kind of medical service. Worse, some faculty mem-bers tend to denigrate the role of such physicians.

There are exceptions, but in the typical medical school hospital, the student does not see a normal range of patients, but a highly selected and specialized sample. In practice, patients seek help for a wide range of ailments, from the merely inconvenient to the crippling and fatal. In the typical medical school hospital, most cases are on referral because of acute conditions that require spe-cialized or round-the-clock attention. In practice, contact may continue over many years, allowing a full, rewarding experience of successful management of health problems over a considerable period of time. In the hospital, contact is likely to be restricted to a few days.

The university hospital type of medical service is essential, and every stu-dent should be acquainted with it. But if this is the only type he sees, if only the hospital-based, acute, disease-oriented kind of practice is held before him as a model, it is little wonder that the interest in comprehensive medicine many students bring to medical school gets blunted and forgotten by the time they are ready to seek internships and residencies.

True enough, preceptorship programs give a few students realistic oppor-tunities to observe family practice, and practically all medical schools devote the major part of a year (usually the senior year) to teaching in the outpatient clinics on ambulatory patients, but this teaching program is given less empha-sis than are others. The low status accorded the outpatient clinic naturally leads the student to the belief that ambulatory medicine is relatively unim-portant.

To inspire young physicians to enter the practice of comprehensive medicine and to educate them appropriately will require major changes in faculty, facil-ities, and attitudes. Merely adding a service of comprehensive medicine will not be enough, for everyone else would then relax and there would be little if any improvement over the present outpatient clinics.

A much more sweeping change is necessary. Continuing, comprehensive care should be a central focus of medical school organization, planning, and clinical teaching. Right at the beginning of the student's introduction to clinical medicine he should begin to realize, and his teachers should emphasize, that illness is usually not an isolated event in a localized part of the body, but is a change in a complex, integrated human being who lives and works in a particular social and family setting, who has a biological-psychological-social history. In this complex history are to be found the interacting factors that determine the nature of his illness, and in his future the effects of the illness are likely to continue to be manifest. Of course the student will not understand all of the subtleties involved—no one does—but this kind of emphasis at this early stage will start to demonstrate how essential in patient care are the concepts of continuity and comprehensiveness. Early emphasis on these concepts will help put into proper perspective the relation of specialized services and particular illnesses to the patient's continuing welfare.

The word *clinic* is inadequate for the program we have in mind, for *clinic* is sometimes used to indicate a medical facility that serves only outpatients. Similarly, *service* may be misinterpreted, for that term is sometimes restricted to the medical services rendered to hospitalized patients. We mean both. The program we recommend as a central focus for the education of primary physicians will service outpatients—and thus be a *clinic*—and when necessary will take those same patients into the hospital—and thus be a *service.* In the following discussion we will call it a *program* or a *service.* Either term will mean the kind of combined clinic and service just described.

The new service will have to have budget, staff, quarters, outpatient facilities, and hospital beds. At its head should be a physician whose central interest is in comprehensive medical care, and on the staff should be other clinical professors and physicians of like interests. Collectively they will assume much of the responsibility for planning, management, patient care, and education.

But responsibility should not rest exclusively with the new service. Its central educational importance requires corporate faculty or staff responsibility, endorsement, and support in developing the teaching program and in maintaining effective integration with other hospital services. Specialists from other services will be required as consultants and part-time participants in the comprehensive program. When necessary, members of the staff will admit patients to the hospital just as do physicians on other services. The hospital beds available to the comprehensive service should not, however, be isolated or distinct from the beds used by other services. The staff members of the comprehensive service will be fully qualified to handle the problems that require hospitalization for some of their patients. In other cases, the services of surgeons, pediatricians, psychiatrists, or other specialists will be required. In either situation, the primary physician and the residents involved should be able to follow the patient throughout the period of hospitalization, even though major responsibility is, for a time, transferred to some other specialist. Continuity before, during, and after hospitalization is part of the responsibility of the primary physician and an essential part of the education of the resident. The achievement of these conditions may require modifications in the customs of some teaching hospitals, and will certainly require the hospital staff as a corporate whole to accept a considerable measure of responsibility for the comprehensive service.

A diverse patient population will be necessary. Patients should not be restricted to those who come by referral, but must include those who come voluntarily, for the educational program will require a patient population that covers the whole age range and a wide range of socioeconomic and educational levels. In the course of time, such patients will display the whole gamut of problems from the common and minor to the most unusual and complicated.

Such services would provide the very best setting in which to introduce the medical school student to the practice of medicine. A clerkship served in this setting would give him opportunities to see a variety of patients with a variety of problems, to follow patients over a considerable period of time, to see comprehensive medicine practiced at a high level of excellence, to observe the work of the different specialists, and to see how their specialized talents can be brought together to contribute to the welfare of the patient.

At the graduate level, students who aspire to careers as primary physicians would find in these programs excellent opportunities for a portion of their residency training. Moreover, the hospitals that establish these programs will present an example of one staff working regularly, continuously, and cooperatively with the staffs of other services. This example should be a good opening wedge in bringing about a greater amount of consultation and a greater degree of corporate responsibility for educational planning. Graduate medical education generally would profit from such a change.

We know of no medical school or teaching hospital that now offers a comprehensive care service of as high quality as we recommend, or one that constitutes as central and important a part of the teaching program. Such services should be established as quickly as possible. It should be recognized from the outset that they are to provide model, exemplary medical services for educational purposes. In size, they should be no larger than is necessary to fulfill these demonstration and educational functions.

We have been warned that some local physicians and medical societies would oppose the establishment of comprehensive-care services, because medical centers would be in direct competition with private physicians. To an extent they would and must be. Yet we think the difficulties can be diminished by careful planning and advance "selling" of the ways in which these services will improve the education of primary physicians. Moreover, effective teaching will usually require the collaboration of some local physicians who are willing and qualified to devote a part of their time to education.

Adjustments will also be necessary on the part of faculty and staff members, for both in university medical centers and in other teaching hospitals many private patients are not used for educational purposes. We believe they should be.

Clearly there will be problems and economic questions to consider. They must be anticipated and—insofar as possible—resolved in advance, for the establishment of model programs offering comprehensive care to a patient population diverse in kind, but limited to the size needed for teaching purposes, is an essential step towards interesting students in this kind of practice and towards giving them an opportunity to experience its problems and its satisfactions. If we provide students with models of high quality, we can expect a reasonable number of them to set their own sights on this type of practice. This urgent educational need is of such importance as to outweigh any minor infringement upon private practice.

These model programs will probably take diverse forms. Initially all will be educational experiments. They should be closely watched and carefully reported, as are any good experiments, so that medical schools and teaching hospitals will be helped to adopt those forms of organization and methods of education that work most effectively.

## GRADUATE PROGRAMS FOR PRIMARY PHYSICIANS

The primary content of graduate education for comprehensive care should consist of medicine, psychiatry, pediatrics, medical gynecology, and preventive medicine. The Commission has five recommendations to make.

> First, simple rotation among several services, in the manner of the classical rotating internship—even though extending over a longer period of time—will not be sufficient. Knowledge and skill in the several areas are essential, but the teaching should stress continuing and comprehensive patient responsibility rather than the episodic handling of acute conditions in the several areas.

Accomplishment of this objective will require joint planning by representatives of the several services, supervision under the direction of senior staff members whose responsibilities and authority cover the entire area rather than individual services, and comprehensive planning through the entire period of graduate medical education.

The method of organization, the time order of different parts of the educational program, and other details will surely vary, but several general principles will have to be observed.

Part of the graduate period should be spent in other specialized services, particularly internal medicine. This experience will provide essential education in the concepts and techniques of areas of medicine in which he must be soundly educated if he is to fulfill his responsibilities as a primary physician and is to earn and merit the respect of physicians in other specialties. Moreover, experience in the specialized services will foster collaboration, as a resident and later, with members of those specialties.

Part of the period of graduate education should be spent in a comprehensive and continuing care service of the kind described earlier. Experience in this service will allow the resident to work with a variety of patients over extended periods of time, to get an overall knowledge of patients' health rather than of short periods of illness, to follow the same patients into and out of the hospital, to integrate and apply knowledge and concepts learned during portions of his graduate period spent in the specialized medical services, and to assume gradually increasing responsibility for medical welfare of his patients.

Although previous experience with preceptorships has usually been unsatisfactory, we believe that it may be possible and practical in some cases to arrange for a portion of the graduate period to be spent in a well-supervised preceptorship in a group practice. This arrangement, however, would provide the young physician with realistic and valuable experience only if the group were willing and qualified to assume serious educational responsibilities. Such an arrangement may never become a frequent one, for private groups are normally not organized for educational purposes. Nevertheless, some so situated as to be able to collaborate effectively with a school of medicine or teaching hospital may wish to participate in the education of primary physicians. Good opportunities of this kind should be seized, and a variety of experimental programs should be tried.

If the residency is to be spent partly in specialized medical services, partly in the comprehensive care service, and perhaps partly in a preceptorship in a group practice, collaborative planning and supervision of the program will be essential. Corporate responsibility will be necessary to ensure that residents have continuing responsibility during a patient's outpatient and hospitalized periods, that the specialized services make their portion of the residency maximally effective in contributing to the resident's education, and that the portions of the residency program spent in different settings be properly articulated. Again, this means that the institution must accept responsibility. Failure of the program can be guaranteed if responsibility is turned over entirely to a new and segregated service that is merely added to the present organization.

Second, some experience in the handling of emergency cases and knowledge of the specialized care required before and following surgery should be included.

The amount and nature of surgical experience is probably the most contentious question in the training of a primary physician. Some general practitioners who hope their area and traditions will develop into a higher form of comprehensive medical care wish to include at least enough training in surgery to enable management of real surgical emergencies. In an emergency, any physician will do what he feels is required, and if that means surgery, he will do the best he can. But under ordinary circumstances, with the primary physician working as a member of a group, he will not need to act as a surgeon. If as a student and during his graduate years he has had appropriate experience in the operating room and with surgical patients, he will have learned much about preoperative and postoperative care and the emergency handling of trauma. He will have a sophisticated knowledge of many conditions that require consultation with a surgeon and that may call for surgical treatment. But he will not be trained as a surgeon and should not expect to act as one.

Third, there should be taught a new body of knowledge in addition to the medical specialties that constitute the bulk of the program.

It is difficult to define this body of knowledge, for it is not yet adequately developed. By analogy with biology, it would include the medical counterparts of ecology, evolution, and fundamental theory rather than the specifics of molecular biology, virology, or the physiology of individual organs.

The young physician preparing himself to offer continuing, comprehensive care needs to know people as well as their tissues and organs, medical histories and relationships as well as individual disease states, medical ecology as well as symptomatology. Work in psychiatry would give him some of this background, and so would some materials from sociology and public health—for example, information on the interrelations of families and illness. But it is not possible to be specific about content, organization, or degree of emphasis, for there has not been sufficient experience with the teaching of the medical applications of these topics, nor is there agreement upon the degrees of relevance of all of the things that might be included.

Much can be learned from patients through working with them on a variety of problems over a period of time. The good primary physicians now in practice have acquired much of their skill and wisdom from experience, or from intuition. What is needed—and what the medical schools and teaching hospitals must try to develop—is a body of information and general principles concerning man as a whole and man in society that will provide an intellectual framework into which the lessons of practical experience can be fitted. This background will be partly biological, but partly it will be social and humanistic, for it will deal with man as a total, complex, integrated, social being.

This background is not now well developed. Clearly, there must be a considerable amount of experimentation on the part of schools of medicine and teaching hospitals in efforts to arrive at the most satisfactory subject matter and methods of teaching. The immediately important thing is to have a clear and definite resolve to impart this new body of knowledge. The rest will follow.

Moreover, there will be opportunities that should be grasped to compare the students who are attracted to comprehensive medicine and do well in it with the students who prefer and excel in the other specialties. It is quite possible that comprehensive medicine will have greater appeal to the more humanistically inclined students and those who prefer the behavioral sciences, while those who find greater satisfaction as undergraduates in physics, chemistry, or biology are more likely to want to enter the traditional specialties. If some such difference should be found to be significant, the implications for admissions policy would be obvious.

> Fourth, there should be opportunities for individual variations in the graduate program.

The concept of comprehensive, continuing care leaves room for a variety of shadings of interest and special competence; the graduates of these programs are not to be stereotyped duplicates of each other. Although all primary physicians will be qualified to render continuing and comprehensive care, the dividing lines separating the problems and patients for which a given physician will retain full responsibility from those he will refer to a colleague will vary substantially. If one primary physician has a greater than usual interest in psychosomatic and social problems and another in renal physiology and pathology, the development of those interests will be assets to the groups or clinics in which they collaborate.

Medical educators who are interested in comprehensive care will find many opportunities to experiment on methods of education for this kind of practice and on the means by which comprehensive medical service can best be organized and provided. There are opportunities for research, and for the benefits to patients, students, and faculty that derive from research, in comprehensive medicine just as there are in other specialties.

> Fifth, the level of training should be on a par with that of other specialties. A two-year graduate program is insufficient.

It follows that there should be a specialty board, certification examinations, and diplomate status for physicians highly qualified in comprehensive care. In terms of responsibility, length of training, and position in the medical hierarchy, the examinations, privileges, and accouterments of specialization are indicated.

A new board might be established to certify primary physicians. One of the existing boards might assume this responsibility. Or perhaps a different arrangement would be superior to either of these possibilities. The primary physician will be a functional specialist rather than a subject-matter or technique specialist. It may therefore seem desirable that he be given recognition by joint action of several existing boards or by an agency different from the traditional boards. Instead of trying to solve this problem now, we leave it to the Commission on Graduate Medical Education. . . .

The result of these educational changes should be a growing corps of physicians who qualitatively are the peers of their classmates who chose surgery or some other specialty. The difference will be in the form rather than the level of practice and responsibility. Having a greater breadth of medical interest, they will normally be the first professional contact for a new patient and the continuing point of contact for an old one. To a greater extent than their more narrowly specialized colleagues, they will be diagnosticians and medical coordinators, to whom the primary question will not be, "What can I personally do to be of most help to this patient?" but, "What can I do and what need I arrange to have done by others that will be of most help to this patient?"

It should be clearly recognized that a major, costly, national effort will be needed to educate primary physicians of the quality and in the number needed to provide comprehensive and continuing care to a population reaching up toward 300 million by the time any substantial number can be prepared for practice. The changes in medical attitudes and the changes in schools of medicine and teaching hospitals will require radical breaks with past traditions. To make these breaks precipitously is too much to expect of many hospitals and schools of medicine, but others have already demonstrated their interest. We wish to encourage some medical schools and teaching hospitals to pioneer. Others will follow. Success can be achieved if the faculties and staffs unite in the thoughtful development and support of the necessary educational programs, and if they enlist the cooperation of the ablest practitioners of medicine in carrying them out.

## THE PRACTICE OF COMPREHENSIVE HEALTH CARE

If the number of physicians preparing themselves for comprehensive medicine is to increase markedly, obviously there must be opportunities for esteemed and rewarding practice. This problem, however, will not be a serious one if the changes considered in the preceding sections can be made, for the demand for such physicians is great.

The ideal place for a primary physician is in group practice. Practice within a group will encourage the use of specialized colleagues for help in diagnosis or treatment. Group practice will give the patient the advantages of continuing contact with a physician who knows him and his medical history, combined with the advantages of access to a wider array of skills and facilities whenever they are needed.

There is no reason to expect that all primary physicians will be identical in training or interest. Those who feel so inclined can provide comprehensive care to their own patients and offer more specialized services to others. Thus, one physician might be the group's expert on gastrointestinal problems and another be the expert on virology. Depending upon the size of the group and the interests of its members, there will be room for a reasonable range of variation among those rendering comprehensive care.

Group practice will also benefit the primary physician himself. He will have the intellectual stimulation of working daily with other physicians with knowledge and interests that complement his own. Like his colleagues, he will benefit from the quality control exercised by able peers. And he will have greater opportunity to take leave for vacations or for special or refresher courses, while his patients are cared for by other members of the group.

Primary physicians would be fully qualified to admit to hospital medical services and should have the same kind of admitting privileges as do present-day specialists. Moreover, through membership on hospital review committees (such as the tissue committee, the medical audit committee, or the hospital utilization committee), they should have a particularly valuable influence in helping to bring about better coordination among the hospital's medical and surgical services.

Men of this stamp are of such value in group practice that there should be no difficulty in convincing students that rewarding opportunities lie ahead for any who wish to prepare themselves for careers as primary physicians.

## COMBINED ACTION

The three difficulties that have stood in the way of the more widespread practice of comprehensive medicine—low status, lack of an appropriate educational concept and accordingly of educational opportunities, and conditions of practice—have reinforced each other.

These have been real barriers to entrance upon a career of comprehensive medical service, but surely they can be overcome. To a large extent they have developed because of the specialization and fragmentation of practice brought about by greatly increased knowledge and the mastery of new skills and new techniques. Now, in order to bring medicine's enhanced diagnostic and therapeutic powers fully to the benefit of society, it is necessary to have many physicians who can put medicine together again.

# CHAPTER TWENTY-THREE

# The Education of Physicians for Primary Care (Excerpt)

## *The Elements of a Successful Program*

### Joel J. Alpert, M.D.; Evan Charney, M.D.
### 1973

In light of the historical trends we have outlined and the programs we have reviewed, what can we recommend so that more physicians will be trained who are prepared to practice competent primary care? Of equal importance, can the education insure that most will adapt to, and some lead in, the evolution of primary care practice during their own careers?

We feel confident in the validity of our proposals as they concern educational programs as a result of our own personal experiences. But why limit ourselves to this level of discussion? Let us see how the history of medical education has been influenced by actions and events occurring at much broader levels—within the entire medical school, the practicing profession, the public funding agencies, and the climate and priorities of the time.

We can begin arbitrarily with the Flexner report. It led to a decision to link medical school and university in the 1910-to-1920 period and fostered the subsequent growth and organization of the medical specialties. Consider these extrinsic factors affecting medical education: the limitation on the number of medical student positions during the 1940s and 1950s, the enormous Federal investment in biomedical research in the 1950s and 1960s, the growth of consumerism and the pressure to admit "minority" students in the 1970s. These are all examples of actions largely emanating from forces outside medical education itself—through, significantly, interacting with persons within the educational system—which have had as much impact on shaping the kind of doctor

This chapter originally appeared as Alpert JJ, Charney E. *The Education of Physicians for Primary Care.* Washington, DC: U.S. Department of Health, Education and Welfare; 1973:5–9, 49–63. HRA 74–3113.

who now enters practice as any set of curriculum changes, special programs, or charismatic instructors.

If another example of the influence of public policy on medical education is needed, we should consider the cutbacks in federal funding of biomedical research during the period, 1969 to 1970. Faculty and schools whose income was largely derived from this source—in increasing annual increments—were rudely awakened to the fact that this was not "natural law" but reflected political skills and realities as much as the importance and worth of the research itself. So it will be with the present "natural law" that medical schools turn out large numbers of practitioners and do it immediately.

Medical educators will, therefore, need to be more actively involved in the political processes that influence medical care organization in general and medical education in particular, if their influence is to count. Although we do not possess the knowledge for elaborating on the tactics of this point, we are quite convinced of the correctness of the strategy. This involvement can be at the local and State levels by regional planning and by developing communication with elected representatives. At a national level, spokesmen for medical education—the Association of American Medical Colleges and the professional societies—already have contact with Congressmen directly or through registered lobbyists. These efforts should be understood, supported by the membership, and expanded if possible. Recent events clearly indicate that government support of medical education is changing. It is the responsibility of medical educators to attempt to influence so that the inevitable strings attached to this funding are not tangled, as so often happens, in an irrational fashion.

At the medical school level, a major task of all concerned individuals is to determine exactly where the responsibility for primary care education should lie. Just as medical education and medical research must compete for finite resources at the public level, so primary care must compete for finite educational resources at the medical school level. Part of the failure to accord primary care education a high enough priority in that it is not been the main commitment of any one department within the school. When the time comes to select the medical students, to divide up the curriculum, to select the resident staff, and to outline their program obligations, no one speaks loudly and consistently enough for the needs of the student who will enter primary care. There are exceptions to this, of course; as with "comprehensive medicine," most faculty members think about the problem some of the time. The major clinical departments—particularly internal medicine and pediatrics—have just enough interest in this issue, so that they are often unwilling to relinquish the responsibility to a new department of family medicine, but not enough to develop effective education efforts themselves. The Pellegrino Committee spoke to the issue as follows:

> Inevitably this vexing question will arise: which department should teach the generalist function? . . . In some instances a department of general practice might well be contemplated; in others, the department of medicine, pediatrics or community medicine might take the lead. An interdisciplinary program calling on all departments, but totally dependent on no single one of them might be the optimal solution.[1]

Our feeling is that public pressure may help to force the issue. Outside funds earmarked for primary care education may serve as the necessary stimulus for the medical school to define where its primary care commitments lie. Without intending to equivocate, however, there is danger in imposing too precipitous or too rigid a solution. The "correct" primary care practice model still remains unresolved, although there are probably several satisfactory ones. It would be a mistake to insist on a single template at this time, for the situation at each medical school varies enormously with interested and capable people located in various clinical departments and in the Dean's Office. Moreover, medical schools have the responsibility to evaluate those programs developed in primary care to provide needed data about the pathways traveled.

With these cautions in mind, we suggest steps to be taken at two levels. First, at the National level, those professional organizations that represent medical educators should begin a more active discussion of the problem, both internally and with representatives of other generalist and specialty groups. This need is particularly apparent in internal medicine and pediatrics; their obligations to primary care education and practice and, specifically, their relationship to family medicine should be defined more precisely. Do they wish largely to relinquish their role in primary care to family medicine—the most radical and least likely solution, though possibly the most rational one? Given the great size and diversity of practice in our country, it is more likely that several coexisting patterns will emerge. Indeed, some variation may be desirable, inasmuch as present evidence for the clear superiority of one pattern or the other is lacking. Nevertheless, national education and practice groups must spell out their positions, with the implications of those positions for student education well elaborated. For example, if internal medicine wishes to retain its current *de facto* primary care obligation, how will it help insure that the majority of its trainees do enter primary practice and, just as important, are well prepared for their career? If internal medicine opts to defer to family medicine in this matter, how will it limit its recruitment of medical students to the minority required for consultant work?

Along with this "vertical" debate, a similar "horizontal" discussion should take place within each medical school. Here, two pertinent decisions are to be made. Which department or interdisciplinary division shall "hold the primary care contract," and what are the obligations of the other clinical departments to primary care? All medical school departments ought to have a stake in any program that accounts for the majority of its graduates—assuming the physician retains his role in primary care. Moreover, each department should state its policy and program at the undergraduate, residency, and continuing-education levels for the advice and discussion of the medical school as a whole. As for other departmental obligations, we have in mind those specialties with important but presently ill-defined roles in primary care, such as psychiatry, obstetrics/gynecology, and community medicine. For example, in our review of liaison programs between psychiatry and medicine, we note that psychiatrists rarely have accepted the challenge of developing a body of knowledge and technique appropriate to primary care. Most often, they selected items from general psychiatric theory and practice and adapted them for consultant purposes, rather than developing ideas from the viewpoint of a primary care participant. Moreover, models that have been developed in these programs are more appropriate to a hospital inpatient or outpatient setting, rather than to primary care.

The establishment of a special clinic within a health center is not what we have in mind either. Although there is a place for such clinics, they do not address the issue of major concern. The question is not what the usefulness is in a health center of an adolescent or an orthopedic clinic, but rather what the implications of orthopedic or adolescent medicine are for the organization and practice of primary care. The latter is a much broader and more difficult charge that must be accepted by specialty divisions within schools of medicine if new knowledge is to develop. Much of the problem stems from the facts that we do not, at present, know the answers and that the specialties have been more concerned with elaborating their own discrete areas rather than attending to the needs of the generalist. Once again, this points out the need for research and evaluation. In addition, the very real service and education obligations of the specialties have rarely left sufficient time or physical energy, much less the intellectual energy, for the investment required in developing primary care programs. We see this as a job for the primary and the consultant departments to undertake together. There are persons within the specialties who would find such questions challenging, and they should be encouraged to develop their ideas within the primary care educational setting. It will be necessary to secure sources of funding directly for this task without attaching it so tightly to service demands that, again, a makeshift model is constructed.

In addition to developing and defining its relationship with other departments within the medical school, the unit responsible for primary care needs to establish ties with those involved in other health science fields, particularly in nursing and social service education. At present the relative roles of the physician, nurse, and social worker in primary care is in flux; but communication among these disciplines is essential as new programs develop. Although physicians often prefer to devise model programs without the advice and participation of these allied health professionals, the limitations of such an approach become evident when attempts are made to expand the program beyond the local level. The fact of the matter is that primary medicine does have ill-defined borders with consultant specialties, on the one hand, and with allied health professions, on the other. Although this makes for organizational complexity, it would be better to recognize and legitimize these relationships overtly rather than to develop programs in isolation.

With these broad charges in mind, let us turn now to specific elements within educational programs for primary care. Even with a supportive public climate, allocated funds, and a committed medical school administration and faculty, the quality of any program will be influenced by a number of internal factors. Hansen and Reeb have outlined a very complete curriculum for primary care education.[2] However, in translating their material into a viable program for student and house staff education, attention to the components of the system is of equal importance. As we have noted earlier, many of the programs reviewed herein have shared identifiable and common internal problems that have compromised their educational effectiveness; and, so, attention to these elements may be useful.

Specifically, these elements or ingredients of any program are the students, the faculty, the patients, the curriculum structure, and the setting. They are all interconnected, each affecting the other to form the "learning environment." There is value, however, in considering them separately, in turn, while recognizing that they form an integral pattern within the larger setting of medical education.

# THE STUDENTS

Whatever the other characteristics of the educational program are, they must all funnel into and be processed by the student, the "final common pathway" and a most important ingredient in education. We have discussed student selection of a medical career and correlates of their success during training in an earlier section, but would here stress several aspects of central importance to primary medicine. These are the attraction and selection of suitable candidates, the concept of student readiness and maturity for various aspects of the program, and the responsibility of the student for his own education.

In general, there has been more work toward correlating test performance and personality of medical school applicants with how they behave during medical school and residency than with how they behave in practice. The reasons for this are understandable: although performance during medical education is only an intermediate or process variable, it is the medical faculty's measure of a student's development. Besides, the performance of students in course work appears easier to measure than how they do in practice, where agreed criteria of adequate performance are still lacking. Unfortunately, the correlation of standardized preadmission tests, like the Medical College Admission Test (MCAT) with performance in medical school is not good, much less with performance in residency and practice. Nevertheless, in the absence of demonstrated validity of other measures, admissions committees still lean heavily on demonstrated science skills in their applicants.[3]

Student personalities are fairly well established and conform generally to specific patterns by the time of admission to medical school. It is hardly likely that all with above-average academic ability and a strong natural science background will be more productive and satisfied in careers as primary care physicians than as competent specialists. We need to identify those personal qualities that prove to be valuable assets in primary practice, and here the data is woefully inadequate. The task might properly begin with an attempt to define certain desirable qualities in all those who have entered medical careers. Jeffreys[4] has outlined seven "ideal characteristics" of a doctor as follows:

1. Above-average academic ability, in order to understand the scientific basis of medicine and acquire the diagnostic and therapeutic skills to apply it;

2. Above-average ability to sustain concentrated study;

3. Well-developed humanistic values, including willingness to forego personal comfort and postpone gratification in order to meet health priorities;

4. Willingness to make decisions and carry responsibility;

5. Physical energy and emotional stability;

6. Interpersonal skills, including sensitivity to the needs of others;

7. Capacity to teach, especially in face-to-face clinical settings.

There may be other characteristics that are highly desirable for the practice of primary medicine. For example, Mechanic identified a set of attitudes and orientations that distinguished satisfied from dissatisfied general practitioners in Great Britain. Satisfied doctors "tend to accept more readily than discontented doctors the personal and social aspects of medicine and . . . in contrast to dissatisfied doctors they report that they prefer to work with illness complicated by emotional factors and with patients who question them and ask for more detailed examinations."[5] On the other hand, work from our own country suggests that students who now select general practice as a career share certain characteristics as a group—most of them not what one would consider very desirable—low academic performance, low scores on measures of "theoretical interest," low intrinsic motivation, and high authoritarianism.[6-8] What this may indicate, however, are selective features within the educational structure that propel students with these qualities away from the specialties and therefore toward general practice. The inducement to students with above-average achievement levels to choose specialty careers by specialty faculty is obviously a strong influence.

It may be fairly argued that qualities desirable in a primary care practitioner may not be easy to define, much less measure, and that attitude and personality measurement are not sophisticated or refined enough to be useful. The reality is that some standards are used already and that there is considerable reason to question their appropriateness. Although there is evidence that the student's clinical competence in practice derives from a combination of his personality and background with the length and quality of his training,[9] there is need for more research on the former.

Our recommendation is that attention now be directed to defining qualities that correlate with satisfaction and performance in practice and to devising methods for measuring these qualities. The concept of peer review in primary care may provide an entering wedge into the definition of clinical competence. The process of attending to selection of students for primary care is, itself, likely to be a beneficial one, even if solid techniques are slower to evolve. With a department or division within the medical school responsible for primary care, this would be an appropriate topic for research and a high priority for admissions committees.

A second concept involves the students' readiness for various aspects of the curriculum. Haggerty[10] suggests a bimodal curve of activity in community programs for educational purposes—high in medical school and late residency, low in the internship year when the students deal with acute illness management. The danger of an approach that omits primary care at the internship stage is that the powerful "imprinting" of the internship experience may be difficult to reverse.[11] Again there are few data on which to base a judgment. It does seem logical, however, to argue that all the content areas in primary care cannot be learned equally well at any given stage of training. Areas involving behavioral or social aspects of care are often attractive and pertinent to the student in the late stages of his education, particularly in practice,[12] when they have not proven to be so earlier. Part of this effect may relate to factors of setting, curriculum, and faculty priorities to be discussed; but "mutual-participation" medicine may require a more mature person that "active-passive" medicine does.[13] Dealing with patient problems that require sharing responsibility for management between therapist and patient calls for a degree of security and clinical judgment in the doctor that needs nurture and time to evolve. Therefore, efforts need to be made to integrate practitioners into educational programs, so that they may continue and deepen their skills.

According to many practitioners, a full-time practice gives them insufficient time for participating in continuing education programs. Also, not being able to get coverage of their practice during an extended absence poses an additional problem. Although a decrease in their income would undoubtedly be a deterrent, time and coverage problems are considered crucial. Here, the university can play an active role. Involvement of practitioners in programs of collaborative research[10] can be achieved if secretarial and research assistant support for the practitioner is provided, a relatively modest expense that saves his time. Involvement in longitudinal behavioral "workshops" and preceptorships should also serve to forge links between the medical center and practice that are educational in themselves and can serve as the basis for further sabbatical-type arrangements. Judicious use of new allied health manpower can also be time-saving. If the addition of nurse practitioners enables pediatricians to care for the same patient population with 25 percent less physician-time involved,[14] this, in effect, can free the time of one practitioner in a four-man group practice. The staff might elect to use this "bonus" to develop rotating educational leave program. Some would argue that such an arrangement would defeat the main purpose of the employment of allied health professionals, namely the ability of the same number of physicians to handle an increased patient case-load. On the other hand, there may be long-term benefit in having arrangements to attract and retain more candidates in primary care, especially if they are given the opportunity of periodic release time for study and change of pace.

Part of the income for the practitioner during his sabbatical may be derived from involvement in certain hospital-based ambulatory programs that complement his skills in practice; e.g., working several half-days in a referral diagnostic unit or in a community-based consultation program in mental retardation, cerebral palsy, or school health. However, direct grants to supplement these fellowships will be required as well. Insofar as these programs are oriented toward improving skills appropriate to primary care practice rather than toward wooing the practitioner into a specialist career, they should be encouraged. Again, sponsorship of these postgraduate programs by the primary care unit should help insure that their focus is indeed appropriate. We wish to emphasize that these suggestions are meant more as a stimulus to thought and initiative rather than as a blueprint for specific actions. Ideally, the educational experience should be tailored to the student's level of skills and maturity.

A final consideration should be given to the responsibility of the student for his own education. Millis observes that graduate medical programs "seem to be training (to form or habituate) but ought to be an education (to develop, cultivate, expand)."[15] Central to this distinction is the assumption that a student should be responsible for his own learning throughout his professional career, an avowed goal of all medical education. We believe that the best way to strengthen this assumption is to encourage this self-teaching pattern, while he is still in an educational setting. The rapid trend for more elective studies within medical school is consistent with this goal, but this has been less true of the residency period. In large part, this reflects that ambivalent position of graduate medical education that is a shared responsibility of the hospital, with its heavy service obligation, and the university, whose primary mission is education. The graduate medical student—the resident—must be given the opportunity to create and be responsible for his own education to a greater degree—in a sense, given the right to experiment. The Family Medicine Residency at the University of Miami is a good example of this innovation.[16] Presently, the only way this can be accomplished is to limit the student's service burden to some degree or limit the time now spent in subspecialty education. The utter dependence of most university hospitals on house staff for patient care conflicts with this goal. For example, how can a resident work with a migrant worker group trying to determine its own health needs and, at the same time, deal with the never-ending flow of patients in the emergency department?

We do not advocate the abandonment of clinical responsibility by house staff. On the contrary, this responsibility is an essential ingredient in their education and must be retained. But we must be cognizant of an imbalance existing in many residency programs that is detrimental to the student. Obviously, he must learn his responsibility to the individual sick and needy patient. He also needs the chance to learn his responsibility to the sick and needy community and to define his own role in that community as well. This learning process requires time and experience.

How can time be secured for elective programs within the constraints of an already crowded schedule? Several mechanisms might be considered: first, effective use of technicians and physician assistants who are now part of the hospital setting and also should be maximally utilized to save the resident's time. For example, residents need not perform routine laboratory tests such as collecting blood samples and setting up intravenous infusions, which now are increasingly carried out by technicians. Infant and adult intensive care units, premature nurseries, burn units and other specialty wards now function largely—some would say more effectively—with technician and nurse manpower with the advantage of greater personnel stability than rotating house staff. As hospital specialty care becomes more technologically complex rather than "intuitive," it is increasingly amenable to direction by a specialist physician with technician assistance. At the primary care level, growing evidence that nurse practitioners can assume portions of the traditional physician role lends support to selective apportionment of the student's time in those areas as well. Moreover, at current house staff salary levels, there is less financial inducement to consider the resident a source of cheap labor.

A second and probably more important approach requires that specialty services be more selective in the experience they provide the resident headed for primary care. While we consider it valuable for the student to be intimately

involved in the complex care of the critically ill patient during part of his education, it is difficult to justify the extensive time required for such care in some
internal medicine and pediatric training at present. In part, this reflects the dual
responsibility of both departments for preparing both primary practitioners and
consultants. But, in this combined program, the primary care trainee is shortchanged. Whereas his basic education is finished at the end of residency, most
consultant specialists will have time for the sharpening of their skills during a
fellowship.

Certainly most of the techniques now taught for managing specialty disease
will change within a very few years, in many cases before the student sees
another case in practice. The major justification for his participation must be in
coming to understand the approach of the specialist, in sensing the potentiali-
ties and limitations of his field and in learning what will happen to patients he
refers. While the multiplicity of specialty areas are inherently interesting disciplines themselves, on balance the student may benefit more from time spent in
programs that direct his energy to primary care problem areas. Of course, the
student requires sufficient time in the specialties, so that he may accurately
identify a patient's need for the specialist referral and also learn how the specialist's skills are best adapted to primary care practice.

In short, we suggest "buying time" for elective experiences by maximizing
use of technician and allied health manpower as well as specialty trainees,
rather than automatically staffing expanded specialty and ambulatory services
with primary care students. The value of each segment of the program must be
justified on educational grounds.

Much of the success of the specialty aspects of the residency relates to the
caliber of the consultants as teachers, quite apart from the applicability of their
teaching to primary care. The challenge faced by primary care programs is that
they need to create stimulating and challenging research and educational projects that are as attractive as those of the specialties. This leads to a consideration of the role of the faculty, a second ingredient in the educational
structure.

# THE FACULTY

"Do as I say, not as I do" can be as fallacious in primary care education as it is
in child rearing. For example, the University of Rochester offered a two-year
rotating internship between 1949 and 1961, one purpose of which was to train
the physician for general practice. In a follow-up study, Romano observed that
only seven percent of the trainees, in fact, ended up in general practice.[17] The
program consisted solely of rotations through specialty services, with no

general practitioners at all on the faculty. In fairness to what was felt to be a successful program, a second goal was the provision of a "broader base for the specialist." Outcomes such as these suggest the important influence of the faculty as role models.

It may seem a truism to state that a good program requires good faculty, so let us be more specific. A review of several programs in "comprehensive medicine" reveal faculty who are not engaged in primary practice, either never having done so or having ceased to do so. It would certainly seem incongruous if cardiologists or endocrinologists taught their skills to students and house staff without themselves practicing their disciplines. In the occasional instance where this situation does occur, students are quick to perceive the inconsistency. It seems to imply that primary medical practice is a less demanding or involved field, which can be adequately taught by specialists or nonpractitioners. The impact of this nonverbal communication is not lost on the student. We do not mean to imply that an administrator, a researcher, or indeed an ex-practitioner has no place in primary care education programs. Rather, we suggest that a program with few actual practitioners resembles that description of William Jennings Bryan, when he was likened to the River Platte: one mile wide at the mouth and one foot deep.

A common assumption in many programs is that primary care education requires no special faculty, that subspecialist faculty alone are competent to train the generalist. This assumes that primary care practice is equal to the sum of several specialists' practices. The experience of the Rochester two-year internship suggests otherwise. That is, given the opportunity in such settings, students will opt for specialty careers. Indeed, the current scarcity of primary care practitioners being graduated from our programs is sufficient evidence that specialty oriented training will produce specialty oriented practitioners in an open market setting. What is more difficult to demonstrate is that pediatricians and internists who do end up in primary care practice—the majority—have been shortchanged in their education and would have been better prepared by primary care faculty. Our impression is that, even if the specialist practitioner is an effective teacher, the disadvantages of inappropriate patients, curriculum, and setting within which he functions militate against the educational experience being a sufficient one for primary care.

One problem in faculty selection involves the issue of academic rank and promotion. Should primary care teachers be judged on the same basis as their clinical and basic research colleagues—the quantity and quality of their research, participation in learned societies, teaching responsibilities and skills? This is part of the larger issue of the relative merits of teaching versus research that concerns most university faculties, but it should not present any special or unique problems for primary medicine.

In general, we see three kinds of faculty involved in primary care training—two of them being part-time appointments and one, full-time. Part-time faculty are those whose major source of income and fringe benefits derive from the practice of medicine. One group has a level of involvement typical of most part-time faculty: they participate in some clinical teaching or preceptorships, attend ward rounds, and supervise outpatient clinics. These activities have been performed in the past in return for staff privileges and, generally, are not salaried.

A second group of part-time faculty consists of those who wish to be involved in more extensive primary care education and so reserve a portion of their time—on the order of two or three one-half days weekly—for supervision and involvement with students at various levels. This group should be selected carefully for their teaching skills and be reimbursed for their time. They should be able to supervise the student's development of clinical skills in primary care, which includes interview technique, diagnosis and management of the range of problems commonly seen in practice, rapport with coprofessional, and the techniques of research in practice. For these faculty, university promotion or fringe benefits properly applied are not a central issue. They are working part-time at a job that complements and enriches their practice, and they are remunerated accordingly.

Can funds be obtained for this level of faculty work and from what source? We do not have a ready answer at a time when funding medical education is a complex situation influenced by categorical programs and shifting government priorities. If each part-time physician is paid approximately $5,000 annually for two one-half days per week—in addition to "homework" required, then the equivalent of one full-time position can be used to obtain five or six committed faculty located in various settings in the community. The value of this group both as role models for the students and as advocates for the needs of primary practice within the faculty would be considerable.

The third group of primary care faculty are those with full-time appointments. They direct the educational and research efforts as their principal work, and they practice to the degree necessary to maintain and develop competence and to achieve their educational and research goals. This group is closely identified with the general functions of the medical school and should be promoted and judged on the same basis as their clinical department colleagues. These are the faculty who must carry out the needed research and evaluation in primary care. There is a good supply of faculty in the first two groups, and there appear to be sufficient numbers of students who are attracted to these roles in primary care education to permit the development of a competent total faculty over the next several years. However, this will require the development of special programs to train the faculty, which should be a high-priority matter for private and public funding agencies.

# THE PATIENTS

Although in some ways difficult to separate from the setting, the patients in a primary care program need to have certain characteristics for the program to achieve its aim. For example, variations in age, education, occupation, racial and ethnic background, as well as the living environment—rural, urban, or suburban—all influence patients' medical care behavior, needs, and demands. In addition, particular disease patterns and their prevalence within the population need to be considered. There may be reason to oversample some kinds of patients for the program on any one of these bases. While any hundred families will provide the student abundant experience in the management of common respiratory and gastrointestinal infections, they are less likely to provide experience with long-term management of some chronic diseases, such as diabetes. If the student's experience were otherwise limited to hospitalized patients with ketoacidosis, he would be unlikely to learn the primary care role with such patients. In other words, there is value in allocating the patient load to achieve a distribution of cases that may not otherwise be achieved. Yet this expedient has generally proven a difficult undertaking in the university medical center.

Practically speaking, it is not possible for each student to work with a full spectrum of patient, disease, and setting. In general, it is easier to add patients with selected disease characteristics, who are already concentrated at a university medical center, than it is to provide each student with patients from a range of environmental backgrounds. These cases can represent the oversampling of medical conditions or of well children for longitudinal growth and development observation that students should be in contact with over long periods of time.

An example of how a program might operate at a graduate level would be as follows: Interns are encouraged to select patients to be cared for over the next few years from among those seen during ward or outpatient rotations who either have no identified source of primary care or where arrangements satisfactory to patient and primary care provider can be arranged. Some guidelines may be obtained from dental education where students have to complete a quota of certain restrictions and procedures before being considered well-rounded in his practice. Faculty supervision is required to help him select appropriate numbers and types of cases. If the internship has a large time commitment to acute block rotations, most trainees will not be able to manage and learn from a large continuity panel of patients. There is great individual variation in the interests and capacities of interns and, hence, value in combining good faculty supervision with maximum responsibility by the intern. Essential are adequate supportive services such as secretary answering service, appointment scheduling, nursing, and social work; these can make the difference between a successful or a frustrating experience for patient and student.

In addition, during the resident's subsequent years, he works with one of the ongoing primary care units with which the university has an affiliation. The variations in these units depend on the location of the medical center. In very large urban centers, it may be more difficult to provide the range of setting that may be practical in a smaller city, where exurban or rural settings can be arranged that are within 30 minutes driving distance. However, variation in social class—particularly, with neighborhood health center and private group practice affiliations—would certainly be possible in most cities. Two or three one-half days per week over a year's time can be adequate for the resident to learn the style of the practice and the needs and habits of the patient population. In other words, he may have one single panel of continuity patients, if the primary care setting is located in the hospital as well; or they may be located in two sites. Through periodic formal conferences, simple research projects, and informal communication, experiences of all the residents can be shared. If each program has faculty members who themselves are practicing, then patients may be returned to their full-time care after the student leaves. In practice, many will be satisfied to have another resident, especially if their right to change physicians is known to them and respected. In addition, the presence of allied health professionals—particularly, nurses, lends an important stability and ongoing continuity to the patient's care.

Finally, patients as "whole people" and as "consumers" are more of an influential factor in primary medicine than is true for secondary or tertiary care. Like it or not, the complexities of the disease and the technology of care occupy more of the time and energy of the consultant than they do that of the primary care doctor. Primary care education should allow the trainee to shape his own definition of how a physician relates to the community or, at least, to begin to think along these lines. This is far better done by experience than by lecture. For example, the student ought to see and work with a program's consumer group (Does it have one?) or have the chance to become involved in school health programs, health education, or social action efforts. Students ought to have the opportunity of working with patients or community groups during various phases of a health program's development—its inception and planning, the identification of new service needs, ongoing health education. The essential ingredient here is that the student is involved at a time of experimentation or flux so that he comes to know the processes of change, conflict, and planning as a participant.[18] These are the most difficult kinds of educational experiences to program, and integrating them into a curriculum while respecting the needs of patient, students, faculty, and university can be a trying experience. Avoiding such conflict altogether has its price as well—in the production and endorsement of the "uninvolved" physician.

Although concern has been expressed about the acceptability of medical students by patients in the primary care sector, our experience has shown that, with tact and honesty, patients of all economic classes accept the physician-in-training if they are assured that he is adequately supervised and if their right to change physicians is respected.

In summary, primary education programs ideally should introduce the student to a variety of patients in a variety of roles. The program should itself direct or be affiliated with primary care units, with organizational and patient diversity, at different levels of development. It should function as a laboratory with case material for primary care study—just as patients with different kinds of heart lesions make up the caseload of a cardiology trainee. If primary care education is indeed the major mission of the department, then this approach is a natural one; i.e., core training in primary care with specialty experience selectively added and not the reverse.

# CURRICULUM TIME

There must be adequate time devoted to primary care education, but perhaps more important is that this time be arranged appropriately within the larger curriculum for both medical student and graduate. It is essential to match the "natural history" of the clinical problem to be studied with the student's time allotment. By natural history, we mean the time it takes for key elements of the problem to become detectable or symptomatic, evolve through critical phases, and either stabilize or be resolved in some fashion. The student needs to experience these critical phases himself. So, for example, the natural history of an episode of pneumonia or otitis media lasts a few days or a few weeks in most cases. If students only see such cases for a few minutes in an emergency room setting, they may miss the fact that not all cases are resolved in the same fashion and that patients they themselves have carefully instructed in drug-taking and symptomatic care frequently ignore all such advice and break return appointments. Usually this continuity of care can be arranged by allowing the student to see his own patients in follow-up and by having an assignment that lasts on the order of a month. Similarly, inasmuch as the average acute hospital stay is of approximately one week's duration, rotations of a month or two on an inpatient service usually provide the student with a good grasp of the course and the crises of most acute hospitalizations.

However, many important clinical content areas in primary care take a good deal longer to make their natural history evident, and failure to take account of this can lead both to inadequate education and inadequate care. For example, Brook and colleagues evaluated the follow-up care of 403 patients discharged from the Baltimore City Hospital. Despite adequate inpatient care by university house staff, one-third of the patients had poor subsequent medical care, even with the use of minimal criteria of evaluation.[19] The fact that members of the house staff do not often learn what happens to chronic disease patients after discharge can lead to a distorted perspective in the trainee as well as to inadequate medical practice. Another example of inadequate experience with natural history leading to inappropriate practice can be seen in the advice given to new mothers by hospital nursery personnel. Although most nurses are quite competent at identifying and caring for the sick neonate, their suggestions to mothers at discharge about such common problems as breast feeding often suffer from lack of further contact with the family over the first few months of life. Similarly, one might speculate that liberal visiting hours for hospitalized children took so long to gain acceptance, because hospital staff in large measure were unaware of the reaction to hospitalization that is displayed for months afterward by some young children.

Table 23.1 suggests how a number of clinical topics in primary care can be divided into short—one day to one month, intermediate—two weeks to three months, and long-term—two months to several years categories, based on their natural history. The list is meant to illustrate the concept rather than be exhaustive. These categories overlap in time, as indicated; and their separation is, to an extent, arbitrary.

Medical education cannot provide the student with experience in every problem he will face in practice; but it does need to convey to him a sense of how a range of problems arises, evolves, and is resolved, so that he does not assume an opportunistic, short-term view. Moreover, these content areas cannot all be experienced in one year. Some require more clinical maturity and readiness in the student if they are to have their maximum impact.

In general, programs for both medical school and house staff training have emphasized block, short-term experiences at the expense of longitudinal ones. We would point out that this has been detrimental to subspecialist as well as to primary care education, insofar as since the management of one chronic disease patient over time, for example, is not the educational equivalent of managing several such patients through acute crisis episodes. Both experiences have educational value.

Developing a curriculum with this concept in mind poses a number of practical problems. Who manages the acute intensive care patients when the trainee leaves the ward to see his long-term patients? Who sees the long-term patient when the trainee is detained by a crisis on the ward? One solution is to work in pairs or teams as the students did in practice; another is to assign nurse practitioners to the trainees in the same way dental assistants are assigned to dental students in their training. The same team functions together for three to six months. How is continuity meshed with rotation through other services or other hospitals? Equally difficult for students, particularly at earlier stages of development, is the problem of coping with the change of pace required in moving from acute care, when the basic need is to extract information quickly, to the

**Table 23.1. "Natural History"[a] of Primary Care Content Areas.**

| Short-Term (1 day to 1 month) | Intermediate (2 weeks to 3 months) | Long-Term (2 months to years) |
|---|---|---|
| 1. Most medical and surgical emergencies | 1. Acute or presenting phase of some chronic disease[b] | 1. The family (patient) as the focus, the disease as the episode. Sociology of the family |
| 2. Common infections | a. congenital abnormalities | 2. Most chronic diseases |
| a. pharyngitis | b. diabetes | a. asthma |
| b. otitis media | c. asthma | b. cerebral palsy |
| c. gastroenteritis | d. leukemia | c. mental retardation |
| d. upper- and lower-respiratory infections | 2. Certain behavioral disorders | d. psychosis and neurosis |
| 3. Average acute hospitalization | a. child rearing conflicts | e. diabetes |
| 4. Minor surgical trauma | b. school adjustment problems | 3. Growth and development of children |
| 5. Relationship with the patient which asks why he comes and what needs the professional must meet | c. some marital conflicts | 4. Working as a coprofessional team member |
| | 3. Recurrent abdominal pain | 5. Design and implementation of a patient care research project |
| | 4. Cardiovascular disorder (acute phase), infarction, hypertension, congestive heart failure | 6. A working relation repeated between professional and consumer |
| | 5. Observation of the "milieu of practice," the life-style of the practitioner | |
| | 6. Learning to work on a hierarchically organized team | |
| | 7. Observation of the "milieu" of patient care research. The techniques of research procedures | |

[a]"Natural history": The time it takes for the problem to become detectable or for symptoms to evolve through critical phases and either stabilize or be resolved.

[b]Although this does not define the condition's entire "natural history" it does indicate the duration it usually takes for the condition to be diagnosed and initial management pattern established.

management of long-term problems where a different interview manner and relationship with the patient is required. The trainee may find it difficult to shift his mental gears without grinding his teeth.

During medical school and residency, the student has not been shown that these different situations may require different or more flexible techniques of patient workup. Indeed, except for the work of Weed,[20] medicine has been slow to develop such tools itself. The student soon learns that his all-purpose, complete "New Patient Workup" rarely fits the clinical situation. Moreover, there is insufficient guidance to help him devise a suitable model for the more common brief-but-long-term contact he will have with patients.

Our suggestion is to construct a curriculum by first determining the actual content material to be learned; next, setting priorities within those content areas; third, deciding how intensive and extensive the learning experience must be to match these content areas; and fourth, specifying that stage of student maturation when the material is most appropriate. Finally, the curriculum should be shaped to meet all these needs. It is far less rational to first decide what service commitments exist and then assign students to fit those needs, as occurs in house staff programs. Undergraduates should begin medical school with exposure to and contact with patients whose needs are in the primary care area. Residency should include initial involvement in a primary care setting as a beginning for a longitudinal experience.

# THE SETTING

The setting of the primary care education program—specifically its size, organization, and relationship to secondary and tertiary care systems and to the patient population—is the last of our ingredients and a crucial one for the success of the program. We refer here to the "style" of the setting as well as to its formal organizational and physical aspects. Specifically, what kinds of problems are considered important or trivial by the staff? How well do physicians and allied professionals communicate with each other? How isolated or integrated is the program from the problems of the community?

For example, evidence was cited earlier about impact of work setting on performance of those in practice. No less significant is this influence in educational programs. Using National Board Examination scores as criteria, Levit and colleagues showed that interns in hospital programs with a full complement of house staff demonstrate greater gains in clinical competence after one year than those in hospitals that do not fill internship positions, regardless of the intern's competence on entry to the program.[21]

In a discussion of educational programs for primary care, Hansen notes, "When primary care responsibilities or functions compete with consultant or tertiary care responsibilities, the primary care functions are consistently underrated by both teacher and student."[22] Although this may reflect qualities of the teacher and student, we believe that the observation holds true largely due to the influence of the setting. If the style, pace, location, and organization is not basically concerned with primary care, and it is seen only as an unwanted but necessary chore, then teacher and student will not be concerned either. It is as impractical to demonstrate primary care practice within most university hospital settings as it is to teach techniques of gall bladder surgery in a neighborhood health center. One of the reasons for the success of the Kansas rural preceptor program[23,24] was the chance for the "student to participate almost totally in a 'medical way of life' and identify with the preceptor in many ways."[25] This is a clear indicator of the impact of the setting on education.

Learning how to diagnose and manage psychological problems has been a particularly vexing and difficult problem in the education of the general physician. A major factor in this difficulty has been the inappropriateness of the setting of the program. Although exemplary techniques of interviewing patients in the hospital[26] or of socially oriented ward rounds[27] have been described, their success seems in large part to stem from the enthusiasm or skill of an instructor. When this is missing, the programs are less successful; and when the original staff changes, the technique is abandoned altogether.

Ward attending rounds, for example, often omit discussion of the social or psychological aspects of the case and, in fact, often ignore the patient altogether. "Give us the lab results and we will do the job" conveys the spirit. Payson and Barchas observed that regular attending physicians spent less than a fifth of their time with the patient during rounds; and most of that one-fifth was spent dealing with physical factors. They concluded that there was "less emphasis on bedside demonstration of individual or personal aspects of medical care than most attending physicians realized. Rounds appeared to show how senior physicians arrive at decisions and relate case findings to medical theory. They did not emphasize the physician's approach to the patient and the establishment of the doctor-patient relationship."[28] As one attending physician stated with candor, "I never discuss what I feel uncertain about. I try to limit my comments to the aspects of scientific medicine that I feel expert in."[28] And at times, inappropriate decisions are made by physicians due to missing psychological information.[29]

Our reaction is not to point with horror at such incidents, but to admit the basic validity of these observations. If we wish to teach about social and psychological factors, this is probably best done where the setting, among other factors, is appropriate. In the instance of inpatient rounds, the curriculum time may not permit the student to unravel the psychological factors that have led to the hospitalization nor to the sequelae after discharge. The setting maximizes acute organic medicine, and the student responds accordingly. In a sense, for him to dwell on social and psychological factors may be unproductive. He would need the time and facilities to follow all his patients, a practical impossibility when the next case of cardiac failure or meningitis is arriving from the emergency department. The student is most likely to learn how to elicit, to appreciate, and to utilize social and psychological data when the curriculum permits long-term contact with and responsibility for some patients and when the setting prompts him to consider such problems as pertinent. However, the curriculum, including attending rounds, is not so fixed that the human aspects of care cannot be included.

Our recommendation, then, is that university schools of medicine become involved in primary care settings and that they conduct their educational and research business in settings either purposely built or within existing practices adapted to meet educational needs. We use the term "involved" advisedly. Obtaining a balance between just enough involvement to insure that the experience is educationally valuable, but not so much that the service burdens are overwhelming is easier said than done. We have been critical in the past of some earlier "comprehensive clinic" programs, largely because they are unrepresentative of primary care. However, investing all the effort of a school into a single large health center practice in order to achieve "reality" has its own drawbacks. It will demonstrate only one kind of practice organization with one kind of patient population, and it will assume a service burden not easily or ethically terminated at a later date if the situation should change. In short, one large "model program" may absorb faculty time and allegiance to a degree that may limit flexibility and preclude the change for continuing experimentation and "tinkering" that should characterize a laboratory setting. As another alternative, new programs might consider the following approach as another.

The university sponsors a teaching practice of no more than several hundred families—large enough to have an air of reality and small enough to ensure that all of the practitioners (other than the students) can be full-time faculty. The allied health professional staff are chosen for their teaching as well as their practice skills. The practice is housed in or very close to the main teaching hospital in order to facilitate integration with inpatient and subspecialty education. However, it is sufficiently independent of the hospital so that professional roles, record systems, patient intake procedures, and other matters can be changed without conflict with existing hospital policies. Within the practice are the "overrepresented" patients suggested earlier. This kind of program sacrifices the reality of practice to a degree because heavy educational priorities—i.e., supervised interviewing and consultation with faculty—preclude concentrating on high-volume patient flow and efficiency to the degree required in practice. In general, this is the model most common in the new family medicine programs, and it contains many elements of the earlier Family Care Programs.

Complementing the above program are relationships, developed slowly and selectively over several years with existing or new group practices, health centers, or solo practitioners. The university "contracts," as described earlier, for the teaching time of some part-time faculty within these practices. Responsibility for service does not depend here on the students to the degree that it does in the hospital program. Programs are selected for affiliation not only because they exemplify quality care, but also because they offer diversity in setting or clientele. This would represent a contemporary application of the preceptorship.

During elective portions of the curriculum, medical students and house staff work with consumer or practice units at varying stages of program development. Commitment for service or involvement is limited to that student group's tenure for the most part. In some instances, more permanent affiliations characteristic of the first two groups of programs may evolve.

We have cautioned against the problem of excessive service obligations incurred in the hospital as a result of the need to find financial support for the resident, and we would not like to see primary care programs end up with the same conflict. Our point is that resident staff are capable of providing high-quality primary care service under supervision in the same way they provide service in the secondary and tertiary care settings. If income from these sources is available, it should be utilized. Ideally, direct funds for education are needed as well, to avoid sole dependence on this one source of income.

A significant handicap in the development of new primary care programs is the obligation to meet service needs that already exist in the hospital inpatient and outpatient department. Most programs will have to contend with this reality in addition to fashioning new models. Existing hospital organization and the traditional clinic system constitute formidable barriers to change.

We have suggested that judicious use of allied health manpower, and greater selectivity in the involvement of trainees in specialty services are required. However, the hospital ambulatory services pose a special problem. The number of patient visits has increased rapidly in most urban locales over the past decade. In addition, the responsibility for clinic management has usually fallen to those on the faculty who are most closely allied with primary care education, absorbing all their teaching and administrative energies in less than ideal settings. In fact, hospital outpatient and emergency departments increasingly provide the first contact portion of primary care to the community as the supply of general practitioners dwindles, and trainees are involved in a large share of that work. A vicious cycle ensues. Fewer generalists in practice mean more people using hospital ambulatory service. In response to this demand from the community, hospitals modernize and expand their facilities and, thereby, attract even more patients. What has evolved is an *ad hoc* pattern of medical care, facilitated in part by the availability of hospital-based trainee manpower. We consider this an inappropriate, short-term response to a long-term need. Indeed, insofar as it endorses short-order emergency room care as the primary practice model, it may have serious long-term consequences. Although this is one solution to the primary care problem, it is not the only one. By investing our trainee manpower in the operation of this model, we limit our option to support and develop others. Equally important, the student confronted with an unsatisfying model of care will be convinced that primary care or what he sees of it is the last thing he wishes to practice.

What can be recommended to resolve the conflict between new program needs and old program demands? First of all, we would emphasize that the problem is not likely to be solved unless we educate more primary care practitioners, a goal to which this monograph is devoted. In the meantime, two approaches are suggested:

Where educational programs are already responsible for significant ambulatory care service, the caseload should be analyzed into its component parts. These usually involve some combination of emergency medical and surgical services, short-term consultation, long-term management of chronic disease, and primary care. These separate functions each lend themselves to different organizational structures and staffing patterns. For example, emergency care needs rapid patient intake and processing facilities, specialized nurse and technician manpower, easy access to surgical and medical specialty consultation, and relatively expensive equipment.

Short-term consultation service requires a good prior sorting system, so that efficient use is made of subspecialist time. The unit stresses good working knowledge of an integration with community health resources, particularly for primary care and chronic disease, so that effective and pragmatic recommendations for follow-up care can be made. Access by the patient is indirect, through primary care resources in the community. The pace of the unit is slower and more capable of regulation.

Long-term management of selected chronic disease involves active participation of the patient in planning his care. Efficiency and speed in patient flow are less vital than a staff that is sensitive to the support-and-caring aspects of medicine.

Primary care embodies aspects of all of these, but it especially stresses easy access for the patient and a staff that has the capability and skills of outreach and follow-up in the community, rather than the highly technical skill required for emergency care or the in-depth knowledge of certain diseases required in chronic illness management. If the entire outpatient service is not large, several of these functions can, of course, be combined successfully by one well-trained and flexible staff. Student physicians who staff several of these services simultaneously often have a difficult time shifting roles, especially if the support staff structure is not designed to meet the needs of the service required.

In short, a good deal more than the "diagnosis-prescription" function of the physician is required to carry out these several tasks successfully, and some reorganization of the services based on patient need would improve the quality of service and the efficiency of the staff.

With the other ambulatory functions separated out, the needs of those using the service for primary care should then be defined accurately. Who are the patients? Where do they come from? Are there actually several different populations using the service for somewhat different purposes—suburbanites for occasional care when their doctor is unavailable or others for all their health needs? What other resources are available? Finally, should an attempt be made within the hospital setting to provide care in a setting more suitable for service and education? This last point requires some difficult decisions. A proportion of emergency room users may not be able to tolerate a long-term, intimate relationship with a health program, which is why they use the emergency facilities in the first place. They may resist being incorporated into a "model practice." Although this is an interesting group to study and to learn more about, they are frustrating to physicians in training and to experienced physicians as well. Having a mature group of full-time faculty and allied professionals share their care can enable students to live with and learn from the rejection they encounter at times. Our recommendation here is to aim for some kind of patient diversity if at all possible. Multiproblem, disorganized families should be part of any teaching program, because they are a part of the reality of practice or should be. They should not, however, be the only group involved in the teaching program. Until adequate primary care resources are available in the community, some programs may have to live with two standards of care provided: a more complete service to a selected group in a longitudinal teaching program and first-contact service on an episodic basis to others.

As a more adequate, long-term solution to the problem, medical education personnel should participate with area-wide health planning units to encourage and stimulate the development of adequate primary care education and service programs outside of the hospital. Planning agencies should be educated to the need for allied health manpower training tied into stable primary care settings. For example, the integration of public health resources now involved in some aspects of primary care such as well-child conferences and visiting nurse services with existing or planned primary care practices may stretch the resources and capabilities of both. In Great Britain, the attachment of health visitors and district nurses (public health nurses) to general practice groups has been accomplished in more than one-half of physician practices with evidence of benefit to patients and providers.[30,31]

While the problem of ambulatory service demands in hospitals is a growing one, we would hope that a combination of more rational, community-wide planning for primary care needs of the total population, adequate funding through a national health insurance scheme, and an increased output of primary care personnel in more effective organizations will be sufficient to reverse the current trend toward inappropriate use of facilities.

# CONCLUSION

If a rapid increase in the number of primary care practitioners is the paramount objective of the Federal Government, we acknowledge that influences outside the medical education system may be all that is required to effect such a change. A shift in terms of financial support to education directed specifically to this end—namely, incentives for the production of primary care physicians, changes in the medical practice system, and some limitation on the availability of sub-specialty careers—would probably have the desired effect. Our strong preference, however, is that not only more practitioners be prepared, but also that they be better educated for their practice. To accomplish this aim, changes within medical education are needed as well.

At the national level, professional societies should enter into discussion with family medicine representatives on their relative roles and obligations in primary care. The implications of any decisions for manpower recruitment and education must be spelled out.

The university should acknowledge its role in coordinating primary care education at the medical school and at graduate and continuing education levels. Such coordination should be accomplished in conjunction with those representing the public and the practicing professions.

The medical school must set as a priority the development of criteria for selecting students who will be suitable candidates for careers in primary medicine practice.

Within each medical school, a department or division responsible for primary care education should be identified or developed. This department should have the responsibility to develop an overall program for primary care education at the undergraduate and graduate levels. It has a particular responsibility to devise continuing education programs that will link the practitioner and the educational unit. Extended leave educational programs for practitioners, collaborative research effort with physicians in practice, and part-time faculty roles should be particularly encouraged. Research and evaluation must be an important activity of the academic medical center in primary care.

The obligations of medical school specialty departments to primary care education must be further defined. These departments in the past have correctly considered the development of their own disciplines as a priority. However, at present, there is an important gap between specialty medicine's body of knowledge and technique and the application of this knowledge at the primary care level. The fact that most physicians in training will end up in primary care practice—short of a major revolution in the way medicine is practiced—underscores the importance of utilizing appropriate aspects of all of medicine to primary care practice.

The university should develop sites for primary care education under its own auspices. These will require a variety of contractual relations, ranging from ownership and direction to short-term and loose affiliations for educational purposes only. In selecting programs to establish or to affiliate with, a diversity of patient population and practice organizations should be sought. These settings together should be considered a part of the university medical effort. They should be closely integrated with the hospital, but continue to remain independent.

In short, all components of the medical education process, which includes the medical school, its parent university, and the teaching hospital, have important work to do. At present, there is a good deal of uncertainty as to how we ought to provide high-quality medical care to our Nation. On the other hand, the uncertainty provides a climate that favors change and in which the education of the primary physician can be reshaped and improved dramatically.

## Notes

1. Pellegrino E, et al. Planning for comprehensive and continuing care of patients through education. *J Med Educ*. 1968;43: 751.

2. Hansen MF, Reeb KG. The outline of a curriculum. *J Med Educ*. 1970;45:1007.

3. Rutstein D. Physicians for Americans: two medical curricula. *J Med Educ*. 1961;36:129.

4. Jeffreys M. Factors determining the choice of medicine as a career. Paper presented at the World Health Organization Conference on Selection of Students for Medical Education, Bern, Switzerland, 1971.

5. Mechanic D. General practice in England and Wales: results from a survey of a national sample of general practitioners. *Med Care*. 1968;6:245.

6. Sanazaro P. Research in medical education: exploratory analysis of a black box. *Ann NY Acad Sci*. 1965;128:519.

7. Monk MA, Terris M. Factors in student choice of general or specialty practice. *N Engl J Med*. 1956;255:1135.

8. Coker RE, Greenberg BG, Kosa J. Authoritarianism and Machiavellianism among medical students. *J Med Educ*. 1965;40:1075.

9. Lyden F, Geiger HJ, Peterson OL. *The Training of Good Physicians*. Cambridge, Mass: Harvard University Press; 1968.

10. Haggerty RJ. The university and primary medical care. *N Engl J Med*. 1969;281:416.

11. Mumford E. *Interns: From Students to Physicians.* Cambridge, Mass: Harvard University Press; 1970.

12. Sumpter EA, Friedman SB. Workshop dealing with emotional problems: one method of preventing the "dissatisfied pediatrician syndrome." *Clin Pediatr.* 1968;7:149.

13. Szasz TS, Hollender MH. A contribution to the philosophy of medicine. *Arch Intern Med.* 1956;97:585.

14. Charney E, Kitzman, H. The child health nurse (pediatric nurse practitioner) in private practice: a controlled trial. *N Engl J Med.* 1971;285:1353.

15. Millis JS. Objectives of residency training. *Can Med Assoc J.* 1969;100:599.

16. Carmichael L, Shore W, Frey J. Teaching ambulatory pediatrics in family health care programs. Workshop presented at the 12th annual meeting of the Ambulatory Pediatric Association, May 23, 1972.

17. Romano J. Study of a two-year rotating internship, University of Rochester Medical Center, 1949–61. *JAMA.* 1964;189:283.

18. Dixon JP. Teaching physicians to be agents of social change. *Arch Environ Health.* 1965;10:713.

19. Brook RH, Appel FA, Avery C, Orman N, Stevenson RL. Effectiveness of inpatient follow-up care. *N Engl J Med.* 1971;285:1509.

20. Weed L. *Medical Records, Medical Education, and Patient Care.* Cleveland: Press of Case Western Reserve; 1969.

21. Levit EJ, Schumacher CF, Hubbard JP. The effect of characteristics of hospitals in relation to the caliber of interns obtained and the competence of interns after 1 year of training. *J Med Educ.* 1963;28:909.

22. Hansen MF. An educational program for primary care. *J Med Educ.* 1970;45:1001.

23. Dimond E. The general practitioner and the medical school. *JAMA.* 1954;156:95.

24. Rising JD. The rural preceptorship. *J Kans Med Soc.* 1962;68:81.

25. White KL. General practice in the U.S. *J Med Educ.* 1964;39:333.

26. Engel G. Care and feeding of the medical student. *JAMA.* 1971;215:1135.

27. Bates B. Comprehensive medicine: a conference approach. *J Med Educ.* 1965;40:778.

28. Payson HE, Barchas JD. A time study of medical teaching rounds. *N Eng; J Med.* 1965;273:1468.

29. Duff RS, Hollingshead AB. *Sickness and Society.* New York: Harper & Row; 1968.

30. Ambler M, Anderson J, Black M, et al. Attachment of local health authority staff to general practices. *Medical Officer.* May 1965:295.

31. McGregor A. Total attachment of community nurses to general practices. *Br Med J.* 1969;2: 291.

# CHAPTER TWENTY-FOUR

# Residency Training in Internal Medicine: Time for a Change?

Steven A. Schroeder, M.D.; Jonathan A. Showstack, M.P.H.;
Barbara Gerbert, Ph.D.
1986

The existence of internal medicine as a specialty with its own certifying board dates back to 1936, and for years this field has been regarded by many as the most challenging, comprehensive, and exciting of all the medical specialties. Flexible enough to adapt to the proliferation of its subspecialties without becoming balkanized (as has surgery), internal medicine has met the challenge of the scientific and technologic explosion after World War II. Its training programs, which have featured a hospital-based educational model, have traditionally attracted many of the medical students with the best academic records. Within academic health centers, departments of internal medicine have been recognized as the flagship units, and the reputations of many medical schools have soared or plummeted with the reputation of their department of medicine. In short, internal medicine has been seen as the specialty that has most effectively integrated the science and art of medicine.

There is concern today, however, that internal medicine stands at a critical juncture. By hewing to a training model that was historically appropriate but now may need reassessment, its programs are in danger of becoming less relevant to the practice of medicine in the decades ahead. Although there is not a consensus that internal medicine is in trouble, evidence suggests that it is time to reassess the philosophy and structure of its graduate medical educational programs, especially residency training. To some extent anecdotal, this evidence includes reports that the brightest medical school graduates are increasingly turning away from internal medicine and selecting such fields as ophthalmol-

This chapter originally appeared as Schroeder SA, Showstack JA, Gerbert B. Residency training in internal medicine: time for a change? *Ann Intern Med.* 1986;104(4):554-561. Copyright © 1986, American College of Physicians–American Society of Internal Medicine. Reprinted with permission.

ogy, radiology, and anesthesiology;[1] that many graduates of internal medicine residencies are electing to pursue careers in radiology, dermatology, anesthesiology, critical care, or emergency medicine rather than internal medicine; and that graduates who remain in internal medicine criticize their training programs as not having prepared them sufficiently to practice as internists.[2-5]

To a degree, these problems may merely reflect trends in the organization, financing, and content of medicine that are beyond the capability of internal medicine programs to redress. The thesis of this analysis, however, is that dramatic changes are occurring in the practice of internal medicine that require revising internal medicine training. In particular, the shift of much internal medicine practice from hospital to ambulatory settings, the increasing demands for internists to provide perioperative consultation, and the probability that most internists—subspecialists as well as generalists—will provide general medical care call into question the educational validity of the traditional hospital-based training.

# THE TRADITIONAL MODEL OF INTERNAL MEDICINE TRAINING

Except for the period between 1970 and 1977, when many residents bound for internal medicine subspecialties were permitted to "short track" after only 2 years of residency training, eligibility for the internal medicine certifying examination has required 3 years of training in an accredited program. The first year characteristically involves intensive experience in the care of hospitalized patients on general medicine and subspecialty services, in the coronary and intensive care units, and in the emergency room. Many programs also include a half-day per week in the continuous care of outpatients. Although the special requirements of the American Board of Internal Medicine state that "the continuity experience should be at least a half-day per week,"[6] apparently many programs still defer this experience until the second year.

The second and third years feature increasing responsibility for more patients on general medicine and subspecialty wards. These rotations are interspersed with time in special care units as well as in block rotations in internal medicine subspecialties. Subspecialty rotations characteristically involve responding to requests for consultation from within the entire hospital, exposure to the technologies of that subspecialty (for example, liver biopsy, upper gastrointestinal endoscopy, sigmoidoscopy, and colonoscopy), and participating in the subspecialty outpatient clinic. Overall, we estimate that, including continuity care, only about 15% of the time of internal medicine residents is spent in ambulatory care (excluding time in the emergency room).

During the past decade, a variant of this model has emerged, the primary care general internal medicine residency track, sponsored initially by The Robert

Wood Johnson Foundation and more recently by the Bureau of Health Professions, Department of Health and Human Services. These programs require a minimum of 25% of the 3 years be spent in the continuing ambulatory care of a group of patients, as well as additional ambulatory time spent in the internal medicine subspecialties and those epidemiologically relevant, non-internal-medicine specialties such as dermatology, office gynecology, and office orthopedics. They also feature more exposure to the social and psychologic aspects of patient care, placing more stress on the recognition and treatment of depression and somatization disorders, on achieving skills in interviewing and in motivating patient compliance and changes in lifestyle, and on understanding the interactions among illness, stress, and personality. Few such programs exist, however; in 1984 there were only about 50 primary care medicine programs, accounting for about 5% of all internal medicine residency positions.[7]

The traditional internal medicine model of intensive and graduated hospital experience has been durable, and for good reason: it provides exposure to the very sickest patients, concentrates patients with severe disease in a convenient time and spatial framework, uses faculty time efficiently, and has heretofore been paid as a part of a hospital's routine costs. Concentrating on care of the very sick accomplishes several important educational objectives. It ensures that trainees will be confident and competent in the face of catastrophic illness, provides a sound foundation in pathophysiology, and motivates residents to prevent illness as well as to detect and treat it at the earliest possible stage. Our concern, however, is that the cumulative effects of changes in the practice of internal medicine threaten the relevance of the traditional model, and that residency programs must adapt to these changing patterns or risk becoming obsolete.

# MEDICAL PRACTICE AND INTERNAL MEDICINE TRAINING

The model of internal medicine residency training has remained relatively constant despite recent dramatic changes in the practice of medicine. Consequently, unintended changes in the residency have resulted, and further ones can be projected.

## Recent Changes

Declining length of hospital episodes, increasing intensity of hospital care, a shift of important diagnostic and management decisions from the hospital to the office setting, an increasing proportion of internal medicine admissions at teaching hospitals for specific invasive procedures, continued evolution of hospitals into surgical institutions, the increasing burden of chronic illness (particularly among the elderly), and the impending oversupply of physicians and especially subspecialists are all recent changes in internal medicine practice.

These trends, which result from powerful economic, demographic, and technologic forces, are creating major changes in clinical practice that have profound educational implications.

**Declining Length of Hospital Stay.** Patients in the United States are hospitalized for shorter periods than are patients in other Western industrialized countries.[8] This trend has accelerated recently because of mounting pressures for cost containment and the move toward fixed-price payment for hospital care. For example, the average length of stay for all patients decreased from 7.82 days in 1970 to 6.67 in 1984, a 15% decline. For Medicare patients, the drop was even more dramatic, from 12.6 to 7.4 days, a 41% decrease. The decreasing length of stay for Medicare patients has been accelerated by recent legislative changes in the ways hospitals are paid; fully one third of the decline in length of stay over the past 15 years has occurred in the last 2 years.[9] Moreover, length of stay will probably continue to decrease.

The decline in length of hospital stay has several educational consequences. As patients who can receive care elsewhere leave the hospital, the residency experience comes to concentrate on a sicker and more disabled group of patients. The decreasing length of stay reduces the time available for residents to interact with those patients and inhibits full appreciation of the natural history of disease, the psychosocial aspects of illness, the rehabilitative process, and the long-term effects of therapeutic interventions.[10] It thereby impairs the ability of residents to know how their patients' diseases affect their lives, thus isolating residents from information essential for good diagnostic and therapeutic decisions.

**Increasing Use of the Intensive Care Unit.** To accommodate the needs of those patients who remain in the hospital, many of whom need support of multiple organ systems, intensive care units have proliferated.[11] Today, about one in eight teaching hospital beds is in an intensive care unit, and the percentage is much higher in some hospitals.[12]

A vivid example of how the change in the nature of hospitalized patients distorts graduate medical education is pediatrics, where the neonatal intensive care unit has been one of the fastest growing pediatric services in major teaching hospitals. To provide around-the-clock coverage for these precariously ill infants, pediatric residency programs began assigning more time to rotations in neonatal intensive care units. Finally, in 1978 the National Pediatric Task Force[13] was forced to recommend limiting this experience to a maximum of 6 months of the 36-month residency period. This recommendation was later adopted by the pediatric residency review committee.

For internal medicine residents, more exposure to intensive care brings greater technical proficiency in those procedures required for the care of patients who need assistance with vital functions. It also means adjusting to a patient population that has a very guarded prognosis. It is not clear that further intensive care experience will bring commensurate educational benefits.

**The Locus of Critical Decisions Shifts out of the Hospital.** The increasing sophistication of diagnostic and therapeutic technologies means that many crucial patient management decisions are no longer made in the hospital. Hospitalizations for the purpose of making a diagnosis are less necessary as sophisticated noninvasive imaging and other techniques permit extensive diagnostic evaluation of ambulatory patients. Similarly, increasingly powerful therapeutic agents permit effective treatment in the ambulatory setting. New cases of diabetes (except those in patients with flagrant ketoacidosis), hyper- and hypothyroidism, adrenal insufficiency and Cushing's disease, renal failure, cancer, inflammatory bowel disease, pneumonia, and heart failure are now frequently diagnosed and treated in the ambulatory setting. Furthermore, many of the acute exacerbations of chronic diseases are now managed effectively without hospitalization. Critical decisions about changing therapy for ambulatory patients with rheumatoid arthritis, inflammatory bowel disease, cancer, angina, diabetes, and respiratory illness are made daily by internal medicine subspecialists and generalists without residents being exposed to any of these patients in the hospital.

Consequently, hospital-based residents tend to see those patients who do not respond to multiple therapies, such as those with refractory asthma or those who comply poorly with their medication schedule and are hospitalized for emergency care (for example, those with severe asthma, gastrointestinal bleeding, or the complications of alcoholism and drug addiction). At the same time, residents are deprived of the opportunity to think through a diagnostic or treatment approach to many of the most remediable problems. Hospital internal medicine services are increasingly becoming a place for the desperately ill, terminally ill, elderly, demented, or those in need of specific procedures.

**Increasing Admissions for Specific Procedures.** As the subspecialties of internal medicine continue to develop their diagnostic technologies, more of a subspecialist's practice will consist of doing procedures. Even though many of these procedures can be done in the office, some still require hospitalization. In many major teaching hospitals, an increasingly common reason for admission to the medical service is to do coronary arteriography, endoscopic retrograde cholangiopancreatography, electrophysiologic studies of the cardiac conduction system, or other procedures. At the University of California, San Francisco, Hospital, approximately 25% of all medical admissions are for such procedures (Fitz G, personal communication). These studies are almost always elective, the decision to do them having already been made in the office by the attending subspecialist or even by the referring primary physician. Often these patients are admitted in the evening, have their procedures the following morning, and are discharged that afternoon or early the next day.

How much this "revolving door" experience adds to the residency learning process is unclear. A more optimal pattern would be for the resident to participate in the decision to do the procedure and then to evaluate the effect of test results on subsequent management. Unfortunately, this pattern, which would require an integrated educational experience, that emphasizes continuity between ambulatory and hospital care, is missing from all but a few internal medicine training programs.

**The Hospital as a Surgical Institution.** In many hospitals, especially academic centers, an increasing proportion of admissions and occupied beds is being devoted to surgery, often for patients with multiple chronic illnesses.[14] Pressures to reduce hospital stays have transferred the site of preoperative evaluation from the hospital to the office setting. In addition, more surgery is being done on an outpatient or "come and go" basis.

The educational implications of these changes are that, as in the past, internists will be called on to manage patients with chronic medical illness; now, however, the patient will be awaiting surgery or recovering from it. An ideal accommodation would be to shift some hospital training from traditional medical services to a surgical consultation rotation. This shift, however, involves some loss of territory for the department of medicine, loss of autonomy for the resident, and acculturation by the resident to the different social organization of the surgical team. Nevertheless, it appears to be responsive to the educational needs of internal medicine residents preparing for future practice.

## Future Trends

A review of the past 75 years shows how difficult it is to predict the future need for physicians. Scientific advances and unforeseen epidemics may change medical practice in unexpected ways. Who could have predicted how the development of antibiotics would alter the practice of otorhinolaryngologists, the bulk of whose operations once consisted of tonsillectomy and adenoidectomy or mastoidectomy, or how the discovery of antituberculosis drugs would affect the practice of chest physicians? Recent immunologic and chemotherapeutic breakthroughs have profoundly changed the subspecialties of oncology and infectious diseases, and no one could have predicted the epidemic of the acquired immunodeficiency syndrome. Nevertheless, at least four current trends in medical care promise to be enduring and to have important consequences for the practice of internal medicine.

**Changing Patterns of Internal Medicine Practice.** We may expect the acute-care hospital to become increasingly a site for surgical treatment, certain diagnostic procedures, treatment of certain complications of chronic illnesses, and care for the desperately ill. Admission for the purpose of diagnosis will become more rare, and those admitted for the treatment of acute and chronic illnesses will have more intense treatment at the beginning of the hospitalization and then will be discharged to home or convalescent facilities as soon as feasible. The result will be further compression and intensification of care, such that entire hospitals may come to resemble what is currently the intensive care unit. Patterns of care will thus diverge from the office practice of internal medicine, and internists will be more split into those who are dominantly hospital based (for example, infectious disease, critical care, and coronary care specialists) and those who are not (for example, rheumatologists, endocrinologists, and generalists). Three distinct patterns of internal medicine practice may emerge: the hospital-based critical care subspecialist, the predominantly procedure-oriented subspecialist, and the office-based specialist and generalist. (Obviously there will be some flexibility in these patterns, with the first group having limited office hours and the last performing some consultative and primary care for hospitalized patients.)

**Demographic Changes.** The familiar litany of the demographics of aging need not be repeated. The increasing proportions of the population who are over age 65, 75, and 85, combined with the recent dramatic declines in age-specific mortality rates for the elderly, mean that more of internists' time and effort will be devoted to the care of elderly patients with chronic illnesses. Internists already see more older patients than do other physicians. In 1981, about 71% of visits to internists were by patients aged 45 or older, compared with less than 40% for other specialists.[15] As the population changes, more and more of an internist's practice will consist of treating the elderly. Care of the elderly will include not only the traditional sites of office and hospital but also institutional settings and the home.

The Federated Council for Internal Medicine has recently recognized deficiencies in residency training in geriatric medicine and has made several recommendations to improve teaching of geriatrics to residents.[16] Because medical manpower trends and economics make it unlikely that internal medicine will abandon the care of the elderly to geriatricians, it seems obvious that internal medicine training must ensure acquisition of those skills and experiences necessary to practice geriatric medicine. These include knowledge about specific diseases and conditions with high prevalence in the elderly, such as dementia, incontinence, insomnia, osteoporosis, and falls; a better understanding of certain general principles such as clinical pharmacology, sexuality, psychogeriatrics, and bioethics; a greater knowledge of resources needed for the homebound and institutionalized elderly; and the attitudes, knowledge, and skills that will permit the physician to function as an advocate for the elderly.

**Managed Systems of Care.** Another important trend is the growth of managed systems of care, such as health maintenance organizations and corporate medicine. Spurred by continued preoccupation with medical costs and by the political strategy of placing physicians at financial risk to motivate them to contain costs, enrollment in health maintenance organizations has grown by over 20% per year recently, and it has been estimated that 55 million people will belong to such organizations by the year 1993.[17] Physician-staffing patterns in health maintenance organizations differ from those in fee-for-service settings in two important ways. First, health maintenance organizations employ far fewer physicians per population—approximately 1/1,000 patients as opposed to 1.9 in the country as a whole.[7] Second, about 60% of physicians in health maintenance organizations are generalists, as opposed to only about 25% in the United States.[7,8] How these two trends in physician staffing of health maintenance organizations will affect the total numbers of internists needed is unclear, but they suggest a need to shift the current specialist-to-generalist ratio within internal medicine. Whether health maintenance organizations choose to have their generalist care provided mainly by generalists or whether they will depend more on internal medicine subspecialists to provide generalist care, the implications for training are that most internists will need to function at least partly as generalists and therefore will need to learn generalist skills, especially in ambulatory care.

**Physician Oversupply.** The impending oversupply of physicians in subspecialty fields has important implications for internal medicine training.[7,8,18] Because most internal medicine subspecialists will find it difficult to sustain a purely subspecialty practice, they will be compelled, at least for economic reasons, to function to some degree as generalists.[7,19] To do so, they will need to care for those problems that, on an epidemiologic basis, are usually seen by the generalist physician. Thus, room must be made in the residency program for training in dermatology, office gynecology, office orthopedics, and, most importantly, psychosocial aspects of care.

In summary, to prepare internists for future practice, more training will be needed in surgical consultation, ambulatory care, general internal medicine, and geriatric medicine. However, some distinguished internal medicine educators believe that immersion in the care of patients with severe illness is the optimal training experience, that many other aspects of an internist's practice can be learned "on the job" after residency training, and that substituting ambulatory care for hospital training would only dilute the residency experience.[20] These assertions seem at variance with any other professional apprenticeship experience and contradicted by reports of recent graduates; it is doubtful that the current model of internal medicine training can resist at least some modifications.

# GAPS IN CURRENT INTERNAL MEDICINE RESIDENCY TRAINING

Because so much of the current internal medicine residency occurs in the teaching hospital, residents gain excellent experience in care of the seriously ill patient. Unfortunately, the rapid development of technology to monitor and treat patients with serious illness on the wards and within the intensive care unit means that much of the technology that is learned in residency may quickly become obsolete. In addition, few internists, except for cardiologists, critical care specialists, and those who will provide perioperative care for surgical patients, will spend much actual practice time within intensive care units, simply because such patients are relatively infrequent in a population-based practice or even in most referral practices. Thus, while learning the principles of managing critically ill patients is essential to internal medicine training, this activity may be relatively overrepresented in most residencies.

Residents enrolled in traditional hospital-based residencies are in danger of inadequate experience in other areas. As outlined in Table 24.1, deficiencies

**Table 24.1. Deficient Areas in Internal Medicine Training.**

*General areas*

- Sense of the natural history of chronic diseases
- Decision making in diagnostic situations
- Management decisions in chronic illnesses
- Underexposure to generic issues of ambulatory care:
  Behavioral medicine
  Patient compliance and behavior modification
  Screening and monitoring
  Cost-benefit issues, including case management principles
  Decision analysis
  Principles of geriatrics
  Practice management

*Specific content areas for general internists*

- Office dermatology
- Office gynecology
- Office orthopedics
- Psychiatry (excluding acute schizophrenia and severe depression)
- Other non-internal-medicine specialties (office ophthalmology, otorhinolaryingology)
- Geriatric medicine
- Bioethics

include both general and specific areas relevant to the practicing internist. The changes in hospital care mix described earlier jeopardize the resident's full understanding of the natural history of chronic diseases and prevent participation in many diagnostic and management decisions crucial to the care of chronically ill patients.[21]

In addition, many process skills essential to the practice of internal medicine in ambulatory settings are either not taught at all or are taught in insufficient amounts. These process skills include understanding behavioral, social, and psychologic medicine; patient compliance; health promotion and disease prevention; principles of screening and monitoring; decision analysis; cost-benefit assessment; medical ethics; care of the elderly; and principles of practice management. Furthermore, some other specific skills are currently absent from most internal medicine residency programs. We know from practice surveys that the generalist physician sees many patients with problems in the domains of dermatology, office gynecology, office orthopedics, and psychiatry.[15] yet few residents acquire experience in these areas. A curriculum in geriatrics should be part of the training of every internist, as should study of the principles and resource inventories of services for long-term care of the home-bound or institutionalized elderly patient. Finally, for those generalists who will function as "gate-keepers" or case managers within organized systems of care, their case-manager function could be enhanced by including education about epidemiologic principles of medicine as well as grounding in medical economics, bioethics, medical-legal issues, and organizational theory.[22]

# LESSONS FROM OTHER SPECIALTIES

Because the educational impact of the changing practice of medicine has not been limited to internal medicine, the response of several other specialties is instructive. When a surgical residency review committee accredits a residency program, it also decides how many residents that program can sustain per year of training. In addition to evaluating the competence of the surgical faculty, the committee reviews the volume of selected procedures and the degree of major responsibility assumed as the resident progresses through the program. The review committee also specifies a minimum number of procedures to be performed. For example, in general surgery, there is a minimum of 150 procedures in the senior residency year. The thoracic surgery committee is even more explicit; it stipulates minimum numbers per resident by type of procedure, for example, 30 myocardial revascularizations and 40 operations involving the lungs and chest wall.[6]

Conscious of the need to maintain a balanced clinical experience, program directors of surgical residencies often must affiliate with community hospitals to provide an educational experience that will comply with certification criteria of the residency review committee and surgical board. In contrast, the internal medicine residency review committee and certifying board are silent regarding the appropriate number and mix of diagnoses for trainees. Not surprisingly, given the inherent administrative and economic difficulties in affiliating with other hospitals, internal medicine program directors have not felt a strong need to monitor, or change, patient volume or case mix. Thus, they have tended to structure their residency rotations according to the service needs of their institutions, rather than on ideal or abstract educational considerations.

Of all the specialties, pediatrics may most resemble internal medicine in its residency experience and its attempt to produce both subspecialists and generalists. The hospital experience of pediatric residents, however, is even less similar to subsequent practice: hospitalized pediatric patients tend to be seriously ill neonates; children with severe chronic diseases such as cystic fibrosis, leukemia, and nephrosis; and children with congenital anomalies. Because of these patterns, Charney[23] has speculated that the residency experience in pediatrics may be more unlike subsequent practice than is true for any other specialty.

Despite this disparity between what pediatric residents do in the hospital and their subsequent practice patterns, the pediatric residency review committee has established two guidelines to make the residency experience as germane as possible. First, as mentioned earlier, the committee has limited the amount of time spent in the neonatal intensive care unit to a maximum of 6 months during the 3 years of residency.[6] Second, they require substantial continuity time in the ambulatory setting as well as encourage up to 2 months of office preceptorships in the second or third residency year.[6] In addition, pediatrics has been more receptive to primary care tracks than has internal medicine. In 1983, 12% of all pediatric residents were enrolled in primary care programs, compared with only 5% of internal medicine residents.[7]

Finally, a new specialty of family practice has emphasized education in model family-practice units. The guidelines of the family-practice residency review committee are explicit about the curriculum and staffing of such units, the amount of time spent each year, and the ways to integrate gerontology, human behavior and psychiatry, and community medicine experiences into the residency.[6]

## RESPONDING TO THE CHALLENGE

How can internal medicine residencies respond to these changes? Successful adaptation will involve specific adjustments in residency design as well as some enabling structural steps (see Table 24.2).

**Table 24.2. Ingredients for Reform of Internal Medicine Training**

*Specific suggestions*

- Shift some training from hospital to ambulatory setting.

- Shift some hospital training from medicine to surgical services.

- Add clinical content areas (see Table 24.1).

*Enabling steps*

- Ensure full funding for residency time spent in ambulatory settings.

- Make payment of physicians more technology neutral.

- The internal medicine residency review committee must recognize ambulatory training as educationally valid.

- Change emphasis in the certifying examination of the American Board of Internal Medicine.

- Consider a fourth year for generalists.

- Reduce subspecialty rotations for residents entering fellowships.

- Individual programs and the internal medicine residency review committee should monitor the educational experiences of residents.

- New hospital affiliations should be considered to achieve clinical balance.

- Provide better educational integration between subspecialty medical clinics and hospital services.

## Specific Suggestions

We have highlighted specific areas in residency training that need to be adjusted, most of which are encompassed by moving some of the training from hospital medical services to surgical services or into the ambulatory care sector. If more time is to be spent in perioperative and ambulatory care, then either the duration of residency training will have to increase or time spent in the traditional medical ward and intensive care unit will have to decrease. In considering these two options, it would be useful to know the incremental contribution to learning of time spent in hospital rotations during the 36 months of residency. Unfortunately, no such data exist. Two types of evidence suggest, however, that hospital training can be decreased without impairing clinical competence.

First, in hospitals where two types of internal medicine residencies coexist, residents who spend substantially less time in inpatient settings have been evaluated as being equally or more clinically skilled, do equally well on the Part III examination of the National Board of Medical Examiners and are recognized as more interested in psychologic and social issues.[24-26] Unfortunately, we cannot compare scores for these two groups on the certifying examination of the American Board of Internal Medicine, because the Board does not record the type of program completed by candidates. Anecdotally, there appears to be a very high and similar pass rate by both groups at those academic teaching hospitals with both types of programs.

Second, a recent survey of 61 graduates of the traditional internal medicine program at Boston University has assessed the appropriateness of residency training.[5] The graduates' responses indicate excessive time in doing technical procedures and insufficient time in "allied medical disciplines" (ambulatory medicine, geriatric medicine, office gynecology, psychiatry, orthopedics, and so on), "areas related to the practice of medicine" (practice management, ethics, cost containment), and "basic skills and knowledge" (interpersonal skills, history taking, continuing care).[5] Other surveys have presented similar results.[2,3]

Shifting some internal medicine training from hospital medical services to surgical services and ambulatory settings will not be easy. For such changes to occur, adjustments must be made in how residents are paid, in accreditation and certification processes, and in how departments of internal medicine conceptualize and organize their clinical and educational programs.

## Enabling Steps

Although increased training in ambulatory care may be desirable, current financing arrangements for residencies make changes of this type difficult at best. Today, third-party reimbursement pays for the time residents spend in the hospital but often does not pay for time spent in ambulatory settings, especially settings not affiliated directly with a hospital. Furthermore, even when health insurance pays for residency training in ambulatory settings, the pro-technology, pro-procedure bias in physician reimbursement makes it easier to pay for faculty who are teaching (and performing procedures) in the hospital than for those teaching in outpatient departments.[27]

These disincentives for ambulatory teaching can be changed in two ways. First, hospitals should be reimbursed equally whether residents are in hospital or ambulatory settings. This issue is addressed very differently by current financing proposals for graduate medical education. At one extreme, the Secretary of the Department of Health and Human Services has recommended that time spent by residents in ambulatory settings be excluded from the Medicare reimbursement formulas for indirect medical education. On the other hand, Congressman Henry Waxman has proposed a formula whereby hospitals would be paid at a higher rate for residents in the primary care specialties than for surgical specialties, and hospital and outpatient training would be treated equally. Another way to encourage ambulatory teaching would be to decrease the discrepancy in physician payment between technology-intensive and time-intensive activities.

Several other important structural changes must also occur. The internal medicine residency review committee has recently indicated its concern about the educational validity of internal medicine residency programs in which residents spend more than 25% of their time in ambulatory medicine; they fear that such an experience would dilute the more intensive hospital-based learning.[28] The evidence presented above, however, shows little scientific justification for that concern.

Even if the internal medicine residency review committee permits increased ambulatory training, program directors and residents will resist such a shift unless the content of the certifying examination of the American Board of Internal Medicine reflects a similar change in emphasis. Although no published analysis exists of content of recent certifying examinations, the American College of Physicians publishes its Medical Knowledge Self-Assessment Program (MKSAP), a syllabus that draws extensively on specialists who also prepare questions for the certifying examination. The last edition, MKSAP VI,[29] devoted sections to endocrinology and metabolism, gastroenterology, clinical pharmacology, hematology, oncology, allergy and immunology, infectious disease, rheumatology, dermatology, neurology, pulmonary diseases, cardiovascular diseases, and nephrology. A new feature of MKSAP VI was a section entitled Selected Topics in Internal Medicine, which was devoted to topics "relevant to the practice of general internal medicine." This section included material on the periodic health examination, nutrition, advice to travelers, perioperative evaluation, psychiatry for the internist, geriatrics, and emergency care. The section covered 15 of the 574 pages in the entire syllabus.[29] The certifying examination of the American Board of Internal Medicine devotes about 8% of its questions to non-internal-medicine disciplines, mainly neurology and dermatology (Blank L, personal communication). Although some content on ambulatory care exists, most text and questions focus on hospital care and ignore non-internal-medicine areas other than neurology and dermatology. The legitimacy of generalist ambulatory training will remain in doubt unless that experience is validated by inclusion of appropriate content in the certifying examination.

Another issue raised by the proposed new content areas shown in Table 24.1 is whether the duration of internal medicine residency training should be increased from 3 to 4 years. Abundant precedent exists for lengthening the residency training period. General surgery, anesthesiology, radiology, and pathology have all recently added an extra year, and even internal medicine has practically eliminated its short-track provision that permitted future subspecialists to take only 2 years of residency training. Perhaps those destined to practice general internal medicine should have a required fourth year, and those who pursue subspecialty fellowships could have less consultation time in their residency so that they may prepare themselves to be part-time general internists. Because we cannot resolve this issue scientifically until the optimal time period of residency training is known, perhaps the effects of additional training should be tested in some experimental pilot programs.

Many university teaching hospitals have become so specialized that they provide an unbalanced educational experience. If this imbalance cannot be remedied by rotations in Veterans Administration or county hospitals (either because those hospitals lack certain "core" experiences or because affiliation with those institutions is not possible), then programs should seek affiliation with other hospitals. It will not be possible, however, to assess systematically the balance of clinical experience until programs begin to monitor the clinical experience of their trainees. We suggest that the internal medicine residency review committee begin such a process.

If new hospital rotations are needed to restore educational balance, program affiliation agreements must resolve issues such as who is to pay resident stipends and the salaries of their teachers, how to ensure quality of education, and what should be the proper balance between the rights of private physicians and the need for trainees to have meaningful responsibility for patient management. Finally, for residents to derive maximal benefit from caring for patients with chronic illness, including those patients who may undergo diagnostic procedures, there must be better coordination between subspecialty outpatient care and inpatient training experiences.

# CONCLUSION

Advocating more internal medicine training in the ambulatory setting is easier than constructing such experiences that are financially viable and educationally stimulating and that provide patient care of quality sufficient to compete with community physicians. A recent evaluation of 15 general internal medicine group practices in leading teaching hospitals has documented that many of these practices frequently fell short of ideal standards.[30] Clearly current physician and hospital payment schemes pose major financial disincentives for teaching programs in ambulatory settings, and as suggested by Kosecoff and associates,[30] the current structure of academic health centers may also inhibit the optimal performance of ambulatory practices.

Despite the barriers to changing the process and content of internal medicine residency programs, we contend that such reforms are needed. The evolution of the practice of medicine has produced major changes in the character of the educational experience in teaching hospitals. Demographic, economic, and political projections promise continued change in the years to come. As much as internal medicine educators might wish to preserve the old model, to do so may be a disservice to trainees and to the public that the trainees will serve. Furthermore, the current debate about how to pay for graduate medical education creates a window in time during which changes may be more easily implemented.[31]

Some reforms called for in this article would be relatively easy to implement; others will require more fundamental changes in how residents are taught, how they and their teachers are paid, and how they prepare for the board certification examination, as well as in how residency programs are accredited. Such changes will not be accomplished without a concerted, integrated plan developed by both the leaders of graduate medical education in internal medicine and those who set national policy on health manpower.

# Notes

1. Petersdorf RG. Alan Gregg Memorial Lecture: managing the revolution in medical care. *J Med Educ.* 1984;59:79–90.

2. Kantor SM, Griner PF. Educational needs in general internal medicine as perceived by prior residents. *J Med Educ.* 1981;56(9 pt 1):748–756.

3. Boyce-Smith G, Zier B, Deller JJ Jr. Deficiencies in the training of internists: results of a survey. *West J Med.* 1977;127:450–452.

4. McCue JD. Training internists: insights from private practice. *Am J Med.* 1981;71:475–479.

5. Kern DC, Parrino TA, Korst DR. The lasting value of clinical skills. *JAMA.* 1985;254:70–76.

6. American Medical Association. *1984–1985 Directory of Residency Training Programs.* Chicago: American Medical Association; 1984:35.

7. Schroeder SA. The making of a medical generalist. *Health Aff (Millwood).* 1985;4:22–46.

8. Schroeder SA. Western European responses to physician oversupply: lessons for the United States. *JAMA.* 1984;252:373–384.

9. National Hospital Association. *National Hospital Panel Survey Report.* Chicago: American Hospital Association; 1984.

10. Rabkin MT. The SAG index. *N Engl J Med.* 1982;307:1350–1351.

11. Myers LP, Schroeder SA, Chapman SA, Leong J. What's so special about special care? *Inquiry.* 1984;21:113–127.

12. Schroeder SA. A comparison of Western European and U.S. university hospitals: a case report from Leuven, West Berlin, Leiden, London, and San Francisco. *JAMA.* 1984;252:240–246.

13. Task Force on Pediatric Education. *The Future of Pediatric Education.* Evanston, Ill: American Academy of Pediatrics; 1978.

14. Sloan FA, Perrin JM, Valvona J. The teaching hospital's growing surgical caseload. *JAMA.* 1985;254:376–382.

15. Cypress BK. *Patterns of Ambulatory Care in Internal Medicine: the National Ambulatory Care Survey.* Hyattsville, Md: National Center for Health Statistics; 1984. DHEW Publication no. (PHS)84-1741 (*Vital and Health Statistics;* series 13, no. 80).

16. Geriatric medicine: a statement from the Federated Council for Internal Medicine. *Ann Intern Med.* 1981;95:372–376.

17. Coker W. Quoted in: Riffer J. Alternate delivery. *Hospitals.* 1984;58:52–54.

18. Health Resources Administration. *Summary Report of the Graduate Medical Education National Advisory Committee to the Secretary, Department of Health and Human Services.* Hyattsville, Md: Department of Health and Human Services; 1980. DHHS Publication no. (HRA) 81:656.

19. Aiken LH, Lewis CE, Craig J, Mendenhall RC, Blendon RJ, Rogers DE. The contribution of specialists to the delivery of primary care: a new perspective. *N Engl J Med.* 1979;300:1363–1369.

20. Barondess JA. The training of the internist: with some messages from practice. *Ann Intern Med.* 1979;90:412–417.

21. Rabkin MT. The teaching hospital and medical education: one-room schoolhouse, multiversity, or dinosaur? *J Med Educ.* 1985;60:92–97.

22. Eisenberg JM. The internist as gatekeeper: preparing for a new role. *Ann Intern Med.* 1985;102:537–543.

23. Charney E. The status of graduate education: pediatrics. In: *Future Developments in Primary Care Graduate Medical Education.* Washington, DC: Public Health Service; 1985:16–18.

24. Rosinski EF, Dagenais F. *Non–Family Medicine Resident Training for Primary Care: A Comparative Evaluation of Federally and Non–Federally Supported Primary Care–Oriented Medical Residency Programs: Final Report.* Washington, DC: Department of Health, Education, and Welfare; 1980. Contract no. HRA 232-278-0115.

25. Rosinski EF, Dagenais F. A comparison of primary care residents with conventional internal medicine and pediatric residents. *West J Med.* 1981;135:245–247.

26. Ramsdell JW, Berry CC. Evaluation of general and traditional internal medicine residencies utilizing a medical records audit based on educational objectives. *Med Care.* 1983;21:1144–1153.

27. Almy TP. The role of the primary care physician in the health care "industry." *N Engl J Med.* 1981;304:225–228.

28. Wartman S. The RRC and the "25 percent rule" [editorial]. *SREP-CIM Newsletter.* January-February 1985:2–3.

29. American College of Physicians. *Medical Knowledge Self-Assessment Program VI.* Philadelphia: American College of Physicians; 1982.

30. Kosecoff J, Fink A, Brook RH, et al. General medical care and the education of internists in university hospitals: an evaluation of the teaching hospital general medicine group practice program. *Ann Intern Med.* 1985;102:250–257.

31. Iglehart JK. Difficult times ahead for graduate medical education. *N Engl J Med.* 1985;312:1400–1404.

# The Education of Pediatricians for Primary Care: The Score After Two Score Years

Evan Charney, M.D.
1995

In a 1973 monograph on the education of physicians for primary care, Joel Alpert and I wrote, "There are two interrelated and serious problems in our present educational structure—not enough physicians enter primary care and those who do so are not adequately prepared for the job."[1] Twenty years and many task forces and exhortatory editorials later, much the same could be said. But that conclusion would not be entirely fair: changes have indeed occurred in the subsequent two score years.

There is now clear consensus that a strong primary care system should be the linchpin of our nation's health care system, with 50% to 60% of physicians as generalists,[2,3] and the medical profession has at least professed to agree with that strategy.[4] Family medicine has grown from a frail newborn to a lusty adolescent, occupying a grown-up seat at the primary care table: 13.2% of American medical school graduates were matched into family practice residencies in 1994, the highest percentage in a decade.[5] Internal medicine has firmly, if belatedly, pledged its commitment to generalism[6] and obstetrics/gynecology has claimed a seat as well.[7]

On the other hand, in that same 20-year period the proportion of generalists has shrunk from 43% to 33% of the physician work force,[8] a substantial and growing minority of our population lack easy access to quality primary care, and our undergraduate and graduate medical education system, like a large battleship, has only barely begun to alter course in response to changed curricular compass settings.

---

How well has pediatrics addressed the issue of primary care education over the past two decades? We wrote in 1973 that "a kind of schizophrenia exists about primary care education within traditional pediatrics and internal medicine—a split allegiance to consultative and primary medicine. Although many departments verbalize the importance of primary care programs for their trainees, their effort remains invested on the ward. These fields do have a dual responsibility and it has been difficult in practice to integrate these often conflicting obligations."[1] That statement still rings true. In fact, the obligations to the care of complexly ill patients on critical care units have markedly increased in the intervening years, further emphasizing the disparity between the educational content of the inpatient experience during residency and the content of clinical practice.[9,10]

On a positive note, however, there are clear indicators of pediatrics' commitment to generalism in practice and ongoing efforts to translate that commitment to our graduate education curriculum. For example, the guidelines for pediatric residency training have been progressively revised over 20 years to strengthen residency education in general pediatrics. An explanation of how these guidelines (called program requirements) are established may be helpful: program requirements are drafted by the Residency Review Committee for pediatrics (RRC) and revised approximately every 5 years. They are approved by the Accreditation Council for Graduate Medical Education, a voluntary body comprised of five sponsoring organizations. The pediatric RRC has ten members, three each appointed for 6-year terms by the American Academy of Pediatrics, the American Board of Pediatrics, and the American Medical Association and a tenth pediatric resident member appointed for a 2-year term.

The RRC program requirements for pediatrics published in 1974 were two paragraphs in length with few details about curricular content and no duration of training specified. In 1978 the Academy of Pediatrics' Task Force on Pediatric Education published its report that identified inadequacies in the residency curriculum and recommended requiring 3 years of general pediatric training, limiting time spent in subspecialties, and expanding experiences in behavioral pediatrics, chronic disease, and adolescent medicine.[11] The 1978 pediatric RRC guidelines for the first time mandated a 3-year residency, identified a "commitment to primary care," and recommended 6 months of ambulatory experience. In 1980 a continuity clinic experience was first "suggested."

Guidelines written as suggestions can only guide: in 1984 Weinberger and Oski found little change in pediatric residency training programs, with only one-half of surveyed residencies requiring experience in child development, behavior, and adolescent medicine.[12]

In 1985 the pediatric RRC guidelines mandated experiences in adolescent medicine, child development, care of the handicapped child, and "continuous care of a group of patients throughout the three-year training," and the 1990 guidelines reaffirmed three core years in general pediatrics, required a weekly continuity clinic and more structured adolescent medicine and behavior/development experiences.

The revised program requirements now being proposed to take that commitment a step forward: the goal of pediatric residency training is clearly identified as the preparation of residents to be competent general pediatricians. The educational content in primary care practice, behavior/development, and adolescent medicine are broadened and more clearly delineated, and community-based experiences to teach trainees about the advocacy role of the pediatrician are now required. Moreover, the intent of subspecialty experiences is specifically directed to what the general pediatrician needs to know. This is consistent with the 1992 RRC pediatric special requirements for all subspecialty fellowships, which emphasize the consultant role of the pediatric subspecialist.

That residency programs have sometimes had difficulty instituting these directives is perhaps understandable: pediatric residencies are all hospital-sponsored, and the need for trainees to staff burgeoning critical care services can be a potent force for program directors to contend with, especially so since the majority of faculty are themselves involved in the care of these tertiary center patients. The schizophrenia (more charitably, the dual responsibility) of being a primary care and a consultant discipline persists.

There are other indicators that pediatrics remains firmly within the primary care fold. In a 1994 position paper on graduate education, the Federation of Pediatric Organizations (which represents both the practicing and academic communities) restated its belief that "Pediatricians are the most appropriate providers of primary care for infants, children and adolescents."[13] At present, 60% of residency graduates directly enter primary care practice, a figure that has remained stable over the past decade.[13] It is also reassuring that we remain a popular career choice among students: approximately 10% of American medical school graduates have chosen pediatrics each year for the past decade.[5] To be sure, our success in attracting trainees is largely attributable to the increasing proportion of women in medical school who still find pediatrics an attractive career choice. In contrast, internal medicine has attracted fewer graduates over that time, the majority of whom have sought subspecialty careers.[5,8] I believe the balance between generalists and specialists in pediatrics to be more appropriate: 40% of pediatricians enter subspecialty fields, a reasonable proportion, especially given the fact that a significant number of children are provided primary care by family physicians.

Despite this strong commitment to primary care, pediatrics faces challenging issues in general pediatric practice and in education. For example, I believe we need to better define (for ourselves and for the public) how pediatricians differ from family physicians in providing primary care to children, acknowledging that there is a place for both disciplines.

In reality, the role of the practicing pediatrician varies considerably, depending on practice location. General pediatricians located at a distance from tertiary centers, in addition to their primary care role, provide an important secondary care function consulting to family practitioners and community hospitals and providing a linkage to pediatric subspecialists at referral centers.[14] However, in metropolitan areas where pediatric subspecialists are readily available. I'm not sure we've demonstrated that our vastly more sophisticated training is put to use in practice. If pediatricians routinely refer to subspecialists children with uncomplicated seizures, chronic constipation, behavioral and developmental problems, we weaken our claim to primary in primary care. Admittedly, until now the reimbursement structure in practice has been a barrier, rewarding brief visits and early referral and "punishing" more comprehensive management of these problems by the generalist. The current managed care mantra to refer fewer cases may actually provide the mandate to expand the role of the primary pediatrician. The challenge will be to restructure practice to allow time for an expanded secondary care role, while remaining cost-effective: admittedly easier to say than to do.

The new RRC guidelines should encourage a dialogue between subspecialists and generalists about the appropriate boundary between primary and consultant care, of particular relevance if practicing pediatricians will be expected to do more. Of course, subspecialists need to believe that primary care pediatricians are competent to manage more complex disease, and we sometimes convey mixed messages during training in that regard. If residents see only neurologists managing children with seizures, endocrinologists managing children with diabetes, and psychiatrists managing those with behavioral problems, that sends a powerful message about how medicine should be practiced.

In summary, there are interesting questions to answer about how we practice general pediatrics and how we educate residents and it is important to address both questions together. If we teach residents to manage more complex problems in training, but do not allow them to do so in the real world, we invite frustration. If we extend primary care pediatrics more deeply into secondary care, but have not provided residents with the appropriate training, we will be guilty of educational malpractice.

In 1994 the prognosis for primary care pediatrics is excellent. Although many of the issues of 20 years ago are still with us, pediatrics has considerably strengthened its subspecialty capability over that time while retraining and nurturing our commitment to the generalist role.

# Notes

1. Alpert JJ, Charney E. *The Education of Physicians for Primary Care.* Washington, DC: U.S. Department of Health, Education, and Welfare, Public Health Service; 1973. DHEW Publication No (HRA) 74-7113.

2. Council on Graduate Medical Education. *Third Report: Improving Access to Health Care Through Physician Workforce Reform: Directions for the 21st Century.* Rockville, Md: U.S. Department of Health and Human Services, Public Health Service, Health Resources and Services Administration; 1992.

3. Physician Payment Review Commission. *Annual Report to Congress.* Washington, DC: Council on Graduate Medical Education; 1993

4. Association of American Medical Colleges. AAMC policy on the generalist physician. *Acad Med.* 1993;68:1.

5. National Resident Matching Program. *Data, March 1994.* Washington, DC: National Resident Matching Program; 1994.

6. Kimball, JR, Young PR. A statement on the generalist physician from the American Boards of Family Practice and Internal Medicine. *JAMA.* 1994;271:315–316.

7. Horton JA, Cruess DR, Pearse WH. Primary and preventive care services provided by obstetrician-gynecologists. *Obstet Gynecol.* 1993;82:723–726.

8. Alpert JJ, Friedman RH, Green LA. Education of generalists: three times a century is all we get! J Gen Intern Med. 1994;9(4 Suppl 1):S4–S6.

9. Bryke CR, Tunnessen WW Jr, Scully TJ, Oski FA. Pediatric residencies: differences between 1959/60 and 1984/85. *Pediatrics.* 1988;82:752–755.

10. Reuben DB, McCue JD, Gerbert B. The residency-practice training mismatch: a primary care education dilemma. *Arch Intern Med.* 1988; 148:914–919.

11. American Academy of Pediatrics Task Force on Pediatric Education. *The Future of Pediatric Education.* Evanston, Ill: American Academy of Pediatrics; 1978.

12. Weinberger HL, Oski FA. A survey of pediatric resident training programs 5 years after the Task Force Report. *Pediatrics.* 1984;74:523–526.

13. Task Force on Graduate Medical Education Reform. Graduate medical education and pediatric workforce issues and principles. *Pediatrics.* 1994;93:1018–1020.

14. Charney E. Secondary care: the role of the community hospital in pediatrics. *Am J Dis Child.* 1983;137:902–906.

# Sustaining the Development of Primary Care in Academic Medicine

Thomas S. Inui, M.D.; W. T. Williams Jr., M.D.; Leslie Goode;
Ron J. Anderson, M.D.; Karyn N. Bhak; John D. Forsyth;
John J. Hutton; Andrew G. Wallace M.D.;
Robert M. Daugherty Jr., M.D., Ph.D.
1998

Medical schools are complex organizations with three primary missions: education, research, and patient care. Although medical schools are not the only institutions that conduct research and patient care, they are the only ones that award the MD degree to students who have been prepared for residency training and eventual practice as physicians. This mission is also the "common denominator" function of all schools of medicine, no matter how substantially they may differ in other ways, such as their levels of focus on research, their relationships to governments, and their niches in the health care marketplace.

The MD is a professional degree. Conferring it implies that the graduate has acquired the foundation of knowledge, skills, and values that a physician must have to assume meaningful responsibility for the care of patients. The principal aim of the medical school curriculum is to make it possible for students to acquire that foundation, whatever their eventual choices of disciplines as specialists or generalists. Our thesis in this article is that schools of medicine, in order to succeed in their unique, core mission of educating physicians, will require a significant educational resource package—personnel, clinical programs, courses, and supportive infrastructure for teaching and learning—*in primary care*.

These primary care resources will be critical for two distinct reasons: (1) adequate educational experience in clinical medicine will require substantial participation in care in settings principally devoted to primary care, and (2) the competencies that form the core objectives for the general education of all physicians are also the fundamentals of effective primary care. In medical school environments, often dominated by basic science, subspecialized practice, and high technologies, how can such primary care resources be developed and sustained?

In this article, we summarize our thinking about the above-mentioned issues. As members of one of the six subgroups of the Advisory Panel on the Mission and Organization of Medical Schools (APMOMS) sponsored by the Association of American Medical Colleges (AAMC), we were charged to explore the strategies and resources required for medical schools to fulfill their roles in generalist education and primary care more effectively. We revised the group's original name, Nurturing the Development of Primary Care, and instead called it Sustaining the Development of Academic Primary Care (hereafter called "the Primary Care Work Group"). This change was to reflect our common belief that primary care should have an enduring position of strength in all medical schools and that it should not be considered an add-on that is merely tolerated, or even nurtured in a permanent position of dependency, merely for reasons of political or financial expediency. In all of our discussions, we attempted to take a future orientation, imagining the type of environment and demands today's students are likely to face throughout their careers, the kinds of changes in medical care delivery future physicians will deal with, and the responsibilities incumbent on future physicians as advocates of the health of the public.

We have not revisited the workforce debate that has preoccupied U.S. academic medicine in recent years, although we are well aware that policymakers and leaders in academic medicine have participated in discussions of, and witnessed intense discussion by others of, the merits of producing more primary care providers.[1-9] Our working group did not extend or resolve that debate. Our view is that whether or not the country needs a greater number of primary care providers, and whether or not medical schools are appropriately responding to those needs at present, all future physicians need a sound general medical education. Given the direction of change in the provision of medical care—which is creating a more central role for primary care and is shifting care from hospitals to ambulatory care settings—a general medical education will require enhanced resources in primary care. Such resources may be on campus, may be elsewhere but sponsored by the medical school, or may be a community resource used by the medical school.

We begin with an examination of definitions, particularly an explanation of the meanings of "primary care" and "generalism." We then discuss in detail the relevance of primary care to the medical school's curriculum and educational goals. We examine the key issues and a variety of changes that are needed to allow primary care to take its central place in the medical school. Our article concludes with a summary and recommendations for medical schools and the AAMC.

# DEFINING PRIMARY CARE AND GENERALISM

Do "primary care" and "generalist medicine" denote the same set of activities or do the terms reflect important differences? This question has been a central issue in many ongoing discussions about the nation's future health care needs, including those focused on the number of primary care providers and the adequacy of their preparation.[1,7-14] It is, then, not surprising that we of the Primary Care Work Group committed time to debating this issue, and we considered our own resolution of the question to be something of a "watershed" from which other conclusions and observations flowed.

Historical definitions of the functions of primary care and generalist physicians have usually made room for several types of physicians (at least general internists, general pediatricians, and family practitioners, but even obstetrician-gynecologists and liaison psychiatrists). In the final analysis the understanding of primary care in these efforts has not been driven so much by physicians' subdiscipline differences as by consideration of levels of care (first contact versus referral), setting (community- versus hospital-based), and descriptions of certain other qualities of care (accessible, comprehensive, continuous). In the context of integrated delivery systems or in descriptions of physicians' functions in certain varieties of insurance and care financing schemes, primary care has also sometimes been depicted as a strategy for organizing health care.

The results of this ongoing definitional discourse are clearly visible in some of the most recent descriptions of the key attributes of primary care. A 1993 draft report of the Ad Hoc Committee on Generalism to the Executive Committee for the Accreditation Council for Graduate Medical Education (ACGME), for example, presented the following working definition of generalist physicians:

> Generalist physicians provide person-centered, continuing, comprehensive care
> to a population unselected by disease or organ system. In addition, generalist
> physicians identify and coordinate other care needed by their patients.[15]

In 1994, the Institute of Medicine (IOM) Committee on the Future of Primary Care, after considerable exploration and deliberation, published the following definition of primary care:

> Primary care is the provision of integrated, accessible health care services by
> clinicians who are accountable for addressing a large majority of personal health
> care needs, developing a sustained partnership with patients, and practicing in
> the context of family and community.[16]

Clearly, these descriptions do not adequately distinguish between generalism and primary care. Whether discussing generalism or primary care, groups of experts have centered their discussion on a limited set of descriptors of care, including accessibility, comprehensiveness, integration, coordination, and continuity. We of the Primary Care Work Group, building upon previous definitions and embracing a future orientation, created the following clearer working definition of primary care as a context for our subsequent discussions and conclusions:

> Primary care is the provision of comprehensive health care services to a defined population by health professionals who address a majority of personal health needs, develop a longitudinal partnership with patients, and provide medical care, prevention, and health promotion in the context of the family and community.

Several features of this definition deserve highlighting. First, we draw a distinction between generalism and primary care. In the most basic terms, generalism is the specialty of medicine practiced by generalist physicians who, both by training and inclination, are the principal providers of general medical services for the populations they serve. The generalists among today's physicians are trained in general internal medicine, general pediatrics, family medicine, and the nonsurgical "women's health care" domain of obstetrics and gynecology.

By contrast, we define primary care as a function. With an eye to the future of organized medical care in integrated systems, we envision the primary care function as one likely to require the coordination and integration of a complex of services rendered by a variety of health professionals, some trained as generalists and others as subspecialists. For example, for certain patients at certain points in time, a psychiatrist or oncologist may contribute substantively to the primary care function. In addition, other clinicians—for example, nurses—will participate in the primary care function. Within a (formally or informally) organized system of care, generalist physicians will serve as the primary care team leaders. Moreover, generalist physicians are usually the most significant contributors to the primary care function. Other types of clinicians may participate in the primary care function to varying degrees by providing critical services to patients under circumstances that require a range of expertise.

A noteworthy feature of our definition is the reference to a defined population. This concept is increasingly part of health care practiced inside systems that serve the needs of "covered lives," enrolled plan members, or even persons inside a specific geographic catchment area. The reference to health professionals in our definition acknowledges that the function of primary care often requires teamwork among physicians, nurse clinicians, social workers, clinical pharmacists, and others.

Other key aspects of our definition are the references to comprehensiveness and longitudinality. By comprehensiveness, we mean broad scope of services; longitudinality refers to the assumption of responsibility for a patient over time.

These characteristics distinguish primary care from other types of care (e.g., episodes of care focused on the resolution of intercurrent, urgent, or emergent problems). Primary care addresses a full spectrum of care for health risks, chronic conditions, and episodes of illnesses. In an ideal situation, primary care involves a partnership between health professionals and patients and also explicit attention to patients' families and communities. Many of the most important health care or prevention aspects of primary care are carried out most effectively through meaningful relationships joining health professionals and patients, grounded in the patients' social contexts.

Our work group's emphasis on primary care as a shared function and our attention to an organizational context incorporates themes developed by earlier consensus groups and recognizes emerging roles for physicians and other health care providers in current and projected health care delivery systems. In our view, to operate most successfully, the function of primary care will need to become an essential element of health care delivery systems for general populations. We hope that our readers understand that our intent was to ground our observations and recommendations in the reality of emerging systems. Our statement is not a political one and not intended to placate those in all specialties of medicine. In short, we have attempted to envision the likely future of medical care, the place of the primary care function within it, and the challenges facing medical school leaders to anchor primary care in their institutions.

The *function* concept of primary care assumes the existence of an organized system of health care in which various clinicians work together to contribute to the needs of patients over time. In most cases, such as densely populated urban or suburban centers, the system will be formally organized. In rural locations, or areas with limited numbers of people and health care providers, a de facto organized system can exist. Whether formally or informally organized, the system and physicians (principally generalists) together will fulfill the "accountability" criteria included in the IOM's definition. Shared accountability by individual physicians and the overall system, including the patient, emphasizes the actions of physicians as well as the context of the health care system in which the physicians work. In other words, responsibility for the effectiveness, quality, and comprehensiveness of the health care delivered is not assigned to either the physician or the system solely, but is jointly shared. Rather, the individual physician is most directly accountable to the patient, and the system is responsible for ensuring that resources are available to enable clinicians to carry out their work. Physicians and systems of care are *interdependent;* neither can succeed without the other. The primary care function cuts across various populations of patients, providers, types of treatment, levels of intervention, and locations of service delivery. It also emphasizes the importance of the multidisciplinary contributions to the system as a whole.

# MEDICAL SCHOOLS' RESPONSIBILITY FOR THE GENERAL EDUCATION OF PHYSICIANS

Medical schools should strive to graduate "undifferentiated" (general) physicians who have solid grounding in the fundamental features of medical science and modern practice, including ambulatory care experience. Graduates should be adequately prepared to pursue further training for any medical career, including a generalist's career. Strengthening the core curriculum for the preparation of future generalists strengthens the learning experience for any student in a school of medicine. Because a generalist core curriculum emphasizes foundational skills for future physicians of all varieties, it also strengthens the position of primary care in the school.

Emphasizing the importance of the undifferentiated graduate is not meant to support the status quo or to suggest that schools need not develop or strengthen programs that prepare students for generalist careers in primary care. We do not, however, support the creation of specific school-by-school targets to produce certain percentages of primary care physicians. Instead, the emphasis on the undifferentiated graduate provides a framework for further deliberations about what knowledge, attitudes, and skills are fundamental to all physicians. Course by course, faculty should be prepared to decide what every physician should know (about cellular biology, epidemiology, surgery, psychiatry, etc.) and should be able to do before being granted an MD degree. We of the Primary Care Work Group maintain that such deliberations would simultaneously result in strengthening the portion of the curriculum that is particularly relevant to generalism. Such deliberations would also highlight the importance of sustaining the development of academic resources in primary care settings, such as community clinics and private physicians' offices.

As a byproduct of this emphasis on strengthening the general education of all physicians, schools of medicine are likely to enhance the prospects that their students will choose generalist careers in greater numbers. Students would see generalism and primary care as valued by faculty, other mentors, and the institution itself, as judged through the lens of the school's educational policies and behaviors. Enhanced development of related curriculum and support for scholarly activities are two important domains within which institutions can demonstrate a commitment to primary care. If through the educational experience, students acquire greater personal knowledge of the demands and rewards of generalism, they will be well positioned to make better informed and professionally responsible career decisions. Only by exposure to generalist role models will students have all the information they need to make well-founded assessments about career choices.

# FOSTERING ACADEMIC EMPHASIS ON PRIMARY CARE

## Operational Emphasis

Reaffirming the status of the MD degree as a general professional degree and thereby emphasizing the centrality of a generalist curriculum will require that medical schools integrate this goal into their missions and strategic plans. It will also require the anchoring of medical schools' primary care faculty and clinical operations in both organizational and curricular terms. That process underscores the need to address fundamental operational issues in medical schools that include

- Developing the necessary commitment to generalist education, in the context of the school's unique history, missions, and limited resources;

- Developing adequate ambulatory, longitudinal, and primary care experiences; and

- Encouraging faculty, particularly basic science and subspecialist faculty, to support curricular change that emphasizes the knowledge, skills, and attitudes necessary to deliver primary care.

Raising the image and status of primary care in the medical school environment is imperative and should be central to the process of educating students and delivering patient care. The concept of primary care as a core function of physicians is consistent with long-held views about the goals of undergraduate medical education—that all physicians, regardless of specialty choice, require a common foundation of knowledge, attitudes, and skills.[17] This view should persist in the future, particularly as the health care delivery system continues to change.

## Organizational Emphasis

The recent focus on producing generalist physicians and concurrent changes in the modes of medical practice has served as a catalyst for medical schools to examine their "classrooms." The modern classroom is expanding to include numerous settings. Dramatic changes in the organization, financing, and delivery of medical care emphasize the need to expose learners to ambulatory care settings, particularly those that foster primary care and managed care educational experiences. While ambulatory care settings may be the most appropriate place to carry out primary care education, experiences in these settings are not necessarily the equivalent of primary care experiences. Similarly, while the insurance product referred to as "managed care" is a financing mechanism of significance that students and residents need to understand, simple exposure to managed care of this variety does not equal or supplant the need for exposure to primary and ambulatory care, in managed care delivery systems and other venues.

A medical school's participation in the formation or ongoing operation of a health care system offers advantages for economic survival, including sustaining a broad base of clinical activities to help support the costs of education and clinical research. Affiliations and partnerships with such systems may integrate a school's education, research, and service missions into the macro (or external) structure of a clinical network. Affiliations and participation in primary care networks also offer schools and students the new environments needed to complement existing sites for medical education. For long-term viability of academic programs, affiliations and networks should be recognized as primary care *education networks;* these are different from clinical referral networks, which are intended to provide only a patient base to support the school's subspecialists. The school need neither own nor operate such a system to secure a place for academic activities, but it will need a system of care that can be held accountable for educational performance and may need a defined source of expanded clinical practice revenue to support the costs of medical education in a competitive marketplace.[18] Linkages with managed care organizations and other community provider groups for teaching experiences are also relevant to a wide variety of legal, financial, and management aims of today's schools of medicine.

## Medical Education and Clinical Delivery Systems

To sustain high quality in academics and patient care in the restructuring medical care marketplace, many schools will need to be substantially involved in a patient care network of teaching sites and care delivery sites. The integrated delivery system and its enrolled population add value to education. In order to seriously discuss joint ventures or partnerships for education, schools must persuade health care systems that networks also derive benefits from a relationship with a medical school.[19] Common challenges to building educational programs in distributed delivery systems include the lack of predeveloped teaching sites, the lack of faculty skilled in teaching in primary care and community settings, and the lack of money to pay for improving these circumstances.[20,21] We address resource needs and financing in more detail in later sections of this article.

Successful negotiations between schools and clinical delivery systems must involve explicit understandings about acceptance of the academic mission, revenues to support education, and accountability that is cost- and quality-driven. A formal affiliation agreement or inter-organizational memorandum of understanding may be required to secure a significant, long-term working arrangement. The medical school and care delivery system may also, together, need to put in place an administration to oversee the conduct of academic affairs in the affiliated care delivery system. The network will develop de facto distributed teaching settings, with faculty and resources committed to the educational mission. There should be an overall system commitment to teaching and scholarship, even though teaching may occur in only select sites within the system. For purposes of quality and economy, certain sites should have some teaching present at all times, or become permanent teaching sites. Establishing some permanent teaching sites will facilitate students' exposure to good patient care, good teaching, and equivalent learning experiences at geographically distinct sites. Other primary care sites may involve teaching on a less frequent or less intensive basis—for example, they may offer initial clinical experiences for first-year students.

While initial thinking about introducing students into a care delivery system is typically dominated by concerns about added costs, in an academic primary care network, students can also function as part of the health care delivery team. To explain the added value of training students in community-based or nontraditional settings, medical schools need to be aware of how an educational mission can enhance service delivery. Preceptors will influence students' types and levels of involvement, and thus the value of the training component. How preceptors design the educational experience will have a major bearing on the students' value to the clinical enterprise. For example, students can enhance communication with patients by extending the amount of time devoted to discussing the value of preventive care. Similarly, students can conduct periodic health reviews or visits to assess the safety of elderly patients' homes. Such activities simultaneously develop students' skills and increase the effectiveness of the services to patients. The presence of students may stimulate clinical faculty to stay up-to-date in innovations in clinical therapeutics, which will help improve the quality of care and the capacity of a system of care to move practitioners toward the best practices quickly. Creating opportunities to teach may enhance the ability of care delivery systems to recruit and retain able clinicians. Other values of such partnerships to care delivery systems may be

- An "insider's position" in recruiting trainees to their workforce;
- Marketing potential in using the university name;
- Decreased employee training costs because there is a built-in educational infrastructure; and
- Ability to meet patients' preferences for board-certified physicians and the latest advances in medicine.

Despite such advantages, schools may need to support dedicated time for physicians who participate in teaching activities or supplement the system in other ways to meet efficiency demands.

## Academic Administrative Structures

In an effort to sustain the development of primary care, many schools have made changes in their statements of missions and goals, including statements directly alluding to support for primary care or generalism. In recent years, schools have also made administrative, organizational, and programmatic changes. Most schools have established some type of administrative infrastructure (usually through departments, divisions, or centers) with the authority to design, implement, and evaluate a generalist curriculum and related clinical experiences. These and other schools have appointed a person with administrative responsibility for coordinating primary care activities and communication across departments. The position may include overseeing the education and service integration of primary care service networks. Other schools have established a center or an office of generalist medical education and charged the entity with that function.

The importance of role models and mentors in medical education is well known. Many schools have increased students' exposure to generalist physicians by increasing the numbers of generalist faculty and community-based physicians who serve as preceptors, career counselors, mentors, and instructors, particularly in the preclinical years. To organize these faculty and coordinate students' educational experiences, most schools have developed structural units for primary care physicians, and some institutions offer primary care residency programs.

Each institution must take local factors into account when deciding on administrative structures and how to organize primary care activities. A physician's professional identity and career advancement are generally structured around departments; the emerging delivery system, on the other hand, has a stronger orientation toward functions. The goal for a structural entity should be to coordinate the full array of primary education and academic activities, including research and clinical program planning. The responsibilities of such an entity should include clinically relevant research. A research presence provides the benefits of educating students in a spirit of inquiry, and research itself helps prevent the "fossilizing" of health care practice. Income from extramurally supported research can create sustainable financing for academic generalist programs.

In sorting through organizational and administrative issues and options, the ultimate goal for all schools should be to join the various interests of all medical specialties relevant to primary care in a manner that serves both the academic and the clinical missions. Organizational changes are likely to require commensurate resource development and support. The APMOMS Working Group on Adapting to Resource Constraints recommended that medical schools develop working environments for implementing flexible generalist curricula.[21] We strongly endorse that recommendation.

# ENSURING GENERALISM'S IMPORTANCE IN THE CURRICULUM

Curricular modifications related to fostering generalist competencies for medical practice should be understood to be enhancements of the overall quality of medical students' education, not solely or even primarily a means of increasing the number of students choosing careers as generalists. Medical schools should aim to produce graduates who are fully prepared to enter residency training in any specialty and who have acquired a sound general foundation for practice now and in the future. Graduates should have strong leadership, communication, and learning skills and a clear understanding of physicians' roles in an evolving health care system.

## Relevant Topics

As an accrediting body, the Liaison Committee on Medical Education (LCME) has commented on medical students' education in ambulatory and primary care. The LCME's "Standards for Accreditation of Medical Education Programs Leading to the M.D. Degree" states that "instruction and experience in patient care must be provided in both ambulatory and hospital settings. All schools must offer a core curriculum in primary care, utilizing the disciplines or multidisciplinary approaches involved in such care. Clinical education programs involving patients should include disciplines such as family medicine, internal medicine, obstetrics and gynecology, pediatrics, psychiatry, and surgery."[22] We note the important distinctions between the "must" and "should" portions of this LCME statement. The LCME emphasizes the need to have primary care and ambulatory care in the curriculum, and that the content is more important than distinctions about which department sponsors or participates in ambulatory and primary care education.

In addition to the LCME standards, much has been written about designing the medical school curriculum to stress the learning, knowledge, and skills considered relevant to the education of generalists.[23-26] The articles underscore a generic, core content of objectives that are relevant to all medical specialties. This core is viewed as the foundation of the medical students' curriculum, designed to produce an undifferentiated physician. Recognizing that decisions about curriculum reside in each school individually, the literature comments on general content areas for medical students. In some cases the content should be mastered; in other cases exposure to or familiarity with the content area is a more reasonable expectation. Examples (but not an exhaustive list) of the content areas and skills are

- Understanding of basic human biology, what is known and not known, and how to apply this knowledge to the analysis of a clinical problem;
- Ability to detect, diagnose, and effectively manage common acute and chronic medical conditions;
- Understanding of the principles of longitudinal care;
- Ability to detect and manage health risk problems;
- Understanding of the application and importance of health promotion and disease prevention;
- Effective interpersonal communication skills, including an ability and desire to share responsibilities and decision making with patients, families, and other clinical team members;
- Ability to lead a team of health professionals in their care for a population;
- Knowledge of how to coordinate aspects of care, including the use of technology;
- Ability to utilize available resources, including those from other health care professionals and the community;
- Good judgment regarding timeliness and appropriateness of referrals to specialists;
- Understanding of the ethical duties and responsibilities of the physician–patient relationship;
- Appreciation of the psychosocial aspects of disease;
- Awareness of the principles of quality improvement and of managed care systems and their practice objectives;
- Competency in the use of clinical and management information systems; and
- Appropriate understanding of clinical epidemiology, evidence-based medicine, and medical informatics in order to evaluate relevant medical literature.

These domains of knowledge, skills, and values form the foundation of the general education of a physician. Although many schools have begun to reorient their curricula to increase the number of graduates who will choose generalist careers, the real challenge for medical schools is to embed generalist concepts into the curriculum and in the educational environment and to prepare all graduates for lifelong learning in an evolving health care system. Faculty and other leaders at each school will determine to what degree their students should acquire the basic competencies during their tenure as undergraduates. Challenges involve developing specific educational goals and curriculum content, developing faculty, evaluating off-site faculty, and orchestrating a critical process that facilitates students' learning from peers as well as from their faculty teachers. Through the Group on Educational Affairs, the AAMC has undertaken a project, the Medical Schools Objective Project, to develop a national framework within which to clarify the content of a sound curriculum for the general education of medical students.[27] We support the development and relevance of this project to the work of sustaining the development of primary care in medical schools.

## New Venues, Courses, and Other Structural Changes

Medical schools may have to develop new sites of education to ensure that a student's experiences meet overall program goals. General ambulatory care experiences require special coordination and new central resources to maintain quality and consistency. For example, both the University of Illinois at Chicago and the University of California, Los Angeles, UCLA School of Medicine have constructed sets of core cases and prepared standardized patients to ensure that all students will have exposure to such problems and critical incident cases.

Longitudinal experiences, not now a required component of the clinical curriculum in a large majority of medical schools, will be critical to developing basic competencies and an understanding of the role of primary care providers. Longitudinal experiences will help students learn the difference between managing an acute illness in an acute care setting and managing the ongoing chronic illness in an ambulatory care setting. Like all competencies, the location of longitudinal experiences is less important than the content of the experiences.

Both longitudinal and acute care should take place in settings where physicians and other health professionals practice. Such environments offer rich opportunities for students to observe a team culture, or the complementary contributions of various clinicians to the primary care function. These environments also raise the possibility of including other health professionals (at a cost lower than the cost of physician faculty) as teachers in appropriate portions of medical students' education. The total experience should provide students a positive view of collaboration as the best way to manage many patients.

The types and levels of interaction between students and residents in ambulatory care settings will not be what they are in inpatient settings. Ambulatory care experiences will require lower student-to-faculty ratios and will increase demands on teachers. For example, ambulatory and primary care settings will likely require faculty members to teach and practice without the presence of residents. Resources and new designs for ambulatory care sessions will be necessary to enable instructors to teach effectively while also providing adequate ambulatory care.

# DEVELOPING FACULTY AND OTHER RESOURCES IN PRIMARY CARE

## Developing Faculty

For medical schools to create high-quality and effective educational programs in the practice areas and settings cited above, faculty development will require significant enhancement. Schools will need to identify the appropriate school-based and community-based faculty and develop their skills and support systems for teaching in ambulatory care settings. Support systems would include academic tracks, information and communication systems, clinical updates in course material designed for clinician teachers, teaching-skills workshops for new and continuing faculty, support resources for faculty and students in problematic situations, and support for remote literature searching. Investment in these individuals and their supporting resources should result in consistent performance of teaching of high quality across diverse settings.

Like all clinical faculty, generalists face challenging demands to serve as teachers, role models, and mentors. At the same time, they are asked to develop their scholarly endeavors and to provide clinical service. In the future, the "triple threat" faculty member, one who is involved in education, research, and patient care, may no longer be a realistic model.[21,28] Most clinical faculty will probably concentrate on roles such as teacher–clinician or clinical researcher–teacher. As primary care is the core of the medical student curriculum, generalist faculty will carry major teaching responsibilities and be challenged to balance practice and/or research with teaching responsibilities. Core support for those who carry the teaching mission will need to be secured within medical schools' operating budgets if these faculty are to succeed in their work. Especially since generalist faculty are in relatively low-income practice specialties, it will not be possible for them to generate income that supports their time as both clinicians and teachers.

Understanding the medical school's educational objectives and program goals will be essential to plan clinical delivery system schedules and for faculty time management. In general, attending physicians and preceptors, whether full- or part-time, community-based, or within the ambulatory care sector of the academic health center, should try to incorporate students into their practices. Although the content, format, and site will vary by school, primary care physicians who participate in teaching should

- Offer students exposure to their practices and practice management;
- Provide timely support to students for patients and academic inquiries;
- Ensure that course aims are explicit and met;

- Give and receive feedback; and
- Understand the school's evaluation process.

For faculty development, it will be necessary to create rewards to recruit and retain appropriate full-time and community-based faculty. Such rewards should include timely progress on an academic track that is appropriate for clinician–teachers. If such a track does not exist, a school will need to decide whether sufficient flexibility is present within existing tracks to accommodate significant numbers of clinician–teachers, or carry out the work of faculty consensus-building to create a new track. Not all tracks will lead to tenure. Differing tracks, however, will allow faculty to be recognized and valued for excellence in the varying types of work, acknowledging that the traditional "triple threat" is no longer an appropriate prototype for most members of the modern medical school faculty. While the landmarks for achievement may differ across tracks, high standards will prevail in each track if faculty are rewarded for attention to excellence, productivity, and being appropriate role models. While all review processes for all faculty should address teaching excellence, it may be expected that clinician–teacher faculty will distinguish themselves in their domain of academic achievement, by their excellence as model clinicians, and as leaders of programs of education and clinical practice in primary care.

Persons and policies related to faculty development should recognize the need for increasing the number of generalist physicians on the full-time faculty. Resources to support such faculty will promote primary-care–related scholarly activities, such as health services and outcomes research, and instruction in cost-effective teaching. Building a rigorous and prestigious scholarly agenda for generalist faculty will require both institutional and public support.

The individual faculty physician should be encouraged to make teaching part of a career. To improve the quality and efficiency of teaching and make participation in education more attractive to community-based faculty, the school should encourage teaching physicians' interest in a long-term teaching commitment. School leaders should evaluate and offer resources such as literature searching, clinical and educational consultation, continuing medical education (CME), time on campus (weekend advances or sabbaticals), locum tenens coverage, and opportunities for research in the ambulatory care setting. Medical schools might also offer preceptors specific CME courses that focus on developing teaching and evaluation skills.

## Making Teaching Resources Available

While faculty development models may differ for full-time academic and part-time or volunteer faculty, all require institutional support to foster a sense of connection to the system, provide technical assistance, and supply basic materials. Schools should make teaching resources available to all full-time faculty, appropriate residents, and community preceptors.

Modules for ambulatory care and generalist experiences, as well as shared curricular materials, are examples of content-related teaching resources. The participation in primary care education of numerous, diverse faculty at many sites increases the importance of sharing standardized materials. Coordination will facilitate all students' receiving fundamental information and achieving consistency among their experiences. Faculty will need to adapt standardized materials to make them relevant to the structure and patient mix of the training site. A balance of learning objectives must be achieved at each site, requiring educational experiences focused on a variety of topics ranging from epidemiology to pathophysiology. At each site and on behalf of the course overall, faculty will need to determine the relative roles of generalists and specialists in co-teaching specific course content.

In addition to providing resource materials and access to information, schools should offer specific sessions to help faculty and preceptors prepare for teaching. Sessions led by physicians and professional educators would involve an orientation to the program and curriculum, a preview of problems educators are likely to face, guidance on providing feedback to students, standards for evaluating students' performances, and advice on supporting students who encounter difficulty. Preceptors should understand the type of case mix desirable for students' development and how to impart to students the evidence base that supports observed practice patterns. Quality measures, as described below, will be necessary to assure consistency or equivalency in the teaching done at different sites by different preceptors.

Good development of resource materials implies planning and requires expertise and evaluation. A number of national resources provide specific information and references on developments and results in education research, including the AAMC, through the Group on Educational Affairs (GEA), the annual conference on Research in Medical Education (RIME); various professional societies, such as clerkship director groups; the newly formed Society of Researchers in Medical Education; two centers funded by the Health Resources and Services Administration (HRSA) at the University of North Carolina and the University of Washington; and various foundation-supported institutes and projects. These sources can help administrators and faculty build a primary care program for a medical school. The key to taking advantage of this expertise is to prepare the information so that it captures the attention of deans and other medical school decision makers.

## Creating a Research Agenda

Clinicians often practice with a limited evidence base to make scientific decisions about basic care. The development of a faculty enterprise in primary care creates rich opportunities for scholarly activity dealing with questions of medical practice in primary care, an open agenda for research in many schools of medicine.

A second research agenda involves research in education. Clearly, despite the impressive contributions made so far in this area, there is an unmet need for discovering which educational methods are most effective in the education of medical students in various content areas and settings. Given the current rapid evolution of the medical marketplace, it is also noteworthy that in September 1995 the AAMC and HRSA held a joint conference to develop a list of priority issues for research in education in managed care.[29] From the perspective of that conference, research priorities include how to define the competencies of an undifferentiated physician graduate and how to involve stakeholders in educational activities.

# FINANCING

The importance of sustainable financing for the development of primary care in medical schools cannot be overstated. Heightened attention to generalist education and to education in ambulatory settings calls for significant resources. We do not comment on the resources needed to finance a comprehensive primary care delivery network—rather, we focus on the portion of the challenge directly related to the support of academic missions.

We note a lack of reliable data from which to draw conclusions about financing needs. The work of the AAMC Task Force on Medical School Financing has contributed to the knowledge base, particularly with respect to the cost of medical students' education.[30] However, we agree with the members of that task force that it is not easy to quantify the cost of education, particularly as schools arrange for increased student experiences in ambulatory care settings. We recommend that the AAMC conduct or sponsor a study of the costs of teaching in the ambulatory setting, and we affirm the importance of collecting, analyzing, and disseminating such data to assist medical school leaders in program and financial planning.

Many medical schools' planning efforts reveal growing acknowledgment of modest decreases in productivity in ambulatory care settings when medical students are present. In most situations, hard dollar support will be necessary to finance medical students' education in these settings. Achieving maximum efficiency for the dedicated dollars points to the need to develop dedicated sites and teachers to carry out primary care and ambulatory care education. Payment of faculty is the most sensitive variable in the equation of financing ambulatory-based primary care education. For full-time faculty, some combination of base pay plus a variable component for attaining specific goals seems most reasonable. For part-time faculty, the situation is more complicated. Staff at the

University of Nevada conducted a brief survey in October 1994 to ascertain how various schools had approached the issue of payment for preceptors.[31] Of the eight schools interviewed, five paid preceptors and all eight offered non-payment incentives. Sources of funds to support the payments included state dollars, federal grants, Area Health Education Center programs, and clinical income. Non-payment incentives included discounts on CME and other university events or products (tickets, bookstore purchases, etc.), awards banquets, access to consults and online information, and faculty development courses. There are numerous in-kind services of value that schools can offer community-based faculty. In addition to those mentioned in the survey, many medical schools could offer management service organization benefits to physicians who serve on the faculty or to the organizations where they work. Such benefits encourage participation in education activities and help offset the costs of lowered productivity. Finally, we recommend that the AAMC develop a project that will provide information and possible strategies for supporting preceptors. In addition to human costs, greater work is required to understand the facility (and other) costs of supporting primary care activities.

# DEVELOPING OUTCOME MEASURES

If a thoroughgoing effort is made to inculcate a generalist curriculum into the learning experiences of all physicians at a medical school, how can school faculty and leaders know whether the net effect of such educational change improves the quality of medical education and prepares graduates to understand the marketplace and the evolving health care delivery system? Residency falls between medical school and entry into the practicing workforce. What quality indicators should be measured to determine a medical school graduate's readiness to enter a residency and to move toward independent practice?

The first step in measurement and evaluation—defining educational objectives or competencies—is a daunting task for faculty. Examples of objectives related to both primary care and medicine as a general degree include increasing the students' knowledge of chronic disease in stages; observing and analyzing patient and clinician interaction; and understanding how interdisciplinary teams deliver care and how various types of physicians develop and disseminate a specific area of expertise. Measurement tools for student performance in such complex domains commonly rely on faculty ratings.

Objectives-based performance indicators, where students demonstrate skills, can supplement faculty assessments. Performance-based standardized evaluation systems will become increasingly important as students move into decentralized sites. General examinations will help calibrate variances in faculty rating systems. Student logs can help assess whether students have seen an appropriate mix of patients. To help assess the quality of the educational experience in a particular site, schools should routinely ask students to complete evaluations of faculty and sites in ambulatory care clerkships, compile these evaluations to build a normative database for ratings, and take all available opportunities (educational sites visits, direct observation of faculty performance, peer evaluations, etc.) to validate the evaluations by the students. Systematic feedback from residency programs on the readiness of graduates for their responsibilities as interns, especially in those areas that the medical school has highlighted as core generalist competencies, will be another available source of salient evaluation information.

Most schools are at the beginning stages of evaluating whether students acquire the knowledge and skills needed in ambulatory care settings. Measures, such as patient logs and standardized patients, are mostly used to record students' experiences rather than to evaluate skills particular to ambulatory care settings. The Robert Wood Johnson Generalist Initiative has helped support such projects. For example, at SUNY–Buffalo, students' experiences are monitored through the use of patient-encounter logs. These experiences are categorized and compared for each of the generalist specialties. Standardized patients may be used in the future as an assessment tool, as they are used presently as a learning tool. An assessment of students' knowledge, skills, and attitudes at the end of the third year, according to each school's educational objectives, will allow students to use the fourth year as a resource to learn what they have not encountered earlier. This approach may not be feasible for schools that do not have an ambulatory care rotation in the fourth year.

# SUMMARY AND RECOMMENDATIONS

We, as members of the APMOMS Working Group on Sustaining the Development of Academic Primary Care, maintain that primary care is a function that should be central to the medical school's mission. The function should cut across traditional departmental boundaries and be part of the school's central focus on graduating, non-differentiated, generalist physicians capable of advancing to any specialty. Accepting these premises has implications for both medical schools and the AAMC.

## Recommendations for Medical Schools

Medical schools' commitment to primary care should be deep and far-reaching. It should be evident in institutional mission and strategic planning, curricular development, faculty and resource development, new outcome standards for assurance of quality in primary education, and financial policy. Our recommendations for medical schools follow.

### Institutional Mission and Planning

- Medical schools should incorporate the concepts of primary care and generalism into their central missions, establishing needed infrastructure for the oversight and management of these mission programs.

- Medical schools should seek alliances with appropriate clinical services networks, including HMOs and other major health care delivery systems.

- Medical schools should retain the responsibility for, and protect the integrity of, academic missions within service affiliations.

### Curriculum

- Medical schools should adopt curricula centered on teaching generalist competencies.

- Medical schools should find or develop appropriate ambulatory teaching settings, including a significant resource in primary care settings.

- Medical schools should develop, in either ownership or partnership arrangements, the appropriate mix of medical school campus faculty and community-based faculty to carry out their primary care mission.

### Faculty and Resource Development

- Medical schools should develop appropriate resources to assure that primary care faculty receive professional development and career support, including appropriate academic appointment and promotion tracks and incentive systems for academic functions.

- Medical schools should develop teaching resources to help students achieve the core competencies fostered by the generalist curriculum.

- Medical schools should encourage the development of primary care research and research about how to achieve the most effective primary care education.

### Measurement

- Medical schools should develop evaluation and monitoring systems to assure that all graduates successfully acquire generalist competencies.

### Finance

- Medical schools should assure that adequate financing is available to support the generalist education of medical students, wherever this mission is carried out, including in extended primary care networks.

## Recommendations for the AAMC

We also identified recommendations for the AAMC, in its role as a champion for medical education and as a forum for innovation, to promote the role of the primary care function in medical schools.

- The AAMC should enhance efforts to spotlight generalism and primary care in regional and national forums.

- The AAMC should reaffirm support for projects on organizational models, generalist curriculum objectives, and opportunities for research in primary care settings.

- The AAMC should conduct surveys and develop a clearinghouse to disseminate the best educational practices, information about the impact of innovative policies, organizational performance benchmarks, and information about pathfinder programs in generalism and primary care education, including (1) workshops to showcase innovations and best practices in primary care teaching and research; and (2) appropriate awards or programs for excellence in primary care to recognize innovative schools, faculty, programs and/or graduates.

- The AAMC should lead in the development of projects to assess costs of undergraduate medical education in all settings.

- The AAMC should advocate that there be increased public and private resources to support scholarly activity in primary care and research in primary care education.

- The AAMC should provide consultative resources and facilitate inter-school exchange to schools trying to promote primary care.

- The AAMC should facilitate professional development programs for leaders of primary care functions.

## Notes

1. Cooper RA. Seeking a balanced physician workforce for the twenty-first century. *JAMA.* 1994;272:680–687.

2. Council on Graduate Medical Education. *Third Report: Improving Access to Health Care Through Physician Workforce Reform: Directions for the 21st Century.* Hyattsville, Md: U.S. Department of Health and Human Services; 1992.

3. Council on Graduate Medical Education. *Fourth Report: Recommendations to Improve Access to Care Through Physician Workforce Reform: Directions for the 21st Century.* Hyattsville, Md: U.S. Department of Health and Human Services; 1994.

4. Hart LG, Wagner E, Pirzada S, Nelson AF, Rosenblatt RA. Physician staffing ratios in staff-model HMOs: a cautionary tale. *Health Aff.* 1997;16:55–70.

5. Kindig DA. Counting generalist physicians. *JAMA*. 1994;271:1505–1507.

6. Rivo ML, Kindig DA. A report card on the physician workforce in the United States. *N Engl J Med*. 1996;334:892–896.

7. Schroeder SA. The latest forecast: managed care collides with physician supply. *JAMA*. 1994;272:239–240.

8. Weiner JP. Forecasting the effects of health reform on the U.S. physician workforce requirements. *JAMA*. 1994;272:222–230.

9. Whitcomb ME. A cross-national comparison of generalist physician workforce data. *JAMA*. 1996;274:692–695.

10. AAMC policy on the generalist physician. *Acad Med*. 1993;68:681–686.

11. Graduate Medical Education National Advisory Committee. *Summary Report to the Secretary of Health and Human Services*. Washington, DC: U.S. Department of Health and Human Services, Health Resources Administration; 1981.

12. Lohr KN, Vanselow NA, Detmer DE, eds. *The Nation's Physician Workforce: Options for Balancing Supply and Requirements*. Washington, DC: National Academy Press; 1996.

13. Petersdorf RG. The doctor is in. *Acad Med*. 1993;68:113–117.

14. Pew Health Professions Commission. *Critical Challenges: Revitalizing the Health Professions for the Twenty-First Century*. San Francisco: University of California, San Francisco, Center for the Health Professions; 1995.

15. Draft Report of the Ad Hoc Committee on Generalism to the Executive Committee for the Accreditation Council for Graduate Medical Education [unpublished]. Chicago: Accreditation Council for Graduate Medical Education; 1993.

16. Donaldson MS, Yordy KD, Vanselow NA, eds. *Defining Primary Care: An Interim Report*. Washington, DC: National Academy Press; 1994.

17. Muller S, chairman. Physicians for the twenty-first century: report of the Project on the General Professional Education of the Physician and College Preparation for Medicine. *J Med Educ*. 1984;59(11 Pt 2).

18. Culbertson RA, Goode LD, Dickler RM. Organizational models for medical school relationships to the clinical enterprise. *Acad Med*. 1996;71:1258–1274.

19. Council on Graduate Medical Education. *Sixth Report: Managed Health Care: Implications for the Physician Workforce and Medical Education*. Hyattsville, Md: U.S. Department of Health and Human Services; 1995.

20. Veloski J, Barzansky B, Nash DB, Stevens DP. Medical student education in managed care settings: beyond HMOs. *JAMA*. 1996;276:667–671.

21. Houpt JL, Goode LD, Anderson RJ, et al. How medical schools can maintain quality while adapting to resource constraints. *Acad Med*. 1997;72:180–185.

22. Association of American Medical Colleges and the American Medical Association. *Functions and Structures of a Medical School: Accreditation and the Liaison Committee on Medical Education: Standards for Accreditation of Medical Education Pro-*

*grams Leading to the M.D. Degree.* Washington, DC: Association of American Medical Colleges and the American Medical Association; 1993:13–14.

23. Group Health Association of America. *Primary Care Physicians: Recommendations to Reform Medical Education to Increase the Supply of Physicians Trained to Practice in Managed Care.* Washington, DC: Group Health Association of America; undated.

24. Noble J, Bithoney W, MacDonald P, et al. The core content of generalist curriculum for general internal medicine, family practice, and pediatrics. *J Gen Intern Med.* 1994;9(4 Suppl 1):S31–S42.

25. O'Neil E. Education as part of the health care solution: strategies from the Pew Health Professions Commission. *JAMA.* 1992;268:1146–1148.

26. Rubenstein LV, Fink A, Gelberg L, et al. Evaluation generalist education programs: a conceptual framework. *J Gen Intern Med.* 1994;9(4 Suppl 1):S64–S72.

27. Association of American Medical Colleges. *Report I: Learning Objectives for Medical Student Education: Guidelines for Medical Schools: Medical Schools Objectives Project.* Washington, DC: Association of American Medical Colleges; 1998.

28. Pellegrin KL, Arana GW. Why the triple-threat approach threatens the viability of academic medical centers. *Acad Med.* 1997;73:123–125.

29. Sanderson SC. Conference challenges traditional thinking in medical education. *AAMC Reporter.* 1995;5(2):6,7.

30. Association of American Medical Colleges. *The Financing of Medical Schools. A Report of the AAMC Task Force on Medical School Financing.* Washington, DC: Association of American Medical Colleges; 1996.

31. Conaboy K, Assistant Dean for Planning and Development, University of Nevada School of Medicine, Reno. Personal communication; 1995.

# Abstracts from the Literature

## Education and Training

## BOOKS AND REPORTS

Council on Graduate Medical Education. *Second Report: The Financial Status of Teaching Hospitals and the Underrepresentation of Minorities in Medicine.* Rockville, Md: U.S. Department of Health and Human Services; 1990.

Council on Graduate Medical Education. *Sixth Report: Managed Health Care: Implications for the Physician Workforce and Medical Education.* Rockville, Md: U.S. Department of Health and Human Services; 1995.

Council on Graduate Medical Education. *Seventh Report. Physician Workforce Funding Recommendations for Department of Health and Human Services' Programs.* Rockville, Md: U.S. Department of Health and Human Services; 1995.

Council on Graduate Medical Education. *Ninth Report: Graduate Medical Education Consortia: Changing the Governance of Graduate Medical Education to Achieve Physician Workforce Objectives.* Rockville, Md: U.S. Department of Health and Human Services; 1997.

Council on Graduate Medical Education. *Eleventh Report: International Medical Graduates, the Physician Workforce, and GME Payment Reform.* Rockville, Md: U.S. Department of Health and Human Services; 1998.

Council on Graduate Medical Education. *Thirteenth Report: Physician Education for a Changing Health Care Environment.* Rockville, Md: U.S. Department of Health and Human Services; 1999.

Council on Graduate Medical Education. *Fifteenth Report. Financing Graduate Medical Education in a Changing Health Care Environment.* Rockville, Md: U.S. Department of Health and Human Services; 2000.

Institute of Primary Care. *Proceedings, October 6–8, 1974.* Washington, DC: Association of American Medical Colleges; 1974.   The Institute of Primary Care, the first AAMC-sponsored institute, was conceived as a forum to focus on the issues surrounding the education of physicians for careers in primary care. The program included a consideration of how physicians relate to other health professions. Sessions covered the following topics: issues in primary care (the academic and policy perspective); organization of model systems for primary care practice and education; education of new health practitioners; graduate physician training in primary care; and new directions in health science education.

Institute of Medicine. *Primary Care Physicians: Financing Their Graduate Medical Education in Ambulatory Settings.* Washington, DC: National Academy Press; 1989.

National Commission on Community Health Services. *Health Is a Community Affair.* Cambridge, Mass: Harvard University Press; 1966.   This report called for the education of a "personal physician who is the central point for integration and continuity of all medical and medically related services to the patient."

Pew Health Professions Commission. *Survey of Practitioners' Perception of Their Education: Summary of Findings.* San Francisco: University of California, San Francisco, Center for the Health Professions; 1991.   Conducted by Louis Harris and Associates in February-March 1991.

Pew Health Professions Commission. *Contemporary Issues in Health Professions' Education and Workforce Reform.* San Francisco: University of California, San Francisco, Center for the Health Professions; 1993.

Pew Health Professions Commission. *Innovative Programs in Health Professions' Education.* San Francisco: University of California, San Francisco, Center for the Health Professions; 1994.

Pew Health Professions Commission. *Physician Retraining as a Strategy to Enhance the Primary Care Workforce.* San Francisco: University of California, San Francisco, Center for the Health Professions; 1994.

Pew Health Professions Commission. *Retraining Specialist Physicians in Primary Care: Conference Proceedings.* San Francisco: University of California, San Francisco, Center for the Health Professions; 1994.

Pew Health Professions Commission. *Health Professions Education and Managed Care: Challenges and Necessary Responses.* San Francisco: University of California, San Francisco, Center for the Health Professions; 1995.

Pew Health Professions Commission. *Beyond the Balanced Budget Act of 1997: Strengthening the Federal GME Policy Task Force.* San Francisco: University of California, San Francisco, Center for the Health Professions; 1998.

# ARTICLES

Alpert JJ. Graduate education for primary care: problems and issues. *J Med Educ.* 1975;50(12):123–128.   This article examines the problems and issues that must be considered in developing primary care graduate education. The author identifies five elements: (1) the setting, (2) the patients, (3) the curriculum, (4) the students, (5) the faculty. He goes on to discuss the disciplines most often identified with primary care programs—internal medicine, pediatrics, and family medicine—and to bring the pressing issues into sharper focus. He concludes by recognizing the importance of specialty boards and suggesting that they could prove to be both a stimulus as well as an obstacle to the development of programs.

Alpert JJ. Primary care: the future for pediatric education. *Pediatrics.* 1990;86:653–659. This article reviews the history of the primary care crisis; revisits the definition of primary care; and, through identification of critical issues, presents a primary care educational agenda for the 1990s. The author suggests that pediatrics is at a crossroads regarding primary care, as powerful social and economic forces affect today's major pediatric care problems. Historically, the pediatric curriculum has been organ and disease based. In the future, it must have a stronger behavioral component emphasizing continuity of care. The future curriculum must include training in the care of hospitalized children, chronically ill children, and adolescents; use of computers and other communication aids; direct physician-patient communication skills, health maintenance counseling; and practice and risk management. The author concludes with reference to the advocacy that must be expected from the primary care pediatrician. He refers to large scale medical and social issues, such as AIDS and poverty that need to be addressed, and the necessity of adopting a national health insurance program.

Alpert JJ, Bauchner H, Pelton SI, et al. Career choice in one general pediatric Title VII–supported residency. *Arch Pediatr Adolesc Med.* 1995;149:1019–1021.   This article considers grants awarded through Title VII of the Public Health Service Act supporting primary care residency training for family practice, general pediatrics, and general internal medicine. A pediatric program at Boston City Hospital and Boston University School of Medicine, in operation since 1976, is examined. Based on questionnaires sent out to trainees one year out of training beginning in 1978 and a 1992 survey of trainees who spent 2 years in training, 66% of the respondents reported careers in generalist pediatrics, 27% were pediatric subspecialists and 7%

had other careers. The study findings confirmed the conclusion that a primary care program can support residents who wish to pursue generalist careers.

Bass JL, Mehta KA, Alpert JJ, Pelton S. Residency training in community pediatrics. *Pediatr Educ.* 1981;20:249–253. The Department of Pediatrics at Framingham Union Hospital, a Boston University affiliate, developed a resident's rotation in community pediatrics, including assignments to preschool and school settings, private pediatric offices, and in-hospital responsibilities. After 14 rotations, analysis of program content, as well as resident and community response, showed the experience to be a practical, workable model for incorporating community pediatrics into residency training.

Baldwin CD, Levine HG, McCormick DP. Meeting the faculty development needs of generalist physicians in academia. *Acad Med.* 1995;70(1 Suppl):S97–S103. As a means to assisting the development of the academic environments of generalist faculty members, the authors conducted a needs assessment that included two thirds of the generalist faculty members in family medicine, internal medicine, and pediatrics at the University of Texas Medical Branch, Galveston, Texas. The participants identified three global needs requiring significant change: (1) better understanding of and rewards for their academic activities, (2) better networking with each other and with non-generalists, and (3) more control over their time and responsibilities. Individual needs were diverse but emphasized teaching and career building skills. The authors recommend building project-oriented teams that collectively develop skills in strategic planning and project management, political negotiation and public relations, and creative use of institutional support systems.

Brooks WB, Orgren R, Wallace AG. Institutional change: embracing the initiative to train more generalists. *Acad Med.* 1999;74(1Suppl):S3–S8. In 1994, Dartmouth Medical School received a Generalist Physician Initiative (GPI) grant from The Robert Wood Johnson Foundation. This article describes the institutional change at the school, noting that while the context in which GPI was launched was receptive, the grant enabled Dartmouth to accelerate institutional changes that were already underway. Dartmouth used an approach to change that worked and, as such, the principles it employed should be generalizable to other schools. Key among these principles were capitalizing on a sense of urgency for change, creating and empowering a guiding coalition, developing and communicating the vision, generating short-term wins, consolidating gains, and anchoring new approaches to the existing institutional culture. Changes are described in the areas of admission and recruitment, undergraduate and graduate medical education, and supporting community practice and shortcomings in developing the program are also described.

Charney E. Internal medicine and pediatric residency education for primary care. *J Med Educ.* 1975;50(12):129–136. This article reviews a number of the new primary educational efforts in internal medicine and pediatric programs. The author considers the model practice goals, the issues and problems related to faculty, and the different curricula types and concludes that department of medicine and pediatrics are attempting to develop attractive and competitive residencies.

Charney E. Medical education in the community: the primary care setting as laboratory and training site. *Pediatr Ann.* 1994;23:664–668. This article on pediatric education in an ambulatory setting outlines some assumptions about residency education in general, expands on what is meant by the term *ambulatory setting,* describes the content of what can be taught in one of those settings—the community-based primary care practice—and suggests some strategies to make that a successful educational experience. The underlying assumption is that if pediatricians are to remain central to the provision of primary care, then the study and teaching of primary care must be central to the educational mission of academic departments of pediatrics.

Christiansen RG, Johnson LP, Boyd GE, Koepshall JE, Sutton K. A proposal for a combined family practice–internal medicine residency. *JAMA.* 1986;255:2628–2630. Both family practice and internal medicine currently train graduates for primary care. A single, four-year program is proposed that combines the strengths of family practice and internal medicine, incorporates community needs into the curriculum, and addresses the physician's changed role in a revolutionized health care provision system. Specific training recommendations and the societal and professional advantages of such a program are detailed.

De Witt DE, Curtis JR, Burke W. What influences career choices among graduates of a primary care training program? *J Gen Intern Med.* 1998;13:257–261. The objective of this study was to identify factors that influence primary care residents to become generalists or specialists. 88 internal medicine residency graduates who completed training between 1979 and 1993 were surveyed and interviewed. Although 82% of the participating graduates reported themselves very committed to primary care at the beginning of residency, only 68% pursued generalist careers. Factors influencing career choice that were more important to generalists than specialists included breadth of knowledge used in primary care practice, breadth of clinical problems in practice, and opportunity for continuity of care. Although salary was rated as "not important," 50% of generalists and specialists advocated increased salaries for generalists. Other promoting factors included mentors, increased prestige for generalists, community based training, lifestyle changes, and decreased paperwork. 73% of participants felt that it was easier to be a specialist than a generalist.

Eisenberg JM. Postgraduate training for general practice in the U.K. *J Med Educ.* 1979;54:314–322. This article considers postgraduate training for primary care practice in the United Kingdom. Trainees may enter a three-year program of coordinated inpatient and outpatient training or may select a series of independent posts. The author notes a curious emphasis on inpatient experience, especially as British general practitioners rarely treat patients in a hospital setting. In their outpatient experiences, trainees are provided with little variety in their instructors, practice settings, and medical problems. With a better understanding of training for primary care medicine in the UK, those planning American primary care training may avoid problems and incorporate some of the attributes of the British system for general practice.

Eisenberg JM. How can we pay for graduate medical education in ambulatory care? *N Engl J Med.* 1989;320:1525–1531. This article explores the financing of ambulatory care education for residents and suggests ways to reconcile the disparity between the educational needs of future physicians and the activities they are paid to perform. It looks at Medicare as an important source of funding but also stresses the need to consider alternatives such as HMOs, income of physicians, and federal grant programs. Other options include redirecting support from Medicaid and the Veterans Administration and using legislative, regulatory and marketplace initiatives to make funding available.

Freeman J, Cash C, Yonke A, Roe B, Foley R. A longitudinal primary care program in an urban public medical school: three years of experience. *Acad Med.* 1995;70(1 Suppl):S64–S68. This article discusses the experience of the University of Illinois at Chicago's College of Medicine with implementing a pilot generalist program. Various features of the program make it an interesting case study: it is inter-disciplinary, comprising pediatricians, general internists, and family practitioners; students join the program in the autumn of their first year; and it is changing from a voluntary to a required course of study. The difficulties and procedures in adopting this kind of program in a traditional medical school are discussed.

Friedman RH, Alpert JJ, Green LA. Strengthening academic generalist departments and divisions. *J Gen Intern Med.* 1994;9(1 Suppl):S90–S98. This article discusses how academic departments of family medicine and divisions of general internal medicine and general pediatrics have an important role in generalist medical education. The major organizational issues facing these units concern institutional influence, faculty development, role in medical education, research productivity, financial stability, and clinical responsibilities. These factors should be understood in order for medical schools to achieve the societal goal of producing generalist physicians.

Friedman RH, Pozen JT, Rosencrans LA, Eisenberg JM, Gertman PM. General internal medicine in academic medical centers: their emergence and functions. *Ann Intern Med.* 1982;96:233–238. General internal medicine units were established to meet institutional needs for primary care internal medicine teachers and clinicians. By the end of the 1970s, they had achieved major administrative and staffing responsibility for a wide variety of general education and service activities. This article concludes that the scope of general internal medicine units goes beyond the narrow definition of primary care internal medicine, to include activities traditionally considered those of the entire department of medicine. The article is based on a 1979 survey of chiefs of general internal medicine units.

Glasser M, Stearns J, McCord R. Defining a generalist education: an idea whose time is still coming. *Acad Med.* 1995;70(1 Suppl):S69–S74. Generalist physician trainees must develop the appropriate skills, knowledge and attitudes to understand patients' specific expectations, address wellness as well as illness, be familiar with concepts of clinical epidemiology, concentrate on interpersonal communication, and strive to control costs. This article examines the experience at The University of

Illinois College of Medicine in Rockford, which was established to provide community-based medical education. Beginning in the second year, all Rockford students have extensive experience in a community health center. The Rockford program has shown that the entire curriculum must give uncompromising support for generalist education. All primary care faculty must have a common knowledge base in the theory and practice of generalist medicine, and the shift to generalist education will require shifts in attitude and behavior throughout the academic medical community and the institution.

Graber DR, Bellack JP, Musham C, O'Neil EH. Academic deans' views on curriculum content in medical schools. *Acad Med.* 1997;72:901–907. Deans of 85 schools affiliated with the Association of American Medical Colleges and 15 schools associated with the American Association of Colleges of Osteopathy responded to a survey questionnaire to determine which of 33 topics they considered worthy of greater emphasis in medical curricula. "Effective patient provider relationships/communication," "outpatient/ambulatory care," "health promotion/disease promotion," had the three highest means ratings for ideal emphasis for allopathic school deans. "Primary care," "professional values," and "use of electronic information systems," also had high mean ratings. "Primary care," "outpatient/ambulatory care," and "health promotion/disease prevention," had the highest mean ratings for ideal emphasis by the osteopathic school deans. The study concludes that changes in health care delivery and an increasing generalist orientation are influencing deans' perspectives on needed curriculum changes, and there appears to be considerable support for a curriculum that will foster a broader, more humanistic role for physicians.

Greenlick MR. Educating physicians for population-based clinical practice. *JAMA.* 1992;267:1645–1648. The author contends that the traditional one-to-one physician-patient role obligations should be expanded to include a set of "one-to-one" physician-population obligations. The latter includes three components: (1) a resource allocation component, (2) a component focusing on the epidemiological nature of clinical practice, and (3) a component focusing on members of the population who are not regularly attended to within the normal context of physician care. These obligations are discussed in turn, and the author concludes by arguing for a population-based clinical practice model of medical education.

Haggerty R J. Community pediatrics. *N Engl J Med.* 1968;278:15–21. Community pediatrics is a new term distinctive from comprehensive pediatrics by its concern for all children in the community—not merely those who come for medical care. It particularly addresses the needs of children who do not receive adequate medical care. It is also concerned with providing adequate manpower to meet the needs of the community as well as quantity and quality of service. In this article, some of the community pediatric programs in which the University of Rochester is engaged are outlined in order to illustrate the role of the university department in this new field.

Haggerty RJ. The university and primary medical care. *N Engl J Med.* 1969;218: 416–422.   This article suggests that primary medical-care programs are legitimate and central concerns of every university medical school. Sufficient engagement in the community to learn how better to meet the needs of large numbers of patients who are now without care is necessary, but over-commitment to service programs should be avoided. The role of the university is to develop new programs, study them, and teach within them. Health service research offers an intellectually rewarding and academically legitimate field for faculty members engaged in this area. They should use the knowledge developed in such research to help forge public policy for health.

Hauer KE, Flanders SA, Wachter RM. Training future hospitalists. *West J Med.* 1999;171:367-370.   The rapid growth in hospitalists presents residents in internal medicine with a new career option as a hospitalist-based generalist physician. As well as being clinically competent in inpatient care, hospitalists should understand managed care, health care delivery systems, quality improvement, practice guidelines, subacute care, and end-of-life care. The internal residency program at University of California, San Francisco has developed a hospital medical residency program that includes exposure to hospitalist practices and continuity of care. Residents also carry out independent research or quality improvement projects, participate in a didactic curriculum, and complete a group project developing a hypothetical hospitalist system.

Inui TS. Reform in medical education: a health of the public perspective. *Acad Med.* 1996;71(1 Suppl):S119–S121.   The author suggests that the appearance of three factors may be responsible for the substantial remodeling of medical theory and practice in the late 20th century, and may act as the underlying paradigm for medical education: (1) a social consensus that the rate of rise of expenditures for medical care needs to abate; (2) the increase in the prevalence of managed care; and (3) the emergence of integrated delivery systems for managed care. He observes that to function within this new paradigm, medical education must give students preparation in "new" special competencies. These include: information management; care resource management; integration of guidelines and clinical judgment; enhanced relationships between clinician-patient, clinician-clinician and clinician-community; and expanded teamwork going beyond the clinical team to managers, for example, or informatics specialists. The synthesis of all these competencies is best described as "managing to optimal outcomes."

Jacoby I, Gary NE, Meyer GS, et al. Retraining physicians for primary care: a study of physicians' perspectives and program development. *JAMA.* 1997;277:1569–1573. The objectives of this study were to determine the number and kinds of programs that medical schools and managed care programs offer or plan to offer to retrain physician specialists to practice primary care medicine and to discover physician attitudes toward retraining. A survey was mailed to 126 medical schools and the 19 largest managed care organizations. Physicians' attitudes towards retraining were elicited from 3 geographically diverse focus groups. Selected specialists were polled through the national survey of the American Medical Association's Socio-Economic Monitoring System to ascertain the demand for retraining. The study found that the majority of institutions contacted perceived a need for retraining but few programs have been established. Physicians preferred programs that would expand their patient base, maintain the practice population, be inexpensive and close to home, and provide hands-on training in the eventual practice environment. They also preferred a goal-oriented part-time retraining program in a large group practice or managed care setting that would allow them to practice their specialty while retraining. The authors conclude that physician interest and program availability for retraining remains low.

Levine MD, Robertson LS, Alpert JJ. A descriptive study of a pediatric internship. *Pediatrics*. 1969;44:986–990. The patient content of a pediatric internship was studied. While 60% of the internship is spent on inpatient services, almost 90% of the defined patient contact occurs in an ambulatory setting. The intern was more likely to provide care to advantaged families in the inpatient services. In the paper, the development of a teaching program in the ambulatory services is suggested as an essential part of pediatric education.

Linzer M, Salvin T, Mutha S, et al. Admission, recruitment, and retention: finding and keeping the generalist-oriented student. *J Gen Intern Med*. 1994;9(1 Suppl):S14–S23. As the country strives to produce larger numbers of generalist physicians, considerable controversy has arisen over whether or not generalist applicants can be identified, recruited, and influenced to keep generalist-oriented commitment throughout medical training. The authors present data to show that: (1) pre-admission programs can help to identify generalist-oriented students; (2) characteristics determined at admission to medical school are predictive of future generalist career choice; (3) current in-patient oriented training programs strongly push students away from a primary care career; (4) women are more likely than men to choose generalist careers, primarily because of those careers' interpersonal orientation; and (5) residency training programs are able to select applicants likely to become generalists. Therefore, to produce more generalists, attempts should be made to encourage generalist-oriented students to enter medical schools and to revise curricula to focus on outpatient settings in which students can establish effective and satisfying relationships with patients. These strategies are most likely to be successful if enacted within the context of governmental and medical school-based changes that allow for more reimbursement and respect for the generalist disciplines.

Lynch DC, Newton DA, Grayson MS, Whitley TW. Influence of medical school on medical students' opinions about primary care. *Acad Med*. 1998;73:433–435. The purpose of this study was to compare first- and fourth-year medical students' opinions about primary care practice. Medical students at New York Medical College and East Carolina University School of Medicine were given a self-administered questionnaire about professional aspects of primary care practice. In all, 639 (79%)

of the first year students and 396 (67%) of the fourth year students returned completed questionnaires. The first year students interested in primary care careers were significantly more likely than students interested in non-primary care careers to believe that primary care practice has more prestige, has more intellectual stimulation, needs a large knowledge base, and involves work that is more important than that of non-primary care physicians, and were significantly more likely to disagree with the assertion that in primary care practice, physicians have more control over their working hours. The comparison of the first and fourth-year students indicated that the fourth-year students were significantly more likely to believe that primary care practice has more intellectual stimulation, needs a large knowledge base, and requires knowledge that non-primary care practice may not; they were also significantly more likely to disagree with the assertions that primary care practice is adequately compensated, has more prestige, and allows more control over working hours. The authors conclude that students' positive perceptions about primary care practice may change as realistic perceptions about the professional demands on primary care physicians develop during medical school.

Martini CJM, Veloski J, Barzansky B, Xu G, Fields S. Medical school and student characteristics that influence choosing a generalist career. *JAMA*. 1994;272:661–668. The objective of this study was to identify predictors in medical schools that can be manipulated to affect the proportion of graduates entering general practice. Based on studies of medical schools and practicing generalist physicians, surveys of MD- granting and DO-granting medical schools, site visits to nine schools with a high proportion of graduates becoming generalist physicians, and a national sampling of MD and DO generalist physicians, the authors found that institutional mission, certain admissions policies, characteristics of entering students, and the presence of a primary care-oriented curriculum explained the statistically significant variation in the number of physicians choosing generalist careers. Personal social values was the individual characteristic that most strongly influenced graduates' career choice.

Mathieu OR Jr, Alpert JJ. Residency training in general pediatrics: the role of federal funding. *Am J Dis Child*. 1987;141:754–775. This study addresses the issue of why residency programs are hesitant to accept Title VII of the Public Health Service Act of 1976 funding. Based on a mailed survey completed by 130 pediatric residency training programs (22 of which were receiving Title VII funding), the authors found that 55% of the large programs (over 30 residents) had applied for federal funds compared with 33% of the medium sized programs (15–30 residents) and 24% of the small programs (under 15 residents). The most cited reason for failure to apply for funding was an unwillingness to finance resident positions with grant funds. The second most cited reason was the inconsistency between primary care training requirements and departmental goals. The requirement of 25% continuity ranked third among reasons. 90% of the programs surveyed, whether funded or not, included curricula in developmental and behavioral pediatrics. In addition, pediatric programs that were receiving Title VII funds reported more use of out-of-hospital teaching sites than non-funded programs.

Mathieu OR Jr, Alpert JJ, Pelton, SI. Residency training in general pediatrics: career direction of primary care graduates. *Am J Dis Child.* 1989;143:217–219. A pediatric primary care program was developed and established at Boston City Hospital in 1974. From 1974–1979 the program had a primary care track and a traditional track. After 1979 pediatrics continued as a primary care program for all residents. From 1977, questionnaires were sent annually to program graduates. The responses to the questionnaires showed that 80% of the initial primary care cohorts chose primary care careers compared with 52% of the traditional track cohorts and that 16% of the primary care cohorts reported themselves to be in subspecialty careers compared to 34.8% of the traditional track residents. Of the 1979–84 primary care cohorts, 78.5% were in general pediatrics and 20% had chosen subspecialty careers. Only three of the 60 graduates from the original primary care cohort had changed career between 1983 and 1987. The study provides additional data that primary care residency programs have achieved the goal of educating pediatricians to pursue careers as generalists.

Matson CC, Ullian JA, Boisaubin EV. Integrating early clinical experience curricula at two medical schools: lessons learned from The Robert Wood Johnson Foundation's Generalist Physician Initiative. *Acad Med.* 1999;74(1 Suppl):S53–S58. The University of Texas Medical Branch and Eastern Virginia Medical School created community based generalist clinical experiences early in the first two years of medical school as part of The Robert Wood Johnson Foundation's Generalist Physician Initiative. The article describes the experiences and related curricula, outlining the common elements and differing approaches at the two institutions. The authors evaluate the success of the programs and discuss nine lessons learned. They conclude that early clinical experience with generalist physicians is an important element of generalist curriculum reform.

Newton DA, Grayson MS, Whitley TW. What predicts medical school career choice? *J Gen Intern Med.* 1998;13:200–203. The literature on medical student career choice has identified several influences that can be categorized as student demographics, medical school characteristics, students' perceptions of specialty characteristics, and student-held values. A model was used that included demographics, medical school, and student-rated influences as a proxy for perceptions and values to determine their relative contribution to student career choice, for three consecutive cohorts of senior medical students attending two schools. The model identified a positive relationship between choice of primary care career and both student-rated influences and one student demographic characteristic, but not between career choice and school attended. Variables positively correlated with primary care career choice were related to working with people and marital status. Negatively correlated variables were related to income and prestige.

Odegaard CE, Inui TS. A 1992 manifesto for primary physicians. *Pharos Alpha Omega Alpha Hono Med Soc.* 1992;55(3):2–6. This article refers to Abraham Flexner's report of 1910. Even Flexner, in 1910, suggested that there should be more than a biological base for the physician's treatment of a patient. The authors discuss the importance of all physicians having some degree of knowledge broader than that currently provided by the established biomedical traditions. Expanding psychosocial understanding of patients is particularly important to the primary care physician. The authors suggest that if the small number of physicians that favor interdisciplinary development is to expand, it will need funding support for increased networking among themselves from innovative foundations, private and public.

Peinado SC, Eisenberg JM. Financing graduate medical education in primary care: options for change. *J Fam Pract.* 1990;31:637–644. This article provides an analysis of the alternatives for changing graduate medical education (GME) financing to aid primary care. Alternative sources of funding for primary care GME include changes in Medicare payments, increased categorical GME funding, ambulatory payment, and grants; commitments from future employers; and redistribution of current funds. One option for spending these funds to aid primary care programs is to divide the sources in three ways: on a per-resident basis, by competitive grants, or by incentives for primary care education.

Perkins I, Vale DJ, Graham MS. Partnerships in primary health care. *Nurs Health Care Perspect.* 2001;22:20–25. This article describes the process of curriculum change in a baccalaureate nursing program and the design of a competency-oriented learning system in primary health care, community focused nursing education. The first priority, the identification of issues and trends in health care and nursing education, was accomplished through a critical review of the literature. The next priority in the assessment process, was to determine the competencies necessary for beginning practitioners of nursing in community-focused settings.

Perkoff GT. Teaching clinical medicine in the ambulatory setting: an idea whose time may have finally come. *N Engl J Med.* 1986;314:27–31. In this article, early attempts to teach clinical medicine in ambulatory-care settings are reviewed and pitfalls identified that new efforts in this direction should avoid. Inpatient and ambulatory-care teaching are compared as a basis for understanding the educational goals that can be achieved more easily in each setting. In addition, recommendations are made about major changes in the flow and use of clinical-practice funds and hospital payments, so that they can become possible sources of financing and organization of an expanded effort to teach in ambulatory-care settings.

Petersdorf RG, Turner KS. Medical education in the 1990s—and beyond: a view from the United States. *Acad Med.* 1995;70(Suppl):S41–S47. This article reviews the standard US medical school curriculum and discusses suggestions for change. The authors suggest that medical education must become more student- and learning-oriented, must place more emphasis on primary care, and must use new settings for education. They also examine the reasons that medical schools fail in their education mission.

Rivo ML, Saultz JW, Wartman SA, De Witt TG. Defining the generalist physician's training. *JAMA*. 1994;271:1499–1504. The objective of this study was to determine the extent to which various specialties prepare residents in the broad competencies required for primary care practice, and to propose guidelines for improving generalist physician training. From a variety of data sources, the authors identified the common conditions and diagnoses that broadly trained generalist physicians could be expected to manage in primary care practice. They then compiled a list of 60 requisite residency training components grouped according to seven practice criteria for generalist physicians. The study found that almost all of the 60 generalist training components were required by family practice (95%), internal medicine (91%), and pediatrics (91%) compared with emergency medicine (42%), and obstetrics and gynecology (47%). Family practice, internal medicine, and pediatric residencies also require lengthy, well-defined continuity-of-care experience. To train competent generalist physicians, the authors recommend that residency programs require training in 90% or more of the 60 components, 50% or more of the components in each of the seven categories, and a continuity-of-care experience for a panel of patients during at least 10% of the entire residency period.

Rosenblatt RA, Alpert JJ. The effect of a course in family medicine on future career choice: a long-range follow-up of a controlled experiment in medical education. *J Fam Pract*. 1979;8:87–91. In this article, the career choices and professional behavior of three cohorts of students who participated in a family medicine program were studied by mail questionnaire. Cohort I was randomly selected for the course; unselected classmates were used as controls. Cohort II and Cohort III were volunteers; alphabetically adjacent classmates were used as a comparison group. The results suggest that the impact of a given medical school course on future behavior must be evaluated in the context of general medical school orientation and societal trends extraneous to the school itself.

Rubenstein LV, Fink A, Gelberg L, et al. Evaluating generalist education programs: a conceptual framework. *J Gen Intern Med*. 1994;9(1 Suppl):S64–S71. This article provides and applies a conceptual framework and a list of guiding principles for the evaluation of generalist education programs. The authors then explore evaluation design based on key generalist competencies agreed upon by pediatricians, general internists and family practitioners and consider the implications of undertaking an evaluation.

Schatz IJ, Realini JP, Charney E. Family practice, internal medicine and pediatrics as partners in education of generalists. *Acad Med*. 1996;71:35–39. The generalist of the future will play an integral role in the health care delivery system, yet the three specialties, family medicine, internal medicine and pediatrics, have developed and functioned along separate tracks. This article calls for the specialties to operate collaboratively in developing new graduate medical education programs that are sufficiently flexible to meet whatever emerges in the future. The article suggests that a substantial part of the training should be generic and interchangeable among the three specialties. They must begin to "train physicians to provide continuing, comprehensive and coordinated medical care to a population undifferentiated by gender, disease or organ system," as urged by the American Boards of Family Practice and Internal Medicine.

Scherger JE, Rucker L, Morrison EH, Cygan R, Hubbell A. The primary care specialties working together: a model of success in an academic environment. *Acad Med.* 2000;75:693–698.   Academic leaders at the University of California at Irvine (UCI) have developed a collaborative model in which faculty in family medicine, general internal medicine and general pediatrics cooperate extensively in research and patient care. The University has appointed an associate dean for primary care who leads the UCI Primary Care Coalition, reflecting and promoting the inter-specialty cooperation. This does not represent a move towards a generic primary care specialty. Generalist disciplines have preserved their individuality. Yet, collaboration has allowed primary care faculty to share resources, a research infrastructure, and clinical systems, thus avoiding duplicative use of valuable resources while maximizing collective negotiating abilities and mutual success.

Schroeder SA. Expanding the site of clinical education: moving beyond the hospital walls. *J Gen Intern Med.* 1988;3(Suppl):S5–S14.   This article describes the profound changes that have taken place in the content of hospital practice up to the 1980s, and how these changes threaten the relevance of the traditional hospital-based model for clinical education. The author argues that unless the current model can adjust, it will become decreasingly relevant. The article reviews briefly how the current model became so entrenched, describes the nature of the forces that threaten it, and examines the barriers to shifting education outside the hospital. The author concludes by noting that to some extent the case for reform of clinical teaching is hampered by the paucity of good evaluation data on medical education.

Schwenk TL, Detmer DE. Whither primary care in the academic health science center? *J Fam Pract.* 1986;23:489–493.   This article describes the current relationship between primary care and the academic medical center, contributions that primary care can make to the medical center, and the benefits that would accrue to both the center and primary care should a closer working relationship develop. The benefits include increased outpatient volume and revenue, a more balanced inpatient mix, better primary medical care education, an enhanced community reputation, and a greater influence by primary care on medical center policies. Published and personal case study experiences that show some of the potential problems with a closer working relationship are also described.

Schwenk TL, Sheets KJ, Marquez JT, et al. Where, how, and from whom do family practice residents learn? A multisite analysis. *J Fam Med.* 1997;19:265–268.   This article presents the results of a multi-site study of 2,481 teacher-learner events reported by family practice residents in four separate training programs. The events were characterized by location, activity and teacher. Hospital-based direct patient care under the supervision of a non-family practice specialist was the most frequent type of educational experience in three years. Learning in the outpatient setting with another specialist matched, or in some cases, exceeded that with a family physician. The authors observe that the study raises important issues regarding the type and nature of educational influences on family practice physicians. Of greatest concern, is the absence of role modeling and direct teaching by family practice specialists.

Urbina C, Hickey M, McHarney Brown C, Duban S, Kaufman A. Innovative generalist programs: academic health centers respond to the shortage of generalist physicians. *J Gen Intern Med.* 1994;9(1 Suppl):S81–S89.   Academic health care centers are increasingly exploring innovative ways to increase the supply of generalist physicians. The authors review successful innovations at academic health centers in recruitment and admissions, undergraduate medical education, residency training, and practice support. Successful recruitment of generalist-oriented applicants requires identification and tracking of rural, minority, and other special groups of students at high school and college levels. Academic health centers that provide early, sustained, community-based, ambulatory experiences for medical students and residents encourage trainees to maintain and choose generalist careers. Finally, academic health centers that link with community providers and with state government encourage the retention of generalist physicians through continuing education and teaching networks.

Valente E, Wyatt SM, Moy E, et al. Market influences on internal medicine residents' decisions to subspecialize. *Ann Intern Med.* 1998;128:915–921.   The study attempted to determine whether market forces, as exemplified by managed care penetration into an area where the residents trained, was associated with a decreased likelihood that general internal medicine graduates pursued subspecialty training. Based on a study of the career paths of 2,263 US medical school graduates who completed general internal medicine residency training in 1993, the authors found that graduates of US medical schools completing general internal medicine training in areas with high HMO penetration were significantly less likely to subspecialize. However, the influence of market forces is small compared with the effects of age and gender.

Weil PA, Schleiter MK, Tarlov AR. National Study of Internal Medicine Manpower V: comparison of residents in internal medicine—future generalists and subspecialists. *Ann Intern Med.* 1981;94:678–690.   Questionnaire III of the National Study of Internal Medicine Manpower was directed to a random sample of residents and subspecialty fellows. Residents were classified according to whether they sought careers predominantly as general internists (49%) or subspecialty internists (51%) and the two groups were compared. Future generalists tended to be non-Jewish, to have incurred higher debts, and to have trained in medical schools in the states where they grew up. They were attracted to their work because of the ability to remain independent. Future subspecialists intended to have academic careers and locate in the larger cities. Although subspecialists expected greater financial rewards, neither group selected their field on this basis.

Weissert CS, Silberman SL. Sending a policy signal: state legislatures, medical schools, and primary care mandates. *J Health Polit Policy Law.* 1998;23:743–770. In the past few years, eleven states have directed their medical schools to produce more primary care practitioners or to change the training of physicians to make careers in primary care more attractive to medical students. This article outlines the progress and politics of the states' desire to hold medical schools accountable for producing more primary care practitioners. The authors find that the laws were not stringent or particularly onerous; they contained many loopholes and no real sanctions. They were important, however, in the message they conveyed.

Weitekamp MR, Ziegenfuss JT. Academic health centers and HMOs: a systems perspective on collaboration in training generalist physicians and advancing mutual interests. *Acad Med.* 1995;70(1Suppl):S47–S53. Academic health centers (AHCs) and health maintenance organizations (HMOs) often hold each other at arm's length because of fundamental organizational differences. AHCs view HMOs as too intrusive in the clinical management of patients and too concerned with the bottom line. HMOs view AHCs as organizationally fragmented and expensive in providing health care services. This authors used an organizational systems model to examine the AHCs and HMOs in order to identify common needs, mutual interests, areas for potential collaboration, and bridging strategies. These include health care systems development, professional education, information management systems, and health services research. As the financing and delivery of health care continue to change, both organizations have much to gain from collaboration.

Young LE. Education and roles of personal physicians in medical practice. *JAMA.* 1964;187:927–933. In this article, the author considers the education and roles of personal physicians in medical practice. He defines the scope of responsibilities of the personal physician and discusses the differing roles of the general practitioner, the family physician, the pediatrician, and the internist. Based on his experience as Chairman of the Department of Medicine at the University of Rochester, the author offers suggestions about appropriate ways to structure undergraduate medical education and residency training in order to educate personal physicians, i.e., physicians who provide comprehensive medical care of their patients.

# CHAPTER TWENTY-SEVEN

# Influencing Academic Health Centers

## The Robert Wood Johnson Foundation Experience

Lewis G. Sandy, M.D., M.B.A.; Richard Reynolds, M.D.

1999

A cademic health centers,[1] or AHCs, are an American success story. The envy of the world, AHCs have created an explosion of knowledge in both basic biomedical science and clinical research. AHCs are also the locus of training for the next generation of physicians, nurses, pharmacists, and other health professionals, and they run the specialty and subspecialty training programs that create the practitioners of the most advanced medical care in the world. Not only are AHCs uniquely American in their grand scale and aspirations, they have developed a quintessential American trajectory, reflecting the American faith in technology, a can-do spirit, and even a bit of the Wild West.

Before World War II, AHCs were relatively modest in scope, had a main emphasis on education and research, and by contemporary terms were modest clinical enterprises. In the 1930s and '40s, the scientific era of medicine began to flourish, with the discovery of insulin, the initial success of antibiotics, and new technologies such as blood transfusion. World War II catalyzed further advances in medicine and surgery, and it was logical to believe that more research would produce effective treatments for cancer, heart disease, and other killers. Also, the success of the Manhattan Project, which led to the rapid development of the atomic bomb, suggested that combining world-class talent with modern facilities and generous financial support could lead to similar success in conquering disease.

After the war, the expansion of the National Institutes of Health, or NIH, and further advances in medical science provided fertile soil for accelerated growth.

In the 1960s, the creation of the Medicare program and its support for graduate medical education, coupled with the national mood of faith in science and technology that led to continued increases in funding for the NIH, created further support for specialty training and research and continued expansions of the clinical enterprise. AHCs began to develop such technologies as intensive care units, burn centers, heart transplant programs, and comprehensive cancer centers. Academic health physicians became household names and even celebrities— Denton Cooley, Michael De Bakey—and the nation's AHCs enjoyed unparalleled prestige, power, and influence.

In that context, the relationship of AHCs to The Robert Wood Johnson Foundation was initiated. When the Foundation became a national philanthropy in 1972, AHCs were viewed as the center of the health and health care universe. It was only logical that the leadership of the Foundation should be sought from that sector, and David Rogers, a former chairman of medicine at Vanderbilt and dean of the Johns Hopkins University School of Medicine, was recruited as the Foundation's first president.

Although the new president was a rising leader in academic medicine, the Foundation's initial view was that what was needed to improve health and health care was not perfectly congruent with the activities of AHCs. The Foundation's staff and board felt that there was an imperfect fit between the mission of AHCs and the needs of the nation. Although not denying the importance and the value of specialty training and practice, the Foundation felt that the declining interest in primary care and the need for a health care workforce that could care for a population's health needs were critical issues not being addressed by AHC leaders. The application of epidemiological principles to health care itself, or health services research, did not find a natural home either in AHCs or in the NIH. Public health, cleaved from medicine earlier in the century, had minimal input into the training of the nation's health care workforce. At the same time, the policy environment, seven years after the passage of Medicare and Medicaid legislation, looked promising for the extension of health entitlement programs to the rest of the population.

Most of David Rogers's academic colleagues thought he would use the Foundation's funds to support biomedical research. Rogers noted, however, that the NIH was putting billions of dollars into research funding, compared with the Foundation's $50 million grant-making capacity at that time. The Foundation thought more leverage could be gained by fostering the public and community responsibility of AHCs. Rogers was strongly criticized by his colleagues for this move. It did, however, represent his own beliefs about what AHCs should do. From that beginning, then, emerged a series of Foundation grants and programs with the aim of influencing academic medicine. What follows is a decade-to-decade analysis of these efforts, their achievements, limitations, and lessons.

# EARLY EFFORTS: THE 1970s

In our view, two additional strategic factors also influenced the relationship of the Foundation to AHCs: first, the recognized position of the AHCs as the leadership institutions in health care, and, second, the desire to work with the nation's leading people and institutions to ensure quality grant making. The more pragmatic requirement of initiating grant making expeditiously was also an important, but secondary, consideration.

The earliest grants made by The Robert Wood Johnson Foundation (see Figure 27.1), then, supported people. It made a series of awards to provide scholarships for medical and dental students, and adopted the Clinical Scholars Program, which had been started by the Carnegie Corporation and the Commonwealth Fund to provide training opportunities in the social, behavioral, and management sciences and other nonbiomedical disciplines for postresidency physicians. This strategy not only met the pragmatic requirements of the time but also was consistent with an academically oriented worldview of change. In brief, this view held that leaders of AHCs were masters of their fate, and had the power and the influence to mold their institutional agendas as they saw fit. Therefore, an appropriate philanthropic strategy was to shape and influence the next generation of leaders in the areas of primary care, public health, and health services research.

A second dimension of the strategy is what we term the augmentation strategy—that is, building new programs on an existing base. In an expansive time of funding for health care, this was reasonable and logical. It also minimized resistance within AHCs: Why not continue to train specialists and also add new primary care residency programs? Why not train baccalaureate nurses and also develop the new nurse practitioner model? With this approach, the Foundation supported the Primary Care Residency Program and the Nurse Faculty Development Program to develop primary care capacity in medicine and pediatrics, and to build capacity for training nurse practitioners. The Foundation also authorized the Teaching Hospital Group Practice Program to help reorganize academic general internal medicine into a model that reflected the primary care principles of continuity, coordination, and access.

The Foundation's investment in primary care residency programs in the 1970s fit the augmentation model to a T. The clear expectation at the time was that the demonstration and training programs funded by the Foundation would be sustained by federal or institutional support, or both. In fact, most of the residency programs funded by the Foundation continued with new federal grant support, and the teaching hospital group practice model became the norm as well. However, the Foundation-supported attempt by the Johns Hopkins University to create a new kind of provider, a health associate, did not succeed.

**Figure 27.1.** RWJF-Authorized AHC Programs in the 1970s (millions of dollars).

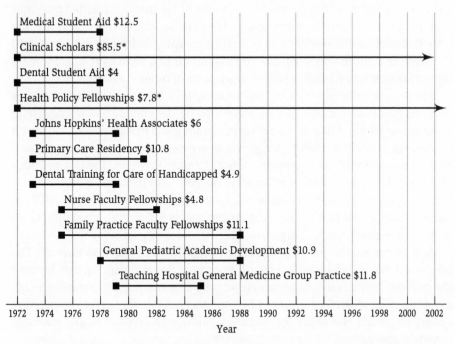

*Note:* Dollars are for sites only and do not include administrative and evaluation costs. An arrow indicates that not all sites have been awarded grants. Dollars indicate the total authorization. An asterisk indicates that decisions about possible additional funding will be made at a later date.

Beginning in 1973, the Foundation provided five years of support to Johns Hopkins to establish an institution that would train these health associates. This program did not survive the combination of a budget crisis at the university, a lack of clarity over the differences between health associates and physician assistants and nurse practitioners, and the lack of continued funding either from the Foundation or from the federal government.

A third dimension of the initial strategy was investment in faculty development. The Robert Wood Johnson Foundation not only invested in the Clinical Scholars Program but also launched programs to support faculty development in the emerging discipline of family medicine and, subsequently, in general pediatrics. The Foundation also initiated the Health Policy Fellows program, which it continues to support. The original purpose of this program was to train future leaders of AHCs in the politics of health care and health policy making at the federal level by offering mid-career academics the opportunity to work for a year in a Washington legislative or executive office.

## Assessment

Did the Foundation's strategy work? Yes, in the sense that it supported programs that attracted talented young people at elite institutions and promulgated the importance of health services research, primary care, and public health. Yes, in the sense that these efforts got the Foundation off to a solid start in grant making and demonstrated that it was an institution of quality and rigor.

Did these efforts significantly influence AHCs? The hope at that time was that, over a decade or two, people supported by the Foundation would rise to prominence within AHCs and steer them toward goals that advanced the health of the public. AHCs did begin grudgingly to accept health services research and clinical epidemiology as legitimate areas of inquiry. However, the Health Policy Fellows had limited impact in influencing the course of their home AHCs. It was becoming clear that the Fellows were not senior enough within their AHCs to initiate change, and that, in any case, single agents for change faced difficulties in altering well-entrenched organizational behavior of AHCs.

And, of course, the policy environment itself did not behave as forecast. The nation did not expand national health insurance nor did primary care become the national norm. Federal support for primary care training programs, although institutionalizing the Foundation's investments, may have masked underlying economic trends and other forces that continued to favor specialty training, research, and care.

For example, it became increasingly clear that the health care financing environment strongly encouraged specialty care and training as opposed to primary care. Medicare, Medicaid, and generous third-party payments for clinical care provided the monetary fuel for huge increases in the clinical enterprises of AHCs. Faculty members could both raise AHC revenue and increase their own productivity by developing clinical and research fellowships, with explicit support by Medicare graduate medical education funding and NIH funding. In turn, this federally funded group of trainees created a local workforce to develop new and ever-expanding clinical programs that would raise further revenue for subsequent expansion. This "positive-feedback" loop led to a tenfold expansion of medical school clinical faculty, from 7,200 in 1961 to 73,400 in 1995, with an accompanying fourfold expansion, from 4,000 to 16,600, in basic science faculty and only a doubling of medical school enrollment.[2] Medical school clinical revenues grew from 5 percent of total medical school support in 1961 to 49 percent of total support in 1995, while federal support has progressively declined to around 20 percent of total support. This increasing reliance on growing clinical revenues and on the specialty training and delivery infrastructure necessary to sustain growth, combined with the protechnology bias in fee-for-service reimbursement, has accounted for AHCs' consistent emphasis on specialist training and on high-technology care delivery as opposed to primary care. It also helps explain why issues important to the population's health—public health, substance abuse, universal access to care, behavioral change—have not been priorities for AHCs.

# THE 1980s

As the 1980s began, AHCs were strong, growing, and relatively autonomous. Yet a few ominous clouds began to appear on the horizon. Medicare's Diagnostic Related Group Reimbursement was the first significant change to the reimbursement of usual, customary, and reasonable costs that had fed the growth of fee-for-service medicine practiced at academic medical centers. Although teaching hospitals managed the transition without incident (and even profited), this change was a harbinger of a more fundamental restructuring of health care financing. Health-care costs were continuing to escalate, and academic centers increasingly began to experience adverse effects of their expanded specialty training programs. Many of these trainees, upon finishing their fellowships, promptly set up competitive programs in their local markets.

Nevertheless, the Foundation's strategy of investing in people and in augmenting academic programs seemed quite solid. Graduates of the Clinical Scholars Program were obtaining notable positions in medical schools and were ascending the academic ladder. By the early nineties, the majority of the leaders of divisions of general internal medicine were former clinical scholars. The faculty development programs were also bearing fruit, yielding new leadership in family medicine and general pediatrics.

Given this solid track record, the Foundation's strategy was to stay the course (see Figure 27.2 for a summary of Foundation programs supported in the 1980s). In 1982, it supported the Dental Services Research Program and the Clinical Nurse Scholars Program, which essentially applied the idea of the physician-oriented Clinical Scholars Program to dentistry and nursing.

The Foundation also began to focus attention on curricular change within medical schools. The rapid development of molecular and cellular biology was transforming basic science and raising questions about the educational focus of academic departments' teaching of medical students. More than ever there was need to integrate the teaching of basic science and clinical training throughout the four years of medical school. New pedagogy such as computer-assisted learning and the use of surrogate patients was rapidly evolving. Behavioral, social, probabilistic, and information sciences were deemed as important as the traditional basic science in the general education of medical students. With the current emphasis on general medicine, the establishment of ambulatory practice sites for training in prevention and primary care made sense.

**Figure 27.2.** RWJF-Authorized AHC Programs in the 1980s (millions of dollars).

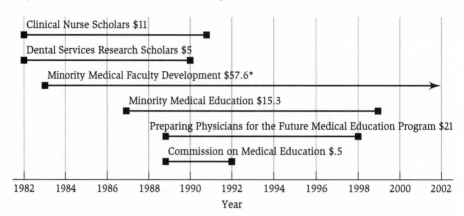

*Note:* Dollars are for sites only and do not include administrative and evaluation costs. An arrow indicates that not all sites have been awarded grants. Dollars shown equal the total authorization. An asterisk indicates that decisions about possible additional funding will be made at a later date.

The Foundation was repeatedly asked to fund another Flexner Report. Since its publication in 1910, the Flexner Report has shaped medical education for most of the twentieth century. Though the report had had a major impact on medical education, its postulates were thought now to be archaic and even an impediment to needed change. The Foundation's response was to support an extensive survey of medical educators. A majority of respondents indicated a need for "fundamental changes" and "thorough reform" in medical education. Against this background the Foundation initiated two programs—the Commission on Medical Education: The Science of Medical Practice, and Preparing Physicians for the Future: A Program in Medical Education.

The recommendations of the commission included the integration of basic and clinical sciences, the need for students to have a better comprehension of the role of behavioral and social aspects of disease, the expansion of clinical training into ambulatory care sites, and a medical school governance to make curriculum change feasible. These were thought to be modest in scope, and all had been already noted by previous commissions or task forces. The thrust of the commission's report, however, was to challenge the departmental segmentation and control of the curriculum and to suggest that medical education could be improved from its present status.

What was different from earlier efforts at curricular reform, however, was that the Foundation followed through with the Program in Medical Education that was designed to support the implementation of the commission's recommendations for curricular change, something no other task force or commission had done.

Rather than just tinkering with the existing scheme of medical education, the Foundation supported eight schools through the Program in Medical Education over a five-year period to make fundamental changes in their curriculum in keeping with the commission's recommendations. An extensive evaluation indicated that they were successful in doing this. The continuation of these changes remains to be seen, but the initial indications are promising.

## Assessment

Through its various programs, the Foundation succeeded in supporting new kinds of medical school faculty. Reforms in medical education also proved to be successful,[3] but the Foundation's catalytic role is less clear. One might reasonably view the Foundation's role as one of facilitating trends that already existed rather than creating any fundamental shifts.[4] Perhaps even more significant is the Foundation's sustained investment in scholarship in the areas of health services research, clinical epidemiology, biomedical ethics, and other disciplines. This extensive and continuing investment, which occurred through both explicit training programs and Foundation research initiatives and demonstration programs on specific topics, has had the effect of legitimizing these disciplines within AHCs. This effect, which may transcend individual programs and eras, may be the Foundation's most lasting contribution to academic health centers.

The Foundation's success in creating new kinds of academic physicians did not extend to dentistry and nursing. As one of us has argued elsewhere,[5] the Clinical Nurse Scholars program may have been terminated prematurely. Additionally, the disparate paths available in nursing education may have made efforts at change significantly more difficult. Dental education was buffeted by forces—including falling student demand for dental education and a reduction of dental diseases such as caries—more powerful than those areas of the Foundation's modest investment. Perhaps the clearest example of philanthropic impact was the Program for Training Dentists in the Care of Handicapped Patients, which led to widespread curricular reform in this area.

The Foundation's mixed record in the areas of nursing and other health professions may reflect a profound ambivalence about power within AHCs. Although the notion was never explicitly articulated, it was generally believed at the Foundation that the major source of power and influence within AHCs was the medical school and its leadership. Egalitarian impulses contributed to the desire to work across a variety of disciplines, but the tension between egalitarian desire and the search for leverage may have contributed to the Foundation's limited impact beyond medicine.

# THE 1990s

By the early nineties, the prevailing winds of change had increased to near-hurricane force. Health care costs had continued to rise, and, in certain areas of the country, managed care growth had begun to affect the clinical operations of academic health centers significantly. For example, contracts for managed care patients were not as lucrative and limited AHCs' ability to cross-subsidize teaching, research, and indigent care. Interest in primary care among medical students and faculty fell dramatically,[6] and academic health centers continued to expand their clinical programs to support the service requirements of expanding specialty training programs and to increase clinical revenue. The number of medical school clinical faculty, for example, increased 11.9 percent from 1992–93 to 1994–95 alone.[7]

Ultimately more disturbing for AHCs, however, was the gradual erosion of their place at the center of power and influence in health care. By training too many specialists (who in turn set up competing tertiary-care programs), AHCs lost their natural monopoly on specialty care. The growth of managed care created powerful new corporations in the health care arena—organizations with no special reverence for the products and the values intrinsic to AHCs. Many AHCs neglected community concerns, and were viewed as arrogant and insular institutions. Finally, the dramatic growth of overall health care spending led to a continued monetarization of the health care sector,[8] with the ascension of economics, business, and politics over medicine. With such developments in mind, the Foundation created a new generation of programs that were, perhaps paradoxically, both more ambitious and more circumscribed than previous efforts (see Figure 27.3).

First, the Foundation developed programs to encourage medical schools to shift their educational focus toward generalism and away from a predominance of specialists. This move away from a strategy of augmentation was quite explicit, for example, in the Generalist Physician Initiative, whose program guidelines insisted on fundamental changes in the school's overall admission process, curriculum, and career path of graduates to encourage generalism. This ambitious program was launched in parallel with a more traditional faculty development program, the Generalist Physician Faculty Scholars Program, and a generalist-oriented research program, the Generalist Provider Research Initiative.

Second, the Foundation's programs to encourage generalism had another thrust—that is, the beginning of an outside-in strategy. Previous efforts to influence AHCs through direct grants to individual agents of change within institutions evolved into grants to support the effort both of AHCs and of potentially influential partners outside the AHCs. For example, the Generalist Physician Ini-

**Figure 27.3.** RWJF-Authorized AHC Programs in the 1990s (millions of dollars).

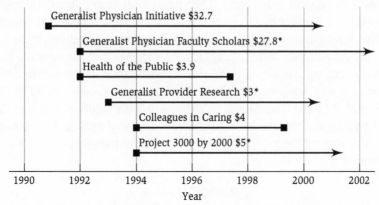

*Note:* Dollars are for sites only and do not include administrative and evaluation costs. An arrow indicates that not all sites have been awarded grants. Dollars indicate the total authorization. An asterisk indicates that decisions about possible additional funding will be made at a later date.

tiative insisted that AHCs have external partners such as HMOs, group practices, or insurers. Early experience in the program suggests that these partners have a considerable influence in the production of generalists, in pointing out deficiencies in the preclinical and clinical curricula, and in highlighting the "hidden curriculum"[9] of academia that encourages excessive specialization and expensive care. The Generalist Provider Research Initiative supports policy and analytic studies in generalism, but also serves as a way to provide information to shape the policy levers that affect specialty choice.

Third, the Foundation provided support to the Health of the Public Program. This program was designed to encourage AHCs to come up with new ideas for their mission and functions, so that teaching, research, and care would be aligned to better meet the needs of the health of defined populations, such as the community surrounding the AHC. The initial two phases of the Health of the Public Program had been supported by the Rockefeller Foundation and the Pew Charitable Trusts. The Robert Wood Johnson Foundation, in collaboration with Pew, funded a third phase to extend and institutionalize the community partnerships and curricular reforms.

Another target of Foundation grant making to influence AHCs in the 1990s included better matching of supply and demand for nurses. The Colleagues in Caring program was designed to bring together employers of nurses—such as hospitals, clinics, home health providers—with educational institutions to plan more rational responses to the way the market operates.

Finally, the Foundation has continued and expanded its support for educating minorities in the health professions. The Minority Medical Education Program, the Minority Medical Faculty Development Program, and other efforts reflect the Foundation's long-standing and continuing commitment to diversity in these professions. An analysis of demographic data suggests that the nation's health workforce is getting less diverse and less representative of the nation overall. The Association of American Medical Colleges' program called 3000 by 2000, partially funded by the Foundation, recognizes that the solution to this problem lies in expanding the pipeline by investing in educational programs in secondary schools, and even earlier, to enlarge the pool of minorities that enter the health professions.

## Assessment

Although current Foundation efforts are ambitious in their goals, they are more modest in their ability to change the overall course and nature of AHCs. As the twentieth century draws to a close, AHCs are enormous engines of clinical care, training, and research, fueled by public and private reimbursement, the NIH and other research funders, and federal and state subsidies for graduate medical education. In spite of the concerns about the effect of marketplace changes and managed care growth on AHCs, most are fiscally and programmatically robust, continue to expand, and have yet to undergo a critical reexamination of their mission and function. The Health of the Public Program, for example, was successful in articulating the argument for a new vision of academic health centers and in supporting a number of important local efforts at curricular reform and community service. But it lacked sufficient leverage to affect the way AHCs responded to enormous economic and market forces. The Health of the Public grants were modest, often funding only one faculty member at an institution, with limited funds to support innovative programs beyond their initiation. Even larger-scale Foundation investments, such as the Generalist Physician Initiative, are seeing positive trends emanating more from market forces than from direct program effects. In addition, the institutional tendency remains to add on programs rather than fundamentally change core activities.

The Foundation itself has evolved as well. From an initial emphasis on health care institutions and health care delivery, it is currently supporting a widened array of programs and projects that are tackling the challenging issues of substance abuse at the community level, enhancing consumer-directed approaches to care for the disabled, and integration of housing and social services, to name just a few. Many of these efforts are quite remote from AHCs, and efforts to influence AHCs are now probably best viewed as one of a number of areas of Foundation action rather than as a central thrust.

# THE FUTURE

Given this experience, what is The Robert Wood Johnson Foundation's current approach to AHCs? First, in addition to continuing the generalist programs developed in the 1990s, the Foundation is investing in an effort to encourage a long-range strategic assessment of the mission and the function of the AHCs. The Forum on the Future of Academic Medicine, sponsored by the Association of American Medical Colleges, is bringing together leaders of AHCs with leaders from outside health and health care to debate the mission, the function, and the role of AHCs in the twenty-first century. The Forum has already identified important areas for further work, such as a better understanding of AHC financial affairs and the need for leadership development. Work in these areas may hold great promise. In parallel, the Commonwealth Fund's Commission on Academic Medicine is contributing important policy analysis to the field, and helping to focus attention on the question of how best to support the mission of AHCs in the current turbulent environment.

Second, the Foundation, with Pew, is supporting a transformation of the Health of the Public Program into a sustainable network. Third, the Foundation is supporting a new nurse executive leadership program, which, although not exclusively focused on academic nursing, will identify and help develop the next generation of nursing leadership. Finally, the Foundation continues to support scholarly endeavors in the areas of health care organization and finance, home care, substance abuse policy, and others that help influence the direction of research within AHCs.

# LESSONS LEARNED

After twenty-five years of grant-making experience, a number of lessons have emerged.

- First, investments in people pay off. Clinical Scholars, for example, now hold a variety of leadership positions in AHCs, in government, and in the private sector. In part, this may be because of the Foundation's sustained commitment to the program over twenty-five years, and the fact that approximately 750 Clinical Scholars have been trained, more than 60 percent of whom remain in academe. Although fellowship programs are expensive, supporting bright young people early in their career may be a more effective institutional change strategy than direct institutional grants.

- Second, AHCs, like most academic institutions, do not follow a logical, planned process of change. As is true of most complex systems, AHCs react to a variety of external changes—political, economic, social, and scientific. For example, the postwar environment encouraged a dramatic growth in specialty training and research, and today managed care is encouraging joint ventures, mergers, and other changes in the clinical systems of care in AHCs. Efforts to influence AHCs may perhaps best be accomplished by shaping those broader social and economic forces, as well as by supporting talented individuals through training and research programs.

• Third, both a strategy of augmentation and one of fundamental change can work, with appropriate targeting and resources. An augmentation strategy can succeed if funding can be sustained over time, and a strategy of fundamental change can work if it is targeted to a fairly specific area and sufficient resources are committed.

• Fourth, it is important to work with both elite and nonelite AHCs, although it may be appropriate to pursue different strategies for each. For example, an augmentation strategy is most appropriate for elite institutions, where adding a new program to a premiere institution enhances the program's visibility. But a fundamental change strategy has a greater chance of succeeding in a nonelite setting, where barriers to reform may be fewer and where there may be greater interest in moving the institution in new directions.

• Finally, the role of philanthropy in influencing large and powerful institutions should be kept in proper perspective. Unlike earlier in the century, when philanthropic resources were a much larger fraction of resources devoted to academia, modern AHCs are multibillion-dollar enterprises. Multimillion-dollar foundation grants, although welcome, cannot by themselves transform AHCs or their directions.

For the Foundation, whose mission is to improve health and health care for all Americans, AHCs have a special role and place. Their role in creating new knowledge, in providing advanced care and specialty training, and in educating the next generation of health professionals is unquestioned. Their role in improving community health, in caring for the underserved, and in being held accountable for societal goals is undergoing vigorous debate. In addition, the commitment of the AHCs to diversity is undergoing both internal and societal challenges at a time when such a commitment is needed more than ever. Nevertheless, AHCs remain in large part a public trust[10] and should be held accountable for their contributions to the society's health. By investing in people, by identifying and shaping those forces that have an impact on AHCs, and by carefully targeting philanthropic investment in the right areas at the right time, The Robert Wood Johnson Foundation continues to seek to influence AHCs to improve health and health care for the American people.

As the twenty-first century draws near, perhaps what is needed is a new concept of the AHC and its function and purpose. A soul-searching look at mission, at function, and at structure may help catalyze creative responses to the future that are not merely reactive but make a compelling case for continued public trust, support, and acclaim.

## Notes

1. According to the Association of Academic Health Centers, AHCs vary in their organization and structure, but all centers include a medical school, at least one other health professional school or program, and one or more owned or affiliated teaching hospitals.

2. D. Korn, "Reengineering Academic Medical Centers: Reengineering Academic Values?" *Academic Medicine* 71(10), Oct. 1996, 1033–1043.

3. An evaluation of the Program in Medical Education by Gordon Moore indicated the funded schools did indeed change, but so did comparison schools. The funded schools felt strongly that the Foundation had made a major impact in updating their curriculum.

4. N. A. Christakis, "The Similarity and Frequency of Proposals to Reform U.S. Medical Education: Constant Concerns," *JAMA* 274(9), Sept. 1995, 706–711.

5. S. L. Isaacs, L. G. Sandy, and S. A. Schroeder, "Grants to Shape the Health Care Workforce: The Robert Wood Johnson Foundation Experience," *Health Affairs* 15(2), Summer 1996, 279–295.

6. J. M. Colwill, "Where Have All the Primary Care Applicants Gone?" *New England Journal of Medicine* 326(5), Feb. 1992, 387–393.

7. J. Y. Krakower, J. Ganem, and P. Jolly, "Review of U.S. Medical School Finances, 1994–1995," *JAMA* 276(9), Sept. 1996, 720–724.

8. E. Ginzberg, "The Monetarization of Medical Care," *New England Journal of Medicine* 310(18), May 1984, 1162–1165.

9. F. W. Hafferty and R. Franks, "The Hidden Curriculum, Ethics Teaching, and the Structure of Medical Education," *Academic Medicine* 69(11), Nov. 1994, 861–871.

10. S. A. Schroeder, J. S. Zones, and J. A. Showstack, "Academic Medicine as a Public Trust," *JAMA* 262(6), Aug. 1989, 803–812.

# Grant Report Summaries from
# The Robert Wood Johnson Foundation

## EVALUATION OF NATIONAL PRIMARY CARE WEEK
## FOR MEDICAL STUDENTS
(last updated August 2001)

### Grantee

American Medical Student Association Foundation (AMSA)

### Summary

This grant from The Robert Wood Johnson Foundation (RWJF) provided support for an evaluation of the 1999 National Primary Care Week (NPCW), held September 27 to October 2, 1999. NPCW, an initiative of the American Medical Student Association Foundation (AMSA), is cosponsored by the Division of Medicine, U.S. Health Resources and Services Administration (HRSA). NPCW educates students and others about primary care and encourages students to pursue this discipline, introduces students to local and national primary care role models, helps students explore career options within primary care, encourages community involvement, and introduces students to policy issues surrounding primary care. An independent national organization, AMSA represents nearly thirty thousand physicians-in-training at 150 allopathic and osteopathic medical schools. Several other organizations, including the American Academy of Family Physicians, the Society of General Internal Medicine, and the Association of American Medical Colleges (AAMC), promoted awareness of NPCW and were represented on a project advisory panel.

AMSA estimated that about 150 different activities took place during NPCW at 118 medical schools throughout the country. Among these were seminars, presentations, and forums (including topics such as pharmaceutical developments, women in medicine, alternative medicine, and the business side of medicine); community clinics (immunization, blood pressure screening); and community health fairs.

AMSA gathered information from participants after the event to gain insights for program improvement and to assess the level of achievement of program objectives. Data were collected from informal telephone conversations between AMSA staff and student coordinators; surveys mailed to students, student leaders, deans, area health education centers (AHECs), and community health leaders (51 percent return rate); and in-depth structured telephone interviews with various student leaders. (AHECs are local health education organizations that coordinate their activities with other local academic institutions and health care agencies.)

The evaluation included the following key findings:

- In general, student leaders spent forty or fewer hours organizing NPCW, with the majority spending fewer than twenty hours.

- The most common obstacles to attracting student participation in NPCW were scheduling issues, balancing schoolwork with NPCW responsibilities, and generating interest among the student body.

- The most frequent suggestion for improving NPCW was to start the planning process earlier.

- Regarding the impact of NPCW on student leaders and participants, the most frequently reported positive responses were being introduced to primary care leaders, learning the role of primary care providers in the community, and increasing understanding of primary care.

The grantee organization made the following recommendations based on evaluation findings:

- Increase the visibility and involvement of AHECs and provide them with the information they need. (AMSA noted that AHECs are good at providing community contact and facilitating community events.)

- Provide guidelines to student leaders on how to accomplish more interdisciplinary activity with other health professions, such as nursing, and more community outreach.

- Create a truly national event through activities such as more work with state governors' offices, gaining full support of the AAMC, and increased distribution to medical schools of the video of the U.S. Surgeon General's announcement of NPCW.

AMS distributed approximately two hundred copies of the twenty-two-page evaluation report to AHECs, dean's offices, and student leaders. HRSA picked up evaluation costs for the 2000 event, which took place October 15–21, 2000.

# PREPARING PHYSICIANS FOR THE FUTURE: A PROGRAM IN MEDICAL EDUCATION

(last updated June 2002)

## Grantees

University of Pennsylvania School of Medicine (Philadelphia)

Harvard Pilgrim Health Care (Boston)

Expansion of Policy Analysis of Medical Education Reform (Boston)

Harvard University School of Public Health (Cambridge, Massachusetts)

University of New Mexico School of Medicine (Albuquerque, New Mexico)

## Summary

Authorized by The Robert Wood Johnson Foundation in 1989, Preparing Physicians for the Future: A Program in Medical Education (PPF) was designed to facilitate major undergraduate curriculum reform in U.S. medical schools. RWJF created PPF, which ran from 1989 to 1998, in response to widespread concern that the growing body of basic science information had created a factual overload in the medical student curriculum and that the primary site of clinical education for medical students—the tertiary care hospital—was no longer providing an adequate learning experience about the course and treatment of disease. This was confirmed by a 1989 Louis Harris and Associates survey (commissioned by the Foundation and summarized in the February 27, 1991, issue of the *Journal of the American Medical Association*) that found that a substantial majority of the leadership of U.S. medical schools believed that medical school curricula were out of step with present-day medical practice and inappropriate for preparing physicians for the twenty-first century.

# SURVEYS OF YOUNG PHYSICIANS ON ESTABLISHING THEIR CAREERS AND PROVIDING CARE IN THE CHANGING MEDICAL MARKETPLACE (1987–1997)

(last updated June 2000)

## Grantees

American Medical Association Foundation (Chicago)

Association of American Medical Colleges (Washington, D.C.)

Georgetown University School of Medicine (Washington, D.C.)

## Summary

This series of grants from The Robert Wood Johnson Foundation funded three national surveys of young allopathic physicians and a smaller national survey of young osteopathic physicians over a ten-year period. The surveys, conducted in 1987, 1991, and 1997, were designed to provide a better understanding of how young physicians were establishing their careers and providing medical care in the face of growing competition, managed care, and other significant changes in the medical marketplace. The first two surveys interviewed approximately six thousand physicians each, while the third, which was cofunded by the federal Agency for Health Care Policy and Research (AHCPR), interviewed about fifteen hundred. Findings highlighted differences in practice patterns based on gender and ethnicity. In particular, the surveys revealed that minority physicians tend to treat a high proportion of patients of their own race or ethnicity, and women and minority physicians are much more likely to serve minority, poor, and Medicaid populations. Practicing under managed care did not have a uniform impact on physician satisfaction, although markets with higher penetration by health maintenance organizations (HMOs) did show higher levels of dissatisfaction. Relatively few physicians reported facing financial incentives to reduce services to patients, but the incentives that do exist may have adverse impacts on the quality of care. Education debt for graduating physicians has risen over time, but few physicians report that debt levels affected their decisions about specialization. The investigators presented their findings at a number of national meetings, including annual meetings of the American Public Health Association and the Association for Health Services Research. Papers have also appeared in the *Journal of the American Medical Association* and *Health Affairs.* Other investigators have conducted additional analyses employing public-use data tapes created under this project. Some of the survey methodology that was developed is being employed in the RWJF's Health Tracking Program, which is monitoring changes within the health care system and how these changes affect people.

# DEVELOPMENT OF A STATEWIDE SYSTEM TO TRACK MEDICAL STUDENTS AND RESIDENTS

(last updated August 1998)

## Grantee

Thomas Jefferson University, Jefferson Medical College (Philadelphia)

## Summary

This grant from The Robert Wood Johnson Foundation supported the Jefferson Medical College and seven other Pennsylvania medical schools to determine the feasibility of developing the Pennsylvania Tracking System (PTS), a uniform statewide system to track the educational and career choices of graduate medical students and residents. This was a cooperative effort with the Pennsylvania

Department of Health. The medical schools' interest in this effort was stimulated by the Commonwealth of Pennsylvania's Generalist Physician Initiative (GPI), which was closely modeled after the Foundation's $32 million Generalist Physician Initiative national program, which had two sites in Pennsylvania, at Pennsylvania State College University of Medicine, in Hershey and the Medical College of Pennsylvania and Hahnemann University in Philadelphia. The team at Jefferson developed the PTS to obtain secondary data from a number of national medical organizations and merge this information with data from eight Pennsylvania medical schools in a single usable format. The PTS longitudinally follows medical students and graduates of the Pennsylvania osteopathic and allopathic medical schools, beginning with background and premedical information, through medical school and residency training, and into practice. At the close of the project, the PTS contained information on eighteen thousand students and graduates, beginning with the entering class of 1982. With the development of the PTS, Pennsylvania has the first statewide tracking system for medical students and residents in the nation. The tracking system, originally undertaken just to monitor the outcomes of the Pennsylvania GPI, broadened its purpose as it was developed to provide a prototype for tracking a wide range of outcomes for medical students. The project team published two articles in *Academic Medicine,* one that details the development of the tracking system and another that presents some initial research on career choices of medical students. Two additional articles have been submitted for publication. The tracking system has been presented at a number of national conferences, including the annual meetings of Research in Medical Education and the Association of American Medical Colleges.

SECTION FIVE

# QUALITY AND COST

# Editors' Introduction to Section Five

As attention to primary care and the need for generalist practitioners grew, a number of different disciplines entered the field. Internal medicine and pediatrics developed generalist tracks; in 1969, family medicine became a recognized specialty. Beyond these so-called generalist disciplines, physicians in specialty practices such as obstetrics-gynecology sometimes held themselves out as offering primary care. The 1960s saw the development of nurse practitioners, physician assistants, and certified nurse-midwives, each of which offered primary care services. The involvement of so many disciplines has raised questions about the quality of care they offer and the cost of providing it. For example, do psychiatrists and generalists provide the same quality of care for patients with depression? Do patients with diabetes receive similar care and have similar outcomes whether they are treated by primary care physicians or specialists? Do nurse practitioners provide the same quality of primary care, at a lower cost, as generalist physicians do? Do nurse practitioners complement or compete with generalist physicians? As the cost of health care rises and concern about quality increases, these questions are as relevant in the 2000s as they were back in the 1960s.

There is a substantial literature on these topics, and we have chosen to break it down into two parts.

Part A examines the quality and the cost of care provided by specialists versus that provided by generalist physicians. Chapter Twenty-Eight is a reprint of "Comparing Generalist and Specialty Care: Discrepancies, Deficiencies, and

Excesses" by Martin Donohoe, a comprehensive review of the evidence published in 1998. The reprint is followed by abstracts of relevant articles, books, and reports.

Part B examines the quality and the cost of care provided by nurse practitioners and other nonphysician practitioners versus that provided by physicians. It begins with Chapter Twenty-Nine, a reprint of "Quality of Patient Care by Nurse Practitioners and Physician's Assistants: A Ten-Year Perspective," by Harold Sox, dating from 1979. Chapter Thirty, a more recent article, published in 2000 by Mary Mundinger and her colleagues, reports on primary care outcomes in patients treated by nurse practitioners or physicians in New York City. This study found that outcomes did not differ whether a nurse practitioner or a physician provided the primary care. This chapter is followed by abstracts of pertinent articles, books, and reports.

During the 1970s and 1980s, The Robert Wood Johnson Foundation played an active role in promoting the development of primary care nurse practitioners and physician assistants. Terrance Keenan explored the Foundation's role in his chapter, "Support of Nurse Practitioners and Physician Assistants," in *To Improve Health and Health Care, 1998–1999: The Robert Wood Johnson Foundation Anthology*, reprinted here as Chapter Thirty-One. It is followed by summaries of grant reports of Robert Wood Johnson Foundation–funded projects.

# PART A

# GENERALISTS AND SPECIALISTS

# CHAPTER TWENTY-EIGHT

# Comparing Generalist and Specialty Care

## Discrepancies, Deficiencies, and Excesses

Martin T. Donohoe, M.D.

1998

This article evaluates the amount and quality of care provided by generalists and specialists, a subject of increasing interest to medical educators, managed care organizations, and the general public. Weaknesses in the knowledge base of practicing physicians are reviewed, and investigations attempting to compare generalist and specialty care for common conditions are described. While some of the differences in quality of care may be due to generalists' knowledge deficits, many are secondary to system factors and most are remediable. Furthermore, disparities between generalist and specialty care likely have less impact on the population's health than the deficiencies all physicians share. After discussing the nature of these deficiencies, I explain how they might be corrected and how generalists and specialists can work together, building on their respective strengths, to improve the quality of health care in this country.

---

# DATA

English-language articles were identified through Medline (1966–present) using the following keywords: *generalist, generalism, (sub)specialist, (sub)specialty, (sub)specialization, consultation, referral,* and *quality of care,* and through the bibliographies of these citations.

For the purposes of this review, *generalists* include general internists, family practitioners, general pediatricians, and general practitioners, although the focus is on problems pertaining to the care of adults. *Specialist* refers to those physicians practicing subspecialties of internal medicine (eg, cardiology or rheumatology) or, when noted, to other specialized fields (eg, psychiatry). Only those studies involving American physicians were evaluated, since generalists in other countries receive less postgraduate training.

# COMPARING GENERALISTS AND SPECIALISTS

For most patients, generalists are the first point of contact with the health care system. They confront a greater variety of illnesses compared with specialists,[1] are more accessible,[2] see more patients per unit of time,[3] charge less for primary care services,[4] and are more likely to provide continuity and comprehensiveness of care.[2] Ideally, generalists treat a wide variety of medical problems; match patients' needs and preferences with the appropriate and judicious use of medical services[5,6]; protect patients from the possible adverse effects of unnecessary care[2,5,6]; decrease health care costs[2,5,6]; and guard against the fragmentation of medical services that results from overspecialization.[7] However, this ideal often does not match reality.

Generalists perform slightly better on standardized tests of general medical knowledge than specialists.[8,9] While there is much room for improvement, they do a little better with respect to test ordering[10,11]; some areas of health promotion and disease prevention[12,13]; risk behavior counseling[12,14]; and the recognition and management of, and willingness to explore and treat, psychosocial problems.[15]

Specialists, due to their advanced education and training, possess in-depth, expert understanding of a limited number of diseases within their respective domains and are qualified to perform many diagnostic and therapeutic procedures not in the repertoire of generalists. Evidence for superior knowledge and practices of specialists in selective diseases is strongest for the care of myocardial infarction and congestive heart failure by cardiologists, depression by psychiatrists, acquired immunodeficiency syndrome (AIDS) and its complications by infectious disease experts, and some rheumatic and musculoskeletal conditions by rheumatologists. Interestingly, myocardial infarction and depression are the diseases for which patients express the least confidence in their primary care providers.[16]

In other areas, however, generalists outperform specialists. For instance, under open-access esophagogastroduodenoscopy, general internists and family physicians did a better job of scheduling patients for appropriate indications than did internal medicine subspecialists.[17] Also, in a prospective observational study,[4] patients with back pain treated by primary care physicians, orthopedic surgeons, and chiropractors all achieved similar functional recovery, return to work, and complete recovery at 6 months; the mean number of radiographs taken and mean total outpatient charges were lowest for primary care physicians.

Specialists provide at least 20% of the primary care delivered in the United States.[18] However, little is known about the quality of generalist care provided by specialists working outside of their particular areas of expertise. Furthermore, specialty care may lead to increased costs of care due to overuse of expensive diagnostic and therapeutic interventions in the absence of any additional health benefits.

# CARDIAC DISEASES

For a prototypical patient with an acute myocardial infarction, Ayanian et al[19] showed that cardiologists were more likely than generalists to use thrombolytic agents to treat acute myocardial infarction and to prescribe b-blockers and aspirin in the postmyocardial infarction setting, all recommended interventions. The cardiologists were less likely to use prophylactic lidocaine, which has been shown to offer no therapeutic benefit,[20] and less likely to use calcium channel blockers, which are potentially harmful.[21] In a retrospective chart review of Medicare patients treated for acute myocardial infarction in 1990, Ayanian et al[22] confirmed that cardiologists were more likely than generalists to prescribe thrombolytic therapy and aspirin but not b-blockers. In a national sample of physicians, Chin et al[23] found that cardiologists were more likely than generalists to appropriately use an angiotensin-converting enzyme inhibitor for a hypothetical patient with congestive heart failure. However, on chart review of patients with congestive heart failure at one academic medical center, only three quarters of eligible patients were taking an angiotensin-converting enzyme inhibitor, and only 60% of these were at doses known to be efficacious.[24] Then, in a recent survey, Jancin[25] found that cardiologists reported greater adherence than generalists to the 1994 Agency for Health Care Policy and Research guidelines for the treatment of congestive heart failure.

Of patients with positive or very positive exercise stress test results who met additional clinical criteria for necessary coronary angiography, Borowsky et al[26] discovered that after adjustment for sociodemographics and clinical presentation, patients with a cardiologist as a regular source of care were more likely than all other patients to have undergone the procedure within 3 and 6 months. On the other hand, Stein et al[27] found that, according to published reports and established practice guidelines, noncardiologists ordered more radionuclide stress tests that were not indicated than did cardiologists. Both groups of physicians, however, overused this test.

In 1 community hospital, Schreiber et al[28] noted that internists were less likely than cardiologists to use aspirin, heparin, and b-blockers in their initial treatment of patients with chest pain. Internists used exercise tests more often for risk stratification and diagnosis; cardiologists performed coronary revascularization procedures 2 to 4 times as often. While patients of cardiologists had a substantially higher prevalence of established coronary artery disease, patients of internists presented more often with atypical chest pain. Even so, there were no significant differences in the incidence of myocardial infarction or in mortality between the 2 groups. It is hard to determine whether cardiologists were overly aggressive in their use of procedures or internists not aggressive enough, although the data on underuse of medications, particularly aspirin, shed a negative light on internists and cardiologists alike. Similarly, Brand et al,[29] analyzing insurance claims for filled prescriptions for the long-term use of b-blockers after acute myocardial infarction, noted that less than 50% of cardiologists' patients were taking b-blockers and that a third of these had contraindications for b-blocker use. Similarly, in the National Registry of Myocardial Infarction,[30] only 36% to 42% of 240989 enrolled patients received b-blockers, while 30% to 40% were given calcium channel blockers.

The more favorable selection of interventions by cardiologists compared with generalists in treating acute myocardial infarction and congestive heart failure may be secondary to differences in frequency of treating myocardial infarctions; inadequate dissemination of guidelines; differences in continuing medical education programs and recertification procedures; generalists' confusion regarding relative vs absolute contraindications; inadequate feedback to generalists regarding clinical practices; and lack of generalists' participation in clinical trials, dissociating them from involvement in the generation of new therapies.[31] Generalists may see more patients who refuse to take certain medications because of potential adverse effects, or more patients who actually experience adverse effects and reactions.[32] This is not likely caused by patients' multiple comorbidities, since patients of cardiologists tend to be sicker and have more underlying medical problems.[33,34] It may result from improper dosing by generalists, although this has not been evaluated.

Since generalists provide more longitudinal care (including the majority of postmyocardial infarction care), they may be more averse to using agents that can cause strokes (thrombolytics) or impotence (b-blockers) because they continue to see the consequences of these adverse effects over the long-term in their patients. Support for this idea comes from an analysis of prescribing patterns, which showed that specialists give greater weighting to the beneficial aspects of antihypertensives, while generalists show greater concern over adverse effects.[35] Furthermore, the benefits of certain commonly used treatments in some circumstances remain controversial, such as the use of b-blockers after myocardial infarction in women, patients younger than 65 years, and those without mechanical or electrical complications.[36] However, others[37] have shown that many generalists have inflated perceptions of cardiovascular risk without treatment and of the benefits of risk-modifying medical treatment. Still, generalists may be slower to adopt new therapies or discard outdated ones secondary to excessive (or, at times, appropriate) caution.

Despite these differences in myocardial infarction and postmyocardial infarction care, McCrory et al[38] found no significant differences in the knowledge and attitudes of generalists and cardiologists regarding anticoagulation for nonvalvular atrial fibrillation in the elderly. In response to vignettes, however, both groups of physicians underused anticoagulation in this group at high risk of thromboembolic stroke. In the Medical Outcomes Study,[39] no specialty differences in 2- and 4-year outcomes of patients with hypertension were discernible. Smaller studies[39,40] have shown that cardiologists and generalists provided similar quality of care for patients with transient ischemic attacks and stroke.

## MENTAL HEALTH DISORDERS

Generalists are not as skillful as psychiatrists at recognizing and treating depression, and they frequently miss clues to suicidal intent.[12,41-44] Inpatients with depression received better management of the psychological aspects of their illnesses (although worse management of the medical aspects) when cared for in psychiatric wards.[45] In the Medical Outcomes Study,[42] psychiatrists' patients had better functional outcomes, largely as a result of more frequent counseling, more appropriate dosing of antidepressants, and less use of potentially harmful minor tranquilizers. Callahan et al[46] found that even when primary care providers were given diagnostic scales and treatment algorithms, fewer than half of the patients they identified with depression actually received treatment. The authors attribute this to patient reluctance to take medicines and to physicians' pessimism regarding the effectiveness of treatments. Compared with psychiatrists, however, generalists see a higher percentage of mildly depressed and less-motivated patients in whom the use of antidepressants may not be as effective.[42] Furthermore, adequately treating anxiety and depression is time and labor intensive,[41] and reimbursement incentives encourage psychiatrists to offer more frequent and longer office visits for counseling.[42]

# HUMAN IMMUNODEFICIENCY VIRUS AND AIDS

In 2 studies, human immunodeficiency virus (HIV)–infected individuals cared for by generalists had higher odds of hospitalization after diagnosis of their seropositivity[47] and significantly shorter survival[48] than those cared for by an AIDS specialist. This may have been due to generalists inappropriately delaying initiation of anti-infective therapy, or to specialists' expertise in detecting AIDS-related complications at an earlier stage or in managing complications on an outpatient basis.[47,49] In recent nationwide surveys, majorities of residents[50] and primary care physicians[51] expressed concerns about the adequacy of their training in AIDS ambulatory care, and more than 80% of primary care physicians believed they lacked information needed to care for patients with those illnesses seen in advanced HIV infection.[51] Generalists failed to discern common HIV-associated lesions when confronted with standardized patients.[52] Even those generalists with more experience managing HIV displayed multiple, significant knowledge gaps surrounding the treatment of *Pneumocystis carinii* pneumonia.[53]

# RHEUMATIC AND MUSCULOSKELETAL DISEASES

In a recent review, Solomon et al[54] concluded that rheumatologists performed arthrocentesis more appropriately than nonrheumatologists for acute monoarthritis and oligoarthritis and produced shorter durations of hospitalization, and that rheumatologists used colchicine during the introduction of urate-lowering therapy for patients with gout more appropriately than generalists. In a retrospective investigation[55] relying on patient recall, the average rate of progression of functional disability secondary to rheumatoid arthritis was substantially lower in those patients followed up regularly by rheumatologists, likely due to the specialists' more intensive use of second-line antirheumatic medications and more frequent joint surgeries. Other aspects of rheumatoid arthritis, such as pain control and psychosocial adjustment, were not evaluated. No consistent differences in outcomes between generalists and rheumatologists for patients with lower back pain have been found.[54]

# OTHER CONDITIONS AND PRACTICES

The strongest data demonstrating the equivalence of quality of care provided by generalists and specialists comes from the Medical Outcomes Study.[39] In this prospective, observational, 4-year investigation in 3 major US cities, no differences in quality of care or adjusted mortality were found for diabetes and hypertension care, other than that endocrinologists, compared with family physicians, achieved better outcomes for diabetic individuals with foot ulcers and infections. Smaller and less well-designed studies have also shown no differences between generalists and specialists in the management of chronic obstructive lung disease[56] and perinatal outcomes.[57]

However, many studies have found superior specialty care in other areas, which may result from greater knowledge and experience. For instance, Fendrick et al[58] surveyed practicing physicians 2 months after a National Institutes of Health Consensus Conference advocated antibiotic therapy for eradication of *Helicobacter pylori* in patients with peptic ulcer disease. Despite a low response rate, more gastroenterologists than generalists were aware of, and had adopted, this practice.

In 1 small retrospective analysis at 2 community hospitals,[59] pulmonologists disagreed with one third of general internists' spirometry interpretations. Much larger investigations have shown that, when compared with accepted management guidelines, pulmonologists and allergists use more appropriate pharmacotherapy for individuals with asthma than do generalists; generalists tended to underuse inhaled corticosteroids and overuse long-term oral corticosteroids, despite the many adverse effects associated with the prolonged use of these drugs, while underusing high-dose corticosteroids for acute exacerbations.[60-62]

In 1 study[63] using a convenience sample of physicians to evaluate patient photographs, dermatologists diagnosed the 10 most common skin conditions more accurately, ordered fewer laboratory tests, and prescribed more appropriate treatment than did family practitioners. In a similar investigation, Dolan et al[64] demonstrated differences in university-based primary care physicians' attitudes toward, behaviors in, and knowledge of skin cancer control, compared with dermatologists. White[65] observed that primary care physicians at 1 clinic underdiagnosed actinic keratoses, using 1 dermatologist's evaluation as a criterion standard.

Clement and Christenson[66] found that surveyed internists and family practitioners used the cytobrush less frequently than gynecologists in the collection of Papanicolaou smears. The authors express concern that this might result in the collection of more false-negative Papanicolaou smears by generalists. Similarly, Starpoli et al[67] found that primary care internal medicine residents at 1 institution often failed to master routine gynecologic skills. In 2 survey studies, general internal medicine residents displayed knowledge[68] and practice[69] deficits surrounding the care of both pregnant and nonpregnant women with diabetes.

In other areas, findings of more appropriate specialty care may have resulted from patient selection. For instance, most generalists and specialists surveyed by Grisso et al[70] advocated exercise and calcium supplementation for postmenopausal women. However, despite the proven benefits of estrogen replacement therapy in this group, in an observational cohort study, Schwartz et al[71] found that only 10% to 15% of general internists and 35% to 45% of gynecologists routinely prescribed estrogen. Those patients cared for by endocrinologists and gynecologists were 2 to 4 times as likely as those of general internists to receive estrogen.[71] Specialists' opinions regarding estrogen replacement therapy may have reflected their heightened awareness of its benefits. Alternatively, patient selection of provider may have affected estrogen prescription rates. Both those patients self-referred to endocrinologists and gynecologists and those patients referred by their primary care physicians (for, say, a low bone density or severe osteoporosis) may have been more likely to choose estrogen replacement therapy for its benefits. The more typical postmenopausal woman seeing a generalist, on the other hand, may have been less willing to assume the possibly slightly increased risk of breast cancer or the inconvenience of vaginal bleeding that can result from taking estrogen.

More effective specialty care may also be the product of more time-, labor-, and financially intensive management by the specialist and his/her ancillary staff. For instance, intensive, multidisciplinary specialty interventions in individuals with severe asthma have been shown to lead to improved pharmacotherapy, fewer emergency department visits, and reduced admission rates, lengths of hospital stay, and overall costs.[62,72–76] In addition to more rational use of antiasthmatic agents by specialists, these studies showed that spending more time to educate patients whose self-management skills were negligible, along with improving provider and ancillary staff availability by telephone and in clinic for minor exacerbations, resulted in better disease control. Similar reasoning may also apply to the improved blood glucose control seen in children attending one diabetes specialty clinic.[77] Even so, the large, prospective, observational Medical Outcomes Study[39] found no meaningful outcome differences between those patients with type 2 diabetes mellitus under the care of a general internist and those under the care of an endocrinologist. However, a claims-based profile of care provided to Medicare patients with diabetes elucidated that while large proportions of individuals with diabetes received few recommended services (eg, hemoglobin $A_{1c}$ measurements, ophthalmologic evaluation, and cholesterol screening), differences between generalists and specialists were not uniformly large.[78]

In a 31-year statistical overview of 10 randomized controlled trials, most of which were conducted outside the United States, Langhorne et al[79] found a trend toward decreased mortality in patients with stroke cared for in a stroke unit, compared with those hospitalized in a general medical ward. Horner et al[80] found a similar difference when comparing the outcomes of patients with stroke treated by neurologists and nonneurologists. These results may reflect neurologists' more appropriate management of cerebrovascular accidents and their complications, more intensive care and rehabilitation provided by nurses and physical and occupational therapists, and better education of patients and their families, but appear to be explained best by neurologists' selection of patients with better initial prognoses.[79-81]

Finally, decreases in mortality in intensive care units with dedicated intensivists[82-84] may result from the specialist's superior knowledge and skills. Alternatively, the constant presence or at least immediate availability of a faculty physician to provide bedside care, the institution of patient care protocols and guidelines, increased teaching of house staff and nurses, the establishment of formal daily work rounds, and increased involvement of allied health workers (eg, physical therapists) may be responsible.

In other instances, within a given organization, superior management of patients by specialists may reflect in part the failure of those specialists to teach their generalist colleagues about properly managing common illnesses (or alternatively, the failure of the generalists to learn from specialists' feedback and education regarding management and consultation). Specialized clinics, such as anticoagulation clinics, can help both generalists and specialists better monitor certain aspects of patients' care.[85]

Only some of the studies discussed were prospective, randomized comparisons,[39,52,72-74] and most did not use adequate risk adjustment.[45,56,81,86] Furthermore, the studies comparing generalists and specialists assessed their adherence to interventions recommended on the basis of expert consensus or, in a few cases, randomized clinical trials (eg, b-blockers following myocardial infarction). However, these process indicators have limitations inherent to the methods by which they were derived, and can change over time as new knowledge is accumulated. Thus, assessing patient outcomes[4,42,47,48,55,72,73,75] may be more valuable than merely comparing the process of generalist vs specialty care. Due to a dearth of data on costs, future studies should include some form of economic analysis.

# DEFICIENCIES AND OVERUTILIZATION COMMON TO ALL PHYSICIANS

While as a group specialists often outperform generalists in some areas of medical practice, this does not imply that any given specialist will provide better care than any particular generalist. Variations in quality of care among generalists and even among specialists are often larger than variations between the 2 groups. Also, while as a group specialists' knowledge base and practice patterns are superior to those of generalists in certain instances, the magnitude of these differences and their overall effects on morbidity and mortality are likely small, compared with the sequelae of deficiencies in disease management and preventive medicine common to all physicians, generalists and specialists alike.

## Deficiencies in Management of Disease

Deficiencies have been documented for the care of hypertension (recognition and treatment),[87,88] atrial fibrillation (knowledge regarding anticoagulation guidelines),[38] congestive heart failure (use of angiotensin-converting enzyme inhibitors),[24] hyperlipidemia (recognition and treatment),[89–91] and myocardial infarction (use of aspirin, thrombolytics, and b-blockers).[22,30,32,92–96] Deficiences have also been noted in the use of endocarditis prophylaxis[97]; in the monitoring of blood glucose control, renal function, and lipid levels in individuals with diabetes[98]; in screening for and recognizing ophthalmic disease in individuals both with and without diabetes[99,100]; for the management of ulcers (treatment of *H pylori*),[101] asthma (use of inhaled corticosteroids),[102] AIDS-associated *P carinii* pneumonia (inappropriate undertreatment),[53] and locoregional breast cancer (use of breast-conserving surgery)[103]; in the care of the dying (attention to end-of-life concerns and remediable suffering),[104,105] and in pain control (dosing of analgesics)[106,107]; and in the recognition of depression,[108] functional disability[109,110] and other psychosocial stressors.[43,111,112] Moreover, Wigton et al[113] surveyed directors of internal medicine programs and found that current residency training does not ensure competency in all the procedures a general internist does in practice.

## Deficiencies in Preventive Care

Equally important are the deficiencies common to all physicians in the provision of preventive care. These include underimmunization; inadequate use of cancer and other screening tests; infrequent, poor health counseling; and inadequate identification and treatment of psychosocial problems. These deficiencies affect all patients and should be particularly distressing to generalists, since they lie in those areas in which generalists have traditionally claimed special expertise.

## Vaccination

Current levels of child and adult vaccination in the United States are less than half the levels in other industrialized countries.[114–116] While this is due in part to poor public awareness and to financial and systems barriers,[117,118] physicians also contribute[119] through missed opportunities,[120,121] failure to administer multiple vaccines during the same visit,[122] inappropriately broadening contraindications to vaccination,[123] and forgetting to assess the vaccination status of patients.[124] Weingarten et al[125] found that primary care physicians grossly overestimated their influenza and pneumococcal vaccination practices when self-report was compared with the medical record.

## Cancer Screening

Physicians also significantly overestimate their performance of common cancer screening tests.[126,127] Deficiencies in performing oral cavity inspections of smokers, rectal examinations, breast examinations, mammography, Papanicolaou smears, breast self-examination teaching, and skin examinations have been extensively documented.[13,64,126,128] These may be due partly to lack of awareness of guidelines, forgetfulness, inconvenience, dislike of performing a procedure, and lack of time.[114,126] In general, tests are used more often to evaluate new patients or those with risk factors for cancer.[127] The elderly, the uninsured, and those of lower socioeconomic status are less likely to receive screening tests, independent of number of physician visits, even in the presence of risk factors.[129–131]

## Substance Abuse

Physicians are frequently unsuccessful in identifying alcohol and drug abuse, despite its high prevalence in both inpatient and outpatient settings.[132] While brief, extensively validated screening tests with good sensitivity and specificity exist and are simple to use, most alcoholics go unrecognized, and, even when diagnosed, are untreated.[133–135]

While up to 80% of physicians may advise smokers to quit, less than half consistently counsel smokers about *how* to quit.[128,136] Few former smokers state that their physician helped them to quit, even though quit attempts are twice as common among tobacco users encouraged by a physician.[137]

## Violence

Physicians frequently fail to identify victims of domestic violence, who represent 10% to 30% of females presenting to emergency departments.[138,139] Even when they recognize abuse, they often provide no treatment, or inappropriate or harmful treatment.[140] Despite mandatory reporting laws, they underrecognize and underreport abuse of the elderly, which has been estimated to affect approximately 10% of Americans older than 65 years.[141]

## Health Counseling

Physicians are frequently neglectful with respect to counseling patients in other areas, including diet,[128,142] exercise,[143] stress reduction, sun exposure,[64] preconception health,[68] breast-feeding,[144] use of seat belts[145] and helmets,[146] and firearm safety.[147]

More than three quarters of parents want physicians to discuss substance abuse, sexuality, mental health issues, nutrition, and general medical issues with their teenagers.[148] Nevertheless, counseling regarding HIV transmission, breast self-examination, and proper diets is infrequently offered during adolescent clinic visits.[149] Many clinicians believe that issues related to sexuality, such as pregnancy, contraception, and premature sexual activity, are less relevant to their adolescent patients than to adolescents in general.[150] They frequently do not assess the sexual orientation nor the potentially risky practices of both their adolescent and adult patients, and often fail to counsel those at high risk about AIDS prevention and safe sex.[151,152] These deficiencies in risk behavior modification are particularly disheartening, given the high prevalence of deleterious health habits and incorrect understanding of sexually transmitted diseases in teenagers, and in view of evidence that advice given to adolescents in clinical settings is likely to be trusted and is often followed.[153,154]

## Psychosocial Factors

In the public's opinion, along with inadequate attention to costs of treatment, physicians' worst deficiencies lie in communication skills and in the recognition and management of psychosocial contributors to health and illness.[16,155] Psychosocial difficulties may prompt up to 50% or more of outpatient generalist visits,[156] and cause as much or even more functional impairment than do strictly physical complaints.[157,158] While most patients want their physicians to assess their functional performance and emotional well-being, a majority report that their physicians rarely or never inquire about these areas.[109] Many believe that physicians do not spend enough time with them, encourage questions, or solicit their opinions; others complain of rushed visits and state that their physicians do not seem to care about their emotional well-being.[159] While most patients prefer to be informed about aspects of their care, many report not getting adequate information about their treatments.[160]

Often, physicians know little about their patients' social histories,[161] and fail to recognize their psychosocial needs[43,112,162] and functional disabilities.[110] At least half, and possibly as many as 90%, of patients with depression in primary care practice remain undetected.[108,163] Even when they are aware of problems, physicians may not intervene appropriately.[164] Some believe that managing psychosocial problems is not their responsibility.[15,165,166]

Physicians often deal poorly with suffering and dying patients, neglecting to provide essential information about cardiopulmonary resuscitation during discussions of code status, or failing to elicit patients' concerns regarding end-of-life issues.[105] They can neglect remediable factors contributing to dying patients' discomfort, such as poor oral hygiene, unquenched thirst, difficulty eating, and lack of personal contact.[104] Many tend to undertreat pain related to malignancies and chronic disease[106,107] and underestimate the effects of nursing home residents' pain and depression on their health status.[167,168]

Yet not all data show that physicians ignore counseling.[169] Those with more positive attitudes toward psychosocial aspects of care offer more empathy and reassurance and ask open-ended questions. In turn, their patients participate more actively in their own care by expressing opinions and asking questions.[170] Furthermore, some patients are unwilling to reveal psychosocial problems or believe that these problems are not something one shares with one's physician.[171,172] Still, the public rates physicians' communication skills poorly; physicians in turn rate their training in counseling skills as inadequate.[16,173,174] And, while they believe that health promotion is important, physicians tend to be pessimistic about their success in working with patients to modify behaviors that affect health.[175,176] Many doubt their competency to deal with psychosocial aspects of care,[177] and up to one third believe that their training to foster wellness and encourage certain preventive behaviors was inadequate.[174] Almost all deans of medical schools have acknowledged that preventive medicine training is underemphasized at their institutions.[178]

## Overutilization

On the other hand, overutilization can also negatively affect quality of care. Overtesting, without an appreciation for the test characteristics, can lead to further unwarranted interventions, including those that may harm the patient either physically or psychologically.[179] This may be true for the rapid, widespread adoption of prostate-specific antigen screening.[180] Overprescribing of potentially inappropriate medications has been documented. In a cross-sectional survey, Wilcox et al[181] found that almost one quarter of community-dwelling elderly were receiving at least one contraindicated prescription drug, placing them at risk for adverse effects such as sedation and cognitive impairment.

On the other hand, high rates of inappropriate care and geographic variation in care patterns that do not affect clinical outcomes have also been extensively documented.[182–192] These may result from excessive test ordering and procedural use by specialists,[6,183] or from differences in payer status,[193,194] resource availability,[195] or local practice styles,[6,190,191] but do not appear to be related to differences in severity of illness.

In cardiology, while certain drugs are clearly underused, coronary angiography and revascularization, expensive and invasive procedures, may be overused. Privately insured patients are more likely to receive angiography, angioplasty, and bypass grafting than Medicaid or uninsured patients.[193] Winslow et al[188,189] found that a substantial proportion of bypass surgeries and endarterectomies were performed for inappropriate reasons. Using RAND criteria, Chassin et al[196] determined that 17% of coronary angiographies and 32% of carotid endarterectomies were inappropriate. Patients in high-use regions of the country were older, had less severe angina, and were treated less intensively medically than patients in low-use sites.[197] Hilborne et al[198] discerned that from one quarter to half of coronary angiograms were performed for uncertain indications.

Blustein[199] found that the availability of cardiac services in the hospital to which patients presented strongly influenced the likelihood of their use in the period following acute myocardial infarction; this was unlikely due to selection bias. Similarly, Every et al[200] discovered that after adjustment for clinical factors, the availability of on-site catheterization facilities was associated with a higher likelihood that a patient would undergo angiography. While no short-term mortality benefit was associated with the greater use of angiography, their study lacked adequate statistical power to detect either short- or long-term mortality benefits.

Thus, overuse of cardiac procedures appears likely. However, others[201,202] have found low rates (approximately 5%) of inappropriate and uncertain coronary angiography and coronary artery bypass grafting in New York State, and Ayanian et al[22] found that Medicare patients in Texas with acute myocardial infarction admitted to hospitals offering coronary angioplasty and bypass surgery had lower adjusted 1-year mortality than patients admitted to other hospitals.

While large US geographic variations in the use of angiography do not correlate with mortality or health-related quality of life,[191] comparisons of the coronary procedure rates in Canada and the United States suggest that the greater rates in the United States may be associated with decreases in anginal symptoms.[203] Even so, Tu et al[204] showed that higher rates of cardiac procedures in the United States, compared with Canada, did not result in better long-term survival rates for elderly patients with acute myocardial infarction. Within the United States, greater physician and hospital experience with cardiovascular procedures leads to better outcomes.[205]

Other procedures may be overused because of broadening of indications, as has been suggested for radiography in lower back pain,[206] for laparoscopic cholecystectomy,[207] and for cesarean delivery and hysterectomies, 15% and 20% of which may be unnecessary, respectively.[184] Using RAND appropriateness criteria on a random sample of elderly patients, Kahn et al[208] concluded that 11% of endoscopies of the upper gastrointestinal tract were performed for equivocal indications, and 17% for inappropriate indications. Interestingly, just as some specialists reach for different technologies first in treating patients, they tend to withdraw these same technologies first when withdrawing care from the terminally ill.[209]

Large geographic variations have also been noted in the use of grafts vs fistulae for patients undergoing hemodialysis.[210] Patients of lower socioeconomic status are more likely to receive a (less appropriate) graft than (the preferred) fistula.

Payment mechanisms may also affect utilization. Patients who receive care in health maintenance organizations are half to one fourth as likely to be operated on as patients in the fee-for-service sector, usually with no major outcome differences.[184] Finally, race may play a role in the differential use of procedures, with seriously ill African Americans less likely to receive major therapeutic interventions than similarly ill white patients.[194,211]

Thus, a number of factors can contribute to overuse, including numbers of specialists, education, differences in local practice styles, uncertainty or skewed beliefs regarding the benefits of an intervention, eagerness to adopt new and unproved tests or procedures, patient race and socioeconomic status, patient choice, and, under fee-for-service, physician financial incentives. With increasing capitation under managed care, the influence of the latter incentive should diminish. Obviously, specialists should not be held responsible entirely for the high-documented rates of inappropriate interventions, since primary care physicians, through the referral process, play some role in determining who eventually receives these interventions. Furthermore, inadequate patient education by physicians and lack of patient involvement in the informed consent process may lead patients to accept more readily procedures they might have refused otherwise.

# CONCLUSIONS

While certain differences point to correctable deficiencies of generalists, these differences are not as striking or clinically important as the deficiencies in disease management, preventive care, and health maintenance common to all physicians. These problems should be particularly distressing to generalists, who claim special interest and expertise in these areas. Furthermore, overuse of diagnostic and therapeutic modalities leads to inappropriate care that increases costs without providing benefit, or, worse, increases risks to patients. Table 28.1 summarizes findings from this review.

Generalists and specialists must work together to effect changes in medical practice and to improve the quality, efficiency, and cost-effectiveness of medical care. To be effective these changes will require the support of payers, such as insurance companies and the government, as well as of managed care organizations.

Likely, the number of generalists will continue to increase and the number of specialists will decrease.[212] Even with today's distribution of physicians, there are not enough specialists (nor financial resources) for every individual with asthma to be cared for by a pulmonologist, or every patient with depression to be followed up by a psychiatrist. Thus, more attention should be paid to minimizing quality-of-care differences for the more common illnesses, eliminating those deficiencies in the provision of preventive care common to all physicians, decreasing unnecessary and inappropriate care, improving the referral process for patients with complicated conditions or those with less common diseases, and promoting comanagement and a teamwork approach to the care of certain kinds of patients.[213] This could be achieved through education and training,

*(continued on page 527)*

**Table 28.1. Quality of Care for Various Specialties.**

| Specialty | Generalists and Specialists | | Specialists Compared With Generalists | Comment | References |
| --- | --- | --- | --- | --- | --- |
| | Deficiencies | Overutilization | | | |
| Cardiology | Use of aspirin, b-blockers, heparin, and thrombolytics in MI | ? Cardiac catheterization and revascularization procedures | More appropriate MI/post-MI knowledge and care | | 19, 22, 25, 27–30, 32, 38, 39, |
| | Anticoagulation for atrial fibrillation | Radionuclide stress tests | Similar care for hypertension, atrial fibrillation, and transient ischemic attacks and strokes | Multiple studies of knowledge base and practice patterns | 87–97, 188, 189, 191, 193, 194, |
| | Endocarditis prophylaxis | Calcium channel blockers, prophylactic lidocaine | ⋯ | ⋯ | 196–204 |
| | Recognition and treatment of hypertension and hyperlipidemia | ⋯ | ⋯ | ⋯ | |
| Mental health disorders | Recognition of depression and suicidality | Benzodiazepines | Psychiatric care more appropriate and more cost-effective | Multiple studies | 12, 41–46 |
| | Use antidepressants at appropriate doses | ⋯ | Worse handling of medical conditions associated with psychiatric illness | ⋯ | |
| | Psychotherapy | ⋯ | ⋯ | ⋯ | |
| HIV/AIDS care | Inadequate education and training | ⋯ | Recognize AIDS-associated illnesses better | ⋯ | 47–51, 53 |
| | | | Patients have better outcomes | Therapies changing rapidly | |
| Rheumatology | ⋯ | ⋯ | More appropriate use of arthocentesis, better care for gout, better functional outcomes in rheumatoid arthritis, no consistent differences for lower back pain outcomes | ⋯ | 54, 55 |
| Pulmonary | Underuse of long-term inhaled corticosteroids and high-dose oral corticosteroids for flares | Long-term oral corticosteroids | ?Better disease control | Multidisciplinary intervention | 56, 59–62, 72–76 |
| | | ⋯ | ± More accurate spirometry interpretations | Small sample | |
| | | | COPD management equivalent | Small study | |

| | Generalists and Specialists | | Specialists Compared | | |
|---|---|---|---|---|---|
| Specialty | Deficiencies | Overutilization | With Generalists | Comment | References |
| Neurology | ... | Carotid endarterectomy | Improved outcome in healthier patients in stroke units | Multidisciplinary intervention, patient selection | 79–81, 188, 189, 196 |
| Endocrinology | Hemoglobin $A_{1c}$, opthalmologic, renal function, and cholesterol screening | ... | Similar quality of diabetes care and mortality, except endocrinologists better for diabetic individuals with foot ulcers | ... | 39, 68, 69, 78, 99, 100 |
| | Internal medicine residents' knowledge of care of pregnant women with diabetes | | ... | | |
| Obstetrics and gynecology | Hormone replacement therapy | Cesarean deliveries, hysterectomies | More patients receiving hormone replacement therapy | Patient selection | 57, 71, 103, 184 |
| | Breast-conserving cancer surgery | ... | Better Papanicolaou smear technique | ... | |
| | | | Perinatal outcomes same | Small study | |
| Gastroenterology | Awareness of the role of *Helicobacter pylori* in peptic ulcer disease | Upper endoscopies | More aware of *H pylori* role and treatment | Studies done soon after guidelines published, inadequate time for dissemination of knowledge to practicing physicians | 17, 58, 207, 208 |
| | ... | ?Laparoscopic cholecystectomies | Generalists order more appropriate endoscopies than nongastroenterology specialists | | |
| Dermatology | Recognition of benign and malignant lesions | Diagnostic tests | Better recognition, more appropriate workup and treatment | ... | 63, 65, 66 |
| | Skin cancer control | ... | Better skin cancer control | ... | |

*(continued)*

**Table 28.1. Quality of Care for Various Specialties.** *(continued)*

| Specialty | Generalists and Specialists | | Specialists Compared | | References |
|---|---|---|---|---|---|
| | Deficiencies | Overutilization | With Generalists | Comment | |
| Orthopedics | ... | Radiography (by orthopedists and chiropractors) | Lower back pain outcomes same, generalists care less expensive | ... | 4, 206 |
| Geriatrics | Care of the dying | Inappropriate, potentially dangerous overmedication | ... | ... | 104, 105, 181 |
| Pain control | Underappreciation of severity, undertreatment | ... | ... | ... | 104, 106, 107, 167, 168 |
| Renal/urology | Fistulae for hemodialysis | Grafts for hemodialysis<br>? Prostrate-specific antigen testing | Socioeconomic, racial differences | ... | 210 |
| Preventive medicine/public health | Immunizations | ... | ± More appropriate test ordering by generalists | Elderly, those of lower socioeconomic status fare worse | 10, 11, 13, 15, 43, 64, 105, 108–112, |
| | Cancer screening | | ... | | 114, 115, 117–121, |
| | Identification and treatment of substance abuse, violence, psychosocial difficulties, and functional impairment | ... | Generalists more willing to treat psychosocial problems | ... | 123, 124, 126–154, |
| | Health counseling | ... | ... | ... | 156–159, 161–166, 173–175 |

*MI indicates myocardial infarction; HIV, human immunodeficiency virus; AIDS, acquired immunodeficiency syndrome; ellipses, not applicable; and COPD, chronic obstructive pulmonary disease.

feedback to providers, evidence-based disease management[214] research, and structural changes in the practice of medicine. Particularly, attention should be paid to improving counseling and screening practices, reversing the decrease in outpatient visit length,[215] defining provider roles, and improving referral utility.[216,217]

# Notes

1. Cave D. Analyzing the content of physicians' medical practices. *J Ambul Care Manage.* 1994;17:15–36.

2. Starfield B. *Primary Care.* New York: Oxford University Press; 1992.

3. Aiken LH, Lewis CE, Craig J, Mendenhall RC, Blendon RJ, Rogers DE. The contribution of specialists to the delivery of primary care. *N Engl J Med.* 1979;300:1363–1370.

4. Carey TS, Garrett J, Jackman A, et al. The outcomes and costs of care for acute low back pain among patients seen by primary care practitioners, chiropractors, and orthopedic surgeons. *N Engl J Med.* 1995;333:913–917.

5. Petersdorf RG, Goitlein L. The future of internal medicine. *Ann Intern Med.* 1993;119:1130–1137.

6. Greenfield S, Nelson E, Zubkoff M. Variations in resource utilization among medical specialties and systems of care: results from the Medical Outcomes Study. *JAMA.* 1992;267:1624–1630.

7. Grumbach K, Bodenheimer T. The organization of health care. *JAMA.* 1995;273:160–167.

8. Carline JD, Inui TS, Larson E, Lo Gerfo J, Ramsey PG. The knowledge base of certified internists: relationships to training, practice type, and other physician characteristics. *Arch Intern Med.* 1989;149:2311–2313.

9. Ramsey PG, Carline JD, Inui TS, et al. Changes over time in the knowledge base of practicing internists. *JAMA.* 1991;266:1103–1107.

10. Manu P, Schwartz S. Patterns of diagnostic testing in the academic setting: the influence of medical attendings' subspecialty training. *Soc Sci Med.* 1983;17:1339–1342.

11. Glassman PA, Kravitz RL, Petersen LP, Rolph JE. Practice style of internists and cardiologists for three scenarios. *J Gen Intern Med.* 1996;11(suppl 1):71.

12. Cantor J, Baker L, Hughes R. Preparedness for practice: young physicians' views of their professional education. *JAMA.* 1993;270:1035–1040.

13. Turner B, Amsel Z, Lustbader E, Schwartz J, Balshem A, Grisso J. Breast cancer screening: effect of physician specialty, practice setting, year of medical school graduation, and sex. *Am J Prev Med.* 1992;8:78–85.

14. Linn L, Yager J. Factors associated with physician recognition and treatment of alcoholism. *N Engl J Med.* 1989;308:97–100.

15. Earp J, Fletcher S, O'Malley M, Fletcher R. Attitudes of internal medicine subspecialty fellows toward primary care. *Ann Intern Med.* 1984;144:329–333.

16. McBride C, Shugars D, Di Matteo R, Lepper H, O'Neil E, Damush T. The physician's role: views of the public and the profession on seven aspects of patient care. *Arch Fam Med.* 1994;3:948–953.

17. Mahajan R, Barthel J, Marshall J. Appropriateness of referrals for open-access endoscopy: how do physicians in different medical specialties do? *Arch Intern Med.* 1996;156:2065–2069.

18. Franks P, Clancy CM, Nutting PA. Gatekeeping revisited: protecting patients from overtreatment [letter]. *N Engl J Med.* 1992;327:424–427.

19. Ayanian JZ, Hauptman P, Guadagnoli E, Antman E, Pashos CL, McNeil BJ. Knowledge and practices of generalist and specialist physicians regarding drug therapy for acute myocardial infarction. *N Engl J Med.* 1994;331:1136–1142.

20. Hine L, Laird N, Hewitt P, Chalmers T. Meta-analytic evidence against prophylactic use of lidocaine in acute myocardial infarction. *Arch Intern Med.* 1989;149:2694–2698.

21. Furberg CD, Psaty BM, Meyer JV. Nifedipine: dose-related increase in mortality in patients with coronary heart disease. *Circulation.* 1995;92:1326–1331.

22. Ayanian JZ, Guadagnoli E, McNeil BJ, Cleary PD. Treatment and outcomes of acute myocardial infarction among patients of cardiologists and generalist physicians. *Arch Intern Med.* 1997;157:2570–2576.

23. Chin MH, Friedmann PD, Cassel CK, Lang RM. Differences in generalist and specialist physicians' knowledge and use of angiotensin-converting enzyme inhibitors for congestive heart failure. *J Gen Intern Med.* 1997;12:523–530.

24. Chin MH, Wang JC, Zhang JX, Lang RM. Utilization and dosing of angiotensin-converting enzyme inhibitors for heart failure: effect of physician specialty and patient characteristics. *J Gen Intern Med.* 1997;12:563–566.

25. Jancin B. Cardiologists outperform generalists for CHF [news report of findings presented at the 1996 Annual Meeting of the American College of Cardiology]. *Internal Medical News.* June 1, 1996:36.

26. Borowsky SJ, Kravitz RL, Laouri M, et al. Effect of physician specialty on use of necessary coronary angiography. *J Am Coll Cardiol.* 1995;26:1484–1491.

27. Stein JH, Uretz EF, Parrillo JE, Barron JT. Cost and appropriateness of radionuclide exercise stress testing by cardiologists and non-cardiologists. *Am J Cardiol.* 1996;77:139–142.

28. Schreiber TL, Elkhatib A, Grines CL, O'Neill WW. Cardiologist versus internist management of patients with unstable angina: treatment patterns and outcomes. *J Am Coll Cardiol.* 1995;26:577–582.

29. Brand DA, Newcomer LN, Freiburger A, Tian H. Cardiologists' practices compared with practice guidelines: use of beta-blockade after acute myocardial infarction. *J Am Coll Cardiol.* 1995;26:1432–1436.

30. Hennekens CH, Albert CM, Godfried SL, Gaziano JM, Buring JE. Adjunctive drug therapy of acute myocardial infarction-evidence from clinical trials. *N Engl J Med.* 1996;22:1660–1667.

31. Doorey A, Michelson E, Topol E. Thrombolytic therapy of acute myocardial infarction: keeping the unfulfilled promises. *JAMA.* 1992;268:3108–3114.

32. Sial S, Malone M, Freeman J, Battiola R, Nachodsky J, Goodwin J. Beta blocker use in the treatment of community hospital patients discharged after myocardial infarction. *J Gen Intern Med.* 1994;9:599–605.

33. De Maria AN, Engle MA, Harrison DC, et al. Managed care involvement by cardiovascular specialists: prevalence, attitudes and influence on practice. *J Am Coll Cardiol.* 1994;23:1245–1253.

34. Kravitz R, Greenfield S, Rogers W, et al. Differences in the mix of patients among medical specialties and systems of care: results from the medical outcomes study. *JAMA.* 1992;267:1617–1623.

35. Knapp D, Oeltjen P. Benefits-to-risk ratio in physician drug selection. *Am J Public Health.* 1972;62:1346–1347.

36. O'Rourke R. Are beta-blockers really underutilized in postinfarction patients? *J Am Coll Cardiol.* 1995;26:1437–1439.

37. Friedmann PD, Brett AS, Mayo-Smith MF. Differences in generalists' and cardiologists' perceptions of cardiovascular risk and the outcomes of preventive therapy in cardiovascular disease. *Ann Intern Med.* 1996;124:414–421.

38. McCrory D, Matchar D, Samsa G, Sanders L, Pritchett E. Physician attitudes about anticoagulation for nonvalvular atrial fibrillation in the elderly. *Arch Intern Med.* 1995;155:277–281.

39. Greenfield S, Rogers W, Magnotich M, Carney MF, Tarlov AR. Outcomes of patients with hypertension and non-insulin–dependent diabetes mellitus treated by different systems specialties: results from the medical outcomes studies. *JAMA.* 1995;274:1436–1444.

40. Garg M, Mulligan J, Gliebe W, Parekh R. Physician specialty, quality and cost of inpatient care. *Soc Sci Med.* 1979;13C:187–190.

41. Eisenberg L. Treating depression and anxiety in primary care: closing the gap between knowledge and practice. *N Engl J Med.* 1992;326:1080–1084.

42. Sturm R, Wells K. How can care for depression become more cost-effective? *JAMA.* 1995;273:51–58.

43. Thompson T, Stoudemire A, Mitchell W, Grant R. Underrecognition of patients' psychosocial distress in a university hospital medical clinic. *Psychiatry.* 1983;140:158–161.

44. Gerber PD, Barrett J, Barrett J, Manheimer E, Whiting R, Smith R. Recognition of depression by internists in primary care: a comparison of internist and "gold standard" psychiatric assessments. *J Gen Intern Med.* 1989;4:7–13.

45. Norquist G, Wells KB, Rogers WH, Davis LM, Kahn K, Brook RH. Quality of care for depressed elderly patients hospitalized in the specialty psychiatric units or general medical wards. *Arch Gen Psychiatry.* 1995;52:695–701.

46. Callahan CM, Dittus RS, Tierney WM. Primary care physicians' medical decision making for late-life depression. *J Gen Intern Med.* 1996;11:218–225.

47. Turner B, McKee L, Fanning T, Markson L. AIDS specialist versus general ambulatory care for advanced HIV infection and impact on hospital use. *Med Care.* 1994;32:902–916.

48. Kitahata M, Koepsell T, Wagner E, Deyo R, Maxwell C, Dodge W. Physicians' experience with acquired immunodeficiency syndrome as a factor in patients' survival. *N Engl J Med.* 1996;334:701–706.

49. Markson L, Cosler L, Turner B. Implications of generalists' slow adoption of zidovudine in clinical practice. *Arch Intern Med.* 1994;154:1497–1504.

50. Hayward R, Shapiro M. A national study of AIDS and residency programs: experiences, concerns, and consequences. *Ann Intern Med.* 1991;114:23–32.

51. Gerbert B, Maguire B, Bleecker T, Coates T, McPhee S. Primary care physicians and AIDS: attitudinal and structural barriers to care. *JAMA.* 1991;266:2837–2842.

52. Paauw DS, Wenrich MD, Curtis JR, Carline JD, Ramsey PG. Ability of primary care physicians to recognize physical findings associated with HIV infection. *JAMA.* 1995;274:1380–1382.

53. Curtis JR, Paauw DS, Wenrich MD, Carline JD, Ramsey PG. Ability of primary care physicians to diagnose and manage *Pneumocystis carinii* pneumonia. *J Gen Intern Med.* 1995;10:395–399.

54. Solomon DH, Bates DW, Panush RS, Katz JN. Costs, outcomes, and patient satisfaction by provider type for patients with rheumatic and musculoskeletal conditions: a critical review of the literature and proposed methodologic standards. *Ann Intern Med.* 1997;127:52–60.

55. Ward M, Leigh J, Fries J. Progression of functional disability in patients with rheumatoid arthritis: associations with rheumatology subspecialty care. *Arch Intern Med.* 1993;153:2229–2237.

56. Strauss M, Conrad D, Lo Gerfo J, Hudson L, Bergner M. Cost and outcome of care for patients with chronic obstructive lung disease. *Med Care.* 1986;24:915–924.

57. Franks P, Eisenger S. Adverse perinatal outcomes: is physician specialty a risk factor? *J Fam Pract.* 1987;24:152–156.

58. Fendrick AM, Hirth RA, Chernew ME. Differences between generalist and specialist physicians regarding *Helicobacter pylori* and peptic ulcer disease. *Am J Gastroenterol.* 1996;91:1544–1548.

59. Hnatiuk O, Moores L, Loughney T, Torrington K. Evaluation of internists' spirometric interpretations. *J Gen Intern Med.* 1996;11:204–208.

60. Kemp J. Approaches to asthma management: realities and recommendations. *Arch Intern Med.* 1993;153:805–812.

61. Horn C, Cochrane G. Management of asthma in general practice. *Respir Med.* 1989;83:67–70.

62. Carpi J. Generalists trail allergists in giving inhaled steroids. *Internal Medical News.* August 15, 1995:1.

63. Clark R, Rietschel R. The cost of initiating appropriate therapy for skin diseases: a comparison of dermatologists and family physicians. *J Am Acad Dermatol.* 1983;9:787–796.

64. Dolan N, Martin G, Robinson J, Rademaker A. Skin cancer control practices among physicians in a university general medicine practice. *J Gen Intern Med.* 1995;10:515–519.

65. White J. Primary care clinicians' performance for detecting actinic keratoses and skin cancer [abstract]. *J Gen Intern Med.* 1995;10(suppl).

66. Clement K, Christenson P. Papanicolaou smear recovery techniques used by primary care physicians. *J Am Board Fam Pract.* 1990;3:253–258.

67. Starpoli C, Moulton A, Cyr M. How well are primary care residents trained in ambulatory gynecology? [abstract]. *J Gen Intern Med.* 1995;10(suppl):94.

68. Conway T, Mason E, Hu T. Attitudes, knowledge, and skills of internal medicine residents regarding pre-conception care. *Acad Med.* 1994;69:389–391.

69. Oberman L. How does your practice compare? *American Medical News.* August 1, 1994:1, 11.

70. Grisso J, Baum C, Turner B. What do physicians in practice do to prevent osteoporosis? *J Bone Miner Res.* 1990;5:213–219.

71. Schwartz M, Anwah I, Levy R. Variations in treatment of postmenopausal osteoporosis. *Clin Orthop.* 1985;182:180–184.

72. Mayo P, Richman J, Harris H. Results of a program to reduce admissions for adult asthma. *Ann Intern Med.* 1990;112:864–871.

73. Zeiger R, Heller S, Mellon M, Wald J, Falkoff R, Schatz M. Facilitated referral to asthma specialist reduces relapse in emergency room visits. *J Allergy Clin Immunol.* 1991;87:1160–1180.

74. Weinberger M. Access to specialty care [letter]. *N Engl J Med.* 1995;332:474.

75. Bucknall C, Robertson C, Moran F, Stevenson R. Differences in hospital asthma management. *Lancet.* 1988;1:748–750.

76. Kassirer J. Access to specialty care. *N Engl J Med.* 1994;331:1151–1153.

77. Bloomfield S, Farquhar J. Is a specialist paediatric diabetic clinic better? *Arch Dis Child.* 1990;65:139–140.

78. Weiner JP, Parente ST, Garnick DW, Fowles J, Lawthers AG, Palmer RH. Variation in office-based quality: a claims-based profile of care provided to Medicare patients with diabetes. *JAMA.* 1995;273:1503–1508.

79. Langhorne P, Williams B, Gilchrist W, Howie K. Do stroke units save lives? *Lancet.* 1993;342:395–398.

80. Horner R, Matchar D, Divine G, Feussner J. Relationship between physician specialty selection and the selection and outcome of ischemic stroke patients. *Health Serv Res.* 1995;30:275–287.

81. Eisenberg J. Commentary: are differences in outcome due to differences in doctors or their patients? *Health Serv Res.* 1995;30:291–294.

82. Brown J, Sullivan G. Effect on ICU mortality of a full-time critical care specialist. *Chest.* 1989;96:127–129.

83. Carson SS, Stocking C, Podsadecki T, et al. Effects of organizational change in the medical intensive care unit of a teaching hospital: a comparison of "open" and "closed" formats. *JAMA.* 1996;276:322–328.

84. Pollack MM, Cuerdon TT, Patel KM, Ruttimann UE, Getson PR, Levetown M. Impact of quality-of-care factors on pediatric intensive care unit mortality. *JAMA.* 1994;272:941–946.

85. Butzlaff ME, Maesner AT, Fuhn SD. Is the quality of anticoagulation management improved with a specialized clinic? *J Gen Intern Med.* 1996;11(suppl 1):44.

86. Storms B, Olden L, Nathan R, Bodman S. Effect of allergy specialist care on the quality of life in patients with asthma. *Ann Allergy Asthma Immunol.* 1995;75(pt 1):491–494.

87. Stockwell S, Madhavan S, Cohen H, Gibson G, Alderman M. The determinants of hypertension awareness, treatment, and control in an insured population. *Am J Public Health.* 1994;84:1768–1774.

88. Siegel D, Lopez J. Trends in antihypertensive drug use in the United States: do the JNC V recommendations affect prescribing. *JAMA.* 1997;278:1745–1748.

89. Schrott HG, Bittner V, Vittinghoff E, Herrington DM, Hulley S. Adherence to National Cholesterol Education Program Treatment goals in postmenopausal women with heart disease: The Heart and Estrogen/Progestin Replacement Study (HERS). *JAMA.* 1997;277:1281–1286.

90. Giles WH, Anda RF, Jones DH, Serdula MK, Merritt RK, De Stefano F. Recent trends in the identification and treatment of high blood cholesterol by physicians: progress and missed opportunities. *JAMA.* 1993;269:1133–1138.

91. Stafford RS, Blumenthal D, Pasternak RC. Variations in cholesterol management practices of U.S. physicians. *J Am Coll Cardiol.* 1997;29:139–146.

92. Meehan T, Hennen J, Radford MJ, Petrillo M, Elstein P, Ballard D. Process and outcome of care for acute myocardial infarction among Medicare beneficiaries in Connecticut: a quality improvement demonstration project. *Ann Intern Med.* 1995;122:928–936.

93. Ellerbeck EF, Jencks S, Radford MJ, et al. Quality of care for Medicare patients with acute myocardial infarction. *JAMA.* 1995;273:1509–1514.

94. Soumerai SB, McLaughlin TJ, Spiegelman D, Hertzmark E, Thibault G, Goldman L. Adverse outcomes of underuse of beta-blockers in elderly survivors of acute myocardial infarction. *JAMA.* 1997;277:115–121.

95. Krumholz HM, Radford MJ, Ellerbeck EF, et al. Aspirin for secondary prevention after acute myocardial infarction in the elderly: prescribed use and outcomes. *Ann Intern Med.* 1996;124:292–298.

96. Saketkhou BB, Conte FJ, Noris M, et al. Emergency department use of aspirin in patients with possible acute myocardial infarction. *Ann Intern Med.* 1997;127:126–129.

97. Durack D. Prevention of infective endocarditis. *N Engl J Med.* 1995;332:38–44.

98. Wisdom K, Fryzek JP, Havstad SL, Anderson RM, Dreiling MC, Tilley BC. Comparison of laboratory test frequency and test results between African-Americans and Caucasians with diabetes: opportunity for improvement—findings from a large urban health maintenance organization. *Diabetes Care.* 1997;20:971–977.

99. Wang F, Ford D, Tielsch JM, Quigley HA, Whelton PK. Undetected eye disease in a primary care clinic population. *Arch Intern Med.* 1994;154:1821–1828.

100. Brechner RJ, Cowie CC, Howie LJ, Herman WH, Will JC, Harris MI. Ophthalmic examination among adults with diagnosed diabetes mellitus. *JAMA.* 1993;270:1714–1718.

101. Boschert S. *H. pylori* left untreated in many ulcer patients. *ACP Observer.* June 1996.

102. Hartert TV, Windom HH, Peebles RS, Freidhoff LR, Togias A. Inadequate outpatient therapy for patients with asthma admitted in two urban hospitals. *Am J Med.* 1996;100:386–394.

103. Lee-Feldstein A, Anton-Culver H, Feldstein PJ. Treatment differences and other prognostic factors related to breast cancer survival: delivery systems and medical outcomes. *JAMA.* 1994;271:1163–1168.

104. Mills M, Davies H, Macrae W. Care of dying patients in a hospital. *Br Med J.* 1994;309:583–586.

105. Tulsky J, Chesney M, Lo B. How do medical residents discuss resuscitation with patients? *J Gen Intern Med.* 1995;10:436–442.

106. American Pain Society Quality of Care Committee. Quality improvement guidelines for the treatment of acute pain and cancer pain. *JAMA.* 1995;274:1874–1880.

107. Sprangers M, Aaronson N. The role of health care providers and significant others in evaluating the quality of life of patients with chronic disease: a review. *J Clin Epidemiol.* 1992;45:743–760.

108. Perez-Stable E, Miranda J, Ying Y. Depression in medical outpatients: underrecognition and misdiagnosis. *Arch Intern Med.* 1990;150:1083–1088.

109. Schor E, Lerner D, Malspeis S. Physicians' assessment of functional health status and well-being. *Arch Intern Med.* 1995;155:309–314.

110. Calkins D, Rubenstein L, Cleary PD, et al. Failure of physicians to recognize functional disability in ambulatory patients. *Ann Intern Med.* 1991;114:451–454.

111. Covinsky K, Goldman L, Cook E, et al. The impact of serious illness on patients' families. *JAMA.* 1994;272:1839–1844.

112. Brody D. Physician recognition of behavioral, psychological, and social aspects of medical care. *Arch Intern Med.* 1980;140:1286–1289.

113. Wigton R, Blank L, Nicolas J, Tape T. Procedural skills training in internal medicine residencies: a survey of program directors. *Ann Intern Med.* 1989;111:932–938.

114. Lurie N, Manning W, Peterson C, Goldberg G, Phelps C, Lillard L. Preventive care: do we practice what we preach? *Am J Public Health.* 1987;77:801–804.

115. Mustin H, Holt V, Connell F. Adequacy of well-child care and immunization in US infants born in 1988. *JAMA.* 1994;272:1111–1115.

116. Abbotts B, Osborn LM. Immunization status and reasons for immunization delay among children using public health immunization clinics. *Am J Dis Child.* 1993;147:965–968.

117. Gardner P, Schaffner W. Immunization of adults. *N Engl J Med.* 1993;328:1252–1258.

118. Centers for Disease Control. Influenza and pneumococcal vaccination coverage levels among persons aged > 65 years: United States, 1973–1993. *MMWR Morb Mortal Wkly Rep.* 1995;44:506–507, 513–515.

119. Brook RH, Fink A, Kosecoff J, et al. Educating physicians and treating patients in the ambulatory care setting. *Ann Intern Med.* 1987;107:392–398.

120. Quick R, Hoge C, Hamilton D, Whitney J, Borges M, Kobayashi J. Underutilization of pneumococcal vaccine in nursing homes in Washington State: report of a serotype-specific outbreak and survey. *Am J Med.* 1993;94:149–152.

121. Wood D, Pereyra M, Halfon N, Hamlin J, Grabowsky M. Vaccination levels in Los Angeles public health centers: the contribution of missed opportunities to vaccinate and other factors. *Am J Public Health.* 1995;85:850–853.

122. Peter G. Childhood immunizations. *N Engl J Med.* 1992;327:1794–1800.

123. Campbell J, Szilagyi P, Rodewald L, Winter N, Humiston S, Roghmann K. Intent to immunize among pediatric and family medicine residents. *Arch Pediatr Adolesc Med.* 1994;148:926–929.

124. Centers for Disease Control and Prevention. Impact of missed opportunities to vaccinate preschool-aged children on vaccination coverage levels: selected U.S. sites, 1991–1992. *MMWR Morb Mortal Wkly Rep.* 1994;43:709–711, 717–718.

125. Weingarten S, Stone E, Hayward R, et al. The adoption of preventive care practice guidelines by primary care physicians: do actions match intentions? *J Gen Intern Med.* 1995;10:138–144.

126. McPhee S, Richard R, Solkowitz S. Performance of cancer screening in a university internal medicine practice: comparison with the 1980 American Cancer Society guidelines. *J Gen Intern Med.* 1986;1:275–281.

127. Montano D, Phillips W. Cancer screening by primary care physicians: a comparison of rates obtained from physician self-report, patient survey, and chart audit. *Am J Public Health.* 1995;85:795–800.

128. Carney P, Dietrich A, Freeman D, Mott L. The periodic health examination provided to asymptomatic older women: an assessment using standardized patients. *Ann Intern Med.* 1993;119:129–135.

129. Weinberger M, Saunders A, Samsa G, et al. Breast cancer screening in older women: practices and barriers reported by primary care physicians. *J Am Geriatr Soc.* 1991;39:22–29.

130. Hayward R, Shapiro M, Freeman H, Corey C. Who gets screened for cervical and breast cancer? results from a new national survey. *Arch Intern Med.* 1988;148:1177–1181.

131. Sloane P. Changes in ambulatory care with patient age: is geriatric care qualitatively different? *Fam Med.* 1991;23:40–43.

132. Simon D, Eley J, Greenberg R, Newman N, Gillespie T, Moore M. A survey of alcohol use in an inner-city ambulatory setting. *J Gen Intern Med.* 1991;6:295–298.

133. Schorling J, Klas P, Willems J, Everett A. Addressing alcohol use among primary care patients: differences between family practice and internal medicine residents. *J Gen Intern Med.* 1994;9:248–254.

134. Wells K, Ware J, Lewis C. Physicians' practices in counseling patients about health habits. *Med Care.* 1984;22:240–246.

135. Moore R, Bone L, Geller G, Mamon J, Stokes E, Levine D. Prevalence, detection, and treatment of alcoholism in hospitalized patients. *JAMA.* 1989;261:403–407.

136. Hollis J, Lichtenstein E, Vogt T, et al. Nurse-assisted counseling for smokers in primary care. *Ann Intern Med.* 1993;118:521–525.

137. Frank E, Winkleby M, Altman D, Rockhill B, Fortman S. Predictors of physicians' smoking cessation advice. *JAMA.* 1991;266:3139–3144.

138. Abbott J, Johnson R, Koziol-McLain J, Lowenstein S. Domestic violence against women: incidence and prevalence in an emergency department population. *JAMA.* 1995;273:1763–1767.

139. McLeer S, Anwar R. The role of the emergency physician in the prevention of domestic violence. *Ann Emerg Med.* 1987;16:1155–1161.

140. Plichta S. The effects of woman abuse on health care utilization and health status: a literature review. *Women's Health Int.* 1992;2:154–163.

141. Lachs M, Pillemer K. Abuse and neglect of elderly persons. *N Engl J Med.* 1995;332:437–443.

142. Glanz K, Tziraki C, Albright C, Fernandes J. Nutrition assessment and counseling practices: attitudes and interests of primary care physicians. *J Gen Intern Med.* 1995;10:89–92.

143. Sherman S, Hershman W. Exercise counseling: how do generalists do? *J Gen Intern Med.* 1993;8:243–248.

144. Freed G, Clark S, Sorenson J, Lohr J, Cefalo R, Curtis P. National assessment of physicians' breast-feeding knowledge, attitudes, training, and experience. *JAMA.* 1995;273:472–476.

145. Lewis C, Clancy C, Leake B, Schwartz S. The counseling practices of internists. *Ann Intern Med.* 1991;114:54–58.

146. Council on Scientific Affairs, American Medical Association. Helmets and preventing motorcycle- and bicycle-related injuries. *JAMA.* 1994;272:1535–1538.

147. Webster D, Wilson M, Duggan A, Pakula L. Firearm injury prevention counseling: a study of pediatricians' beliefs and practices. *Pediatrics.* 1992;89:902–907.

148. Fisher M. Parents' views of adolescent health issues. *Pediatrics.* 1992;90:335–341.

149. Igra V, Millstein S. Current status and approaches to improving preventive services for adolescents. *JAMA.* 1993;269:1408–1412.

150. Fogle S. Pitching prevention: will doctors listen? *J Natl Inst Health Res.* 1991;3:90–92.

151. Gerbert B, Bleecker T, Maguire B, Caspers N. Physicians and AIDS: sexual risk assessment of patients and willingness to treat HIV-infected patients. *J Gen Intern Med.* 1992;7:657–664.

152. Wenrich MD, Curtis JR, Carline JD, Paauw DS, Ramsey PG. HIV risk screening in the primary care setting: assessment of physicians skills. *J Gen Intern Med.* 1997;12:107–113.

153. Mellanby A, Phelps F, Lawrence C, Tripp J. Teenagers and the risks of sexually transmitted diseases: a need for the provision of balanced information. *Genitourin Med.* 1992;68:241–244.

154. Lowenstein S. Injury prevention in primary care. *Ann Intern Med.* 1990;113:261–263.

155. Laine C, Davidoff F, Lewis C, et al. Important elements of outpatient care: a comparison of patients' and physicians' opinions. *Ann Intern Med.* 1996;125:640–645.

156. Stoeckle J, Zola I, Davidson G. The quality and significance of psychological distress in medical patients. *J Chronic Dis.* 1964;17:959–970.

157. Kroenke K, Wood D, Mangelsdorff A, Meier N, Powell J. Chronic fatigue in primary care: prevalence, patient characteristics, and outcome. *JAMA.* 1988;260:929–934.

158. Smith G, Monson R, Ray D. Patients with multiple unexplained symptoms: their characteristics, functional health, and health care utilization. *Arch Intern Med.* 1986;149:69–72.

159. Roter D, Hall J. How is your doctor treating you? *Consumer Reports.* February 1995:81–87.

160. Delbanco TL, Stokes DM, Cleary PD, et al. Medical patients' assessments of their care during hospitalization: insights for internists. *J Gen Intern Med.* 1995;10:679–685.

161. Griffith C, Rich E, Wilson J. Housestaff's knowledge of their patients' social histories. *Acad Med.* 1995;70:64–66.

162. Hickam D, Smith S, Joos S. Natural history and management of psychogenic problems in a general medical clinic [abstract]. *J Gen Intern Med.* 1994;10:56.

163. Wells K, Hays R, Burnam M, Rogers W, Greenfield S, Ware J. Detection of depressive disorder in prepaid fee-for-service practices: results from the Medical Outcomes Study. *JAMA.* 1989;262:925–930.

164. Horwitz S, Leaf P, Leventhal J, Forsyth B, Speechley K. Identification and management of psychosocial and developmental problems in community-based, primary care pediatric practices. *Pediatrics.* 1992;89:480–485.

165. Hull J. Community physicians: perceptions of their role in treating psychiatric disorders. *Int J Psychiatry Med.* 1980–1981;10:9–21.

166. Gropper M. A study of the preferences of family practitioners and other primary care physicians in treating patients' psychosocial problems. *Soc Work Health Care.* 1987;13:75–91.

167. Berlowitz D, Du W, Kazis L, Lewis S. Health-related quality of life of nursing home residents: differences in patient and provider perceptions. *J Am Geriatr Soc.* 1995;43:799–802.

168. Avorn J, Gurwitz J. Drug use in the nursing home. *Ann Intern Med.* 1995;123:194–204.

169. Russell N, Roter D. Health promotion counseling of chronic-disease patients during primary care visits. *Am J Public Health.* 1993;83:979–982.

170. Levinson W, Roter D. Physicians' psychosocial beliefs correlate with their patient communication skills. *J Gen Intern Med.* 1995;10:275–279.

171. Good M, Good B, Cleary PD. Do patients' attitudes influence physician recognition of psychosocial problems in primary care? *J Fam Pract.* 1987;25:53–59.

172. Meyer M. Patients' duties. *J Med Philos.* 1992;17:541–545.

173. Petrozzi M, Rosman H, Nerenz D, Young M. Clinical activities and satisfaction of general internists, cardiologists, and ophthalmologists. *J Gen Intern Med.* 1992;7:363–365.

174. Shugars D, O'Neil E, Bader J, eds. *Healthy America: Practitioners for 2005: an Agenda for U.S. Health Professional Schools.* Durham, NC: Pew Health Professions Commission; 1991.

175. McPhee S, Schroeder SA. Promoting preventive care: changing reimbursement is not enough. *Am J Public Health.* 1987;77:780–781.

176. Moser R, McCance K, Smith K. Results of a national survey of physicians' knowledge and application of prevention capabilities. *Am J Prev Med.* 1991;7:384–390.

177. Eisenthal S, Stoeckle J, Ehrlich C. Orientation of medical residents to the psychological aspects of primary care: influence of training program. *Acad Med.* 1994;69:48–54.

178. Gottlieb L, Holman H. What's preventing more prevention? barriers to development at academic centers. *J Gen Intern Med.* 1992;7:630–635.

179. Mold J, Stein H. The cascade effect in the clinical care of patients. *N Engl J Med.* 1986;314:512–514.

180. Cohen M, Preisser J, Shelton B, Wofford J, McClatchey M, Wolf P. PSA testing:

dissemination of low cost technology in primary care. *J Gen Intern Med.* 1996;11(suppl):81.

181. Wilcox S, Himmelstein D, Woolhandler S. Inappropriate drug prescribing for the community-dwelling elderly. *JAMA.* 1994;272:292–296.

182. Wennberg JE, Freeman JL, Shelton RM, Bubolz TA. Hospital use and mortality among Medicare beneficiaries in Boston and New Haven. *N Engl J Med.* 1989;321:1168–1173.

183. Welch WP, Miller ME, Welch HG, Fisher ES, Wennberg JE. Geographic variation in expenditures for physicians' services in the United States. *N Engl J Med.* 1993;328:621–627.

184. Leape LL. Unnecessary surgery. *Annu Rev Public Health.* 1992;13:363–383.

185. Merrick N, Brook RH, Fink A, Solomon DH. Use of carotid endarterectomy in five California Veterans Administration medical centers. *JAMA.* 1986;256:2531–2535.

186. Greenspan A, Kay H, Berger B, Greenberg R, Greenspan A, Gaughan M. Incidence of unwarranted implantation of permanent cardiac pacemakers in a large medical population. *N Engl J Med.* 1988;318:158–163.

187. Leape LL, Park R, Solomon DH, Chassin MR, Kosecoff J, Brook RH. Does inappropriate use explain small area variations in the use of health care services? *JAMA.* 1990;263:669–672.

188. Winslow C, Solomon DH, Chassin MR, Kosecoff J, Merrick N, Brook RH. The appropriateness of carotid endarterectomy. *N Engl J Med.* 1988;318:721–727.

189. Winslow C, Kosecoff J, Chassin MR, Kanouse D, Brook RH. The appropriateness of performing coronary artery bypass surgery. *JAMA.* 1988;260:505–509.

190. Pilote L, Califf RM, Sapp S, et al. Regional variation across the United States in the management of acute myocardial infarction. *N Engl J Med.* 1995;333:565–572.

191. Guadagnoli E, Hauptman P, Ayanian JZ, Pashos CL, McNeil BJ, Cleary PD. Variation in the use of cardiac procedures after acute myocardial infarction. *N Engl J Med.* 1995;333:573–578.

192. Porreco RP. High cesarean section rate: a new perspective. *Obstet Gynecol.* 1985;65:307–311.

193. Wenneker MB, Weissman JS, Epstein AM. The association of payer with utilization of cardiac procedures in Massachusetts. *JAMA.* 1990;264:1255–1260.

194. Tunis SR, Bass EB, Klag MJ, Steinberg EP. Variation in utilization of procedures for treatment of peripheral arterial disease: a look at patient characteristics. *Arch Intern Med.* 1993;153:991–998.

195. Fisher ES, Wennberg JE, Stukel TA, Sharp SM. Hospital readmission rates for cohorts of Medicare beneficiaries in Boston and New Haven. *N Engl J Med.* 1994;331:989–995.

196. Chassin MR, Kosecoff J, Park R, Winslow C, Kahn K. Does inappropriate use explain geographic variations in the use of health services? *JAMA.* 1987;258:2533–2537.

197. Chassin MR, Kosecoff J, Solomon DH, Brook RH. How coronary angiography is used: clinical determinants of appropriateness. *JAMA.* 1987;258:2543–2547.

198. Hilborne LH, Leape LL, Bernstein SJ, et al. The appropriateness of use of percutaneous transluminal coronary angioplasty in New York State. *JAMA.* 1993;269:761–765.

199. Blustein J. High-technology cardiac procedures: the impact of service availability on service use in New York State. *JAMA.* 1993;270:344–349.

200. Every NR, Larson EB, Litwin PE, et al. The association between on-site cardiac catheterization facilities and the use of coronary angiography after acute myocardial infarction: Myocardial Infarction Triage and Intervention Project Investigators. *N Engl J Med.* 1993;329:546–551.

201. McGlynn EA, Naylor CD, Anderson GM, et al. Comparison of the appropriateness of coronary angiography and coronary artery bypass graft surgery between Canada and New York State. *JAMA.* 1994;272:934–940.

202. Leape LL, Hilborne LH, Park RE, et al. The appropriateness of use of coronary artery bypass graft surgery in New York State. *JAMA.* 1993;269:753–760.

203. Rouleau JL, Moye LA, Pfeffer MA, et al. A comparison of management patterns after acute myocardial infarction in Canada and the United States: The SAVE Investigators. *N Engl J Med.* 1993;328:779–784.

204. Tu JV, Pashos CL, Naylor CD, et al. Use of cardiac procedures and outcomes in elderly patients with myocardial infarction in the United States and Canada. *N Engl J Med.* 1997;336:1500–1505.

205. Hannan EL, Racz M, Ryan TJ, et al. Coronary angioplasty volume: outcome relationships for hospitals and cardiologists. *JAMA.* 1997;277:892–898.

206. Carey TS, Garrett J, NC Back Pain Project. Patterns of ordering diagnostic tests for patients with acute low back pain. *Ann Intern Med.* 1996;125:807–814.

207. Legorreta AP, Silber JH, Costantino GN, Kobylinski RW, Zatz SL. Increased cholecystectomy rate after the introduction of laparoscopic cholecystectomy. *JAMA.* 1993;270:1429–1432.

208. Kahn K, Kosecoff J, Chassin MR, Solomon DH, Brook RH. The use and misuse of upper gastrointestinal endoscopy. *Ann Intern Med.* 1988;109:664–670.

209. Christakis NA, Asch DA. Medical specialists prefer to withdraw familiar technologies when discontinuing life support. *J Gen Intern Med.* 1995;10:491–494.

210. Hirth R, Turenne M, Woods J, et al. Predictors of type of vascular access in hemodialysis patients. *JAMA.* 1996;276:1303–1308.

211. Phillips R, Hamel M, Teno J, et al. Race, resource use, and survival in seriously ill hospitalized adults. *J Gen Intern Med.* 1996;11:387–396.

212. Rivo ML, Kindig DA. A report card on the physician work force in the United States. *N Engl J Med.* 1996;334:892–896.

213. Katon W, Korff MV, Lin E, et al. Collaborative management to achieve treatment guidelines: impact on depression in primary care. *JAMA.* 1995;273:1026–1031.

214. Ellrodt G, Cook DJ, Lee J, Cho M, Hunt D, Weingarten S. Evidence-based disease management. *JAMA*. 1997;278:1687–1692.

215. Wilson A. Consultation length in general practice: a review. *Br J Gen Pract*. 1991;41:119–122.

216. Goldman L, Lee T, Rudd P. Ten commandments for effective consultations. *Arch Intern Med*. 1983;143:1753–1755.

217. Donohoe MT, Kravitz RL, Chandra R, Chen A, Humphries N. Reasons for and avoidability of referrals from generalists to specialists [abstract]. *J Gen Intern Med*. 1996;11(suppl):68.

PART A

# Abstracts from the Literature

*Quality and Costs: Generalists and Specialists*

## BOOKS AND REPORTS

Institute of Medicine. *Advancing the Quality of Health Care: Key Issues and Fundamental Principles. A Policy Statement.* Washington, DC: National Academy Press; 1974.

Institute of Medicine. *Assessing Quality in Health Care: An Evaluation Report.* Washington, DC: National Academy Press 1976.

Institute of Medicine. *Improving Health in the Community: A Role for Performance Monitoring.* Report by a Committee, Division of Health Promotion and Disease Prevention. Durch JS, Bailey LA, Stoto MA, eds. Washington, DC: National Academy Press; 1997.

Institute of Medicine. *Statement on Quality of Care.* Washington, DC: National Academy Press; 1998.

Institute of Medicine. *Measuring the Quality of Health Care.* Washington, DC: National Academy Press; 1999.

Institute of Medicine. *Interpreting the Volume-Outcome Relationship in the Context of Health Care Quality: Workshop Summary.* Washington, DC: National Academy Press; 2000.

Institute of Medicine. *Envisioning the National Health Care Quality Report.* Washington, DC: National Academy Press; 2001.

Institute of Medicine. *Crossing the Quality Chasm: A New Health System for the Twenty-First Century.* Washington, DC: National Academy Press; 2001.

# ARTICLES

Alpert JJ, Robinson LS, Kosa J, Heagarty MC, Haggerty RJ. Delivery of health care for children: report of an experiment. *Pediatrics.* 1976;57:917–930.   This article summarizes an experiment evaluating the effectiveness of primary pediatrics care delivery to a sample of low-income inner-city families. The findings indicate that the effects of primary care compared with episodic care received by the control families were appreciable. These benefits include decreased hospitalizations, operations, illness visits, and appointment breaking; increased health supervision visits, preventive services, and patient satisfactions; and accomplishing these changes at a lower cost. Patient morbidity was not altered. The controlled clinical trial offers the best opportunity to compare different models of primary care.

Ayanian JZ, Guadagnoli E, McNeil BJ, Cleary PD. Treatment and outcomes of acute myocardial infarction among patients of cardiologists and generalist physicians. *Arch Intern Med.* 1997;157:2570–2576.   This study compares treatment and outcomes of acute myocardial infarction (AMI) among patients of cardiologists and generalist physicians. The authors identified attending and consulting physicians, patient characteristics, drugs, procedures, and mortality from the clinical and administrative records of 1,620 Medicare beneficiaries aged 65 to 79 years old who were treated for AMI at 285 hospitals in Texas during 1990. The study found that patients treated by attending cardiologists were younger, had prior congestive heart failure less frequently, and were initially treated in hospitals offering coronary angioplasty or bypass surgery more often than patients treated by attending generalist physicians. Cardiologists used some, but not all, effective drugs more frequently, as well as coronary angiography, and angioplasty. Although the differences were not associated with lower adjusted mortality among cardiologists' patients, cardiologists were more likely to treat patients in hospitals with better outcomes. Future studies should identify organizational factors that improve outcomes of myocardial infarction.

Bertakis KD, Robbins JA. Gatekeeping in primary care: a comparison of internal medicine and family practice. *J Fam Pract.* 1987;24:305–309.   In this study, 520 new patients were randomly and prospectively assigned to receive care in either the internal medicine clinic or the family practice clinic of a large university hospital. After a mean length of care of slightly over 2 years, the charts were reviewed for frequency of visits to primary care providers (internal medicine or family practice), emergency room, acute care clinic, and all clinics other than primary care and for laboratory tests ordered. The study found that frequency of visits to all clinics and broken appointments were significantly higher for patients randomized to the internal medicine clinic. In addition, the median total cost of laboratory testing was significantly higher for patients followed by internal medicine physicians, largely because of higher laboratory charges generated by specialist consultants. Over the study period, internal medicine patients had a significantly higher number of visits to all non-primary care clinics and specifically to dermatology, obstetrics, and gynecology, and general surgery consultant clinics.

Bertakis KD, Robbins JA. Utilization of hospital services: a comparison of internal medicine and family practice. *J Fam Pract.* 1989;28:91–96. In this study, 520 new patients were randomly and prospectively assigned to receive care in the internal medicine clinic or family practice clinic of a large university hospital. Previous analyses of outpatient data demonstrated that the frequency of visits to clinics of primary care, acute care clinic, emergency room, and consultant clinics were all significantly higher for patients randomized to internal medicine compared with family practice. In this study, patients' charts were reviewed for information regarding hospitalization. During the 3.4-year study period, there were a total of 61 hospital admissions for internal medicine (35 of 249 patients) and 58 for family practice (27 of 271 patients). The average total cost of hospitalization for each patient was greater for those randomized to the internal medicine clinic: $7,193 for internal medicine patients as compared to $5,764 for family practice patients. The professional costs per hospitalization showed greater variation: $913 for internal medicine clinic patients and $626 for family practice clinic patients. Internal medicine clinic patients had a longer mean length of hospitalization (7.5 days) compared to 6.3 days for family practice clinic patients. The study concludes that both cost and length of care are less for those followed by the family practice clinic.

Bodenheimer T, Lo B, Casalino L. Primary care physicians should be coordinators, not gatekeepers. *JAMA.* 1999;281:2045–2049. The authors suggest that primary care gatekeeping, in which the goal of the primary care physician (PCP) is to reduce patient referrals to specialists and thereby reduce costs, is not an adequate system to practice medicine. They recommend that PCPs should be transformed from gatekeepers to coordinators of care, in which their goal is to integrate both primary and specialty care to improve quality. Changes in the PCPs daily work process, as well as the referral and payment processes, need to be implemented to reach this goal. The proposed model would eliminate the requirement that referrals to specialists be authorized by the PCP or the managed care organization. Financial incentives would be needed, for example, to encourage PCPs to manage complex cases and to discourage overreferral and underreferral to specialists. Budgeting specialists should control excess costs.

Bodenheimer T, Wagner EH, Grumbach K. Improving primary care for patients with chronic illness: the Chronic Care Model, part 2. *JAMA.* 2002;288:1909–1914. This article reviews research evidence showing to what extent the chronic care model can improve the management of chronic conditions (using diabetes as an example) and reduce health care costs. Thirty-two of 39 studies found that the interventions based on chronic care model components improved at least one process or outcome measure for diabetic patients. Regarding whether chronic care model interventions can reduce costs, 18 of 27 studies concerned with three examples of chronic conditions (congestive heart failure, asthma and diabetes) demonstrated reduced health care costs or lower use of health care services. Even though the chronic care model has the potential to improve care and reduce costs, several obstacles hinder its widespread adoption.

Bowman MA. The quality of care provided by family physicians. *J Fam Pract.* 1989;28:346–355. This article presents a literature review that summarizes the quality of care of family physicians by outcome and process measures. Studies in the literature are perceived to be flawed by methodologic weaknesses, including the frequent lumping of all general and family physicians into one group, and the general lack of description of the physicians involved. Some studies measuring the process of care indicate poorer process by family physicians or general practitioners, such as recording fewer medical process criteria used to measure quality of care. The quality of care by outcome, however, appears to be similar.

Carey TS, Garrett J, Jackman A, et al. The outcomes and costs of care for acute low back pain among patients seen by primary care practitioners, chiropractors, and orthopedic surgeons. *N Engl J Med.* 1995;333:913–917. Patients with back pain receive different care from different types of health practitioners. The object of this study was to determine whether the outcomes of and charges for care differ among primary care practitioners, chiropractors, and orthopedic surgeons. Two hundred and eight practitioners in North Carolina were randomly selected from six strata: urban primary care physicians, rural primary care physicians, urban chiropractors, rural chiropractors, orthopedic surgeons, and primary care providers at a group-model health maintenance organization (HMO). The patients were contacted by telephone periodically for up to 24 weeks to assess functional status, work status, use of health care services, and satisfaction with care received. The study found that the times to functional recovery, return to work, and complete recovery from low back pain were similar among all six groups of practitioners, but there were marked differences in the use of health care services. The mean total estimated outpatient charges were highest for patients seen by surgeons and chiropractors and were lowest for patients seen by HMO and primary care providers. Satisfaction was greatest among the patients who went to chiropractors.

Chen J, Radford MJ, Wang Y, Krumholz HM. Care and outcomes of elderly patients with acute myocardial infarction by physician specialty: the effects of comorbidity and functional limitations. *Am J Med.* 2000;108:460–469. Because some of the survival benefits associated with cardiology care may be due to baseline differences in patient characteristics, this study evaluates how differences in case-mix of comorbid illness and functional limitations may affect the results of studies measuring outcomes between specialty and generalist care. The authors first examined the association of physician specialty with 30-day and 1-year mortality in patients hospitalized for acute myocardial infarction. They then assessed the extent to which this relation was mediated by differences in the use of guideline supported therapies (e.g. aspirin, beta-blockers, repurfusion, angiotensin-converting enzyme inhibitors) or differences in the clinical characteristics of the patients. The study found that after adjustment for the use of guideline supported therapies, differences in 1-year survival between patients treated by cardiologists or general practitioners were not significantly dissimilar from those patients treated by internists.

Chin MH, Zhang JX, Merrell K. Specialty differences in the care of older patients with diabetes. *Med Care.* 2000;38:131–140. The object of this study was to determine differences in health status, quality of care, and resource utilization among older diabetic Medicare patients cared for by endocrinologists, internists, family practitioners, and general practitioners. The authors analyzed 1,637 patients with diabetes over 65 years or older. The study found that compared with patients of family practitioners, patients of endocrinologists and internists had more comorbidity and diabetic complications, but similar health perception and deficiencies in activities of daily living. The patients of endocrinologists also had higher utilization of ophthalmologic screening, lipid testing, and gycosylated hemoglobin measurement than patients of generalist physicians, but similar rates of influenza vaccination. Patients of endocrinologists and internists had higher total reimbursement than those of family practitioners and general practitioners. Patient satisfaction was generally similar. The study concluded that older diabetic patients of endocrinologists had higher utilization of diabetes-specific process of care measures and had similar functional status despite more diabetic complications. However, they received a more costly style of care than patients of family practitioners and general practitioners. Future work needs to explore the optimal coordination of care of diabetic patients among different health practitioners.

Deitrich AJ, Goldberg H. Preventive content of adult primary care: do generalists and subspecialists differ? *Am J Pub Health.* 1984;74:223–227. The authors compared preventive care performed by 20 generalists and 20 subspecialists practicing in Santa Clara and San Mateo Counties, California, by auditing charts of adult primary care patients for compliance with recommendations of the Canadian Task Force on the Periodic Health Examination. Generalists and specialists both provided 49% of recommended preventive services. The two groups did not differ significantly in performance of any individual service. The generalist vs specialist debate assumes that physician's specialty classification is an important predictor of behavior. For the performance of preventive care, this was not true according to the findings of this study.

Engstrom S, Foldevi M, Borgquist L. Is general practice effective? A systematic literature review. *Scand J Prim Health Care.* 2001;19:131–144. The objective of this study was to find evidence of the effectiveness of physicians working in primary care. 45 studies that compared primary care with specialist care were extracted. Outcome measures were health indicators, costs and quality. The study found that primary care contributed to improved public health, as expressed through different health parameters, and a lower utilization of medical care leading to lower costs.

Physicians working in primary care, in comparison with other specialists, took care of many diseases without loss of quality and at lower costs. There are too few studies on how to most effectively organize primary health care.

Fernandez A, Grumbach K, Goiten L, et al. How primary care physicians perceive hospitalists. *Arch Intern Med.* 2000;160:2902–2908.  The objective of this study was to discover how primary care physicians perceive hospitalists: how they affect their practices, their patient relationships, and overall patient care. A mailed survey was sent to a randomly selected group of internists, general pediatricians, and family practitioners practicing in California. Of the 524 respondents (out of 708 that were eligible for the study) 335 had hospitalists available to them and 120 were required to use them for all admissions. Physicians perceived hospitalists as increasing (41%) or not changing (44%) the overall quality of care. 28% of primary care physicians believed that the quality of physician-patient relationship decreased; 69% reported that hospitalists did not affect their income; 53% believed that hospitalists decreased their workload; and 50% believed that they increased practice satisfaction. The study concludes that practicing primary care physicians generally have favorable perceptions of the hospitalist and his or her effect on patients and on their own practice satisfaction, especially in a voluntary hospitalist system. Primary care physicians, particularly internists, are less accepting of mandatory hospitalist systems.

Flocke SA, Orzano J, Selinger A, et al. Does managed care restrictiveness affect the perceived quality of primary care? A report from the Ambulatory Sentinel Practice Network. *J Fam Pract.* 1999;48:762–768.  The purpose of this study was to examine the association of the organizational and financial restrictiveness of managed care plans with important elements of primary care, the patient-clinician relationship, and patient satisfaction. A cross-sectional study of 15 member practices of the Ambulatory Sentinel Practice Network was carried out to represent diverse health care markets. Each practice completed a Managed Care Survey to characterize the degree of restrictiveness for each health care plan. 199 plans were characterized. Then, 1,475 consecutive outpatients completed a patient survey that included: the Components of Primary Care Instrument as a measure of attributes of primary care; a measure of the amount of inconvenience involved with using the health care plan; and the Medical Outcomes Study Visiting Rating Form for assessing patient satisfaction. The results showed that clinicians reports of inconvenience were significantly associated with the financial and organizational restrictiveness scores of plans. There was no association between restrictiveness and patients' reports of multiple aspects in quality of primary care or patient satisfaction with the visit. The authors conclude that physicians and their staff appear to be buffering patients from the potential negative effects of restrictive plans.

Forrest CB, Glade GB, Baker A, et al. The pediatric–specialty care interface: how pediatricians refer children and adolescents to specialty care. *Arch Pediatr Adolesc Med.* 1999;153:705–714.  This article reports on a study of 58,771 patient visits, made to 142 pediatricians in a national primary care practice-based research network to understand how pediatricians refer patients to specialists. The study found that pediatricians referred patients to specialists during 2.3% of office visits. Referrals made during telephone conversations with parents accounted for 27.5% of the whole. The most common reason for a referral was advice on diagnosis or treatment (74.3%). Referrals were made most commonly to surgical sub-specialists (52.3%) followed by medical (27.9%), non physicians (11.4%) and mental health practitioners (8.4%). Physicians requested a consultation with shared management in 75% of cases. Otitis media was the condition referred most often (9.2%). 50 other conditions accounted for another 84.3%. The study concludes that physician training to increase clinical competency in the 50 most commonly referred conditions may be useful. Education regarding the referral process should focus on the respective roles of the referring physician and specialist, particularly as they relate to approaches for co-managing patients.

Forrest CB, Starfield B. The effect of first-contact care with primary care clinicians on ambulatory health care expenditures. *J Fam Pract.* 1996;43:40–48.   This study examined the relationship between first contact care, defined as the use of an identified primary care source for the first visit of an episode, and ambulatory episode-of-care expenditures. The study, using data from the 1987 National Medical Expenditure Survey, found that episodes beginning with a visit to a primary care clinician, as opposed to other sources of care, were associated with reductions in expenditures of 53% overall ($63 vs $134), 62% for acute illness ($62 vs $164), and 20% for preventive care ($64 vs $80). For 23 of the 24 health problems studied, first contact care was associated with reductions in expenditures.

Forrest CB, Starfield B. Entry into primary care and continuity: the effects of access. *Am J Public Health.* 1998;88:1330–1336.   The objective of this study was to examine the relationship between access and use of primary care physicians as sources of first contact and continuity with the medical system. Data from the 1987 National Medical Expenditure Survey were used. The results showed that no after-hours care, longer office waits, and longer travel times reduced the chances of a first contact visit with a primary care physician for acute health problems. Longer appointment waits, no health insurance, and no after-hours care were associated with lower levels of continuity. Generalists provided more first contact care than specialists, largely because of their more accessible practices. These findings provide support for the link between access and care seeking with primary care physicians.

Frances CD, Shlipak MG, Noguchi H, Heidenrich PA, McClellan M. Does physician specialty affect the survival of elderly patients with myocardial infarction? *Health Serv Res.* 2000;35(5 pt 2):1093–1116.   The objective of this study was to determine the effect of treatment by a cardiologist on mortality of elderly patients with acute myocardial infarction (AMI) accounting for both measured confounding using risk-adjustment techniques and residual unmeasured confounding with instrumental variables methods. Hospital records and death records were obtained for 161,558 patients aged 65 and over with AMI admitted to a nonfederal acute care hospital.

The principal measure of significant cardiologist treatment was whether a patient was admitted by a cardiologist. Primary outcomes were 30-day and one-year mortality, and secondary outcomes included treatment with medications and revascularization procedures. The study found no significant incremental mortality benefit associated with treatment by cardiologists and non-cardiologists but did find treatment differences. Patients treated by cardiologists were more likely to undergo revascularization procedures and to receive thrombolytic therapy, aspirin, and calcium channel-blockers, but were less likely to receive beta-blockers.

Franks P, Fiscella K. Primary care physicians and specialists as personal physicians: health care expenditures and mortality experience. *J Fam Pract.* 1998;47:105–109. This article considers whether persons using a primary care physician have lower expenditures and mortality than those using a specialist. Total annual health care expenditure and 5-year mortality experience were examined using data from a nationally representative sample of 13,270 adult respondents to the 1987 National Medical Expenditure Survey. Respondents who reported using a primary care physician compared with those using a specialist had 33% lower annual adjusted health care expenditures, lower adjusted mortality and were more likely to be women, white, live in rural areas, report fewer medical diagnoses and have higher health perceptions. These findings provide evidence for the cost-effective role of the primary care physician.

Go AS, Rao RK, Dauterman KW, Massie BM. A systematic review of the effects of physician specialty on the treatment of coronary disease and heart failure in the United States. *Am J Med.* 2000;108:216–226. The purpose of this study was to assess the effects of physician specialty on the knowledge, management, and outcomes of patients with coronary disease or heart failure. Twenty-four articles met the authors' selection criteria: eight involved knowledge or self-reported practices; 14 described actual practice patterns; and six measured clinical outcomes. Cardiologists were more knowledgeable than generalist physicians about the optimal evaluation and management of coronary disease but not about the use of angiotensin-converting enzyme (ACE) inhibitors for heart failure. Patients with unstable angina or myocardial infarction were more likely to receive proven medical therapies, and possibly had improved outcomes, if cardiologists treated them. The use of lipid lowering drugs after myocardial infarction was also more common among patients of cardiologists. ACE inhibitor use for heart failure was probably greater, and short-term readmission rates were lower in cardiology care. The study concludes that patients with coronary disease or heart failure in the United States who are treated by cardiologists appear more likely to receive evidence-based care and probably have better outcomes. Investigation of collaborative methods of care and innovative efforts to improve the use of proven therapies by physicians are needed.

Goldberg HI, Dietrich AJ. The continuity of care provided to primary care patients: a comparison of family physicians, general internists, and medical subspecialists. *Med Care.* 1985;23:63–73. In this article, a comparison was made between the continuity of care that family physicians, general internists, and medical subspecialists provided to their adult primary care patients. The 40 physicians in the study came from large multispecialty practices. The study found that the three physician types did not differ significantly in the degree of continuity provided, measured by the proportion of total visits to a primary provider. Each type provided approximately 80 percent of its primary care patients' visits. In contrast, the continuity scores of individual physicians ranged widely, from 57 percent to 98 percent. A more detailed exploration of the subspecialists revealed that the lowest levels of continuity were afforded patients with high utilization rates who did not carry a diagnosis in their primary physician's area of subspecialty expertise. The "generalist vs. specialist" debate assumes that a physician's training background is a major determinant in the quality of primary care delivered. This study demonstrated that this supposition was not true for the provision of one aspect of quality—a high level of continuity.

Greenfield S, Kaplan SH, Kahn R, Ninomiya J, Griffith JL. Profiling care provided by different groups of physicians: effects of patient case-mix (bias) and physician-level clustering on quality assessment results. *Ann Intern Med.* 2002;136:111–121. The object of this study was to examine the effect of case-mix bias and physician-level clustering on differences in quality of diabetes care between specialty groups. A retrospective record review was made of both process and outcome measures over one year and a cross-sectional patient survey. The sample included 29 solo and group practice sites in diverse regions of the United States. Of the 29 sites, 15 were endocrinology sites and 14 were primary care sites. After accounting for patient case-mix variables and physician-level clustering, observed differences between specialties were no longer statistically significant for any quality measures except patient satisfaction. The findings underscore the importance of designing physician profiling studies with sufficient power to account for variables.

Greenfield S, Rogers W, Mangotich M, et al. Outcomes of patients with hypertension and non-insulin-dependent diabetes mellitus treated by different systems and specialties: results from the Medical Outcomes Study. *JAMA.* 1995;274:1436–1444. The objective of this study was to compare the outcomes of patients with hypertension and non-insulin-dependent diabetes mellitus (NIDDM) who were cared for in different systems of care. Patients were designated as belonging to one of three systems of care: (1) fee for service; (2) prepaid patients in solo or small single-specialty groups or in large multispecialty groups referred to as independent practice associations; and (3) staff-model health maintenance organizations. The study found no evidence that any one system of care or physician specialty achieved consistently better two- or four-year outcomes than others for patients with NIDDM or hypertension. Moreover, no adjusted mortality differences among systems or among physician specialties were observed in the seven-year follow-up period.

Grumbach K, Selby JV. Outcomes and physician specialty: quality of primary care practice in a large HMO according to physician specialty. *Health Serv Res.*

1999;34:485–502. The objective of this study was to determine whether physician specialty is associated with differences of quality in primary care practice and patient satisfaction in a large, group model HMO based on a cross-sectional patient survey of 10,000 patients in the Kaiser Permanente Medical Care Program in Northern California. The authors observed few differences in the quality of primary care by physician specialty in this setting. It may be that in certain settings, practice organization has more influence than physician specialty on the delivery of primary care.

Harrold LR, Field TS, Gurwitz JH. Knowledge, patterns of care, and outcomes of care for generalist and specialists. *J Gen Intern Med.* 1999;14:499–511. The objective of this study was to evaluate the differences between generalist physicians and specialists in terms of knowledge relative to widely accepted standards of care, patterns of care, and clinical outcomes of care. Relevant English-language articles written between January 1981 and January 1998 were identified through Medline and evaluated. The results showed that in many studies, specialists were reported to be more knowledgeable about conditions encompassed within their specialty. Specialists were more likely to use medications associated with improved survival and to comply with routine health maintenance screening guidelines; they used more resources including diagnostic testing, procedures and longer hospital stays. In a limited number of studies examining the care of patients with acute myocardial infarction, acute non-hemorrhagic stroke, and asthma, specialists had superior outcomes. The authors conclude that more research is needed to examine whether these patterns of care translate into superior outcomes for patients.

Hermann WH. More than provider specialty. *Med Care.* 2000;38:128–130. This article reviews past studies that have compared the differences in quality of care between generalists and specialists. In most studies the differences have not been as striking as the deficiencies common to both types of providers. The author suggests that deficiencies in provider, patient or health system variables can affect quality of care. For example, a busy clinician's oversight to recommend an annual influenza immunization, a patient's lack of knowledge of the need for immunization, and the health care system's inability to identify and contact patients who need a flu shot will almost certainly result in the service not being provided. Increasingly, as we attempt to understand the most appropriate coordination of care for patients with chronic diseases, we must do more to understand and address the complex interplay of provider, patient, and health-system related variables

Ho M, Marger M, Beart J, et al. Is the quality of diabetes care better in a diabetes clinic or in a general medicine clinic? *Diabetes Care.* 1997;20:472–475. The objective of this study was to compare the quality of ambulatory diabetes care delivered by physicians in the diabetes clinic versus the general medicine clinic of a university-affiliated VA Medical Center. 112 patient medical records were examined retrospectively; 56 were cared for in a diabetes clinic and 56 were cared for in the hospital. The results showed that the diabetes clinic performed significantly better than the general medicine center on the following criteria: patients' self monitoring of blood glucose levels; foot examinations; comprehensive eye examinations; a glycated hemoglobin measurement; referrals for diabetic education. The proportion of patients meeting the minimally acceptable levels of quality was better in the diabetes clinic than the general medicine clinic. The study concludes that if patient care is to be shifted from specialists to generalists, the latter must have the knowledge and the resources that they need to deliver acceptable quality of diabetes care.

Jollis JG, De Long ER, Peterson ED, et al. Outcome of acute myocardial infarction according to the specialty of the admitting physician. *N Engl J Med.* 1996;335:1880–1887.   This study considered the outcome of patients with acute myocardial infarction (AMI) according to specialty of the admitting physician. One-year mortality was examined among 8,241 Medicare patients who were hospitalized for AMI in four states during a seven-month period. To determine the generalizability of the authors'findings, insurance claims were also examined and survival data for 220,335 patients for whom there were Medicare claims for hospital care for AMI. The study found that after adjustment for characteristics of patients and hospitals, patients who were admitted to the hospital by a cardiologist were 12 percent less likely to die within one year than those admitted by a primary care physician. Cardiologists also had the highest rate of use of cardiac procedures and medications, including medications that are associated with improved survival.

Lafata JE, Martin S, Morlock R, Divine G, Xi H. Provider type and the receipt of general and diabetes-related preventive health services among patients with diabetes. *Med Care.* 2001;39:491–499.   The objective of this study was to determine the contribution of provider type on receipt of general and diabetes-related preventive health services. Automated clinical and administrative data was used to identify 10,991 adult patients with type 1 and 2 diabetes receiving care from a multi-specialty, salaried group practice and enrolled in a large health maintenance organization between March 1997 and February 1998. The findings revealed that patients seeing an endocrinologist and primary care physician (PCP) were more likely than those seeing endocrinologists alone, to receive glycated hemogolbin testing, lipid testing, mammograms and Pap smears and more likely than those seeing PCPs alone to receive glycated hemoglobin testing, lipid testing, retinal examinations and mammograms. Patients seeing an endocrinologist only were more likely to receive retinal examinations and less likely to receive Pap smears than those seeing PCPs only. The study concluded that no one single care provider type is associated with greater receipt of all recommended services. Instead patients seeing both an endocrinologist and a PCP are more likely to receive recommended services.

Lipkin M Jr. Psychiatry and primary care: two cultures divided by a common cause. *New Dir Ment Health Serv.* 1999;81:7–15.   Primary care, the author notes, is the foundation of the mental health system in the United States. Half of the people with one of the 13 most common mental disorders are cared for by the primary care sector, while only about 20% are cared for in the mental health sector. The public generally prefers to seek care for mental disorders at the primary care physician level. Psychiatrists focus on the sickest patients, and managed care is increasingly restricting access to psychiatrists. Yet problems between primary care physicians and psychiatrists have persisted. These include an inability to understand each other, disrespect, mutual distrust and competition. The author suggests that reconciliation between the two fields is needed, and he suggests ways in which this might be accomplished. One way to diminish the separation between the mental and physical is through mutual participation in training, in both behavioral medicine and primary care disciplines, at pre-clinical and clinical levels. A second technique is to have primary care residents do ambulatory consultations with mental health specialists and psychiatry residents do "real" primary care training instead of excessive inpatient medicine that is now typical.

McBride P, Schrott HG, Plane MB, Underbakke G. Primary care practice adherence to national cholesterol education program guidelines for patients with coronary heart disease. *Arch Intern Med.* 1998;158:1238–1244. Clinical trials demonstrate significant benefit from cholesterol management for patients with cardiovascular disease (CVD). This study examines cholesterol screening and management by primary care physicians to see how closely national screening guidelines were followed in practice. Medical records and patient surveys provided data for 603 patients with CVD, aged 27 to 70 years, from 45 practices in 4 states during 1993 to 1995. Thirty-three percent of patients with CVD were not screened with lipid panels; 45% were not receiving dietary counseling; and 67% were not receiving cholesterol medication. Physician specialty was not associated with differences in treatment, but physicians in practice for fewer years ordered more lipid panels.

McCulloch DK, Price MJ, Hindmarsh M, Wagner EH. A population-based approach to diabetes management in a primary care setting: early results and lessons learned. *Eff Clin Pract.* 1998;1:12–22. The objective of this study was to determine the effect of a multi-faceted program of support on the ability of primary care teams to deliver population-based diabetes care. The setting was a staff model HMO in which more than 200 primary care providers treated approximately 15,000 diabetic patients. The program elements included: 1) a continually updated online registry of diabetic patients; 2) evidence-based guidelines on retinal screening, foot care, screening for microalbuminuria, and glycemic management; 3) improved support for patient self management; 4) practice redesign to encourage group visits for diabetic patients in a primary care setting; and 5) decentralized expertise through a diabetes expert care team. Results showed that patient and provider satisfaction improved steadily. There was interest and increased use of the registry. Rates of retinal eye screening, documented foot examinations, and testing for microalbuminuria and hemoglobin A1c increased substantially. The study concluded that providing support to primary care teams in several key areas, can make a population-based approach to diabetes care a practical reality in the setting of a staff model HMO.

Nash IS, Corrato RR, Dlutowski MJ, O'Connor JP, Nash DB. Generalist vs. specialist care for acute myocardial infection. *Am J Cardiol.* 1999;83:650–654. This study assessed the magnitude and mechanism of the influence of physician specialty on inpatient mortality for acute myocardial infarction (AMI). Using data from the Pennsylvania Health Care Cost Containment Council and elsewhere, the authors found that caseload was significantly higher among cardiologists and was inversely proportionate to inpatient mortality. Mortality models with caseload, but not physician designation or physician designation without caseload, found each predictor statistically significant in the absence of the other. Older patients of physicians with higher caseloads had a lower risk-adjusted inpatient mortality for AMI. This might explain the trend towards better outcomes among patients of cardiologists compared to patients of non-cardiologists.

Renders CM, Valk GD, Griffin SJ, et al. Interventions to improve the management of diabetes in primary care, outpatient, and community settings: a systematic review. *Diabetes Care.* 2001;24:1821–1833.   The objective of this study was to review the effectiveness of interventions targeted at health care professionals and the structure of care, in order to improve the management of diabetes in primary care, outpatient, and community settings. Forty-one controlled trials were reviewed. Multifaceted professional and organizational interventions that facilitated structured and regular review of patients improved the process of care, but the effect on patient outcomes remained less clear because such outcomes were rarely assessed. Adding patient education and enhancing the role of the nurses led to improvements in patient outcomes and the process of care.

Rosser WW. Approach to diagnosis by primary care clinicians and specialists: is there a difference? *J Fam Pract.* 1996;42:139–144.   The Institute of Medicine's Committee on the Future of Primary Care provides a definition of primary care that suggests significant differences between the problem solving approaches of the family physician and those of the specialist. Family physicians address personal health care needs in the context of a sustained partnership with patients, their families and communities; they generally see problems early and on and deal with greater diagnostic uncertainty. In contrast, specialists see illness at a more advanced stage and generally do not deal with problems beyond their discipline. Faced with the same patient problems, family physicians will order fewer tests and procedures than specialists, yet produce identical outcomes. In countries where family physicians provide first access to the health care system, costs are lower and patients report greater satisfaction with their care. The author suggests that mutual respect for the fundamental differences between primary health care and specialist care will lead to improved efficiency and effectiveness in the health care system.

Rothert ML, Rovner DR, Elstein AS, et al. Differences in medical referral decisions for obesity among family practitioners, general internists, and gynecologists. *Med Care.* 1984;22:42–55.   This study explored the variation in the decisions of primary care physicians to refer or not to refer obese patients to an endocrinologist and the principles underlying their decisions. Forty-five physicians (family practitioners, obstetricians, and general internists) made referral judgments on 24 cases and completed a questionnaire. The data indicate that physician characteristics did not explain the differences in decisions to refer. Rather, the results showed that the patient's desire for treatment by an endocrinologist was overwhelmingly the major factor in decisions to refer.

Safran DG, Rogers WH, Tarlov AR, et al. Organizational and financial characteristics of health plans: are they related to primary care performance? *Arch Intern Med.* 2000;160:69–76.   The objective of this study was to compare the primary care received in each of five models of managed care and identify specific characteristics of health plans associated with performance differences. The five models comprised managed indemnity, point of service, network-model health maintenance organizations (HMOs), group model HMOs, and staff model HMOs. Participants completed a validated questionnaire measuring seven defining characteristics of primary care. Senior health plan executives provided information about financial and non-financial features of a plan's contractual arrangements with physicians. The results showed that the managed indemnity system performed most favorably. The point of service and network model HMO equaled the indemnity system on many measures. Staff model HMOs performed least favorably. The study concludes that the current movement towards open-model managed care is consistent with goals for high-quality primary care, but that plans with specific financial and non-financial incentives must continue to be examined.

Safran DG, Tarlov AR, Rogers WH. Primary care performances in fee-for-service and prepaid health care systems: results from the Medical Outcomes Study. *JAMA.* 1994;271:1579–1586.   The aim of this study was to examine differences in the quality of primary care delivered in pre-paid and fee-for-service health care systems. 1,208 patients with chronic disease were studied whose health insurance was through a traditional indemnity fee-for-service plan, an independent practice association (IPA) or a health maintenance organization (HMO). Information obtained from physicians and patients by self administered questionnaires. Seven indicators of quality of primary care were used and measured in each health insurance setting. Results showed that financial access was highest in prepaid systems; organizational access, continuity and accountability highest in FFS; and coordination highest and comprehensiveness lowest in HMOs. The results marked notable differences in quality of care between the three payment systems.

Schneeweiss R, Ellsbury K, Hart LG, Geyman JP. The economic impact and multiplier effect of a family practice clinic on an academic medical center. *JAMA.* 1989;262: 370–375.   Academic medical centers are facing the need to expand their primary care referral base in an increasingly competitive medical environment. This study describes the medical care provided during a one-year period to 6,304 patients registered with a family practice clinic located in an academic medical center. The relative distribution of primary care, secondary referrals, inpatient admissions, and their associated costs are presented. The multiplier effect of the primary care clinic on the academic medical center was substantial. For every $1 billed for ambulatory private care, there was $6.40 billed elsewhere in the system. Each full-time equivalent family physician generated a calculated sum of $784,752 in direct, billed charges for the hospital and $241,276 in professional fees for the other specialty consultants. The cost of supporting a primary care clinic is likely to be more than offset by the revenues generated from the use of the hospital and referral services by patients who received primary care in the primary care setting.

Schroeder SA, Schapiro R. The hospitalist: new boon for internal medicine or retreat from primary care? *Ann Intern Med.* 1999;130(4 pt 2):382–387.   This article discusses some of the potential advantages and disadvantages of the use of hospitalists in the following areas of internal medicine: patient care; administration; clinical practice; and medical education. The new hospitalist practice mode highlights long-standing tensions about the role and direction of internal medicine. The career trajectory of hospitalists will depend on whether burnout is a problem and on whether hospitalists will be able to compete effectively with subspecialists, such as cardiologists and physicians specializing in AIDS. This new field warrants close monitoring not only because of its effect on primary care and medical education, but also because its birth was strongly influenced by financial considerations.

Showstack JA, Katz PP, Weber E. Evaluating the impact of hospitalists. *Ann Intern Med.* 1999;130:376–381.   This article describes key outcomes that need to be assessed and methodological issues that need to be addressed when conducting and interpreting the results of evaluations of the hospitalist model. To provide evidence, quality of care should be evaluated through measurement of outcomes and processes. The research design must distinguish between outcomes that are attributable to the introduction of hospitalists and those attributable to other changes in medical treatments and the organization of care.

Simon GE, Von Korff M, Rutter CM, Peterson DA. Treatment process and outcomes for managed care patients receiving new antidepressants prescriptions from psychiatrists and primary care physicians. *Arch Gen Psych.* 2001;58:395–401.   This study compares baseline characteristics, process of care, and outcomes for managed care patients who receive new antidepressant prescriptions from psychiatrists and primary care physicians. At baseline, psychiatrists' patients reported slightly higher levels of functional impairment and greater prior use of specialty mental health care. During follow-up, psychiatrists' patients made more frequent follow-up visits, and the proportion making three or more visits in 90 days or more was 57% vs 26% for primary care physicians' patients. The proportion receiving antidepressant medication at an adequate dose for 90 days or more was similar (49% vs 48%). The two groups showed similar rate of improvement in all measures of symptom severity and functioning. The study concludes that clinical differences between patients treated by psychiatrists and primary care physicians were modest. Shortcomings in treatment were common in both practices.

Sox HC Jr. The hospitalist model: perspectives of patients, the internist, and internal medicine. *Ann Intern Med.* 1999;130(4 pt 2):368–372.   The use of the hospitalist model has implications for patients, internists, and for the specialty of internal medicine. For patients, the greatest concern is interrupting the continuity of a supportive relationship with a regular physician. For the internist, the hospitalist model could result in excluding them from hospital care and thus depriving them of an important source of professional satisfaction. For the specialty of internal medicine, the mandatory hand-off of the patient to the hospitalist threatens the internist's identity as the physician who cares for the sickest patients in any venue. The author suggests that the hospitalist movement has much to offer, but internal medicine should resist the mandatory hand-off and use the hospitalist's focus on excellent inpatient care to improve the practice of medicine by all internists.

Sox HC Jr. The hospitalist model: proceed with caution. *Healthplan.* 1999;40(6):17–19. In the hospitalist model, physicians transfer complete responsibility for the care of their hospitalized patients to a hospital-based physician. This results in a break in continuity of care for a sick patient, the effects of which are not yet known. The author suggests testing the assumptions about the importance of continuity of care for seriously ill, hospitalized patients. He notes that this testing will involve carefully designed and controlled clinical trials to determine the effects of different degrees of interruption in continuity of care during hospitalization including patient satisfaction, psychological adaptation, physiologic responses, length of stay, discharge planning; post discharge follow-up; morbidity and mortality. Hospitalist programs can be voluntary or mandatory. The author urges internists to resist the mandatory model. For Americans, the freedom to choose a physician when they are sick is an important one. For physicians, relinquishing the patient to the care of another strikes at the very core of the internist's identity as the "go-to" physician for sick, complicated patients.

Starfield B, Holtzman NA, Roland MO, Sibbald B, Harris R, Harris H. Primary care and genetic services: health care in evolution. *Eur J Public Health.* 2002;12:51–56. The demand for services for predicting, diagnosing and managing genetic diseases or diseases with a genetic component is likely to increase faster than the availability of services from medical geneticists and genetic counselors. Health care systems may also impose limitations on referrals to these specialists. If genetic problems are to be identified and excessive referrals avoided, non-geneticist practitioners will have to recognize when genetic problems should be considered and initiate diagnosis and even management. Primary care centered systems offer the greatest potential for maximizing cost effectiveness, by reducing the demand for specialty services not essential for improving health. However, primary care centers may pose a risk of underdetection and undermanagement of genetic problems, if practitioners are not actively supported by information and other educational networks. Several models for dealing with these challenges are presented, including algorithms that aid in recognizing genetic problems.

Wachter RM, Goldman L. The emerging role of "hospitalists" in the American health care system. *N Engl J Med.* 1996;335:514–517. The authors of this article anticipate a rapid growth of a new breed of physician called "hospitalist"—specialists in inpatient medicine—who will become responsible for managing the care of hospitalized patients in the same way that primary care physicians are responsible for managing the care of outpatients. The burgeoning of hospitalists is largely driven by managed care organizations who reward efficient care and place a greater emphasis on high value care, defined as the quality of care divided by its cost. The authors consider what the hospitalist job in academia will look like and the likely effect this new role will have on house staff in internal medicine. The authors conclude that as with any major transition, the medical community must continuously reevaluate the new approach to ensure that any possible discontinuity in care is outweighed by improved clinical outcomes, lower costs, better education for physicians, and greater satisfaction on the part of the patients.

Wachter RM, Goldman L. The hospitalist movement five years later. *JAMA.* 2002;287: 487–494.  The objective of this study was to review data regarding the effect of the hospitalist model of inpatient care on resource use, quality of care, satisfaction and teaching; and to analyze the impact of hospitalists on the health care system. The authors reviewed studies that compared hospitalist care with a control group and noted that most studies found that implementation of hospitalist programs was associated with significant reductions in resource use, usually measured as hospital costs (average decrease, 13.4%) or average length of stay (average decrease, 16.6%). The results on outcomes, such as inpatient mortality and readmission rates, were inconsistent. Patient satisfaction was generally preserved, while limited data supported positive effects on teaching. The authors observe that the clinical use of hospitalists is growing rapidly, and hospitalists are also assuming prominent roles as teachers, researchers, and leaders.

Weiner JP, Parente ST, Garnick DW, Fowles J, Lawthers AG, Palmer R. Variation in office-based quality: a claims-based profile of care provided to Medicare patients with diabetes. *JAMA.* 1995;273:1503–1508.  Based on analyses of services provided in an ambulatory setting in three states (Alabama, Iowa, and Maryland), the authors found that 84% of diabetics did not appear to receive recommended hemoglobin A1c measurement, 54% did not see an ophthalmologist, and 45% received no cholesterol screening. Practice patterns varied considerably across the three states, even after adjustment for patient case mix and physician characteristics. Patients of general practitioners were less likely to meet recommended quality criteria than patients of internists or family practitioners. Patients receiving care from rural practitioners were less likely to receive services, either recommended or not, than those in urban locations. This study underscores the value of practice guideline development and dissemination in the ambulatory setting.

Willison DJ, Soumerai SB, McLaughlin TJ, Gurwitz JH. Consultation between cardiologists and generalists in the management of acute myocardial infarction: implications for quality of care. *Arch Intern Med.* 1998;158:1778–1783.  The objective of this study was to compare the quality of medical care when generalists and cardiologists work separately or together in the management of patients with acute myocardial infarction (AMI). Patients cared for by a cardiologist alone were younger, presented earlier to the hospital, were more likely to be male, had less severe co-morbidity, and were more likely to have an ST elevation of 1mm or more, than the generalists' patients. There was no variation in the use of effective agents between patients cared for by a cardiologist attending physician and a generalist with a consultation by a cardiologist. However, there was a consistent trend towards increased use of aspirin, thrombolytics, and beta-blockers for those in care of both a cardiologist and a generalist, compared with those cared for by a generalist attending physician only. The study concludes that for patients with AMI, consultation between generalists and specialists may improve the quality of care.

# NURSE PRACTITIONERS AND OTHER NONPHYSICIAN PRACTITIONERS

# CHAPTER TWENTY-NINE

# Quality of Patient Care by Nurse Practitioners and Physician's Assistants: A Ten-Year Perspective

Harold C. Sox Jr., M.D.
1979

The major recent development in primary care may be the discovery that appropriately trained nonphysicians can do much of the physician's work with apparent safety and patient satisfaction. When nurse practitioners and physician's assistants were first introduced, their proponents claimed that they would provide welcome help for overworked physicians and improved access to health care for many patients. There was concern, however, that health workers with relatively brief clinical training would not be able to provide good quality patient care, even when closely supervised by physicians. These concerns were expressed in editorial comment[1,2] and were implicit in the appearance of over 40 journal articles reporting observations of patient care given by nurse practitioners and physician's assistants. This review will examine this evidence on the quality of care provided by nurse practitioners and physician's assistants.

We identified 21 studies in which care given by nurse practitioners or physician's assistants was compared with that given by physicians. In reviewing these articles, we shall ask two questions. The first concerns the validity of the evidence: Did the investigators accurately describe what happened and were their conclusions justified? The answer to this question will depend on the adequacy of the study design and the methods used to measure the quality of care. The second question concerns the general implication of the findings: Can the findings be applied to all practitioners and all activities in a primary care practice?

This chapter originally appeared as Sox HC Jr. Quality of patient care by nurse practitioners and physician's assistants: a ten-year perspective. *Ann intern Med*, 1979;91:459–468. Copyright © 1979, American College of Physicians–American Society of Internal Medicine. Reprinted with permission.

The answer to this question will depend on the methods used to select study participants and the scope of activities that were actually observed.

# METHODS

The terms "nurse practitioner" and "physician's assistant" will be used to denote providers who are not physicians but who diagnose and treat illness under the supervision of a physician.

## Study Selection Criteria

To facilitate an orderly review of the literature, minimal criteria for review and methodologic standards were established before the papers were read. Forty-five studies reported between 1967 and early 1978 met the minimal criteria. Each was evaluated for adherence to methodologic standards. One of these standards, the requirement that care by nurse practitioners and physician's assistants be compared to care given concurrently by physicians, was the basis for selecting 21 studies[3-24] for discussion. The other studies[25-47] will not be discussed further. The following were minimal criteria for selecting a study for review.

1. The report was written in English.
2. The practitioners were providing direct primary patient care.
3. The report provided information about at least one of the following measures of the quality of patient care.

*Process of Health Care:* Information about the process of care was accepted as a measure of quality if the actions taken in a provider-patient contact were compared with established standards of care. The medical record was the source of this information unless otherwise noted.

*Outcome of Health Care:* Typical measures of illness outcome used as indices of quality included symptom relief, return to normal activities, and functional status. This information was usually obtained by interviewing the patient some time after the index encounter.

*Patient Satisfaction with Care:* Information about patient satisfaction was obtained by questionnaires that assessed patients' feelings about their care or by observing subsequent behavior that might reflect satisfaction (missed follow-up appointments or use of alternative sources of care).

*Agreement with a Physician:* There were several studies in which nurse practitioner or physician's assistant and physician saw the same patient, and their conclusions and decisions were compared. In these studies, one of the measures of quality was the extent of agreement with the physician. Although it may have been unfair to use perfect agreement with a physician as a standard of care (because the nurse practitioner or physician's assistant could equal but never exceed the physician), patient care by a physician is a widely accepted standard of comparison.

## Methodologic Standards

*Year of Observations:* There have been training and employment opportunities for nurse practitioners and physician's assistants only during the past decade. The breadth of their patient care activities and their acceptance by physicians and patients may have changed significantly during this time. In many states, there have been changes in health practice laws and certification requirements that may have affected both the range of legally sanctioned activities and the quality of practitioners that were entitled to practice. Therefore, a report should indicate when the study was performed.

*Number of Patients:* The number of observations of care is essential information for the assessment of the validity of a study's conclusions.

*Number of Providers:* The larger the number of providers that are studied, the more likely that conclusions based on their activities will apply to other providers.

*Description of Practice Environment:* The report should describe the practices in the study so that the types of practice to which the conclusions apply can be identified. The medical specialty, the method of provider reimbursement, and the form of practice should all be specified.

*Description of Patients:* Medical and demographic information about the patients should be specified.

*Description of Provider Training and Experience:* Because neither the duration nor the content of the training of nurse practitioners or physician's assistants is standardized, reports should specify this information or cite a published source. Reports should also specify how long the nurse practitioner or physician's assistant had been in practice at time of the study.

*Controlled Observations:* Comparison of care by nurse practitioners or physician's assistants and physicians should be based on concurrent observations of care given in the same practice setting.

*Methods of Allocating Patients:* The optimal conditions for comparing nurse practitioners and physician's assistants with physicians occur when the patients they see are alike in all characteristics. To achieve this condition, both providers may see the same patient, as was done in four studies. If they see different patients, random allocation of patients is preferable. Even though identifiable sources of bias might successfully be avoided in a nonrandom allocation procedure, only random allocation of a large sample assures the equitable distribution of all sources of bias, known and unknown, to both experimental groups. Reports should characterize study dropouts to be sure that the patients who remained in the study were comparable. In addition, the pretreatment status of the study groups should be compared.

*Probability That a True Difference Was Overlooked:* When a new method is found by statistical tests of significance to be indistinguishable from a well-accepted standard, it is important to calculate the probability that a true difference did exist but was overlooked. As pointed out by Spitzer and colleagues[4], the results of tests of statistical significance should be expressed in terms of the probability that a true difference of a specified size in either direction has been missed.

# RESULTS

## Assessment of Study Design

The relation between the design characteristics of the 21 controlled studies and the methodologic standards is summarized in Table 29.1. Although none of the studies met all 11 methodologic standards, five of the eight randomized trials and three of the nine nonrandomized studies met at least seven criteria. Most of the studies provided enough information to assess their general application, but it was difficult to assess the validity of the nonrandomized studies because few of them adequately characterized the patients' status before the study.

## Study Characteristics and Results

The characteristics of the study practices and participants, the quality of care measures, and the results are summarized in Tables 29.2, 29.3, and 29.4.

The eight experiments in which patients were randomly allocated to a provider are shown in Table 29.2.[3-11] The subjects were nurses or nurse practitioners in all but one study. In four studies patients of nurse practitioners were more satisfied with their care than patients of physicians[6-8,11] and had better outcomes in one study.[7] In the latter study, however, control patients did not have a regular physician. Otherwise, these experiments revealed no measurable differences in care given by nurse practitioners or physician's assistants as compared with that given by physicians.

The three studies in which a nurse practitioner and a physician evaluated the same patient are summarized in Table 29.3.[12-14] All but one were studies of pediatric practice. The order of seeing the patient was randomized in only one study[14]; in the other two, the physician saw the patient after the nurse practitioner. In a fourth study, four standardized case histories were provided over the telephone by a nurse playing the role of a worried mother.[15] In all of these studies, the two types of providers made essentially the same diagnoses and triage decisions.

There were nine reports[16–24] of studies in which patients were assigned non-randomly to a provider (Table 29.4). There were no significant differences between nurse practitioners or physician's assistants and physicians in the quality of care as measured in these studies. This finding is difficult to interpret because it is difficult to be sure that the two types of providers saw comparable patients. Four of the reports compared some of the characteristics of the patients seen by the two types of providers.[20–22,24] In three of these studies, the patients appeared to be comparable[21,22,24]

# DISCUSSION

In the 21 studies comparing primary ambulatory care by nurse practitioners and physician's assistants with care by physicians, there were essentially no differences between the two types of health provider. Two principal questions may be asked about these studies: (1) Are the findings a valid description of the care in the study practices? (2) Can the findings be applied to other practice settings, other providers, and all primary care activities?

## Validity of Quality of Care Measures

Techniques for measuring the quality of health care are still in an early stage of development and may be too insensitive to detect clinically important differences between practitioners. Therefore, the findings described in these studies should be interpreted with caution. To assess the quality of care, one usually examines how care is given (process measurements)[48] or the results of care (outcome measurements),[49] The outcome of care is a direct reflection of one goal of medical care, which is to assure that the patient gets as well as possible with minimum ill effects. However, factors that are independent of the provision of care may influence outcomes (access to housing, food, medication, or education). Furthermore, since illness often resolves spontaneously, the end result of an illness may not be attributable to the provider of care. These problems are largely avoided by evaluating the process used to care for a patient.

The information that is obtained from the patient, its interpretation, and the action taken constitute the technical content of the process of care. Proposed standards for the technical content of care should be evaluated by prospectively studying how well they predict illness outcomes. Unfortunately, the relation between the process of care and its outcome has begun to be studied only recently. Criteria for defining the technical process of care are widely available,

*(continued on page 568)*

Table 29.1. Relation of Study Design to Methodologic Standards.

| | Random Allocation of Patients | | | | | | | | Patients Seen by Two Types of Provider | | | | Nonrandom Allocation of Patients | | | | | | | | |
|---|---|---|---|---|---|---|---|---|---|---|---|---|---|---|---|---|---|---|---|---|---|---|
| Reference number | 3 | 4, 5 | 6 | 7 | 8 | 9 | 10 | 11 | 12 | 13 | 14 | 15 | 16 | 17 | 18 | 19 | 20 | 21 | 22 | 23 | 24 |
| Measures of quality[a] | O | POS | S | OS | OS | OS | OS | OS | A | A | OA | A | S | S | O | S | OS | P | POS | O | PO |
| Internal validity criteria[b] | | | | | | | | | | | | | | | | | | | | | |
| Random allocation of patients | + | + | + | + | + | + | + | + | – | – | – | – | – | – | – | – | – | – | – | – | – |
| Comparison of patients' pretreatment status | + | + | + | – | + | – | + | + | NA | NA | NA | NA | – | – | – | – | + | + | + | – | + |
| Description of patients who drop out of study | – | + | + | – | + | + | – | – | NA | NA | + | NA | – | – | – | – | – | – | – | – | – |
| Calculation of probability that a true difference was missed | – | + | – | – | – | – | – | – | – | – | – | – | – | + | – | – | – | – | – | – | – |
| Size of patient groups | + | + | + | + | + | + | + | + | + | + | + | NA | – | + | + | + | + | + | + | + | + |

| | Random Allocation of Patients | | | | | | | | Patients Seen by Two Types of Provider | | | | | | | | | | Nonrandom Allocation of Patients | | | | |
|---|---|---|---|---|---|---|---|---|---|---|---|---|---|---|---|---|---|---|---|---|---|---|---|
| Number of internal validity criteria present | 3 | 5 | 4 | 2 | 3 | 3 | 3 | 1 | 1 | 1 | 2 | 0 | 0 | 1 | 1 | 1 | 2 | 2 | 1 | 1 | 2 | 2 | 2 |
| General applicability criteria[b] | | | | | | | | | | | | | | | | | | | | | | | |
| Dates of study | – | + | + | – | + | + | + | + | + | – | + | + | + | + | + | + | + | + | – | – | + | + | + |
| Description of patients | + | + | + | – | + | + | – | + | – | + | + | + | – | + | + | + | + | + | – | – | + | + | – |
| Number of providers | + | + | + | + | + | + | + | + | + | + | + | + | + | + | + | + | + | + | + | + | + | + | + |
| Description of practice | + | + | + | + | + | + | + | + | + | + | – | NA | + | + | + | + | + | + | + | + | + | + | + |
| Description of training | + | + | + | – | + | + | – | + | + | + | – | – | + | + | + | + | + | + | + | + | + | – | – |
| Duration of prior practice experience | – | – | + | – | – | – | – | – | – | + | – | + | + | – | + | + | – | – | + | – | + | + | – |
| Number of criteria present | 4 | 5 | 6 | 2 | 4 | 5 | 5 | 4 | 4 | 4 | 3 | 3 | 4 | 5 | 6 | 4 | 5 | 3 | 4 | 2 | 3 | 6 | 3 |

aP = process of care, O = outcome of care, S = satisfaction with care, A = agreement with physician.

bPlus (+) = present, minus (–) = absent, NA = not applicable because of study design.

**Table 29.2. Studies of Care in Which Patients Were Allocated Randomly to Providers.**

| Study (Number of Providers) | Type of Health Provider (Number of Providers) | Type of Practice (Number of Practices Studied) | Number of Patients (non-MDs Group/ Control Group) | Quality of Care Variables Measured |
|---|---|---|---|---|
| 3 | Nurse practitioner (4); MD (NA) | Municipal hospital medical clinic (2) | 275/275 | Outcome of diabetes care Disease control Missed appointments & clinic dropouts |
| 4, 5 | Nurse practitioners (2); MD (2) | Suburban family practice (2) | 1529/2796 | Process of care for 10 conditions Use of 13 drugs Health, emotional, and social status Dropouts from practice Deaths Satisfaction questionnaire responses |
| 6 | Pediatric nurse practitioner (4); pediatrician (4) | Private pediatric practice (4) | 703/517 | Patient attitude toward provider of well-child care for newborns |
| 7 | Nurse practitioners (2); MDs (NA) | Medical clinic of university hospital (1) and of metropolitan hospital (1) | 33/33 in university hospital and 53/85 in metropolitan hospital | Death Return to work Number of symptoms Missed appointments Attitude toward care Seeking other care |
| 8 | Nurse practitioner (5); MD (internists and general practitioners) (32) | Walk-in clinic of prepaid group practice (1) | 222/197 | Symptom relief Satisfaction with care Revisit with same symptoms |
| 9 | Pediatric nurse practitioners (6); pediatrician (NA) | Prepaid group practice (1) | 474/678 | Well-child care "No show" or cancelled appointments Hospitalization rate Reported frequency of acute and chronic illness Transfer rate between provider type Identification of congenital anomalies |
| 10 | Health assistants (6); internists (5) | Municipal hospital diabetes clinic (1) | 84/53 | Serum glucose Missed follow-up appointments Seeking of other care |
| 11 | RN (5); MD (32) | Prepaid group practice walk-in clinic (1) | 203/193 | Symptom relief Satisfaction questionnaire responses Seeking of other care |

| Study Design | Results | Comment | Study |
|---|---|---|---|
| Patients selected from diabetes clinic; randomly allocated to nurse practitioners or continued care in diabetes clinic | Nurse practitioners = MD (nurse practitioners had less clinic dropouts) | MDs were house staff; no continuity of MD provider in diabetes clinic; MD saw all nurse practitioners' patients | 3 |
| All families randomized to have MD or nurse practitioners as primary provider | Nurse practitioner = MD (in all measures) | Two thirds of nurse practitioners' patient contacts did not involve MD | 4, 5 |
| Newborns randomly assigned to receive care from nurse practitioner/ MD team or from MD alone | More satisfaction with developmental assessment by nurse practitioner, more concern shown by nurse practitioner, and more confidence in MD. Otherwise, equally satisfied with care by nurse practitioner/MD team or by MD alone | | 6 |
| Stable patients with five chronic diseases selected from medical clinic; randomly allocated to nurse practitioners or MD care. Evaluation after 1 year | Patients of nurse practitioners did better than MD patients for all end points except death rate | Not clear if control patients saw same provider at each visit | 7 |
| Walk-in patients with back pain randomly allocated to MD or nurse practitioner | For symptom relief and revisit with same symptom, MD = nurse practitioner; for satisfaction with care, nurse practitioner > MD | Nurse practitioners used back pain algorithm; MDs did not | 8 |
| Newborns randomly assigned to receive well-child care from nurse practitioners or MD; crossover allowed | Nurse practitioner = MD for all measures except more transfers from nurse practitioners to MD than vice versa | | 9 |
| Patients selected as suitable for protocol care; randomly allocated to health assistant and protocol or to MD | Blood sugar increased in MD group and decreased in health assistant and protocol group; MD = health assistant for other measures | Health assistants used a management protocol; MD saw 63% of health assistants' patients | 10 |
| Patients randomized to see MD or RN using management protocol | MD = RN for symptom relief (70%) and seeking other care (20%); RN-protocol > MD for satisfaction questionnaire responses | RN used management protocol; MD saw 45% of RN patients (RN-protocol alone not compared with RN-protocol + MD) | 11 |

*Notes:* MD = physician; NA = not available; RN = registered nurse.

**Table 29.3. Studies of Care in Which Different Providers Evaluated the Same Patient.**

| Study | Type of Health Provider (Number of Providers) | Type of Practice (Number of Practices Studied) | Number of Patients (non-MDs Group/ Control Group) | Quality of Care Variables Measured |
|---|---|---|---|---|
| 12 | Pediatric nurse practitioner (6); pediatrician (6) | Urban university hospital (1) | 113 | Triage of acute illness (severity of illness, need for emergency treatment, roentgenograms, or fever evaluation, disposition of patient) |
| 13 | Child health associate (6); pediatrician (9) | Private pediatric practice (6) | 143 | Diagnosis |
| 14 | RN (1); MD (13) | Student health service (1) | 151 | Errors in data collection Relief of female genitourinary tract symptoms |
| 15 | Child health associate (9); pediatric residents (8) | Not applicable | Four case histories | Triage by telephone Were appropriate questions asked? Was appropriate advice given? |

**Table 29.3. Studies of Care in Which Different Providers Evaluated the Same Patient.** *(continued)*

| Study Design | Results | Comment | Study |
|---|---|---|---|
| Every fourth patient was seen by a nurse practitioner and then by MD independently; each recorded decisions independently; clinic chief served as third observer when MD and nurse practitioner disagreed | Disagreement on 4–21% of patients; overall, no significant differences between nurse practitioner and MD | Nurse practitioner always saw patient first | 12 |
| Patients with acute problems were selected by receptionist to be seen by both child health associate and MD who recorded diagnosis independently | Child health associate = MD (concurrence in 92% of patients) | Study patients selected only when practice not busy; order of seeing patients not randomized | 13 |
| All patients seen by both RN and MD in randomized order; therapy randomized between MD decision and RN-protocol decision | Data collection errors unusual (RN = MD); symptom outcome same for MD decision or RN-protocol decision | RN used management protocol for dysuria and vaginitis | 14 |
| Each participant interrogated a nurse practitioner who simulated the mother in four case histories; panel scored appropriateness of questions and decisions as transcribed from tape recording | Child health associate = MD | Neither type of provider achieved more than 50% of a perfect score | 15 |

*Notes:* MD = physician; RN = registered nurse.

## Table 29.4. Studies of Care in Which Patients Were Allocated Nonrandomly to Providers.

| Study | Type of Health Provider (Number of Providers) | Type of Practice (Number of Practices Studied) | Number of Patients (non-MDs Group/ Control Group) | Quality of Care Variables Measured |
|---|---|---|---|---|
| 16 | Nurse practitioner (4); pediatrician (4) | Private practice (3); emergency room of municipal hospital (1) | Unknown | Patient attitude Sympathy and interest Communication effectiveness Apparent competence |
| 17 | Pediatric nurse practitioner (1); pediatrician (1) | University hospital clinic | 34/45 | Patient satisfaction |
| 18 | Nurse practitioner (3); MD (1) | Private general practice (1) | 286/74 | Accuracy of clinical diagnosis of streptococcal pharyngitis |
| 19 | Nurse practitioner (Primex) (10); MD (10) | Student health (2); solo practitioner (2); community clinics (3); hospital clinics (2); prepaid group practice (1) | 110–442/313–1120 | Patient attitude Access to provider General satisfaction with visit Rapport with provider Satisfaction with physicians and with nurses |
| 20 | Physicians assistant (12); internists and pediatricians (10) | Prepaid group practice | Attitude: 2284 Satisfaction, 1 week: MD, 169; physicians' assistant, 218 Outcome: MD, 584; physician's assistant, 264 | Attitude toward provider at time of visit Satisfaction with care 1 week and 1 month after visit Outcome (discomfort and activity limitation) 1 week and 1 month after visit |
| 21 | Physician's assistants (10); primary care physicians (10) | Rural primary care (10) | 383/406 | Process of care (diagnostic and therapeutic appropriateness) |
| 22 | Physician's assistants (2); faculty and residents (34) | University affiliated family practice center (2) | 146/1655 | Self-reported health status Satisfaction with care Process of care for seven problems; health status was determined on all |
| 23 | Pediatric nurse practitioner (3); pediatrician (3); RN (3); receptionist (3) | University pediatric clinic (1) | 211 (MD); 245 (nurse practitioner); 216 (RN); 216 (receptionist) | Appropriateness of triage referral Waiting time before triage |
| 24 | Physician's assistants (20); MD (20) | Private primary care (20) | Process study: 1005/4599 Outcome study: 540/2403 | Use of appropriate laboratory tests for six common problems Use of appropriate counseling and drugs for four common illnesses Change or maintenance of functional status |

**Table 29.4. Studies of Care in Which Patients Were Allocated Nonrandomly to Providers.** *(continued)*

| Study Design | Results | Comment | Study |
|---|---|---|---|
| Structured interview with parent after provider-child contact | Nurse practitioner = MD | One third of all patients left before being interviewed; no description of method of patient allocation | 16 |
| For 5 weeks, both drop-in and scheduled patients allocated by a not-described mechanism to be seen by nurse practitioner or MD; child's escort was interviewed immediately after | Nurse practitioner = MD | Patients rated general satisfaction on a four-point scale | 17 |
| Patients were seen and cultured by one provider who recorded clinical diagnosis | Nurse practitioner had less clinically negative patients with positive cultures and more clinically positive patients with negative cultures | Assignment of patients unstructured | 18 |
| For 1 week all patients in each site asked to fill out questionnaire | MD = nurse practitioner except that patients of nurse practitioners were relatively dissatisfied with access (waiting) and more satisfied with nurses than patients of MDs | 87% of questionnaires returned; assignment of patients nonrandom; number of respondents varied among various indices of care | 19 |
| In 2-week period, all patients answered questionnaire and a 50% random sample received 1-week telephone follow-up; all patients with medical problems had 1-month mail follow-up; patients assigned to provider with first available appointment | Outcome: physician's assistant > MD<br>Satisfaction: MD > physician's assistant (prior to visit); MD = physicians assistant (after visit) | Outcome differences attributed to appointment system that routed patients with chronic problems to MDs and acutely ill to physician's assistants | 20 |
| Physician observed provider-patient contact and rated severity of patient problem and appropriateness of the action taken | Physician's assistants = MD independently of the severity of the problem | Patient assignment haphazard in five practices; in the other five, physician's assistants saw less complex patients | 21 |
| Patients with an acute illness interviewed before and several weeks after they were seen by an MD or physician's assistant | When outcomes were stratified by type of illness or by entry health status, physician's assistant = MD<br>For process of care scores, physician's assistant = MD | No description of patient allocation method | 22 |
| Survey of triage function by different types of providers | Waiting time and inappropriate referrals: MD = nurse practitioner = RN; receptionists made more inappropriate referrals | No structured method for allocating patients<br>Inappropriate referral defined as more than one MD having to see patient | 23 |
| Survey of patient care by MDs or physician's assistants; for process study, patient contact forms were reviewed; for outcome study, patients were interviewed before and several weeks after being seen by MD or physician's assistant | Process study: small but significant differences favored physician's assistants for 3/10 measures; physician's assistants = MD for others<br>Outcome study: physician's assistants = MD | Patients seen by both MD and physician's assistant were analyzed separately<br>Results independent of time since the completion of physician's assistant training<br>Patient allocation mechanism unknown | 24 |

*Notes:* MD = physician; RN = registered nurse.

but they generally do not reflect the branching nature of the decision-making process.

The art of care is another component of the process of providing health care. It is defined by Brook as the "milieu, manner, and behavior of the provider in delivering care to, and communicating with, the patient."[50] Favorable results attributable to the art of care include compliance with therapeutic and preventive regimens and appropriate use of health care services. Study of the art of health care is also just beginning.[51-56]

**Process of Care.** The process of care was evaluated in eight of the 21 controlled studies, and there were no measurable differences between physician and nurse practitioner or physician's assistant. In four studies, data gathering, triage decisions, and diagnoses by pediatric nurse practitioners were compared to the same processes by physicians who evaluated each patient independently.[12-15] In three studies, the process of care was measured by reviewing medical records and encounter forms for adherence to standards of care for managing common clinical problems.[4,22,24] In one of these studies, there was limited access to clinical information, since the investigators used only information taken from encounter forms.[24] In the randomized trial of the nurse practitioner,[4,5] there was sufficient information to use detailed standards of care. Another study used detailed Professional Standards Review Organization criteria but reviewed too few patient records for any meaningful conclusions.[22]

An entirely different approach was taken by two investigators who observed care given to nonrandomly assigned office patients and used implicit criteria to rate on a numerical scale the severity of a patient's problem and the appropriateness of care.[21] This study is noteworthy because the scores for appropriateness of care were stratified by the severity of illness to detect possible differences that might be seen only in more ill patients. Remarkably, there were no differences. However, there were relatively few complex patients and rather wide interobserver variation in appropriateness scores. With the randomized trial of the nurse practitioner,[4,5] this study provides the strongest evidence that nurse practitioners and physician's assistants can provide office care the process of which is comparable in quality to that used by physicians.

**Outcome of Care.** There were no systematic differences in the outcome of illness in patients of nurse practitioners or physician's assistants and physicians in seven randomized trials[3-5,7-11] and five other studies.[18,20,22-24] This finding does not necessarily mean that care was of equivalent quality. Outcome is most apt to reflect care in seriously ill patients, in whom a favorable outcome requires optimal care and an unfavorable outcome is easily detected. Because most office patients are relatively well, a very large study population is required to include many who are seriously ill. In the randomized trial of the nurse practitioner,[4,5] there were 1,529 patients of nurse practitioners and 2,796 patients of physicians. These two groups of patients had similar outcomes as judged by physical, social, and emotional status at the end of 1 year of study. The proportion of well patients who became disabled and disabled patients who became well was the same for nurse practitioners and physicians.

Other studies reported illness outcome of well-child care,[9] acute minor illness,[8,11,14,18,20,22] and stable chronic diseases.[3,7,10] These latter studies did not achieve ideal conditions for using illness outcome to assess the quality of care. Although office patients of nurse practitioners or physician's assistants appear to have illness outcomes identical to those of patients of physicians, illness outcome was a sensitive measure of quality of care in only one study.[4,5]

**Satisfaction with Care.** In nearly all of these studies, patient satisfaction was used as an index of quality of care. Care given by nurse practitioners and physician's assistants uniformly gave satisfaction that was equal to or greater than satisfaction resulting from care given by physicians. This finding is important, but it should not be overinterpreted. There is little basis for the assumption that patient satisfaction reflects the way care is provided. No studies have tested the hypothesis that provider behavior that maximizes patient satisfaction also leads the patient to work synergistically with the provider to ensure a favorable illness outcome. The patients' knowledge of their disease and medications, the degree of patient compliance with a therapeutic plan, and the concordance between what the provider thinks the patient was told and what the patient remembers are all more direct measures of the "art of patient care" than patient satisfaction. These refined methods were not used in the studies described in this review. Therefore, it is premature to infer equal quality of care from equal patient satisfaction.

Satisfaction with care is a good measure of acceptance by patients, however. These studies indicate a high level of acceptance of nurse practitioners and physician's assistants as providers of primary ambulatory care. With the question of patient acceptance clearly answered, it is time to use sophisticated measures of the "art of patient care" to compare nurse practitioners and physician's assistants with physicians.

## Validity of Study Design

The most important requirement for a valid comparison of nurse practitioners and physician's assistants with physicians is evidence that they cared for similar patients. The most direct way to provide this assurance is to have both providers see the same patient and to compare their independent conclusions. Although direct, this experimental method has serious limitations. First, the normal pattern of practice must be disrupted as most physicians do not usually do a complete, independent assessment of each patient. Second, although useful for assessing the care of a single episode of acute illness, the method is difficult to apply to one of a series of visits for chronic illness, as information gained on previous visits might affect subsequent providers. Third, the method can really only be used to assess the process of care because assignment of credit or blame for illness outcome or changes in patient knowledge of illness would be very difficult with two providers caring for the same patient. Therefore, the four studies summarized in Table 29.3 lead to a limited conclusion: Nurse practitioners and physician's assistants reach similar diagnostic and therapeutic decisions when they both evaluate the same patient with acute illness. Comparing care given by two providers to the same patient is a valid but limited method of assessing the quality of patient care.

When patients are randomly allocated to receive care by either of two types of health provider, the two groups of patients are likely to be the same in the characteristics, known and unknown, that might otherwise bias the comparison. To check this assumption, the frequency of these characteristics in the two groups should be compared, as was done in six of the eight randomized trials. Patients who drop out of the practice or transfer from one provider to the other should be characterized to be sure that their withdrawal does not bias the comparison. Dropouts were characterized in four of the randomized trials.[4,6,8,9] Three studies both compared the pretreatment status of the two experimental groups and characterized patients who dropped out of the study. In these studies, nurse practitioners were indistinguishable from physicians in general ambulatory family practice,[4] care of acute low back pain,[8] and infant well-child care.[6]

The 10 remaining controlled studies comparing nurse practitioners and physician's assistants with physicians were not experiments because the normal methods of allocating patients were not altered to assure a valid comparison. The credibility of these studies depends on the extent of the efforts that were made to describe the clinical and demographic characteristics of the patients. There were five studies that did not compare the pretreatment state of the patients, evaluated a limited range of clinical activities, and used but few methods to assess the quality of care.[16-19,23] In each of the remaining studies, the pretreatment state of the patients was compared, and several different measures of quality of care were used.[20-22,24] In one of these studies, a valid comparison was not possible because the physician's assistants saw a greater proportion of patients with acute minor illness than did the physicians.[20] It is difficult to assess the validity of two other studies because the patients were characterized only by a simple measure of functional status and not by the complexity of their medical problem.[22,24] In the most detailed study, the investigators observed episodes of care and characterized the severity of the clinical problem and the appropriateness of care. The physician's assistants and physicians saw equally difficult patients and, regardless of the severity of the problem, provided care of equal quality.[21] This study of 10 rural practices is the most convincing of the nonexperimental comparisons because there was ample evidence that the comparison was valid.

## General Application of Results

In these studies, nurse practitioners and physician's assistants provided care that was equal in quality to care provided by physicians, at least as measured by the somewhat limited techniques used. The design and execution of some of these studies were sound, and their conclusions seem justified. To what extent can their findings be applied to other providers and the full range of activities in primary care practice? In trying to answer this question, we will discuss only the problems in assuming that the conclusions of these studies apply to an average primary care practice. We will not try to assess the impact of wide deployment of nurse practitioners and physician's assistants because the economic, political, and educational issues related to this question are beyond the scope of this review.

Are nurse practitioners and physician's assistants equally competent? There has been considerable controversy about the relative merits of nurse practitioners and physician's assistants as providers of health care. It would also be important to know if there are measurable differences between physician's assistants with different types of training. Unfortunately, none of these studies helps to resolve these issues. No studies directly compared nurse practitioners and physician's assistants. The only study reporting observations of two types of physician's assistant did not stratify the findings by the type of provider.[21] Thus, there is no direct evidence that all types of nurse practitioners and physician's assistants give care of equivalent quality. Nonetheless, since all of these studies showed equivalent quality of care by physicians and nurse practitioners or physician's assistants, differences between care given by nurse practitioners and physician's assistants are probably small or nonexistent.

Are nurse practitioners and physician's assistants competent in all primary care activities? An important defect of these studies is the failure to observe care under circumstances where differences between physician and nurse practitioner or physician's assistant are most likely to be found. Nurse practitioners and physician's assistants frequently cover emergency rooms, do hospital rounds, and visit nursing homes. In these places, they may initially take sole responsibility for recognizing and managing seriously ill patients. Unfortunately, nearly all of these studies were done in an office setting, in which there are relatively few patients with potentially serious acute illness. To define the limits of safe care by nurse practitioners and physician's assistants, they should be observed while taking the initiative to treat patients in emergency rooms, nursing homes, or hospitals. The conclusions of past studies apply only to office-based care.

Most legal definitions of nurse practitioners and physician's assistants require that they work under the supervision of a physician. However, a large proportion of the care that they give does not involve a physician directly.[4] Nurse practitioners and physician's assistants are often the sole source of coverage of emergency rooms, especially in rural areas. Solo practice by nurse practitioners is legal in some states. None of these studies analyzed the results of solo care separately from care in which a physician provided consultation. There is no basis for extrapolating from these studies to a nurse practitioner or physician's assistant in solo practice.

It is important to be cautious in applying the findings of these studies to the "average practice" because the study practices were probably not representative. None of the reports describes how practices were selected for study, but it is likely that many were chosen because the providers were known to the investigator through prior professional contact. Because a complex experimental design is likely to interfere with normal practice patterns, only a highly motivated physician is likely to volunteer to participate. Furthermore, a comprehensive study design is likely to limit the number of practices that can be studied simultaneously. This problem is illustrated by the best designed and most comprehensive of all these studies, the Burlington randomized trial of the nurse practitioner.[4,5] Only two practices and two nurse practitioners participated in this study, which reached valid conclusions about the efficacy of care given in highly selected practice settings but clearly had limited general application. On the other hand, because the factors that bias the selection of practices favor the selection of above-average practices, the nurse practitioners and physician's assistants were probably compared with primary care physicians of above-average ability. Because the care given by nurse practitioners and physician's assistants was indistinguishable from that by the physicians, it is clear that the quality of care provided by nurse practitioners and physician's assistants may be very good indeed; however, this level of performance may only be possible while they are working with physicians of above-average ability.

# CONCLUSIONS

This review has shown that in these studies the quality of primary ambulatory care given by nurse practitioners and physician's assistants was indistinguishable from that given by physicians. Although there have been 21 controlled studies reported in the past decade, many are of limited usefulness. In fact, only four investigators used detailed quality of care measures, studied general office care, and had patient groups that had been adequately characterized and appeared comparable.[4,21,22,24] Several other studies had clearly comparable patient groups but dealt with a narrow range of patient care activities or measures of care.[3,6,8,10–15] Even in the best of these studies, it is difficult to generalize from the particular study practice to the full range of primary care activities, patients, and practices. There has been very little description of care in emergency rooms, hospital beds, and nursing homes. Differences in care of the infrequent, seriously ill patient may have been overlooked, because measurements of care have not been stratified by the difficulty of the patient's problem. In addition, unbiased methods for allocating patients to a provider are apt to bias the selection of practices toward the unusually cooperative and above-average practice.

Despite the limitations of these studies, the primary care physician has enough information to predict the impact of a nurse practitioner or physician's assistant on the quality of care in a practice. A nurse practitioner or physician's assistant should be well accepted by patients and provide the average office patient with primary care that compares very favorably with care given by the physician. The physician may wish to take extra pains in supervising care for adults seen in emergency rooms, hospital beds, and nursing homes because studies of care given by nurse practitioners and physician's assistants in these settings have not yet been reported.

# Notes

1. Miles DL. Physician's assistants: the evidence is not in. *N Engl J Med.* 1975;293:555–556.

2. Baker AS. Primary care by the nurse. *N Engl J Med.* 1974;290:282–283.

3. Bessman AN. Comparison of medical care in nurse clinician and physician clinics in medical school affiliated hospitals. *J Chron Dis.* 1974;27:115–125.

4. Spitzer WO, Sackett DL, Sibley JC, et al. The Burlington randomized trial of the nurse practitioner. *N Engl J Med.* 1974;290:251–256.

5. Sackett DL, Spitzer WO, Gent M, et al. The Burlington randomized trial of the nurse practitioner: health outcomes of patients. *Ann Intern Med.* 1974;80:137–142.

6. Charney E, Kitzman H. The child-health nurse (pediatric nurse practitioner) in private practice: a controlled trial. *N Engl J Med.* 1971;285:1353–1358.

7. Lewis CE, Resnik BA, Schmidt G, Waxman D. Activities, events and outcomes in ambulatory patient care. *N Engl J Med.* 1969;280:645–649.

8. Greenfield S, Anderson H, Winickoff RN, Morgan A, Komaroff AL. Nurse-protocol management of low back pain: outcomes, patient satisfaction and efficiency of primary care. *West J Med.* 1975;123:350–359.

9. Burnip R, Ericksen R, Barr GD, Shinefield H, Schoen EJ. Well-child care by pediatric nurse practitioners in a large group practice: a controlled study in 1,152 preschool children. *Am J Dis Child.* 1976;130:51–55.

10. Komaroff AL, Black WL, Flatley M, Knopp RH, Reiffen B, Sherman H. Protocols for physician assistants: management of diabetes and hypertension. *New Engl J Med.* 1974;290:307–312.

11. Greenfield S, Komaroff AL, Anderson H. A headache protocol for nurses: effective-

ness and efficacy. *Arch Intern Med.* 1976;136:1111–1116.

12. Russo RM, Gururaj VJ, Bunye AS, Kim YH, Ner S. Triage abilities of nurse practitioner vs. pediatrician. *Am J Dis Child.* 1975;129:673–675.

13. Fine LL, Silver HK. Comparative diagnostic abilities of child health associate interns and practicing pediatricians. *J Pediatr.* 1973:83:332–335.

14. Greenfield S, Friedland G, Scifers S, Rhodes A, Black WL, Komaroff AL: Protocol management of dysuria, urinary frequency, and vaginal discharge. *Ann Intern Med.* 1974;81:452–457.

15. Ott JE, Bellaire J, Machotka P, Moon JB. Patient management by telephone by child health associates and pediatric house officers. *J Med Educ.* 1974;49:596–600.

16. Kahn L, Wirth P. The modification of pediatrician activity following the addition of the pediatric nurse practitioner to the ambulatory care setting: a time-and-motion study. *Pediatrics.* 1975;55:700–708.

17. Skinner EA, Kahn L. A comparison between the pediatric nurse practitioner (PNP) and the pediatric resident in the out-patient department: a pilot study. *Clin Pediatr.* 1972;11:142–147.

18. Merenstein JH, Rogers KD. Streptococcal pharyngitis: early treatment and management by nurse practitioners. *JAMA.* 1974;227:1278–1282.

19. Linn LS. Patient acceptance of the family nurse practitioner. *Med Care.* 1976;14:357–364.

20. Levine DM, Morlock LL, Mushlin AI, Shapiro S, Malitz FE. The role of new health practitioners in a prepaid group practice: provider differences in process and outcomes of medical care. *Med Care.* 1976;14:326–347.

21. Duttera MJ, Harlan WR. Evaluation of physicians assistants in rural primary care. *Arch Intern Med.* 1978;138:224–228.

22. Kane RL, Gardner J, Wright DD, et al. Differences in the outcome of acute episodes of care provided by different types of family practitioners. *J Fam Pract.* 1978;6:133–138.

23. De Angelis C, McHugh M. The effectiveness of various health personnel as triage agents. *J Comm Health.* 1977;2:268–277.

24. Kane RL, Olsen DM, Castle CH. Medex and their physician preceptors: quality of care. *JAMA.* 1976;236:2509–2512.

25. Mackay RC, Alexander DS, Kingsbury LJ. Parents' attitudes towards the nurse as physicians associate in a pediatric practice. *Can J Public Health.* 1973;64:121–132.

26. Flynn BC. The effectiveness of nurse clinicians' service delivery. *Am J Public Health.* 1974;64:604–611.

27. Charles G, Stimson DH, Maurier MD, Good JC. Physician's assistants and clinical algorithms in health care delivery. *Ann Intern Med.* 1974;81:733–739.

28. Spector R, McGrath P, Alpert J, Cohen P, Aikins H. Medical care by nurses in an internal medicine clinic: analysis of quality and its cost. *JAMA.*

1975;232:1234–1237.

29. Greenberg RA, Loda FA, Pickard CG, et al. Primary child health care by family nurse practitioners. *Pediatrics*. 1974;53:900–906.

30. Merenstein JH, Wolfe H, Barker KM. The use of nurse practitioners in a general practice. *Med Care*. 1974;12:445–452.

31. Fairweather JL, Kifolo A. Improvement of patient care in a solo ob-gyn practice by using an RN physician's assistant. *Am J Public Health*. 1972;62:361–363.

32. Dutton CB, Hoffman S, Ryan LK. Nurse practitioners: clinical performance in diagnosis and treatment of urinary tract infection. *NY State J Med*. 1975;75:2424–2427.

33. Adamson TE, Watts PA. Patients' perceptions of maternity nurse practitioners. *Am J Public Health*. 1976;66:585–586.

34. Vickery DM, Liang MH, Collis PB, et al. Physician extenders in walk-in clinics: a prospective evaluation of the AMOSIST program. *Arch Intern Med*. 1975;135:720–725.

35. Clark AB, Dunn M. A nurse clinician's role in the management of hypertension. *Arch Intern Med*. 1976;136:903–904.

36. Gardner HH, Ouimette R. A nurse-physician team approach in a private internal medicine practice. *Arch Intern Med*. 1974;134:956–959.

37. Greenfield S, Bragg FE, McGraith DL, Blackburn J. Upper-respiratory tract complaint protocol for physician-extenders. *Arch Intern Med*. 1974;133:294–299.

38. Machotka P, Ott JE, Moon JB, Silver HK. Competence of child health associates: I. Comparison of their basic science and clinical knowledge with that of medical students and pediatric residents. *Am J Dis Child*. 1973;125:199–203.

39. Horrocks JC, De Dombal FT. Diagnosis of dyspepsia from data collected by a physician's assistant. *Br Med J*. 1975;3:421–423.

40. Nelson EC, Jacobs AR, Johnson KG. Patients' acceptance of physician's assistants. *JAMA*. 1974;228:63–67.

41. Thompson T. The evaluation of physician's assistants in radiology. *Radiology*. 1974;111:603–606.

42. Butler AM, Abrams I, Roessler M, Cutler K. Pediatric nurse-practitioners and screening physical examinations. *Clin Pediatr*. 1969;8:624–628.

43. Duncan B, Smith AN, Silver HK. Comparison of the physical assessment of children by pediatric nurse practitioners and pediatricians. *Am J Public Health*. 1971;61:1170–1176.

44. Chappel JA, Drogos PA. Evaluation of infant health care by a nurse practitioner. *Pediatrics*. 1972;49:871–877.

45. Komaroff AL, Sawayer K, Flatley M, Browne C. Nurse practitioner management of common respiratory and genitourinary infections using protocols. *Nurs Res*. 1976;25:84–89.

46. Winickoff RN, Ronis A, Black WL, Komaroff AL. A protocol for minor respiratory

illness: an evaluation of its use by nurses in a prepaid group practice. *Public Health Rep.* 1977;92:473–480.

47. Komaroff AL, Flatley M, Browne C, Sherman H, Fineberg E, Knopp RH. Quality, efficiency, and cost of a physician-assistant-protocol system for management of diabetes and hypertension. *Diabetes.*1976;25:297–306.

48. Williamson JW. Evaluating quality of patient care: a strategy relating outcome and process assessment. *JAMA.* 1971;218:564–569.

49. Brook RH, Davies-Avery A, Greenfield S, et al. Assessing the quality of medical care using outcome measures: an overview of the method. *Med Care.* 1977;15(suppl):1–84.

50. Brook RH, Williams KN, Davies-Avery A. Quality assurance today and tomorrow: forecast for the future. *Ann Intern Med.* 1976;85:809–817.

51. Ware JE Jr, Wright WR, Snyder MK, Chu GC. Consumer perceptions of health care services: implications for academic medicine. *J Med Educ.* 1975;50:839–848.

52. Hulka BS, Cassel JC, Kupper LL, Burdette JA. Communication, compliance, and concordance between physicians and patients with prescribed medications. *Am J Public Health.* 1976;66:847–853.

53. Hulka BS, Kupper LL, Cassel JC, Babineau RA. Practice characteristics and the quality of primary care: the doctor-patient relationship. *Med Care.* 1975;13:808–820.

54. Ware JE Jr, Snyder MK. Dimensions of patient attitudes regarding doctors and medical care services. *Med Care.* 1975;13:669–682.

55. Sackett DL, Haynes RB, eds. *Compliance with Therapeutic Regimens.* Baltimore, Md: Johns Hopkins University Press; 1976.

56. Hulka BS, Zyzanski SJ, Cassel JC, Thompson SJ. Satisfaction with medical care in a low income population. *J Chron Dis.* 1971;24:661–673.

# Primary Care Outcomes in Patients Treated by Nurse Practitioners or Physicians

*A Randomized Trial*

Mary O. Mundinger, Dr.Ph.; Robert L. Kane, M.D.;
Elizabeth R. Lenz, Ph.D.; Annette M. Totten, MPA; Wei-Yann Tsai, Ph.D.;
Paul D. Cleary, Ph.D.; William T. Friedewald, M.D.;
Albert L. Siu, M.D., MSPH; Michael L. Shelanski, M.D., Ph.D.

2000

The many pressures on the U.S. health care system and greater focus on health promotion and prevention have prompted debates about primary care workforce needs and the roles of various types of health care professionals. As nurse practitioners seek to define their niche in this environment, questions are often raised about their effectiveness and appropriate scope of practice. Several studies conducted during the last 2 decades[1-4] suggest the quality of primary care delivered by nurse practitioners is equal to that of physicians. However, these earlier studies did not directly compare nurse practitioners and physicians in primary care practices that were similar both in terms of responsibilities and patient panels.

Over time, payment policies and state nurse practice acts that constrained the roles of nurse practitioners have changed. In more than half the states, nurse practitioners now practice without any requirement for physician supervision or collaboration, and in all states nurse practitioners have some level of independent authority to prescribe drugs.[5] Additionally, nurse practitioners are now eligible for direct Medicaid reimbursement in every state, direct reimbursement for Medicare Part B services as part of the 1997 Balanced Budget Act,[6] and commercial insurance reimbursement for primary care services within limits of state law. Finally, state law determines whether nurse practitioners are eligible for hospital admitting privileges, either by regulating access at the state level or by allowing local hospital boards to decide. The combination of authority to prescribe drugs, direct reimbursement from most payers, and hospital admitting

This chapter originally appeared as Mundinger MO, Kane RL, Lenz ER, et al. Primary care outcomes in patients treated by nurse practitioners or physicians: a randomized trial. *JAMA.* 2000;283:59–68. Copyright © 2000, American Medical Association. Reprinted with permission.

privileges creates a situation in which nurse practitioners and primary care physicians can have equivalent responsibilities. The present study is a large randomized trial designed to compare patient outcomes for nurse practitioners and physicians functioning equally as primary care providers.

The opportunity to compare the 2 types of providers was made possible by several practice and policy innovations at the Columbia Presbyterian Center of New York Presbyterian Hospital in New York City. In 1993 when the medical center sought to establish new primary care satellite clinics in the community, the nurse practitioner faculty were asked to staff 1 site independently for adult primary care. This exclusively nurse practitioner practice was to be similar to the clinics staffed by physicians. All are located in the same neighborhood, serve primarily families from the Dominican Republic who are eligible for Medicaid, and follow the policies and procedures of the medical center. The nurse practitioner practice, the Center for Advanced Practice, opened in the fall of 1994.

New York State law allows nurse practitioners to practice with a collaboration agreement that requires the physician to respond when the nurse practitioner seeks consultation. Collaboration does not require the collaborating physician to be on site and requires only quarterly meetings to review cases selected by the nurse practitioner and the physician. The state also grants nurse practitioners full authority to prescribe medications, as well as reimbursement by Medicaid at the same rate as physicians. The medical board granted nurse practitioners who were faculty members in the school of nursing hospital admitting privileges, thereby making the basic outpatient services, payment, and provider responsibilities the same in the nurse practitioner and physician primary care practices. Additionally, nurse practitioners and physicians in the study were subject to the same hospital policy on productivity and coverage, and a similar number of patients were scheduled per session in each clinic.

While it has been posited that nurse practitioners have a differentiated practice pattern focused on prevention with lengthier visits,[7] this study was purposely designed to compare nurse practitioners and physicians as primary care providers within a conventional medical care framework in the same medical center, where all other elements of care were identical. Nurse practitioners provided all ambulatory primary care, including 24-hour call, and made independent decisions for referrals to specialists and hospitalizations. The Spanish language ability of the nurse practitioners and physicians was similar, although the physicians had somewhat better Spanish facility on average. All of the nurse practitioners ($n = 7$) and most of the physicians ($n = 11$) had limited knowledge of Spanish, and 6 physicians were either fluent or bilingual. Staff who served as interpreters were available at each study site. The central hypothesis was that the selected outcomes would not differ between the patients of nurse practitioners and physicians.

# METHODS

## Participants and Randomization

Between August 1995 and October 1997, adult patients were recruited consecutively at 1 urgent care center and 2 emergency departments that are part of the medical center. Patients who reported a previous diagnosis of asthma, diabetes, and/or hypertension, regardless of the reason for the urgent visit, were oversampled to create a cohort of patients for whom primary care would have an impact on patient outcomes, as has been postulated in previous studies.[8,9] Patients were screened by bilingual patient recruiters and asked to participate if they had no current primary care provider at the time of recruitment and planned to be in the area for the next 6 months. The study was approved by the institutional review board of Columbia Presbyterian Medical Center. After an oral explanation of the consent form, written informed consent was obtained from each patient (both English and Spanish explanations and forms were available).

Those who provided informed consent were randomly and blindly assigned to either the nurse practitioner or 1 of the physician practices. Different assignment ratios were used during the recruitment period. Initially the ratio was 2:1, with more patients assigned to the nurse practitioner practice, because it opened after the physician practices and was able to accept more new patients. Subsequently, the ratio was changed to 1:1 as the nurse practitioner practice's patient panel increased. Despite this change, the mean number of days between the urgent visit at which patients were recruited and the follow-up appointments was similar (8.6 days for patients assigned to nurse practitioners compared with 8.9 days for patients assigned to physicians).

Recruited patients were then offered the next available appointments at the assigned clinic, and project staff made reminder calls the day before the appointments. Patients who missed their appointment were offered another appointment at the assigned practice. After patients kept their initial appointments, they were considered enrolled in the study and eligible for follow-up data collection.

Patients were told which provider group they were assigned to after randomization, and the type of provider could not be masked during the course of care. Patients who refused to participate or were deemed ineligible for the study were given follow-up primary care appointments by the study recruiters to the same practices. Additionally, during the study period, all practices received new patients from usual sources such as hospital discharges, recommendations from friends and family, referrals from other physicians, direct access by the patients themselves, and advertising. The study did not require a different process of care or documentation for enrolled patients.

At the initial visit, the patients became a part of the nurse practitioner or physician practices' regular patient panel, and all subsequent appointments, care, and treatments were arranged through the practice site of the assigned primary care nurse practitioner or physician. The primary care nurse practitioners and physicians had the same authority to prescribe, consult, refer, and admit patients. Furthermore, they used the same pool of specialists, inpatient units, and emergency departments. No attempt was made to differentiate study patients from other patients in the practice or to influence the practice patterns of the participating nurse practitioners and physicians. However, patients were free to change their source of medical care during the study. Medicaid in New York is currently fee-for-service and patients could go to other providers, go to a specialist directly, or use the emergency department without notifying their primary care provider. Approximately 3% of patients ($n$ = 43) went to another clinic after keeping the first randomly assigned appointment, and 9% ($n$ = 116) went to multiple primary care clinics during the 6-month period.

## Data Collection

At the time of recruitment, patients provided demographic and contact information and completed the Medical Outcomes Study 36-Item Short-Form Health Survey (SF-36). After the initial primary care visit, interviewers contacted the enrolled patients either by telephone or in person, if necessary, to administer a satisfaction questionnaire. Six months after this initial appointment, the enrolled patients were again contacted and asked to complete a second, longer interview. The decision to interview patients 6 months after the initial primary care visit was based on prior survey experience with this patient population.[10] The primary care patients served by the medical center are primarily immigrants and frequently change residences, travel between New York and their countries of origin, and have interruptions in telephone service. Attempts were made to locate all enrolled patients for this follow-up, including those who could not be located for the initial satisfaction interview. At the 6-month interview, the SF-36 and the satisfaction questionnaire were repeated, and additional questions were asked about health services utilization. A research nurse accompanied the interviewers, and for patients who reported a diagnosis of asthma, diabetes, or hypertension, physiologic data were collected.

Data on all health services utilization at the assigned practice and all other medical center sites were obtained from the medical center computer records for both the 6 months prior to recruitment and for 6 months and 1 year after the initial primary care appointment. These data were collected for all patients who were enrolled, including those who could not be located for the 6-month follow-up interview. Utilization data were also available for patients who were recruited but who did not keep their initial primary care appointment and therefore were not enrolled in the study. For these patients, the data were collected for the 6 months prior to recruitment and 6 months and 1 year after the date of the missed appointment they were given at recruitment.

## Main Outcome Measures

The SF-36 was used as a baseline and follow-up measure of health status. This instrument elicits patient responses to 36 questions designed to measure 8 health concepts (general health, physical function, role–physical, role–emotional, social function, bodily pain, vitality, and mental health)[11] or to create 2 summary scores (physical component summary and mental component summary).[12] The origin and logic of the item selection, as well as the psychometrics and tests of clinical validity, have been reported by the survey's developers.[13,14] Additionally, the survey's utility for monitoring general and specific populations, measuring treatment benefits, and comparing the burden of different diseases has been documented in 371 studies published between 1988 and 1996.[15,16] For example, the SF-36 has been used to measure differences in function between chronically ill patients with and without comorbid anxiety disorder;[17] has demonstrated that it can detect changes in health status that correspond to clinical profiles for 4 common conditions;[18] and has shown that it reflects changes in health status that correspond to a predicted clinical course for elective surgery patients.[19]

Patient satisfaction was measured by using "provider-specific" items from a 15-item satisfaction questionnaire used in the Medical Outcomes Study.[20] Three items related to clinic management were included in the survey to provide the medical center administration with information about patients' perceptions of the clinic, but those items were not intended for use in the comparison of providers.

The survey instruments used in the study were written in English and then translated into Spanish. The bilingual members of the study team reviewed the Spanish versions to ensure that the meaning had not been changed. Approximately 80% (78.8% at recruitment and 83.7% at 6 months) of the interviews were conducted in Spanish.

Physiologic measures included disease-specific clinical measurements taken by a research nurse at the time of the 6-month follow-up interview. Blood pressure was determined for patients with hypertension, peak flow for those with asthma, and glycosylated hemoglobin for those with diabetes.

Utilization data included hospitalizations, emergency department visits, urgent care center visits, visits to specialists, and primary care visits within the Columbia Presbyterian Medical Center system. Only visits with a nurse practitioner or physician at a primary care site were counted as primary care. Specialty visits were defined as visits to a medical specialty clinic or specialist physician office. Emergency department and urgent care center visits were combined before analysis.

## Sample Size

Recruitment and enrollment goals were established based on estimates of the sample size needed to detect a difference of 5 points on a 100-point scale for the SF-36 scores on all scales when comparing 2 groups with repeated measures. As the randomization ratio was projected to change during the course of the study with availability of appointments, it was projected that the final ratio between the 2 groups would be 1 patient in the physician group for every 1.5 patients in the nurse practitioner group. The sample size estimates for unequal groups were extrapolated from those presented by the instrument's developer for equal groups, assuming $a$ = .05, 2-tailed $t$ test, and power of 80%. Differences of more than 5 points are considered clinically and socially relevant, according to the guidelines for the interpretation of the survey.[11]

# ANALYSIS

Baseline demographics and health status for the nurse practitioner and physician groups at randomization and following enrollment were compared using $g^2$ and $t$ tests. Ten of the 12 satisfaction questions were factor analyzed (the 11th question that asks whether the patient would recommend the clinic to family and friends was left as a separate item; an item about medication instructions was dropped, as it was not applicable to the majority of respondents who were not prescribed any medications at their first visit). There were 3 factors with eigenvalues greater than 1, indicating that they represented reasonable constructs. The first, "provider attributes" (Cronbach $a$ = .80) rated the provider on technical skills, personal manner, and time spent with the patient on a 5-point scale from poor to excellent. "Overall satisfaction" (Cronbach $a$ = .86) was the factor created from 2 items addressing the quality of care received and overall satisfaction with the visit. The "communications" factor (Cronbach $a$ = .59) combined 5 areas in which patients may have had problems understanding the provider's assessment and advice. Mean scores were computed for each factor.

Using the data collected at recruitment, mean baseline scores on the SF-36 for the scales and summary scores were used to establish the comparability of the nurse practitioner and physician groups in terms of health status. Four types of analyses were conducted using the SF-36 as an outcome measure. The first 2 included $t$ tests to compare mean scores for nurse practitioner and physician patients at 6-month follow-up (both unadjusted and adjusted for baseline demographics and health status) and baseline to 6-month change scores. The third was a subgroup analysis designed to compare the sickest patients. Patients whose baseline score on the physical component summary of the SF-36 was in the bottom quartile (sickest) of the study sample were selected, and 6-month follow-up SF-36 scores were compared using the same analyses used for the total sample.

The fourth analysis classified patients into categories according to the change from baseline to follow-up in each patient's individual scores on the summary measures. This analysis was modeled on a comparison of patients treated in health maintenance organization and fee-for-service systems.[21] The SE of measurement was used to create 3 categories: "same" (change not greater than what would be expected by chance), "better" (improved more than expected), and "worse" (declined more than expected).[12] While these definitions are based on a statistical construct, they provide results that may be more clinically relevant than mean scores or mean change in scores over time. A $g^2$ test was then used to compare the distribution of the nurse practitioner and physician patients among these groups. In addition, the change from baseline to follow-up for the entire sample was compared using paired $t$ tests.

Ranges and mean values for the physiologic measures were obtained, and mean values for the 2 groups were compared using $t$ tests.

For the analyses of health services utilization, data were obtained for 6 months prior to the date of recruitment, 6 months after, and 1 year after the first primary care visit. Neither the recruitment visit nor the assigned primary care visit was included. Comparisons between the nurse practitioner and physician patients' health services utilization after enrollment were made using $g^2$ tests (unadjusted) and Poisson regression (adjusted). To compare the utilization prior to recruitment with that following, signed rank tests were used.

The 159 patients (12.1%) who, after the first visit, either went to a clinic other than the one assigned or to multiple primary care clinics were maintained in the initially assigned group for the analyses, consistent with an intent-to-treat analysis. All analyses were repeated without these 159 patients, and the results were the same.

# RESULTS

## Recruitment, Enrollment, and Loss to Follow-up

Of the 3,397 patients screened and given follow-up appointments, 41.6% were not randomized because they either refused to participate (11.2%) or did not meet the screening criteria (30.4%). Of the 1,981 patients who were randomized, 1,181 (59.6%) were assigned to the nurse practitioner clinic and 800 (40.4%) to the physician clinics. The average age of the randomized patients was 44.4 years and 74.6% were female; 84.9% were Hispanic, 8.8% were black, and 1.1% were white. There were no statistically significant differences in the demographics or health status of the patients randomized to nurse practitioners or physicians (Table 30.1).

**Table 30.1. Randomized and Enrolled Patient Characteristics at Baseline.**

| | Randomized Patients | | | | Enrolled Patients | | | |
|---|---|---|---|---|---|---|---|---|
| | Nurse Practitioner Group (n = 1181) | Physician Group (n = 800) | Comparison | P Value | Nurse Practitioner Group (n = 806) | Physician Group (n = 510) | Comparison | P Value |
| Mean age, y | 44.0 | 44.9 | $t = 1.347$ | .18 | 45.5 | 46.7 | $t = 1.324$ | .19 |
| Female sex, % | 74.2 | 75.3 | $x^2 = 0.291$ | .59 | 75.9 | 78.2 | 0.932 | .33 |
| Race, % | | | | | | | | |
| Hispanic | 88.2 | 87.3 | | | 91.0 | 89.3 | | |
| Black | 8.3 | 10.4 | | | 5.5 | 8.1 | | |
| White | 1.3 | 0.9 | $x^2 = 6.853$ | .14 | 1.5 | 0.8 | $x^2 = 5.675$ | .23 |
| Other | 1.8 | 1.4 | | | 1.7 | 1.8 | | |
| Unknown | 0.4 | 0.0 | | | 0.3 | 0.0 | | |
| Mean No. of days between recruitment and initial appointment | 8.6 | 8.9 | $t = 0.478$ | .63 | 7.9 | 7.5 | $t = -0.709$ | .48 |
| Prevalence of selected chronic conditions, % of patients reporting each condition | | | | | | | | |
| Asthma | 20.2 | 17.6 | $x^2 = 2.10$ | .15 | 17.9 | 16.1 | $x^2 = 0.702$ | .40 |
| Diabetes | 10.2 | 11.8 | $x^2 = 1.25$ | .26 | 11.5 | 14.3 | $x^2 = 2.183$ | .14 |
| Hypertension | 30.0 | 34.1 | $x^2 = 3.79$ | .05 | 33.9 | 38.0 | $x^2 = 2.371$ | .12 |

|  | Randomized Patients | | | | Enrolled Patients | | | |
|---|---|---|---|---|---|---|---|---|
|  | Nurse Practitioner Group (n = 1181) | Physician Group (n = 800) | Comparison | P Value | Nurse Practitioner Group (n = 806) | Physician Group (n = 510) | Comparison | P Value |
| MOS SF-36 subscale scores, mean | | | | | | | | |
| Physical functioning | 63.1 | 61.5 | t = -1.27 | .21 | 61.4 | 59.2 | t = -1.347 | .18 |
| Role-physical | 40.1 | 39.0 | t = -0.554 | .58 | 38.0 | 34.5 | t = -1.402 | .16 |
| Bodily pain | 44.5 | 44.6 | t = 0.032 | .98 | 44.0 | 43.2 | t = -0.416 | .68 |
| General health | 44.5 | 45.8 | t = 1.097 | .27 | 43.7 | 43.4 | t = -0.211 | .83 |
| Vitality | 48.4 | 48.3 | t = -0.016 | .99 | 47.8 | 46.7 | t = -0.827 | .41 |
| Social functioning | 60.0 | 60.0 | t = -0.074 | .94 | 59.3 | 57.8 | t = -0.979 | .33 |
| Role-emotional | 48.5 | 47.4 | t = -0.505 | .61 | 46.9 | 42.3 | t = -1.694 | .09 |
| Mental health | 55.0 | 55.7 | t = 0.603 | .55 | 54.6 | 53.7 | t = -0.608 | .54 |
| Summary scores | | | | | | | | |
| Physical component | 38.4 | 38.0 | t = -0.637 | .52 | 37.9 | 37.2 | t = -1.041 | .30 |
| Mental component | 41.3 | 41.4 | t = 0.222 | .83 | 41.1 | 40.2 | t = -1.135 | .26 |

MOS SF-36 indicates Medical Outcomes Study Short-Form 36.

The 1,316 patients (66.4%) who kept their initial primary care appointments following randomization were considered enrolled in the study. This rate is comparable to the normal rate of appointments (65%) kept at the participating clinics (P. Craig, personal communication, August 4, 1999). Compared with the 665 patients (32.4%) who did not keep their appointments, those who did (the enrolled patients) differed significantly at baseline in several respects. Enrolled patients were older (45.9 vs 41.3 years); a higher proportion were female (76.8% vs 70.2%) and Hispanic (90.3% vs 82.9%); a higher percentage reported a history of 1 or more of the selected chronic conditions (53.7% vs 45.0%); and they had to wait fewer days for their follow-up appointments (7.8 vs 10.7). These findings are consistent with other studies of patient behavior relative to keeping or missing appointments.[22–24]

Our analysis of the data available on patients who did not keep their primary care appointments found no differences in health services utilization after 1 year among the patients assigned to the nurse practitioner group and physician group.

The difference in the retention rates between recruitment and enrollment for the nurse practitioner group (68.2%) and the physician group (63.8%) was statistically significant $\chi^2_1 = 4.3$, $P = .04$). However, neither the patients who enrolled nor those who failed to keep their appointments differed significantly between the nurse practitioner and physician groups in terms of baseline demographics, SF-36 scores, or patient-reported prior diagnosis of the selected chronic conditions (Table 30.1).

Among the nurse practitioner patients, 59% saw the same provider for all primary care visits in the first year after the initial visits compared with 54% of the physician patients, and this difference was not statistically significant $\chi^2_1 = 2.7$, $P = .11$).

Initial satisfaction interviews were completed for 90.3% ($n = 1188$) of all patients who made a first clinic visit (90.8% of the nurse practitioner group and 89.4% of the physician group). Almost 92% of all completed interviews took place within 6 weeks of the initial appointment.

Six-month interviews were completed for 79% of all enrolled patients (80.5% of the nurse practitioner group and 76.7% the physician group). This completion rate is considered high for a transient immigrant population and is comparable to or better than that achieved by other studies in the area served by the medical center. The majority of completed interviews (91.4%) took place between 180 and 240 days after the initial appointment. The most common reasons for loss to follow-up were the inability to locate the patient (65.9%) or that the patient had moved out of the area (17%). A small number of patients (23 [2.8%] in the nurse practitioner group and 16 [3.1%] in the physician group) refused to complete the interview when they were contacted. Five patients (2.9%) were located but were unable to complete the interview due to physical limitations or mental illness, and 3 patients (1.1%) were deceased. Figure 30.1 summarizes the participation rates at each major stage in the study.

**Figure 30.1.** Study Profile.

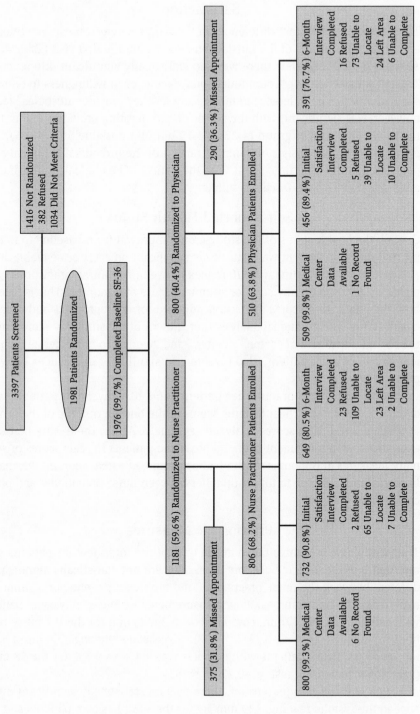

3397 Patients Screened

1416 Not Randomized
382 Refused
1034 Did Not Meet Criteria

1981 Patients Randomized

1976 (99.7%) Completed Baseline SF-36

800 (40.4%) Randomized to Physician

1181 (59.6%) Randomized to Nurse Practitioner

290 (36.3%) Missed Appointment

510 (63.8%) Physician Patients Enrolled

375 (31.8%) Missed Appointment

806 (68.2%) Nurse Practitioner Patients Enrolled

509 (99.8%) Medical Center Data Available
1 No Record Found

456 (89.4%) Initial Satisfaction Interview Completed
5 Refused
39 Unable to Locate
10 Unable to Complete

391 (76.7%) 6-Month Interview Completed
16 Refused
73 Unable to Locate
24 Left Area
6 Unable to Complete

800 (99.3%) Medical Center Data Available
6 No Record Found

732 (90.8%) Initial Satisfaction Interview Completed
2 Refused
65 Unable to Locate
7 Unable to Complete

649 (80.5%) 6-Month Interview Completed
23 Refused
109 Unable to Locate
23 Left Area
2 Unable to Complete

SF-36 indicates Medical Outcomes Study 36-Item Short-Form Health Survey.

## Satisfaction

There were no significant differences in the scores between nurse practitioners and physicians for any of the satisfaction factors after the first visit (Table 30.2). At the 6-month interview there were no statistically significant differences in "overall satisfaction" or "communications" factors or in willingness to refer the clinic to others. The difference in mean score for the "provider attributes" factor, however, was significant, with the physician group rating providers higher than the nurse practitioner group (4.22 vs 4.12 out of a possible 5; $P = .05$). The provider attribute consists of patients' ratings of the providers' technical skill, personal manner, and time spent with the patient. The clinical significance of a 0.1 difference on a 5.0 scale is unlikely.

## Self-Reported Health Status

Overall, the health status of the study group improved from baseline to follow-up, and the improvement was statistically significant on every scale (Table 30.3).

There were no significant differences between the nurse practitioner and physician patients on any scale or summary score at 6 months. This is true for both the unadjusted scores and scores adjusted for demographics and baseline health status. The additional analysis (not shown) of the summary scores, using the change categories of "same," "better," and "worse" to characterize the clinical course of each patient, also revealed no significant differences between provider types.

Finally, 152 nurse practitioner patients and 103 physician patients were defined as the sickest (health status scores in the bottom quartile of the sample at baseline) and their scores analyzed separately. Again, there were no differences between nurse practitioner and physician patients in scale scores or summary measures at 6 months (both unadjusted and adjusted), nor did the change in scores from baseline to follow-up differ between nurse practitioner and physician patient groups.

## Physiologic Measures

The physiologic measures taken at the time of the interview for patients who reported 1 of the selected chronic illnesses were not statistically significantly different between the nurse practitioner and physician patients for asthma and hypertension. The mean peak flow measurements for the 64 physician patients with asthma was 292 L/min, compared with 297 L/min for the 107 nurse practitioner patients ($t$ test $= -0.29$, $P = .77$). Glycosylated hemoglobin mean value for the 46 physician patients with diabetes was 9.4% vs 9.5% for the 58 nurse practitioner patients ($t$ test $= -0.22$, $P = .82$).

For patients with hypertension, there was no statistically significant difference in the systolic reading: 139 mm Hg for the 145 physician patients and 137

**Table 30.2. Patient Satisfaction: Initial Visit and 6-Month Follow-Up Interviews.**

| | Initial Visit | | | | 6-Month Follow-up | | | |
|---|---|---|---|---|---|---|---|---|
| | Nurse Practitioner Group (n = 726) | Physician Group (n = 453) | Comparison | P Value | Nurse Practitioner Group (n = 644) | Physician Group (n = 389) | Comparison | P Value |
| Provider attributes mean score[a] | 4.16 | 4.19 | $t = 0.815$ | .42 | 4.12 | 4.22 | $t = 1.963$ | .05 |
| Overall satisfaction mean score[a] | 4.59 | 4.60 | $t = 0.144$ | .89 | 4.45 | 4.46 | $t = 0.161$ | .87 |
| Problems, % of patients reporting[b] | | | | | | | | |
| 0 | 74.4 | 70.2 | | | 59.1 | 62.7 | | |
| 1 | 15.4 | 18.7 | $x^2 = 2.605$ | .46 | 25.1 | 23.5 | $x^2 = 2.146$ | .54 |
| 2 | 6.5 | 7.2 | | | 10.2 | 7.8 | | |
| 3–5 | 3.7 | 3.9 | | | 5.6 | 5.9 | | |
| % of patients who would recommend clinic to others | 98.7 | 98.2 | $x^2 = 0.544$ | .46 | 95.0 | 95.1 | $x^2 = 0.000$ | .99 |

[a]Calculated from items rated on a 5-point scale, in which 5 is the most positive response.
[b]Percentages may not add to 100% due to rounding.

**Table 30.3. Health Status Based on MOS SF-36 Results.**

| | Comparison of Baseline and 6-Month Scores for Entire Sample (n = 1040) | | | 6-Month Scores for Nurse Practitioner Group (n = 649) and Physician Group (n = 391) | | | | | |
| | | | | Unadjusted Mean Scores | | | Adjusted Mean Scores[a] | | |
| | Baseline | 6 mo | Change (Paired t tests)[b] | Nurse Practitioner Group | Physician Group | Comparison | Nurse Practitioner Group | Physician Group | Comparison[c] |
| --- | --- | --- | --- | --- | --- | --- | --- | --- | --- |
| Physical functioning | 60.30 | 64.26 | t = 4.631 | 64.94 | 62.90 | t = -1.126 P = .26 | 64.21 | 63.78 | t = 0.394 P = .77 |
| Role-physical | 36.06 | 53.31 | t = 10.519 | 53.74 | 52.62 | t = -0.375 P = .71 | 52.92 | 53.38 | t = -0.192 P = .85 |
| Bodily pain | 42.74 | 53.01 | t = 9.133 | 53.66 | 52.07 | t = -0.748 P = .45 | 52.91 | 52.73 | t = 0.092 P = .93 |
| General health | 42.94 | 48.75 | t = 7.662 | 48.79 | 48.67 | t = -0.070 P = .95 | 48.42 | 49.04 | t = -0.454 P = .65 |
| Vitality | 47.02 | 53.45 | t = -7.771 | 53.86 | 52.79 | t = -0.635 P = .53 | 53.27 | 53.38 | t = -0.072 P = .94 |
| Social functioning | 58.51 | 70.47 | t = 12.507 | 70.39 | 70.59 | t = 0.114 P = .91 | 70.25 | 70.70 | t = -0.279 P = .78 |

| | Comparison of Baseline and 6-Month Scores for Entire Sample (n = 1040) | | | 6-Month Scores for Nurse Practitioner Group (n = 649) and Physician Group (n = 391) | | | | | |
| --- | --- | --- | --- | --- | --- | --- | --- | --- | --- |
| | | | | Unadjusted Mean Scores | | | Adjusted Mean Scores[a] | | |
| | Baseline | 6 mo | Change (Paired t tests)[b] | Nurse Practitioner Group | Physician Group | Comparison | Nurse Practitioner Group | Physician Group | Comparison[c] |
| Role-emotional | 44.70 | 56.26 | t = 7.105 | 56.71 | 55.24 | t = -0.488 P = .63 | 55.81 | 56.34 | t = -0.192 P = .85 |
| Mental health | 53.51 | 60.17 | t = 8.177 | 60.75 | 59.45 | t = -0.742 P = .46 | 60.37 | 59.63 | t = 0.491 P = .62 |
| Physical component summary | 37.46 | 40.63 | t = 8.706 | 40.83 | 40.29 | t = -0.728 P = .47 | 40.53 | 40.60 | t = -0.102 P = .92 |
| Mental component summary | 40.56 | 44.58 | t = 9.438 | 44.64 | 44.29 | t = -0.398 P = .69 | 44.55 | 44.48 | t = 0.103 P = .92 |

*Note:* MOS SF-36 indicates Medical Outcomes Study Short-Form 36.

[a]Adjusted for age, sex, baseline MOS subscale scores, and each selected chronic condition.

[b]$P$ values for change are all $< .001$.

[c]Adjusted $t$ test is based on a regression model, with age, sex, baseline MOS subscale scores, and each condition entered as covariates.

mm Hg for the 211 nurse practitioner patients ($t$ test = 1.08, $P$ = .28). The mean diastolic reading, however, was statistically significantly lower for the nurse practitioner patients at 82 mm Hg compared with 85 mm Hg for the physician patients ($t$ test = 2.09, $P$ = .04).

## Utilization

For our comparison of outcomes we analyzed utilization of health care services for nurse practitioner and physician patients who enrolled in the study by keeping their initial primary care appointment. There were no statistically significant differences between the nurse practitioner and physician patients for any category of service during either the first 6 months or the first year after the initial primary care visit for either unadjusted or adjusted use rates (Table 30.4). When the utilization analyses were repeated for the subsets of "sickest" patients as defined in the "Self-Reported Health Status" section above, no differences were found in the health care services utilization between the nurse practitioner and physician patients (Table 30.5). In the 6 months and 1 year after the initial primary care visit, enrolled patients in both groups made significantly more primary care and specialty visits and fewer emergency/urgent visits than in the 6 months prior to recruitment. The percentage of enrolled patients hospitalized was not significantly different for either 6 months or 1 year after the initial primary care appointment.

# COMMENT

This study was designed to compare the effectiveness of nurse practitioners with physicians where both were serving as primary care providers in the same environment with the same authority. The hypothesis predicting similar patient outcomes was strongly supported by the findings of no significant differences in self-reported health status, 2 of the 3 disease-specific physiologic measures, all but 1 of the patient satisfaction factors after 6 months of primary care, and in health services utilization at 6 months and 1 year.

The difference between the nurse practitioner and physician patients' mean ratings of satisfaction with provider attributes was small but statistically significant. It may be attributable to the fact that the nurse practitioner practice was moved to a new site after 2 years and before recruitment and data collection were completed; the physician practices were not moved during the study period. When the "provider attribute" subscale scores for the nurse practitioner and physician patients whose 6-month follow-up period overlapped this move were compared, the ratings by nurse practitioner patients were significantly lower than those of the corresponding physician patients (4.16 vs 4.36; $P$ = .04). There was no significant difference in ratings among patients not affected

**Table 30.4. Utilization of Health Services.**

| | Change for Entire Sample, % | | | 6 Months After Initial Primary Care Visit, % | | | 1 Year After Initial Primary Care Visit, % | | |
|---|---|---|---|---|---|---|---|---|---|
| | 6 mo Prior (N = 1309) | 6 mo After (N = 1309) | Change, z Score[a] (N = 1309) | Nurse Practitioner Group (n = 800) | Physician Group (n = 509) | Comparison | Nurse Practitioner Group (n = 800) | Physician Group (n = 509) | Comparison |
| **Primary care visits** | | | | | | | | | |
| 0 | 88.8 | 21.2 | | 20.6 | 22.2 | | 18.0 | 19.1 | |
| 1 | 5.7 | 22.4 | | 22.6 | 22.0 | | 18.4 | 16.1 | |
| 2 | 2.9 | 17.3 | | 18.0 | 16.3 | $x^2 = 0.059$ | 13.8 | 13.4 | $x^2 = 1.033$ |
| 3 | 2.6 | 13.8 | −26.809 | 14.5 | 12.8 | $P = .81$ | 10.3 | 8.8 | $P = .31$ |
| 4 | 0 | 9.8 | | 9.6 | 10.0 | | 9.3 | 8.8 | |
| 5 | 0 | 6.1 | | 5.3 | 7.5 | | 7.5 | 6.1 | |
| ≥6 | 0 | 9.3 | | 9.4 | 9.2 | | 22.9 | 27.7 | |
| **Specialty visits** | | | | | | | | | |
| 0 | 89.1 | 62.3 | | 61.8 | 63.1 | | 54.5 | 54.8 | |
| 1 | 5.6 | 14.2 | | 13.3 | 15.7 | $x^2 = 0.678$ | 13.9 | 16.5 | $x^2 = 0.265$ |
| 2 | 2.3 | 9.3 | −15.578 | 10.8 | 7.1 | $P = .41$ | 8.9 | 6.3 | $P = .61$ |
| ≥3 | 3.1 | 14.2 | | 14.3 | 14.1 | | 22.8 | 22.4 | |
| **ED and urgent care** | | | | | | | | | |
| 0 | 58.1 | 76.5 | | 77.4 | 75.0 | | 65.8 | 66.2 | |
| 1 | 16.4 | 16.2 | | 15.3 | 17.7 | $x^2 = 0.428$ | 20.4 | 17.7 | $x^2 = 0.286$ |
| 2 | 16.4 | 4.0 | −12.937 | 4.3 | 3.7 | $P = .51$ | 7.4 | 8.6 | $P = .59$ |
| ≥3 | 9.1 | 3.3 | | 3.1 | 3.5 | | 6.5 | 7.5 | |
| **Hospitalizations** | | | | | | | | | |
| 0 | 94.5 | 95.3 | −0.884 | 95.9 | 94.3 | $x^2 = 1.703$ | 91.5 | 90.2 | $x^2 = 0.664$ |
| ≥1 | 5.5 | 4.7 | $P = .38$ | 4.1 | 5.7 | $P = .19$ | 8.5 | 9.8 | $P = .42$ |

*Notes:* Percentages may not add to 100% due to rounding. ED indicates emergency department.

[a]Except for hospitalizations, $P < .001$ for column.

Table 30.5. Subgroup Analyses.

| SF-36 Subscales | Nurse Practitioner Group (n = 152) | Physician Group (n = 103) | Comparison |
|---|---|---|---|
| *6-Month MOS SF-36 Scores for the Sickest Patients, Mean (SD)[a]* | | | |
| Physical functioning | 46.69 (27.05) | 48.17 (27.46) | *t* = 0.425 *P* = .67 |
| Role-physical | 33.55 (42.88) | 32.28 (43.53) | *t* = −0.231 *P* = .82 |
| Bodily pain | 38.10 (29.72) | 39.25 (29.36) | *t* = 0.306 *P* = .76 |
| General health | 38.06 (23.02) | 37.08 (23.48) | *t* = −0.333 *P* = .74 |
| Vitality | 43.06 (25.21) | 42.43 (25.14) | *t* = −0.197 *P* = .84 |
| Social functioning | 62.67 (28.87) | 60.56 (29.33) | *t* = −0.568 *P* = .57 |
| Role-emotional | 42.39 (47.25) | 43.04 (47.06) | *t* = 0.109 *P* = .91 |
| Mental health | 52.56 (28.11) | 50.92 (52.47) | *t* = −4.77 *P* = .63 |
| Physical component summary | 23.71 (3.12) | 23.84 (3.58) | *t* = 0.293 *P* = .77 |
| Mental component summary | 39.57 (13.35) | 40.39 (12.70) | *t* = 0.490 *P* = .63 |

by the move. Additional research will be needed to determine whether this is a persistent difference or if it results from conditions unique to this study.

A statistically significant, but small, difference was discerned in the mean diastolic blood pressure of patients with hypertension, with the nurse practitioner group having a slightly lower average reading at 6 months. Given the size of this change and the lack of differences in self-reported health status, there does not seem to be an obvious reason for this difference.

Although insufficient statistical power to discern differences has been a problem in much of the previous research comparing nurse practitioners and physicians, the sample size in this study was adequate to test the hypothesized

Table 30.5. **Subgroup Analyses.** *(continued)*

| SF-36 Subscales | Nurse Practitioner Group (n = 152) | Physician Group (n = 103) | Comparison |
|---|---|---|---|
| *Health Services Utilization for the Subgroup of "Sicker Patients," No. (%)* | | | |
| | (n = 151) | (n = 101) | |
| **Primary care visits** | | | |
| 0 | 30 (19.9) | 17 (16.8) | |
| 1 | 31 (20.5) | 21 (20.8) | x2 = 0.144 |
| 2 | 27 (17.9) | 21 (20.8) | P = .71 |
| ≥ 3 | 63 (41.7) | 42 (41.6) | |
| **Specialty visits** | | | |
| 0 | 82 (54.3) | 56 (55.4) | |
| 1 | 23 (15.2) | 21 (20.8) | x2 = 0.390 |
| 2 | 20 (13.2) | 8 (7.9) | P = .53 |
| ≥ 3 | 26 (17.2) | 16 (15.8) | |
| **ED and urgent care center visits** | | | |
| 0 | 108 (71.5) | 79 (78.2) | |
| 1 | 28 (18.5) | 17 (16.8) | x2 = 1.81 |
| 2 | 9 (6.0) | 2 (2.0) | P = .18 |
| ≥ 3 | 6 (4.0) | 3 (3.0) | |
| **Hospitalizations** | | | |
| 0 | 142 (94.0) | 99 (96.1) | |
| 1 | 7 (4.6) | 3 (2.9) | x2 = 0.542 |
| 2 | 1 (0.7) | 1 (1.0) | P = .46 |
| 3 | 1 (0.7) | 0 (0) | |

*Notes:* Percentages may not add to 100% due to rounding. MOS SF-36 indicates Medical Outcomes Study Short-Form 36; ED, emergency department.

[a]Selection of "sickest patients" was determined using MOS SF-36 scores using the bottom quartile of the baseline physical component summary. Patients with a score below 28.16 were included.

similarity of nurse practitioner and physician groups. At the end of the study, power calculations were repeated using final sample size and the means and SDs from these data. These revealed that the sample size was adequate to detect differences from baseline to follow-up between the 2 patient groups of less than 5 points for 6 of the 8 scales (3.2 for general health; 3.3 for vitality; 3.4 for mental health; 3.4 for social function; and 4.2 for bodily pain) and less than 6 points on 2 scales (5.9 on role—physical and role—emotional). This magnitude of difference is similar to differences commonly reported in studies comparing groups[21,25] and in studies of change over time within 1 group.[17,26]

There is evidence that the outcome measures chosen were sensitive enough to discern any important differences. The SF-36 is a widely used outcome measure and its sensitivity has been documented in several studies.[11,18,27] In this study, there were sizable and statistically significant changes for both nurse practitioner and physician patients in all scale scores and summary measures from baseline to follow-up. Some improvement would be expected, even over a 6-month period with or without primary care, following the urgent care visits at which subject recruitment occurred; the SF-36 did detect improvement. The utilization indicators are in widespread use in cross-sectional and longitudinal studies. With the exception of number of hospitalizations, which stayed the same in both groups, these measures also changed significantly over time.

Strengths of this study included adequate sample size and the ability to randomize patients to equivalent clinical settings and to providers with equal responsibilities. However, there were also several limitations.

Patients could not be randomized at the point of initial contact with the provider. Because the nurse practitioner and physician practice sites were geographically separate, patients had to be randomized when they were recruited in the emergency department or urgent care center to give them follow-up appointments at various locations with different appointment schedules. This time and location gap likely contributed to the loss of almost one third of the sample between randomization and enrollment. Although this is substantial, it is within the range reported in similar randomized trials.[28]

While the loss rate was significantly different for the nurse practitioner and physician groups, there is no reason to suspect that this represents a systematic violation of the protocol or any compromise of randomization. Patients dropped out before receiving care, and the dropout rate was higher for those assigned to the traditional model of physician care. This suggests that assignment to the new model of nurse practitioner care did not negatively influence patient behavior. There is no evidence of selection bias in that there were no significant differences in demographics, baseline health status, or prerecruitment health services utilization patterns between nurse practitioner and physician randomized patients, for either those who enrolled or those who did not keep their appointments.

A 1-year follow-up for SF-36 and patient satisfaction would have been more useful than taking these measures at 6 months. In part, we believed a population with limited access to health care would show changes in these measures in 6 months. But more influential in the decision regarding follow-up was the knowledge that this population is difficult to track because of changing addresses, changing eligibility for Medicaid, and frequent extended trips out of the country. Although we do have service utilization data for both 6 months and 1 year, data on satisfaction and self-perceived health status were not collected for 1 year.

Finally, the study had some characteristics that limit the generalizability of results. It was conducted in medical center–affiliated, community-based primary care clinics, which may differ from individual providers or small group practices. The providers were faculty from a university medical center, hence were not necessarily typical of those in nonacademic practice settings. The patients were predominantly immigrants from the Dominican Republic who were eligible for Medicaid and many did not speak English. This differs from the setting in which many commercially insured patients receive primary care but does resemble other academic, public and safety net providers, and the Medicaid populations they serve. While the setting and patient population are limitations, they are also what permitted randomized assignment and an environment in which nurse practitioners and physicians were able to function equally as primary care providers. The ability to do this type of study, even in a setting atypical for some patients, adds significant weight to the results from prior studies that have demonstrated the competence of nurse practitioners.

Who provides primary care is an important policy question. As nurse practitioners gain in authority nationally with commercially insured and Medicare populations now accessing nurse practitioner care, additional research should include these populations. As cost and quality issues pervade the public debate on managed care, those who are the first-line health care providers become pivotal resources in the emerging health care system. Nurse practitioners have been evaluated as primary care providers for more than 25 years, but until now no evaluations studied nurse practitioners and physicians in comparable practices using a large-scale, randomized design. The results of this study strongly support the hypothesis that, using the traditional medical model of primary care, patient outcomes for nurse practitioner and physician delivery of primary care do not differ.

## Notes

1. Spitzer WO, Sackett DL, Sibley JC, et al. The Burlington randomized trial of the nurse practitioner. *N Engl J Med.* 1974;290:251–256.

2. Brown SA, Grimes DE. A meta-analysis of nurse practitioners and nurse midwives in primary care. *Nurs Res.* 1995;44:332–339.

3. U.S. Congress, Office of Technology Assessment. *Nurse Practitioners, Physician Assistants, and Certified Nurse-Midwives: A Policy Analysis.* Washington, DC: U.S. Government Printing Office; 1986. Health Technology Case Study 37.

4. Safriet BJ. Health care dollars and regulatory sense. *Yale J Regul.* 1992;9:417–488.

5. Pearson LJ. Annual update of how each state stands on legislative issues affecting advanced nursing practice. *Nurse Pract.* 1999;24:16–19, 23–24, 27–30.

6. The Balanced Budget Act of 1997. Pub L No. 105-33.

7. Mundinger MO. Advanced-practice nursing: good medicine for physicians? *N Engl J Med.* 1994;330:211–214.

8. Bindman AB, Grumbach K, Osmond D, et al. Preventable hospitalizations and access to health care. *JAMA.* 1995;274:305–311.

9. Billings J, Anderson GM, Newman LS. Recent findings on preventable hospitalizations. *Health Aff (Millwood).* 1996;15:239–249.

10. Garfield R, Broe D, Albano B. The role of academic medical centers in delivery of primary care, 1995. *Acad Med.* 1995;70:405–409.

11. Ware JE Jr, Snow K, Kosinski M, Gandek B. *SF-36 Health Survey: Manual and Interpretation Guide.* Boston: New England Medical Center; 1993.

12. Ware JE Jr, Snow K, Kosinski M, Gandek B. *SF-36 Physical and Mental Health Summary Scales: A User's Manual.* Boston: Health Institute, New England Medical Center; 1994.

13. Ware JE Jr, Sherbourne CD. The MOS 36-Item Short-Form Health Survey (SF-36). I: conceptual framework and item selection. *Med Care.* 1992;30:473–483.

14. McHorney CA, Ware JE Jr, Raczek AE. The MOS 36-Item Short-Form Health Survey (SF-36), II: psychometric and clinical tests of validity in measuring physical and mental health constructs. *Med Care.* 1993;31:247–263.

15. Shiely JC, Bayliss M, Keller S, Tsai C, Ware JE Jr. *SF-36 Health Survey Annotated Bibliography: First Edition (1988–1995).* Boston: Health Institute, New England Medical Center; 1996.

16. Tsai C, Bayliss M, Ware JE Jr. *SF-36 Survey Annotated Bibliography: 1996 Supplement.* Boston: New England Medical Center; 1997.

17. Sherbourne CD, Wells KB, Meredith LS, Jackson CA, Camp P. Comorbid anxiety disorder and the functioning and well-being of chronically ill patients of general medical providers. *Arch Gen Psychiatry.* 1996;53:889–895.

18. Garratt AM, Ruta DA, Abdalla MI, Russell IT. SF-36 health survey questionnaire. II: responsiveness to changes in health status in four common clinical conditions. *Qual Health Care.* 1994;3:186–192.

19. Mangione CM, Goldman L, Orav EJ, et al. Health-related quality of life after elective surgery. *J Gen Intern Med.* 1997;12:686–697.

20. Rubin HR, Gandek B, Rogers WH, Kosinski M, McHorney CA, Ware JE Jr. Patients' ratings of outpatient visits in different practice settings: results from the Medical Outcomes Study. *JAMA.* 1993;270:835–840.

21. Ware JE Jr, Bayliss MS, Rogers WH, Kosinski M, Tarlov AR. Differences in 4-year health outcomes for elderly and poor, chronically ill patients treated in HMO and fee-for-service systems. *JAMA.* 1996;276:1039–1047.

22. Deyo RA, Inui TS. Dropouts and broken appointments: a literature review and agenda for future research. *Med Care.* 1980;18:1146–1157.

23. Vikander T, Parnicky K, Demers R, Frisof K, Demers P, Chase N. New-patient no-shows in an urban family practice center. *J Fam Pract.* 1986;22:263–268.

24. Dockerty JD. Outpatient clinic nonarrivals and cancellations. *N Z Med J.* 1992;105:147–149.

25. Kusek JW, Lee JY, Smith DE, et al. Effect of blood pressure control and antihypertensive drug regimen on quality of life. *Control Clin Trials.* 1996;17(suppl 4):40S–46S.

26. Temple PC, Travis B, Sachs L, Strasser S, Choban P, Flancbaum L. Functioning and well-being of patients before and after elective surgical procedures. *J Am Coll Surg.* 1995;181:17–25.

27. Kopjar B. The SF-36 health survey: a valid measure of changes in health status after injury. *Inj Prev.* 1996;2:135–139.

28. Bertakis KD, Callahan EJ, Helms LJ, Azari R, Robbins JA, Miller J. Physician practice styles and patient outcomes. *Med Care.* 1998;36:879–891.

# Abstracts from the Literature

*Quality and Costs: Nurse Practitioners
and Other Nonphysician Practitioners*

## BOOKS AND REPORTS

Institute of Medicine. *Community-Oriented Primary Care: New Directions for Health Services Delivery*. Washington, DC: National Academy Press; 1983. This report presents the papers given at a 1982 Institute of Medicine–sponsored conference on community-oriented primary care (COPC). It contains three parts: first, a consideration of the theoretical issues; second, summaries of 16 case reports illustrating the application of COPC to medical education and health services delivery; and third, a summary of the discussion, conclusions, and suggestions that emerged from the workshops.

Pew Health Professions Commission, Center for the Health Professions, University of California, San Francisco. *Charting a Course for the 21st Century: Physician Assistants and Managed Care*. San Francisco: Pew Health Professions Commission, Center for the Health Professions; 1998. This report provides a comprehensive examination of the status of state laws regulating the practice of physician assistants (PAs), the role of PAs in managed care, the education and training of PAs, and the potential supply and demand for PAs.

U.S. Congress, Office of Technology Assessment. *Nurse Practitioners, Physician Assistants, and Certified Nurse-Midwives: A Policy Analysis*. Washington DC: U.S. Government Printing Office; 1986. The questions that this study attempts to answer are threefold: (1) What contributions do nurse practitioners (NPs), physician assistants (PAs) and certified nurse midwives (CNMs) make in meeting the nation's health care needs? (2) How would changing the method of payment affect the roles that these practitioners would play in the evolving health care system? (3) How would changing the payment method affect health care costs for patients, third party payers, and society? The study focuses on NPs, PAs and CNMs who provide primary care. It suggests that NPs, PAs and CNMs are making important contributions to meeting the nation's health care needs by improving the quality and accessibility of health care services and increasing the productivity of medical practices and institutions. The study finds that NPs, PAs, and CNMs have been willing to locate in rural and inner city areas and that these practitioners will continue to play vital roles in these underserved areas. It concludes that extending financial coverage for NPs, PAs and CNMs would benefit individuals who live in rural areas and inner cities, who reside in nursing homes or receive home care, or who are chronically disabled. Coverage for the services of NPs, PAs and CNMs in at least some settings, could improve health care for segments of the population that are not being served adequately.

# ARTICLES

Cooper RA, Laud P, Craig L, Dietrich BS. Current and projected workforce of nonphysician clinicians. *JAMA*. 1998;280:788–794.   This article examines the current supply and distribution of 10 types of nonphysician clinicians (NPCs)—nurse practitioners (NPs), physician assistants (PAs), nurse-midwives, chiropractors, acupuncturists, naturopaths, optometrists, podiatrists, nurse anesthetists, and clinical nurse specialists—and the rates at which new NCPs are being trained, and the effect on the practice of primary care. Data was collected from professional certifying and other national organizations, schools and colleges, state licensing boards, the internet and previously published studies. The study projects an increment of 68% in NPC supply between 1995 and 2005 to 384,000 (or 132 per 100,000 people). If training continues at the rates projected, NPC supply will grow by an additional 40% between 2005 and 2015, to 540,000 (or 170 per 100,000 people). The greatest growth is projected among those NPCs that provide primary care services. During this time the total physician supply will be at its maximum levels, in a range of 237 to 247 per 100,000. It seems unlikely that the health service will be able to absorb both the number of physicians and NPCs that is projected. To conclude, the authors ask what will the impact of this growth of NPCs be on the demand for physicians and suggest that the answer depends on what kind of services NPCs will provide.

De Angelis, CD. Nurse practitioner redux. *JAMA*. 1994;271:868–871.   This author, a nurse and physician, discusses the history of the nurse practitioner (NP) movement in the context of the proposed health care reform and the need for organized medicine and nursing to work together. She considers the number of NPs who are able to function as generalists, the geographic maldistribution of health care, the cost-effectiveness of using NPs, and the scope and legal implications. She recommends that a national committee composed of physicians and NPs be organized and charged with defining a scope of practice model, delineating the specific roles for NPs and generalist physicians in primary care. She also suggests more studies should be conducted to assess the safety and cost-effectiveness of NPs practicing independently. In the meantime, NPs should work with physicians as teams of interdependent professionals.

Hooker RS, McCaig LF. Use of physician assistants and nurse practitioners in primary care, 1995–1999. *Health Aff.* 2001;20:231–238.   This article analyzes the work of physician assistants (PAs) and nurse practitioners (NPs) in primary care. Primary care physician office encounter data is studied from the 1995–1999 National Ambulatory Medical Care Surveys. About one-quarter of primary care office-based physicians used PAs and/or NPs for an average of 11 percent of visits. The mean age of patients seen by physicians was greater than that for PAs or NPs. NPs provided counseling/education during a higher proportion of visits than did PAs or physicians. Overall, this study suggests that NPs and PAs are providing primary care in a way that is similar to physicians.

Knickman, JR, Lipkin M, Finkler SA, Thomson WG, Kiel J. The potential for using nonphysicians to compensate for the reduced availability of residents. *Acad Med.* 1992;67:429–438.   The article considers the use of non-physicians to compensate for the decreasing number of residents and the decreasing amount of time that residents have in which to carry out their activities. In order to find out how residents spend their time, the authors conducted a time-motion study of 8 internal medicine residents at two urban hospitals in New York City in 1988. The authors classified the possible activities into three categories; (1) those that had to be done by a physician; (2) those that were educational only; (3) those that could be done by a non-physician. The authors analyze and project their data using two models—the traditional model of care where the physician is the primary medical manager of the patient, and an alternative model where a mid-level practitioner, such as a nurse, would perform the day-to-day monitoring of patients. In the traditional model, almost half the activities must be carried out by a physician, meaning that another physician would have to be called if the resident were unavailable. In the alternative model, only around 20 percent of the activities required a physician. The authors give detailed breakdown of their data, estimate the kinds and numbers of non-physician health care professionals necessary to substitute for residents, and review difficulties in implementation.

Lancaster J, Lancaster W, Onega LL. New directions in health care reform: the role of nurse practitioners. *J Bus Res.* 2000;48:207–212.   Managed health care, health maintenance organizations, and other cost containment measures driven by the private sector in conjunction with Congressionally funded initiatives are serving as the guiding forces in health care reform in the US. Within this move towards restructuring health-care services, the role of the nurse practitioner (NPs) is expanding and evolving. NPs provide high-quality, cost-effective, and comprehensive primary care services. Increased use of NPs in disease preventions, illness management, and health education is one way of meeting the health care needs of the US population.

Artificial and politically imposed barriers to effective utilization of NPs should be removed. Innovative strategies for more effective use of nurse practitioners must be identified and implemented.

Riportella-Muller R, Libby D, Kindig DA. The substitution of physician assistants and nurse practitioners for physician residents in teaching hospitals. *Health Aff.* 1995;14:181–191. This study documents features of clinical departments in teaching hospitals that are using physician assistants (PAs) and nurse practitioners (NPs) to perform some tasks previously done by medical or surgical residents. More than 60% of teaching hospital medical directors surveyed, reported experience with substitution in their hospitals. The experience overall appears to be positive; one third of the departments are planning to increase the number of PAs and NPs that they use. The results imply that some of the services in house-staff reductions called for in many physician workforce reform proposals could be provided by alternative health professionals.

Rosenblatt RA, Huard B. The nurse practitioner as a physician substitute in a remote rural community: a case study. *Public Health Rep.* 1979;94:571–575. This article reports the results of an experiment in which a solo physician in an isolated rural community in Oregon was replaced by a solo nurse practitioner in an attempt to provide stable primary care. The study found that the nurse practitioner saw 36% more individual patients in 42% more encounters (600 patients in 1,139 encounters) than the physician (440 patients in 800 separate encounters) during the same time period. The physician saw twice as many new patients as the nurse practitioner. Both practitioners had almost the same percentage of return visits and the same number of encounters outside clinic hours. On an annualized basis the nurse practitioners' charges were $63,000 compared to $42,000 for the physician. The authors cite three major factors contributing to the program's demise: (1) the nurse practitioner's ineligibility for Medicare reimbursement diminished the potential patient population; (2) the opposition of members of the boards of medicine and pharmacy in Oregon to the concept of a new health practitioner led to a 5-month prohibition on the signing of prescriptions by nurse practitioners, and (3) the high cost of obtaining physician supervision that further eroded the financial viability of the clinic.

Stone EL. Nurse practitioners and physician assistants: do they have a role in your practice? *Pediatrics.* 1995;96(Suppl):844–851. During the next decade, pediatricians will confront the difficult challenge of providing quality health care services to more children with increasingly diverse and difficult problems, with no extra funding. This article discusses how pediatric nurse practitioners (PNPs) and some physician assistants (PAs) are being trained to perform health supervision care and to diagnose and treat common illness of children. Substantial evidence suggests that PNPs provide high quality health care services, and that collaborative teams of pediatricians and PNPs can provide high quality, cost effective care to a broader spectrum of children than can be served by either profession alone.

# CHAPTER THIRTY-ONE

# Support of Nurse Practitioners and Physician Assistants

Terrance Keenan

1999

From its inception as a national philanthropy in 1972, The Robert Wood Johnson Foundation has endeavored to establish nurse practitioners and physician assistants as part of the nation's professional workforce in patient care. The Foundation has pursued this goal with persistence, and staked both its hopes and money on a positive outcome. Why did the Foundation make this commitment? Why has this goal remained important to it for so long? A brief account of the Foundation's grant making record concerning nurse practitioners and physician assistants may provide some answers.

Sometimes referred to as "new health professionals" or "mid-level practitioners," members of these two professions have much in common. Working in concert with physicians, practitioners in both domains are qualified to take a complete patient history and give a physical exam; perform or order standard laboratory tests; recognize and interpret abnormal clinical findings; diagnose and treat common illnesses; and give appropriate emergency care. Although both can and do see patients without the presence of a physician (at rural and inner-city satellite clinics, for example), they must have formal arrangements

This chapter originally appeared as Keenan T. Support of nurse practitioners and physician assistants. *To Improve Health and Health Care, 1998–1999* (Chap. 11), San Francisco: Jossey-Bass, 1999. Copyright © 1999, The Robert Wood Johnson Foundation. Reprinted with permission.

for dependable physician backup and referral. Finally, both nurse practitioners and physician assistants are institutionally based. They are employees of hospitals, health centers, HMOs, and solo and group medical practices. These institutions charge for their services, but both nurse practitioners and physician assistants are salaried staff.

As for the differences between the two professions, physician assistants function within the context, the rules, and the norms of medical practice, whereas nurse practitioners define themselves as an integral part of the nursing profession. Physician assistants are licensed by state boards of medical examiners, and they practice under the auspices of physicians as members of a medical provider team. Nurse practitioners are equipped to assume advanced responsibilities analogous to the roles performed by certified nurse midwives, nurse anesthetists, and such clinical nurse specialties as critical care and neonatal intensive care. The scope of practice of nurse practitioners and, usually, their education and certification are defined by state boards of nursing. In some states, however, statutes call for joint regulation by both medical and nursing boards.

Although the differences between nurse practitioners and physician assistants may seem subtle, they have meant that two professions with similar functions could not emerge within a single structural framework but instead required separate and parallel structures and policies for their advancement—a fact that compounded the challenge to The Robert Wood Johnson Foundation in its effort to establish the professions.

The Foundation's emergence as a national philanthropy in the early 1970s occurred at a time when communities across America were losing their general practitioners to retirement and the demand for new doctors in primary care far exceeded the supply. One major Foundation response was a series of initiatives to rebuild the educational and practice infrastructure of primary care medical practice, particularly general internal medicine, pediatrics, and family medicine.

In a corresponding set of initiatives, the Foundation targeted the education and deployment of nurse practitioners and physician assistants. Evidence that nurse practitioners and physician assistants could perform, with equal competence, perhaps 80 percent of the tasks confronting physicians in office practice was a compelling factor in this decision. In addition, they could be prepared for practice in much less time and at a much lower cost than physicians—eighteen months to two years of formal professional training against at least six years for primary care physicians. Moreover, it seemed likely that nurse practitioners and physician assistants, in general, would find greater satisfaction than physicians for their work in underserved communities. Finally, the services rendered by these new providers were more affordable than the services of primary care physicians. In combination, these factors became powerful incentives for a commitment to establishing nurse practitioners and physician assistants as a cardinal feature of patient care in the United States.

# MAKING A BEGINNING

The concept of nurse practitioner originated in the early 1960s, when a few physicians began to expand the clinical skills of their nurses and accept them as full partners in practice coverage. Formal training of nurse practitioners began in 1965 at the University of Colorado Health Sciences Center under a doctor-nurse team in pediatrics—Henry Silver and Loretta Ford. Supported principally by the Commonwealth Fund, this program helped to define the nurse practitioner's functions, relationships with physicians, and the essentials of effective education.

The role of physician assistant had roots in part in the medical corpsmen of the military, many of whom subsequently trained for civilian service in the Medex programs established by such eminent academic health sciences centers as the University of Washington, Seattle. However, the acknowledged pioneer in thinking of physician assistants as a key primary care profession—and in providing educational and practice leadership for its emergence—was the late Dr. Eugene Stead of Duke University. This program, brought to fruition by Dr. Harvey Estes of Duke's Department of Family Practice, has served from its outset as a model of excellence nationwide.

By 1972, when The Robert Wood Johnson Foundation became a national philanthropy, the viability of nurse practitioners and physician assistants as recognized health professionals had thus been tested to some degree. Even so, what was known about these two fields, however promising they seemed, was hardly sufficient to justify the Foundation's vision for their future. There was widespread opposition, from within both organized medicine and the professional nursing establishment. Medical education (as opposed to organized medicine itself) was relatively accepting, and even supportive, of the idea, but nursing education was not. Indeed, the great majority of America's nursing deans were outraged. The issues were largely ideological, and therefore quite volatile and difficult to contest. To many physicians, the concept of the new professionals meant authorizing unprepared and unlicensed medical practice. To many nurses, the concept meant that the nurses would become "physician extenders," and that the profession would lose ground in its struggle to escape subordination to medicine.

Professional resistance to the introduction of the new health professions foreclosed engagement by the federal government and the states. This did not change until the advent of the 1980s.

It might have seemed reasonable to expect that the Foundation, as a new national philanthropy, would be circumspect about addressing controversial issues. But in this case two things argued against that sort of caution. First, the logic of using the two professional fields to expand primary care was intrinsically convincing. Second, several of the staff members had come from funding or service institutions—the Carnegie Corporation, the Commonwealth Fund, Yale—that had participated in the birth of the new professions, and in the face of considerable odds had nurtured them through their infancy. The Robert Wood Johnson Foundation, they believed, could be instrumental in helping the new professions develop into thriving fields. They did not realize at first how difficult this journey would be, or how long it would take.

# FROM EXPERIMENTS TO REALITY

The Foundation's first major thrust consisted of a series of regional demonstrations focused on the in-service training and deployment of nurse practitioners. (The physician assistant profession did not lend itself to in-service training and, early in its history, adopted a quite different and more formal educational strategy.) These five multisite networks, devoted to building physician-nurse practitioner teams, were intended to move these fields from an experimental, single-site stage to patient-care networks covering many sites.

## University of California, Davis

This university provided an environment for demonstrating how a new type of professional could help rural America prevent the decline of its patient care. First, Davis was a land-grant institution that embodied the tradition of community service. Second, the University was the home of a new medical school specifically established to attract and train physicians for practice in rural Northern and Central California. Third, to serve as the prime mover of this mission, Dr. Len Hughes Andrus was recruited from private practice to head the school's Department of Family Practice. Andrus had the trust of the physician community and a sure understanding of the potential of office nurses in sharing the burdens of rural practice.

Together with two nurses—Mary O'Hara-Devereaux and Leona Judson—Andrus quickly organized a training program for family nurse practitioners as an integral component of the department. Over the next several years, this group established a network of primary care practices made up of nurse-physician teams that served locations ranging from small coastal fishing villages to remote mountain valleys. The nurse practitioners were recruited directly from practice, and received instruction at regional hospitals under the direction of circuit-riding faculty from Davis. They then completed their clinical education under physicians in their home towns (often their employers) whom Davis trained and qualified as preceptors.

Davis expanded further by collaborating with an established physician assistant program at Stanford University. Stanford—perhaps the epitome of research-based academic health science centers—had organized a medical residency in family practice in affiliation with several Central California community hospitals. Using this base, Stanford also formed an alliance with a number of California community colleges to establish a physician assistant program. The ingenuity of these measures matched those of the Davis initiative, and the two faculties in family practice came together in the nation's only program to train nurse practitioners and physician assistants as colleagues.

## Utah Valley Hospital, Provo

In the annals of American philanthropy, the Utah Valley Hospital—at Provo, just south of Salt Lake City—has landmark significance. It was one of a dozen or so model community hospitals established by the Commonwealth Fund in the 1930s. The governance, the administration, and the staffing of these institutions became the blueprint for the Hill-Burton legislation enacted by Congress in 1948.

For the small towns scattered across Utah, however, the Hospital's standing as an exemplary community institution had no special meaning. These remote towns—many founded by Mormon pioneers—had no doctors, no nurses, and no ready access to health care. The residents were poor but by no means impoverished. Their land was arable, and was kept productive by irrigation. The men were good hunters and tracked game in the desert hills. People were self-sufficient. They survived by thrift, hard work, and a disciplined love for their families and for one another. With the nearest doctor as distant as two hundred miles, there was no way to manage a medical crisis. For generations, these communities had endured a heavy burden of suffering from illness and injury.

This began to change for the better during the 1970s, when the Utah Valley Hospital administration and medical staff organized a network of rural clinics. Based in the hospital's emergency department, the system consisted of local facilities built by the communities and staffed by family nurse practitioners recruited, trained, and deployed by the department. The nurses were experienced professionals who were eager to assume a new level of responsibility for patient care. Around-the-clock backup support was provided by emergency department physicians. Twice weekly, and sometimes at considerable risk, physicians piloted their own planes to the sites to see patients who, in the nurses' judgment, required their attention.

## Tuskegee Institute

Founded by Booker T. Washington, the Tuskegee Institute in Tuskegee, Alabama, offers young African-Americans across the rural South an opportunity for higher education. The town is also the home of a Veterans Administration hospital, which for many years enabled Tuskegee to attract a physician staff of sufficient size to operate a small community hospital—the John A. Andrew Memorial Hospital.

Under the leadership of Dr. Cornelius Hopper, this community institution became the base for a three-county rural health system employing state-of-the-art communications technology. Local citizens who were trusted and respected throughout their neighborhoods were recruited and trained by Tuskegee to serve as health aides. Stationed in churches and other local institutions, the aides identified people who needed care and scheduled them for visits by a provider team from the Tuskegee-based hospital.

The team traveled to the sites in a specially designed mobile van staffed by a Tuskegee-trained nurse practitioner and a laboratory technician, who doubled as a van driver. The van was outfitted as a mobile medical office, and was linked to its Tuskegee base by phone and fax. This enabled the nurses to communicate readily with Tuskegee physicians, who could fax signed prescriptions and medical information immediately to the vans.

This project died after reductions in federal health spending that began in the 1980s, but it stands as a prototype for the delivery of rural health services that has great potential, especially in the light of the advances that have been made in electronic communications.

## Frontier Nursing Service, Hyden, Kentucky

In 1925, deep in the mountainous terrain of East Kentucky, Mary Breckenridge founded this country's first training and service program in nurse midwifery. Headquartered in Wendover, where she made her home, and using a primitive community hospital in nearby Hyden, the program became renowned as the Frontier Nursing Service, or FNS. The FNS was dedicated to the needs of women and families trapped in a culture of social isolation, and it emerged as a cause among women leaders nationwide. Those who came to the FNS school for training and service were characterized not only by their idealism but also by their stamina and courage. The FNS nurses, stationed in a far-flung network of clinics, visited their patients on horseback—summoned at all hours, braving any weather. Their impact is beyond dispute. The calamitous infant mortality rates of the remote area they served fell dramatically, and in time, the statistics were among the best in the country.

Although FNS nurses had long provided care for all age groups in the families they visited, their training was focused largely on maternity and newborn care.

With the advent of the nurse practitioner movement, the FNS decided that it would be advantageous for its staff and students to have dual training as family nurse practitioners. The Robert Wood Johnson Foundation provided funding to the FNS to develop a curriculum, which was used to train family nurse practitioners. FNS nurses are still stationed in a dispersed clinic network, but the use of jeeps and telephone and radio communications has made their work easier. Also, the FNS now has a new and modern hospital, which has increased the availability of physicians to back up the nurses.

### University of Tennessee Medical Center, Memphis

The Department of Community Medicine, at the University of Tennessee College of Medicine, in Memphis, has a demonstrated ability to attract and hold top clinical faculty. It was built by a visionary chairman, Dr. John Runyon, who believed that the department should function as a community-based clinical service. Not only did the department set out to define community health problems such as hypertension, it also set out to solve them. Concern over these problems prompted Runyon and his colleagues to help initiate a large network of primary care clinics that targeted the city's large African-American community.

This system was a collaborative venture among the medical school, the Memphis City Hospital, and the Memphis-Shelby County Health Department. It consisted of a strategically placed set of comprehensive community health centers, each responsible for a cluster of satellite neighborhood clinics staffed by carefully trained nurse practitioners. The system was coordinated through a central command post based at the hospital. For example, nurses at the satellite posts promptly reported referral requests that had come into their area centers to the central command center. If the referral was not completed in a timely way, corrective action was taken. Managerial steps of this kind assured that this complex urban provider network would remain responsive to the needs of the front-line nurses.

# IMPACT ON THE FOUNDATION'S PROGRAMMING

The Foundation's experience in the 1970s with these five nurse-based community health networks affirmed its confidence that nurse practitioners could play a vital role in the nation's health care, and the Foundation proceeded to promote this role in two areas of special need—emergency services and school health services.

In the first area, the Foundation recognized that emergency department nurses, especially in small rural hospitals, confronted a relentless load of non-emergency health problems. People with all manner of complaints came to emergency rooms. Doctors were rarely there, as they were usually local practitioners on rotating coverage. Thus, nurses had to solve the problems that patients presented.

To equip rural emergency nurses more fully for this responsibility, at the close of the 1980s the Foundation established a multisite program to give them training in primary care. The program was headed by Mildred Fink, nursing director of Allegheny General Hospital in Pittsburgh, which became a regional training site for the area's rural hospitals. Other sites included Herman Hospital in Houston; Maricopa General Hospital in Phoenix; Good Samaritan Hospital in Portland, Oregon; Nebraska Methodist Hospital in Omaha; and the University of Alabama Medical Center in Birmingham.

Each site developed a rigorous curriculum in the basic sciences as well as in clinical reasoning and procedure. Students were enthusiastic about the opportunity for professional growth and learning, but the program failed to find a niche in the health care labor market. It was a casualty not only of hospital cost cutting but also of the hostility of academic nursing, which had no interest in its success.

In school nursing in the early 1980s, the Foundation initiated a training program to enable nurses in elementary schools to provide on-site primary care. The program encompassed thirty-six school districts enrolling 37,000 children in four states—Colorado, New York, North Dakota, and Utah. The program was directed by Catherine De Angelis, a pediatrician with a prior career in nursing. This program was successful as an experiment, but it, too, was a market failure. Costs were higher than school districts were willing to pay, and (with the sole exception of the University of Colorado) the innovation was shunned by academic nursing. In the mid-1980s and into the nineties, the Foundation resumed its investment in nursing in the public schools—this time targeting adolescents.

# CONFRONTING ACADEMIC NURSING

In part because of the apparent success of the regional training and demonstration programs for nurse practitioners, the Foundation was slow to think strategically about how to promote the concept over the long run. The failure of its efforts in emergency care and school health were disappointments that prompted the staff to reconsider the strategy it was pursuing.

What was missing was an authentic educational infrastructure. The Foundation's initial approach was to retrain the existing registered nurse workforce for expanded clinical roles through the engagement and support of physicians. The approach worked, but only in part. It did not enlist the educational and intellectual base of nursing—did not call upon the scientific and scholarly leadership of the profession. The nurse practitioner field, in fact, had no professional home—nowhere to grow a faculty of its own. If it had a future, that future was most uncertain.

When the Foundation made this discovery, it shifted its strategy from in-service training and continuing education to an effort to build clinical primary care nursing into the heart of advanced graduate education in the profession. The change required that the Foundation enlist the participation of academic nursing—especially of nursing deans. Most of them responded negatively.

Yet a handful of leaders on graduate nursing faculties envisioned primary care as an important new scholarly and practice discipline of nursing; they had been trained as nurse practitioners and were emerging as thinkers in this evolving area. They espoused the Foundation's cause and became its allies within academic nursing. This group included, among others, Claire Fagin at the University of Pennsylvania, Ingeborg Mauksch at the University of Missouri at Columbia, Loretta Ford, who had moved from Colorado to Rochester University, and Rheba de Tornyay at the University of Washington (who in 1990 became the Foundation's first female trustee). With their counsel and that of their colleagues, the Foundation made a series of grants to establish new master's-level programs in several primary care domains (adult nursing, pediatric nursing, family nursing) at a number of universities. The recipients included the universities of Indiana, Pace, Pennsylvania, Rochester, Seton Hall, and Washington.

Although these graduate programs did become thriving enterprises that helped win acceptance of the nurse practitioner concept among the profession's academic élite, the Foundation soon realized that the concept could not establish an educational base without qualified faculty members. Recognition of this need led the Foundation to establish the Nurse Faculty Fellowships in Primary Care. The program proved to be a timely initiative that had first-rate leadership. Ingeborg Mauksch served as program director, and Loretta Ford was chairwoman of the program advisory committee. The fellows received their training at one of four university nursing schools—Colorado, Indiana, Maryland, and Rochester. Over five years—1977 to 1982—ninety-nine outstanding young faculty members completed the fellowships, and as a group they made a decisive difference in the ability of nursing education to secure the future of the nurse practitioner field.

Despite its satisfaction with the program and its pride in the fellows, in the final years of the initiative the Foundation's vision for nurse practitioners began to wane. Almost out of nowhere, questions surfaced about the projected demand for nurse practitioners in the health care marketplace. A wave of doubt caused the Foundation to falter, and the fellowships were not continued beyond 1982. No one at the Foundation could predict that in a few years, nurse practitioners would be serving as the cornerstone for a system of adolescent health care based in the public schools. Nor was it foreseen that in the mid-1990s the Foundation would be fostering programs for the joint training of nurse practitioners and physician assistants from defined geographic regions—initiatives similar to the Davis-Stanford project it had funded twenty years before.

## PHYSICIAN ASSISTANTS: BLUEPRINT FOR A NEW PROFESSION

The physician assistant profession emerged more clearly than did the nurse practitioner field. In its early days, its membership established a group to assure professional standards and accountability—the American Academy of Physician Assistants. Similarly, training facilities formed the Association of Physician Assistant Programs as a national accrediting body to guarantee consistency of curricula and educational performance. In addition, a national certification examination was established under the auspices of the National Board of Medical Examiners to establish a level of competence for entry into the profession.

The Robert Wood Johnson Foundation provided startup funding for these efforts. However, although they helped define performance and training standards of the profession, the physician assistant field still faced contention and challenges. State and local medical societies feared the advent of the physician assistant concept, and for years blocked the new profession in several states through their control of state licensing laws. Nevertheless, the profession has prevailed in every state except Mississippi. This is in no small measure due to the fact that a number of preeminent academic medical centers—notably Duke, Stanford, and Yale—took part in the formation of the field.

Although a significant proportion of current training programs—about a fourth of them—are offered at the master's level, physician assistant education has emerged largely as an undergraduate professional major. In the mid-1970s, the Foundation helped to create two early models for this development. The first—which had been funded initially by the Commonwealth Fund—was based at Alderson-Broadus College in Phillipi, West Virginia. The college had a number of features that made it a logical place to undertake this innovation. First, it was the site of a community hospital, so the program had a clinical home. Second, the hospital's key staff was made up of physicians from a multispecialty group practice, the Myers Clinic, in Phillipi. Finally, Hu Myers, chief of the clinic, was a person of exceptional standing and vision. His commitment to physician assistants as first-line providers facilitated the acceptance of the concept by the state and local medical community.

Lake Erie College, in Painesville, Ohio—site of the second program to create an undergraduate professional major with Foundation assistance—had attributes comparable to those of Alderson-Broadus. A small institution for women, it forged a professional training base in health by joining with the nearby Cleveland Clinic. Although the clinic was an acclaimed specialty referral center, it was assuming increasing responsibility for primary care in its community. Physician assistants were seen as a way of helping the clinic fulfill this role. In partnership with Lake Erie College, it initiated a superb program.

Two other model projects funded by the Foundation were intended to train first-line practitioners capable of assuming an expanded level of physician delegation. One project, as noted earlier, was initiated by Henry Silver at the University of Colorado, who (with Loretta Ford) had established the country's first formal nurse practitioner training program. Known as Child Health Advocates, graduates of this new program were especially well equipped for practice in medically underserved areas, which included much of the American hinterland. The program remained small, however, and was not replicated by other universities.

The second advanced-level program financed by the Foundation was designed to train a group known as physician associates. The project was initiated by Johns Hopkins University, which established the School of Health Services as a new academic entity for this purpose. A talented faculty was recruited to launch the school. Leadership included Malcolm Peterson and Archie Golden, members of a young physician team engaging the university in service innovations. On the strength of the apparent commitment from Johns Hopkins, the Foundation invested heavily in this enterprise, but when economic adversity confronted the university its commitment collapsed, and soon after so did the school.

Clearly, the Foundation could have renewed its support and assured the school's survival for a further period. However, it faced the decision that sooner or later confronts every source of venture capital—to continue its funding or not. It elected to cut its losses.

As is evident in the Foundation's history of investing in the development of nurse practitioners and physician assistants, the two fields have simply coexisted and done almost nothing to help each other succeed. True, this observation does not apply to most individual practice sites, where collegiality has a palpable and necessary presence. But it is a characteristic of professional education where there is an immense distance between the faculty of the two fields—and thus no strategic activity to bring them together as a united force working to expand access to patient care services.

To help the professions surmount this structural impasse, the Foundation undertook a six-year program, Partnerships for Training, in 1995. The idea was to build collaborative regional networks among providers and develop training programs that would build a strong areawide workforce in primary care. Twelve planning grants and as many as eight implementation grants were authorized. By the end of 1997, three implementation grants had been made—to the University of Colorado, University of Minnesota, and University of Wisconsin. The networks include certified nurse midwives as well as nurse practitioners and physician assistants. Students are to be recruited locally, and that should help ensure their long-term retention as regional providers. The program is administered by the Association of Academic Health Centers under the direction of Jean Johnson-Paulson, an accomplished nurse clinician who is associate dean of the George Washington University School of Medicine.

# REMAINING CHALLENGES

Over the twenty-five years of its investment in the potential of nurse practitioners and physician assistants, the Foundation has done much to help bring about the progress these fields have made. With the exception of Mississippi, which still does not authorize physician assistants, these new professionals are licensed by all states. Rapid headway is also being made among the states on breaching such remaining barriers as permission to write prescriptions.

Some 24,000 nurse practitioners are now at work, and 28,000 physician assistants have been trained and deployed. Further, an educational infrastructure of two hundred nurse practitioner programs and sixty programs for physician assistants is in place.

Although only about half of each group works in primary care settings, this is still a combined workforce of 25,000 new professionals—a resource equivalent to 12.5 percent of the 200,000 physicians in primary care fields.

The Foundation's early interventions helped to make it safe for the federal government and the states to encourage and fund the nurse practitioner and physician assistance professions. The United States Bureau of Health Professions has played a pivotal role in financing the educational infrastructure these fields have developed.

After twenty-five years of engagement, what lessons have been learned?

First, medical specialties and in-patient practice compete with primary care for the services of nurse practitioners and physician assistants. Surgical specialties attract many of them and hospitals also seek to substitute them for resident physicians.

Second, the geographic distribution of these new professions is governed by their employment base. Inner-city and rural areas have limited health care resources and few jobs for health care professionals. Notwithstanding these limitations, nurse practitioners and physician assistants offer an important resource for undertaking health service initiatives targeted on underserved and at-risk populations. That is the purpose of the regional care networks being instituted under the Foundation's Partnerships in Training Program authorized in 1995.

At-risk population groups in the United States, including the elderly and working poor, are growing. Issues of financing, including health insurance, are dominating the emerging public policy debate surrounding this phenomenon. Ultimately, however, the challenge will be to develop and bring to scale an effective and economical system for assuring health and medical services for these groups. Nurse practitioners and physician assistants are a key to building the workforce called for by this challenge.

# Grant Report Summaries from
# The Robert Wood Johnson Foundation

## EDUCATION OF SOUTHERN POLICYMAKERS ABOUT THE USE OF NURSE PRACTITIONERS

(last updated March 1998)

### Grantee

Council of State Governments (Lexington, Kentucky)

### Summary

The southern states have the highest proportion of citizens living in areas that have a shortage of health professionals. Evidence suggests that certified nurse-midwives, nurse practitioners, and physician assistants can provide high-quality, cost-effective care, but their use is limited in the South. The goals of this grant were to (1) educate southern policymakers about the benefits of using these health professionals, (2) document barriers to practice for these practitioners, (3) help southern states improve the regulatory environment for these practitioners, and (4) act as an information clearinghouse for advocates seeking to expand use of these practitioners. The project conducted a survey of more than eight hundred key stakeholders to document barriers to practice for these health professionals in the South. It also assembled a state-by-state "snapshot" detailing the specific numbers of these practitioners in each state, the educational and training resources available for them, and the current regulatory climate affecting their practice. The project culminated in a sixty-four-page report that was disseminated to more than 3,500 governors, legislators, and policymakers throughout the South. The report concluded that nurse practitioners, certified nurse-midwives, and physician assistants can provide selected medical services equivalent to those provided by primary care physicians and at lower cost. Southern states could improve the health care of women and children, particularly in rural areas, if they made greater use of these practitioners. These health professionals, however, face a number of common barriers to practice in the South, including poor public awareness about their training and scope of practice, exclusion from lists of health providers maintained by managed care companies, and lower Medicaid reimbursement than that offered to physicians who provide the same services. In addition, nurse practitioners and certified nurse-midwives face organized opposition from physicians to their practice.

# EVALUATION OF A NURSE-RUN PRIMARY CARE PRACTICE

(last updated March 2000)

## Grantee

Columbia University School of Nursing (New York, New York)

## Summary

The Robert Wood Johnson Foundation (RWJF) grant supported the development of a plan to evaluate Columbia Advanced Practice Nurse Associates (CAPNA), a nurse practitioner–run primary health care practice based in Manhattan that is sponsored by Columbia University School of Nursing. Since its opening, CAPNA had received significant media attention, including negative comments from physician organizations that objected to nurse practitioners' assuming the role of primary care providers for commercially insured patients. Given the media attention, the innovative nature of this practice, the current public policy discussions surrounding the organization of health care in general, and more specifically, the composition of the primary care workforce, the Columbia University School of Nursing proposed to plan and then implement an evaluation of this practice. The primary purpose of this grant was to pilot-test methods and instruments to allow a subsequent full-scale evaluation of the program that would add to the existing knowledge about nurse practitioners in primary care. The project developed a plan to measure visit-specific satisfaction, established a patient database, selected a methodology for overall evaluation of the project, and set up a scientific advisory board. Because of the scrutiny the practice was receiving, the plan included a quality improvement approach that centered on comparing the practice with established benchmarks or standards and with itself over time. The investigators obtained funding for full evaluation of CAPNA from the W. K. Kellogg Foundation.

# BRIDGE FUNDING FOR THE EVALUATION OF A PRIMARY CARE PRACTICE IN WASHINGTON HEIGHTS

(last updated August 2001)

## Grantee

Columbia University School of Nursing (New York, New York)

## Summary

This grant from The Robert Wood Johnson Foundation (RWJF) provided funding to the Columbia University School of Nursing for Phase II of a study comparing nurse practitioners and physicians as primary care providers. Nurse practitioners serving as primary care providers have the potential to improve access to care, but there is a lack of definitive data on their impact in this role. During Phase I of this study (funded by the New York State Department of Health, the Division of Nursing of the U.S. Department of Health and Human Services, and The Leslie Samuels and Fan Fox Foundation), 1,316 patients were assigned randomly to either a nurse practitioner (NP) or a physician (MD) at Columbia Presbyterian Medical Center. As reported in the *Journal of the American Medical Association,* after one year, no significant differences were found in the health status or health services utilization of patients in the two study groups. Phase II of the study, conducted under this RWJF grant, built on the original project by collecting additional data to see if the findings were maintained over an additional year. The researchers conducted 756 interviews (with 439 NP patients and 318 MD patients from the original study) between April 1998 and December 1999, representing a 66.3 percent response rate. These interviews included questionnaires on health status, specific medical conditions, satisfaction, and health services utilization. The researchers validated health services utilization data with hospital data and some Medicaid data. Researchers found that patients who were assigned to NPs were similar demographically to patients assigned to MDs and that in the year before this data collection, 33.3 percent of patients received care only at the assigned clinic, 6.3 percent received care at the assigned clinic and another provider, 27.1 percent only sought care elsewhere, and 32.4 percent did not seek primary health care at all. After the grant ended, the researchers also analyzed two subsamples of patients who received primary care from the practices to which they were randomly assigned. The researchers concluded that the subsample analyses confirm the preliminary results: in an ambulatory care situation where NPs have the same authority, responsibility, productivity, and administrative requirements as MDs, patient outcomes are comparable.

# ANALYSIS OF NURSE PRACTITIONER
# CLINICAL TRAINING COSTS
(last updated May 2002)

## Grantee
American Association of Colleges of Nursing (Washington, D.C.)

## Summary

This grant from The Robert Wood Johnson Foundation (RWJF) funded the American Association of Colleges of Nursing (AACN) to study the costs of clinical training for nurse practitioners. Managed care organizations are making growing use of nurse practitioners as mainstream primary care providers, and training programs in this field have experienced a brisk growth. Such training includes extensive hands-on experience of at least six hundred hours' supervised by practicing clinicians, and much of it is carried out in nonhospital, ambulatory care settings. Because the advent of managed care is exerting pressures on those settings to reduce expenditures and increase productivity, the cost of teaching time is becoming a contentious issue between nursing schools and their affiliated practice sites. In contrast to the cost of training medical residents, which is underwritten by the federal Medicare program, there is no equivalent source of funding for the clinical training of nurse practitioners, and the real costs remain unknown.

In this project, the AACN reviewed the methodology and results of previous research led by James Boex of Northeastern Ohio Universities College of Medicine, which involved a comprehensive study to ascertain the cost of ambulatory care medical residency training. AACN considered the study's applicability for an assessment of the unique costs, benefits, and quality factors involved in advanced-practice nursing education. To determine the applicability of the Boex model, investigators conducted a literature search, interviewed leaders in nurse practitioner training, convened an advisory committee to investigate the model, and consulted with Boex.

Investigators also conducted research into the feasibility of using electronic personal data assistants (PDAs) to collect information on clinical trainees' and supervisors' activities throughout the day. PDAs, which were used in the original Boex study, are handheld computers that are programmed to signal clinical supervisors or trainees to respond to a series of questions at intermittent intervals. Data collected with the PDAs enables investigators to see how clinical supervisors and students use their time in the ambulatory setting and provides investigators with the data to estimate how time spent teaching students affects the clinicians' productivity. It also provides information on how much clinical care student nurses provide while working in ambulatory settings. A project advisory committee and consultants conducted a review of the PDA program menus and engaged a consultant to complete a reprogramming of the PDA software for use in the study of the cost of training nurse practitioners. A pretest of the revised PDA program was conducted by nurse practitioner preceptors and students at three locations: East Tennessee State University in Johnson City; Northeastern University in Boston; and George Mason University/George Washington University in Fairfax, Virginia, and Washington, D.C., respectively, through the Washington Regional Community Partnership. Subsequently, nurse practitioner preceptors and students at Northeastern University conducted a more extensive pilot test of the modified program. Feedback from participants led to further revisions of the program.

Researchers concluded that the Boex model would be applicable if several modifications were made and an adequate and representative sample were obtained. For instance, they learned that the lack of financial resources available for support of the clinical education of nurse practitioners has created a system in which students are dispersed to a large number of sites with few students at each site. This would require sophisticated methodological modifications for the collection of data across multiple setting types with a small number of students in each of the setting types.

An advisory committee member made a presentation on the project at the 1999 annual meeting of the Harvard Nursing Research Institute. No further work on this project is under way. AACN contributed $12,450 in staff support to the project.

# NAME INDEX

# SUBJECT INDEX

672

This constitutes a continuation of the copyright page.

Abstracts from the Literature are reprinted in this volume with permission
from the following publications and organizations:

Alpert JJ, Friedman RH, Green LA. Education of generalists: three tries a century is all we get! *J Gen Intern Med*. 1994;9(4 Suppl.1):S4–S6. Reprinted with permission from Blackwell Publishing.

Altman DF. Revising the definition of the generalist physician. *Acad Med*. 1995;70:1087–1090. Reprinted by permission.

Association of American Medical Colleges Generalist Physician Task Force. AAMC policy on the generalist physician. *Acad Med*. 1993;68:1–6. Reprinted by permission.

Ayanian JZ, Guadagnoli E, McNeil BJ, Cleary PD. Treatment and outcomes of acute myocardial infarction among patients of cardiologists and generalist physicians. *Arch Intern Med*. 1997;157:2570–2576. Copyright © 1997, American Medical Association. All rights reserved.

Baldwin CD, Levine HG, McCormick DP. Meeting the faculty development needs of generalist physicians in academia. *Acad Med*. 1995;70(1 Suppl):S97–S103. Reprinted by permission.

Block SD, Clark-Chiarelli N, Peters AS, Singer JD. Academia's chilly climate for primary care. *JAMA*. 1996;276:677–682. Copyright © 1996, American Medical Association. All rights reserved.

Bodenheimer T, Lo B, Casalino L. Primary care physicians should be coordinators, not gatekeepers. *JAMA*. 1999;281:2045–2049. Copyright © 1999, American Medical Association. All rights reserved.

Bodenheimer T, Wagner EH, Grumbach K. Improving primary care for patients with chronic illness: the Chronic Care Model, part 2. *JAMA*. 2002;288:1909–1914. Copyright © 2002, American Medical Association. All rights reserved.

Brooks WB, Orgren R, Wallace AG. Institutional change: embracing the initiative to train more generalists. *Acad Med*. 1999;74(1Suppl):S3–S8. Reprinted by permission.

Brown JW, Robertson LS, Kosa J, Alpert JJ. A study of general practice in Massachusetts. *JAMA*. 1971;216:301–306. Copyright © 1971, American Medical Association. All rights reserved.

Budetti PP. Achieving a uniform federal primary care policy: opportunities presented by National Health Reform. *JAMA*. 1993;269:498–501. Copyright © 1993, American Medical Association. All rights reserved.

Chen J, Radford MJ, Wang Y, Krumholz HM. Care and outcomes of elderly patients with acute myocardial infarction by physician specialty: the effects of comorbidity and functional limitations. *Am J Med*. 2000;108:460–469. Used by permission of Elsevier. All rights reserved.

Chin MH, Zhang JX, Merrell K. Specialty differences in the care of older patients with diabetes. *Med Care*. 2000;38:131–140. Reprinted by permission.

Christiansen RG, Johnson LP, Boyd GE, Koepshall JE, Sutton K. A proposal for a combined family practice–internal medicine residency. *JAMA*. 1986;255:2628–2630. Copyright © 1986, American Medical Association. All rights reserved.

Cohen JJ, Whitcomb ME. Are the recommendations of the AAMC's task force on the generalist physician still valid? *Acad Med*. 1997;72:13–16. Reprinted by permission.

Colwill JM, Perkoff GT, Blake RL Jr, Paden C, Beachler M. Modifying the culture of medical education: the first three years of the RWJ Generalist Physician Initiative. *Acad Med*. 1997;72:745–753. Reprinted by permission.

Cooper RA. Perspectives on the physician workforce to the year 2020. *JAMA*. 1995;274:1534–1543. Copyright © 1995, American Medical Association. All rights reserved.

Cooper RA. Seeking a balanced physician workforce for the 21st century. *JAMA*. 1994;272:680–687. Copyright © 1994, American Medical Association. All rights reserved.

Cooper RA, Laud P, Craig L, Dietrich BS. Current and projected workforce of nonphysician clinicians. *JAMA*. 1998;280:788–794. Copyright © 1998, American Medical Association. All rights reserved.

De Angelis, CD. Nurse practitioner redux. *JAMA*. 1994;271:868–871. Copyright © 1994, American Medical Association. All rights reserved.

De Witt DE, Curtis JR, Burke W. What influences career choices among graduates of a primary care training program? *J Gen Intern Med*. 1998;13:257–261. Reprinted with permission from Blackwell Publishing.

Deitrich AJ, Goldberg H. Preventive content of adult primary care: do generalists and subspecialists differ? *Am J Pub Health*. 1984;74:223–227. Reprinted with permission from the American Public Health Association.

Dwinnell B, Adams L. Why we are on the cusp of a generalist crisis. *Acad Med*. 2001;76:707–708. Reprinted by permission.

Eisenberg JM. Cultivating a new field: development of a research program in general internal medicine. *J Gen Intern Med*. 1986;1(4 Suppl):S8–S18. Reprinted with permission from Blackwell Publishing.

Eisenberg JM. Sculpture of a new academic discipline: four faces of academic general internal medicine. *Am J Med*. 1985;78:283–292. Used by permission of Elsevier. All rights reserved.

Engstrom S, Foldevi M, Borgquist L. Is general practice effective? A systematic literature review. *Scand J Prim Health Care*. 2001;19:131–144. Reprinted by permission of Taylor & Francis AS (www.tandf.no/primhealth).

Fernandez A, Grumbach K, Goiten L, et al. How primary care physicians perceive hospitalists. *Arch Intern Med*. 2000;160:2902–2908. Copyright © 2000, American Medical Association. All rights reserved.

Forrest CB, Starfield B. Entry into primary care and continuity: the effects of access. *Am J Public Health*. 1998;88(9):1330–1336. Reprinted with permission from the American Public Health Association.

Frances CD, Shlipak MG, Noguchi H, Heidenrich PA, McClellan M. Does physician specialty affect the survival of elderly patients with myocardial infarction? *Health Serv Res*. 2000;35(5 pt 2):1093–1116. Reprinted with permission from Blackwell Publishing.

Freeman J, Cash C, Yonke A, Roe B, Foley R. A longitudinal primary care program in an urban public medical school: three years of experience. *Acad Med*. 1995;70(1 Suppl):S64–S68. Reprinted by permission.

Friedman RH, Alpert JJ, Green LA. Strengthening academic generalist departments and divisions. *J Gen Intern Med*. 1994;9(1 Suppl):S90–S98. Reprinted with permission from Blackwell Publishing.

Fryer GE, Green LA, Dovey SM, Phillips Rl Jr. The United States relies on family physicians unlike any other specialty. *Am Fam Physician*. 2001;63:1669. Copyright © 2001, American Academy of Family Physicians. All rights reserved.

Geyman JP. Training primary care physicians for the 21st century: alternative scenarios for competitive vs. generic approach. *JAMA*. 1986;255:2631–2635. Copyright © 1986, American Medical Association. All rights reserved.

Glasser M, Stearns J, McCord R. Defining a generalist education: an idea whose time is still coming. *Acad Med*. 1995;70(1 Suppl):S69–S74. Reprinted by permission.

Go AS, Rao RK, Dauterman KW, Massie BM. A systematic review of the effects of physician specialty on the treatment of coronary disease and heart failure in the United States. *Am J Med.* 2000;108:216–226. Used by permission of Elsevier. All rights reserved.

Goldberg HI, Dietrich AJ. The continuity of care provided to primary care patients: a comparison of family physicians, general internists, and medical sub-specialists. *Med Care.* 1985;23:63–73. Reprinted by permission.

Goodman DC, Fisher ES, Bubolz TA, et al. Benchmarking the U.S. physician workforce. *JAMA.* 1996;276:1811–1817. Copyright © 1996, American Medical Association. All rights reserved.

Graber DR, Bellack JP, Musham C, O'Neil EH. Academic deans' views on curriculum content in medical schools. *Acad Med.* 1997;72:901–907. Reprinted by permission.

Green LA. British general practice: a visiting American family medicine resident's view. *J Arkansas Med Soc.* 1977;73:457–461. Reprinted by permission.

Greenfield S, Rogers W, Mangotich M, et al. Outcomes of patients with hypertension and non-insulin-dependent diabetes mellitus treated by different systems and specialties: results from the Medical Outline Study. *JAMA.* 1995;274:1436–1444. Copyright © 1995, American Medical Association. All rights reserved.

Greenlick MR. Educating physicians for population-based clinical practice. *JAMA.* 1992;267:1645–1648. Copyright © 1992, American Medical Association. All rights reserved.

Grumbach K, Selby JV. Outcomes and physician specialty: quality of primary care practice in a large HMO according to physician specialty. *Health Serv Res.* 1999;34:485–502. Reprinted with permission from Blackwell Publishing.

Grumbach K, Selby JV, Damberg C, et al. Resolving the gatekeeper conundrum: what patients value in primary care and referrals to specialists. *JAMA.* 1999;282:261–266. Copyright © 1999, American Medical Association. All rights reserved.

Harrold LR, Field TS, Gurwitz JH. Knowledge, patterns of care, and outcomes of care for generalist and specialists. *J Gen Intern Med.* 1999;14:499–511. Reprinted with permission from Blackwell Publishing.

Hermann WH. More than provider specialty. *Med Care.* 2000;38:128–130. Reprinted by permission.

Ho M, Marger M, Beart J, et al. Is the quality of diabetes care better in a diabetes clinic or in a general medicine clinic? *Diabetes Care.* 1997;20:472–475. Copyright © 1997 American Diabetes Association. From *Diabetes Care,* Vol. 20, 1997; 472–475. Reprinted with permission from The American Diabetes Association.

Igra V, Millstein SG. Current status and approaches to improving preventive services for adolescents. *JAMA.* 1993;269:1408–1412. Copyright © 1993, American Medical Association. All rights reserved.

Inui TS. Reform in medical education: a health of the public perspective. *Acad Med.* 1996;71(1Suppl):S119–S121.

Jacoby I, Gary NE, Meyer GS, et al. Retraining physicians for primary care: a study of physicians' perspectives and program development. *JAMA.* 1997;277:1569–1573. Copyright © 1997, American Medical Association. All rights reserved.

Kindig DA. Counting generalist physicians. *JAMA.* 1994;271:1505–1507. Copyright © 1994, American Medical Association. All rights reserved.

Kindig DA. Policy priorities for rural physician supply. *Acad Med.* 1990;65:S15–S17. Reprinted by permission.

Kindig DA, Libby DL. Domestic production vs. international migration: options for the U.S. physician workforce. *JAMA.* 1996;276:978–982. Copyright © 1996, American Medical Association. All rights reserved.

Kindig DA, Libby DL. How will graduate medical education reform affect specialties and geographic areas? *JAMA.* 1994;272:37–42. Copyright © 1994, American Medical Association. All rights reserved.

Kindig DA, Ricketts TC. Determining adequacy of physicians and nurses for rural populations: background and strategy. *J Rural Health* 1991;7(4 Suppl):313–326. Reprinted by permission.

Knickman, JR, Lipkin M, Finkler SA, Thomson WG, Kiel J. The potential for using nonphysicians to compensate for the reduced availability of residents. *Acad Med.* 1992;67:429–438. Reprinted by permission.

Lafata JE, Martin S, Morlock R, Divine G, Xi H. Provider type and the receipt of general and diabetes-related preventive health services among patients with diabetes. *Med Care.* 2001;39:491–499. Reprinted by permission.

Lancaster J, Lancaster W, Onega LL. New directions in health care reform: the role of nurse practitioners. *J Bus Res.* 2000;48:207–212. Used by permission of Elsevier. All rights reserved.

Leader S, Perales PJ. Provision of primary-preventive health care services by obstetrician-gynecologists. *Obstet Gynecol.* 1995;85:391–395. Used by permission of Elsevier. All rights reserved.

Linzer M, Salvin T, Mutha S, et al. Admission, recruitment, and retention: finding and keeping the generalist-oriented student. *J Gen Intern Med.* 1994;9(1 Suppl):S14–S23. Reprinted with permission from Blackwell Publishing.

Lundberg GD, Lamm RD. Solving our primary care crisis by retraining specialists to gain specific primary care competencies. *JAMA.* 1993;270:380–381. Copyright © 1993, American Medical Association. All rights reserved.

Lynch DC, Newton DA, Grayson MS, Whitley TW. Influence of medical school on medical students' opinions about primary care. *Acad Med.* 1998;73:433–435. Reprinted by permission.

Martini CJM, Veloski J, Barzansky B, Xu G, Fields S. Medical school and student characteristics that influence choosing a generalist career. *JAMA.* 1994;272:661–668. Copyright © 1994, American Medical Association. All rights reserved.

Matson CC, Ullian JA, Boisaubin EV. Integrating early clinical experience curricula at two medical schools: lessons learned from The Robert Wood Johnson Foundation's Generalist Physician Initiative. *Acad Med.* 1999;74(1 Suppl):S53–S58. Reprinted by permission.

McBride P, Schrott HG, Plane MB, Underbakke G. Primary care practice adherence to national cholesterol education program guidelines for patients with coronary heart disease. *Arch Intern Med.* 1998;158:1238–1244. Copyright © 1998, American Medical Association. All rights reserved.

Moore, GT. The case of the disappearing generalist: does it need to be solved? *Milbank Quarterly.* 1992;70(2):361–374. Reprinted by permission of *Milbank Quarterly.*

Moscovice IS, Rosenblatt RA. Rural health care delivery amid federal retrenchment: lessons from The Robert Wood Johnson Foundation's Rural Practice Project. *Am J Public Health.* 1982;72(12):1380–1385. Reprinted with permission from the American Public Health Association.

Nash IS, Corrato RR, Dlutowski MJ, O'Connor JP, Nash DB. Generalist vs. specialist care for acute myocardial infarction. *Am J Cardiol.* 1999;83:650–654. Used by permission of Elsevier. All rights reserved.

Newton DA, Grayson MS, Whitley TW. What predicts medical school career choice? *J Gen Intern Med.* 1998;13:200–203. Reprinted with permission from Blackwell Publishing.

Pellegrino ED. The identity crisis of an ideal. In: Ingelfinger FJ, Relman AS, Finland M, eds., *Controversy in Internal Medicine.* Vol. 2. Philadelphia: Saunders; 1974:41–50. Used by permission of Elsevier. All rights reserved.

Petersdorf RG, Turner KS. Medical education in the 1990s—and beyond: a view from the United States. *Acad Med.* 1995;70(Suppl):S41–S47. Reprinted by permission.

Politzer RM, Hardwick KS, Cultice JM, Bazell C. Eliminating primary care Health Professional Shortage Areas: the impact of Title VII generalist physician education. *J Rural Health.* 1999;15:11–20. Reprinted by permission.

Rabinowitz HK, Diamond JJ, Veloski JJ, Gayle JA. The impact of multiple predictors on generalist physicians' care of underserved populations. *Am J Public Health.* 2000;90:1225–1228. Reprinted with permission from the American Public Health Association.

Renders CM, Valk GD, Griffin SJ, et al. Interventions to improve the management of diabetes in primary care, outpatient, and community settings: a systematic review. *Diabetes Care.* 2001;24:1821–1833. Copyright © 2001 American Diabetes Association. From *Diabetes Care*, Vol. 24, 2001; 1821–1833. Reprinted with permission from The American Diabetes Association.

Rivo ML, Henderson TM, Jackson DM. State legislative strategies to improve the supply and distribution of generalist physicians, 1985–1992. *Am J Public Health.* 1995;85(3):405–407. Reprinted with permission from the American Public Health Association.

Rivo ML, Satcher D. Improving access to health care through physician workforce reform: directions for the 21st century. *JAMA.* 1993;270:1074–1078. Copyright © 1993, American Medical Association. All rights reserved.

Rivo ML, Saultz JW, Wartman SA, De Witt TG. Defining the generalist physician's training. *JAMA.* 1994;271:1499–1504. Copyright © 1994, American Medical Association. All rights reserved.

Robert Graham Center, Policy Studies in Family Practice and Primary Care. The importance of primary care physicians as the usual source of health care in the achievement of prevention goals. *Am Fam Physician.* 2000;62:1968. Copyright © 2000, American Academy of Family Physicians. All rights reserved.

Rosenblatt RA. The potential of the academic medical center to shape policy-oriented rural health research. *Acad Med.* 1991;66:662–667. Reprinted by permission.

Rosenblatt, RA, Whitcomb ME, Cullen TJ, Lishner DM, Hart LG. Which medical schools produce rural physicians? *JAMA.* 1992;268:1559–1565. Copyright © 1992, American Medical Association. All rights reserved.

Rosenblatt RA, Whitcomb ME, Cullen TJ, et al. The effect of federal grants on medical schools' production of primary care physicians. *Am J Public Health.* 1993;83(3):322–328. Reprinted with permission from the American Public Health Association.

Rothert ML, Rovner DR, Elstein AS, et al. Differences in medical referral decisions for obesity among family practitioners, general internists, and gynecologists. *Med Care.* 1984;22:42–55. Reprinted by permission.

Rubenstein LV, Fink A, Gelberg L, et al. Evaluating generalist education programs: a conceptual framework. *J Gen Intern Med.* 1994;9(1 Suppl):S64–S71. Reprinted with permission from Blackwell Publishing.

Safran DG, Rogers WH, Tarlov AR, et al. Organizational and financial characteristics of health plans: are they related to primary care performance? *Arch Intern Med.* 2000;160:69–76. Copyright © 2000, American Medical Association. All rights reserved.

Safran DG, Tarlov AR, Rogers WH. Primary care performances in fee-for-service and prepaid health care systems: results from the Medical Outcomes Study. *JAMA.* 1994;271:1579–1586. Copyright © 1994, American Medical Association. All rights reserved.

Sandy LG, Foster NE, Eisenberg JM. Challenges to generalism: views from the delivery system. *Acad Med.* 1995;70(1Suppl):S44–S46. Reprinted by permission.

Schatz IJ, Realini JP, Charney E. Family practice, internal medicine and pediatrics as partners in education of generalists. *Acad Med.* 1996;71:35–39. Reprinted by permission.

Scherger JE, Rucker L, Morrison EH, Cygan R, Hubbell A. The primary care specialties working together: a model of success in an academic environment. *Acad Med.* 2000;75:693–698. Reprinted by permission.

Schneeweiss R, Ellsbury K, Hart LG, Geyman JP. The economic impact and multiplier effect of a family practice clinic on an academic medical center. *JAMA.* 1989;262:370–375. Copyright © 1989, American Medical Association. All rights reserved.

Schroeder SA. Expanding the site of clinical education: moving beyond the hospital walls. *J Gen Intern Med.* 1988;3(Suppl):S5–S14. Reprinted with permission from Blackwell Publishing.

Schroeder SA. Western European responses to physician oversupply. *JAMA.* 1984;252:373–384. Copyright © 1984, American Medical Association. All rights reserved.

Schroeder SA, Mitchell T. Employment choices in conditions of physician oversupply. *J Gen Intern Med.* 1988;3:25–31. Reprinted with permission from Blackwell Publishing.

Schwenk TL, Woolley RF. The role of the community-oriented primary care physician. *Am J Prev Med.* 1986;2:49–58. Used by permission of Elsevier. All rights reserved.

Simon GE, Von Korff M, Rutter CM, Peterson DA. Treatment process and outcomes for managed care patients receiving new antidepressants prescriptions from psychiatrists and primary care physicians. *Arch Gen Psych.* 2001;58:395–401. Copyright © 2001, American Medical Association. All rights reserved.

Sox HC Jr. Supply, demand, and the workforce of internal medicine. *Am J Med.* 2001;110:745–749. Used by permission of Elsevier. All rights reserved.

Sox HC Jr. The hospitalist model: proceed with caution. *Healthplan.* 1999;40(6):17–19. Reprinted by permission.

Starfield B. Is primary care essential? *Lancet.* 1994;344:1129–1133. Used by permission of Elsevier. All rights reserved.

Starfield B, Holtzman NA, Roland MO, Sibbald B, Harris R, Harris H. Primary care and genetic services: health care in evolution. *Eur J Public Health.* 2002;12(1):51–56. Reprinted by permission of Oxford University Press.

Starfield B, Simpson L. Primary care as part of U.S. health services reform. *JAMA.* 1993;269:3136–3139. Copyright © 1993, American Medical Association. All rights reserved.

Urbina C, Hickey M, McHarney Brown C, Duban S, Kaufman A. Innovative generalist programs: academic health centers respond to the shortage of generalist physicians. *J Gen Intern Med.* 1994;9(1 Suppl):S81–S89. Reprinted with permission from Blackwell Publishing.

Wachter RM, Goldman L. The hospitalist movement five years later. *JAMA.* 2002;287:487–494. Copyright © 2002, American Medical Association. All rights reserved.

Weiner JP. Forecasting the effects of health reform on U.S. physician workforce requirement: evidence from HMO staffing patterns. *JAMA.* 1994;272:222–230. Copyright © 1994, American Medical Association. All rights reserved.

Weiner JP, Parente ST, Garnick DW, Fowles J, Lawthers AG, Palmer R. Variation in office-based quality: a claims-based profile of care provided to Medicare patients with diabetes. *JAMA.* 1995;273:1503–1508. Copyright © 1995, American Medical Association. All rights reserved.

Weissert CS, Silberman SL. Sending a policy signal: state legislatures, medical schools, and primary care mandates. *J Health Polit Policy Law.* 1998;23:743–770. Reprinted by permission.

Weitekamp MR, Ziegenfuss JT. Academic health centers and HMOs: a systems perspective on collaboration in training generalist physicians and advancing mutual interests. *Acad Med.* 1995;70(1Suppl):S47–S53. Reprinted by permission.

Willison DJ, Soumerai SB, McLaughlin TJ, Gurwitz JH. Consultation between cardiologists and generalists in the management of acute myocardial infarction: implications for quality of care. *Arch Intern Med.* 1998;158:1778–1783. Copyright © 1998, American Medical Association. All rights reserved.

Young LE. Education and roles of personal physicians in medical practice. *JAMA.* 1964;187:927–933. Copyright © 1964, American Medical Association. All rights reserved.

Young LE. The broadly based internist as the backbone of medical practice. In: Ingelfinger FJ, Relman AS, Finland M, eds., *Controversy in Internal Medicine.* Vol. 2. Philadelphia: Saunders; 1974:51–63. Used by permission of Elsevier. All rights reserved.